Natural Medicines

Natural Medicines

Clinical Efficacy, Safety and Quality

Edited by

Dilip Ghosh and Pulok K. Mukherjee

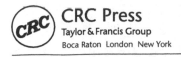

CRC Press is an imprint of the
Taylor & Francis Group, an **informa** business

CRC Press
Taylor & Francis Group
6000 Broken Sound Parkway NW, Suite 300
Boca Raton, FL 33487-2742

First issued in paperback 2021

ISBN 13: 978-1-03-209079-5 (pbk)
ISBN 13: 978-1-138-73306-0 (hbk)

This book contains information obtained from authentic and highly regarded sources. Reasonable efforts have been made to publish reliable data and information, but the author and publisher cannot assume responsibility for the validity of all materials or the consequences of their use. The authors and publishers have attempted to trace the copyright holders of all material reproduced in this publication and apologize to copyright holders if permission to publish in this form has not been obtained. If any copyright material has not been acknowledged please write and let us know so we may rectify in any future reprint.

Library of Congress Cataloging-in-Publication Data

Names: Ghosh, Dilip K., editor. | Mukherjee, Pulok K., editor.
Title: Natural medicines : clinical efficacy, safety and quality / [edited by] Dilip Ghosh and Pulok K. Mukherjee.
Other titles: Natural medicines (Ghosh)
Description: Boca Raton : Taylor & Francis, [2019] | Includes bibliographical references and index.
Identifiers: LCCN 2019005122 | ISBN 9781138733060 (hardback : alk. paper)
Subjects: | MESH: Herbal Medicine--standards | Biological Products--standards | Functional Food--standards | Treatment Outcome
Classification: LCC RS164 | NLM WB 925 | DDC 615.3/21--dc23
LC record available at https://lccn.loc.gov/2019005122

Visit the Taylor & Francis Web site at
http://www.taylorandfrancis.com

and the CRC Press Web site at
http://www.crcpress.com

Publisher's Note
The publisher has gone to great lengths to ensure the quality of this reprint but points out that some imperfections in the original copies may be apparent.

Contents

SECTION I Quality and Chemistry

SECTION II   Safety

SECTION III   Regulation

SECTION IV   Clinical Efficacy

SECTION V   Reviews

Editors

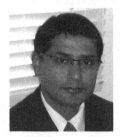

Dilip Ghosh, PhD, FACN, is an international speaker, facilitator and author and Director at NutriConnect & Food Nutrition Partner in Australia; Honorary Ambassador, Global Harmonization Initiative (GHI) and adjunct at NICM, University of Western Sydney. Dr Ghosh is a food/nutritional, nutraceuticals and natural medicine specialist based in Sydney, Australia. He is an advisor and executive board member of Health Foods and Dietary Supplements Association (HADSA), India.

His research interests include oxidative stress, bioactive, clinically proven functional food and natural medicine development, regulatory and scientific aspects of functional foods, nutraceuticals and herbal medicines. He has been involved for a long time in drug development and nutraceutical research and development and its commercialisation, both in academic and industry domains.

Dr Ghosh has published more than 100 papers in peer-reviewed journals, as well as numerous articles in food and nutrition magazines and books. His most recent book is *Pharmaceuticals to Nutraceuticals: A Shift in Disease Prevention* (CRC Press, 2017). Dr Ghosh is review editor for *Frontiers in Nutrigenomics* (2011 to present), the *American Journal of Advanced Food Science and Technology* (2012 to present), the *Journal of Obesity and Metabolic Research* (2013 to present), the *Journal of Bioethics* (2013 to present). He is also an associate editor and member of *Toxicology Mechanisms and Methods*, (2006–2007) and a columnist with *Nutraceuticals World*.

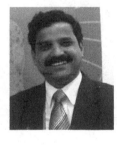

Pulok K. Mukherjee, PhD, FRSC, FNASc, is the Director of the School of Natural Product Studies, Jadavpur University, Kolkata, India, and presently the Head of the Department of Pharmaceutical Technology, JU. His research and academic work highlights traditional medicine inspired by drug discovery from Indian medicinal plants with a major emphasis on validation of Indian medicinal plants, their formulation and standardisation, metabolomic profiling and safety documentation, which are useful bio-prospecting tools for the traditional medicine–based drug discovery programme. He has made several innovative and outstanding contributions in academics and research in the areas of natural product studies, ethnopharmacology and evidence-based validation of herbs used in AYUSH.

Dr Mukherjee is a Fellow of the Royal Society of Chemistry (FRSC), a Fellow of the National Academy of Sciences, India (FNASc) and a Fellow of the West Bengal Academy of Science and Technology. He has been awarded with several laurels from the Government of India and abroad, including the Commonwealth Academic Staff Fellowship from the Association of Commonwealth Universities (ACU), UK; NASI-Reliance Industries Platinum Jubilee Award from the National Academy of Science, India; TATA Innovation Fellowship by the Department of Biotechnology, Government of India; Outstanding Service Award from the Drug Information Association (DIA), USA; Career Award for Young Teacher from All India Council for Technical Education (AICTE), Government of India; BOYSCAST Fellowship from DST, Government of India; Best Pharmaceutical Scientist of the Year, from the Association of Pharmaceutical Teachers' of India (APTI); and many others.

He has to his credit more than 200 publications in peer-reviewed journals and several patents. Dr Mukherjee has authored or edited five books and eighteen book chapters. He is the secretary of the Society for Ethnopharmacology, India (SFE India), working on dissemination of knowledge promotion and development of medicinal plant and ethnopharmacology with the vision of 'Globalizing Local Knowledge – Localizing Global Technology'. Dr Mukherjee is serving as an associate editor of the *Journal of Ethnopharmacology*. He is a member of the editorial board of several other journals including *Phytomedicine, Pharmaceutical Analysis, Synergy, Phytochemical Analysis, Indian Journal of Traditional Knowledge*, the *Journal of Pharma Education and Research*, and others. He is associated as an advisor or member with different organizations and administrative bodies of the Government of India and abroad.

Contributors

Nahla S. Abdel-Azim
Phytochemistry Department
National Research Centre
Giza, Egypt

Sara Abdelfatah
Department of Pharmaceutical Biology
Institute of Pharmacy and Biochemistry
Johannes Gutenberg University
Mainz, Germany

Sabrina Adorisio
Department of Medicine
University of Perugia
Perugia, Italy

Nisar Ahmad
Department of Pharmacy
Abasyn University
Peshawar, Pakistan

Javaid Alam
Drug and Herbal Research Centre
Faculty of Pharmacy
University Kebangsang Malaysia
Kuala Lumpur, Malaysia

Gowhar Ali
Department of Pharmacy
University of Peshawar
Peshawar, Pakistan

Víctor Andrade
Laboratory of Cellular and Molecular
   Biology and Neuroscience
Faculty of Sciences International Centre
   for Biomedicine (ICC)
University of Chile
Santiago, Chile

Dhyan Kusuma Ayuningtyas
Bandung Institute of Technology
Bandung, Indonesia

Subhadip Banerjee
School of Natural Product Studies
Department of Pharmaceutical
   Technology
Jadavpur University
Kolkata, India

Kalpana Bhaskaran
Glycaemic Index Research Unit
Temasek Polytechnic
Singapore

Sayan Biswas
School of Natural Product Studies
Department of Pharmaceutical
   Technology
Jadavpur University
Kolkata, India

Tuhin Kanti Biswas
Department of Kayachikitsa (Medicine)
J.B. Roy State Ayurvedic Medical
   College and Hospital
Kolkata, India

Fernão C. Braga
Department of Pharmaceutical Products
Faculty of Pharmacy
Universidade Federal de Minas Gerais
   (UFMG)
Belo Horizonte, Brazil

Thomas Brendler
Pharmatoka SAS
Rueil-Malmaison, France

Shin Seung Chul
Food Safety Policy Bureau
Ministry of Food and Drug Safety
Chungcheongbuk-do, Korea

Nicole Cortés
Laboratory of Cellular and Molecular Biology
   and Neuroscience
Faculty of Sciences International Centre for
   Biomedicine (ICC)
University of Chile
Santiago, Chile

Steyner F. Côrtes
Department of Pharmacology
Institute of Biological Sciences
Universidade Federal de Minas Gerais
   (UFMG)
Belo Horizonte, Brazil

Bhaskar Das
School of Natural Product Studies
Department of Pharmaceutical Technology
Jadavpur University
Kolkata, India

Neeladrisingha Das
Molecular Endocrinology Laboratory
Department of Biotechnology
Indian Institute of Technology Roorkee
Uttarakhand, India

Abdessamad Debbab
Debbab Med
Munich, Germany

Domenico V. Delfino
Department of Medicine
University of Perugia
Perugia, Italy

Hiteshi Dhami-Shah
Medical Research Centre
Kasturba Health Society
Mumbai, India

Sharanbasappa Durg
Independent Researcher
Bidar, India

Asim K. Duttaroy
Chronic Disease Section
Department of Clinical Nutrition
Faculty of Medicine
University of Oslo
Oslo, Norway

Thomas Efferth
Department of Pharmaceutical Biology
Institute of Pharmacy and Biochemistry
Johannes Gutenberg University
Mainz, Germany

Hesham R. El-Seedi
Division of Pharmacognosy
Department of Medicinal Chemistry
Uppsala University
Uppsala, Sweden

and

Department of Chemistry
Faculty of Science
El-Menoufia University
Shebin El-Kom, Egypt

Abdelsamed I. Elshamy
Natural Compounds Chemistry Department
National Research Centre
Giza, Egypt

and

Faculty of Pharmaceutical Sciences
Tokushima Bunri University
Tokushima, Japan

Arunporn Etherat
Department of Applied Thai Traditional
   Medicine
Faculty of Medicine
Thammasat University
Bangkok, Thailand

Abdel-Razik H. Farrag
Department of Pathology
National Research Centre
Cairo, Egypt

B. Fibrich
University of Pretoria
Pretoria, South Africa

M. Frevel
ENZO Nutraceuticals Limited
Paeroa, New Zealand

Dilip Ghosh
NutriConnect
Sydney, Australia

Debayan Goswami
School of Natural Product Studies
Department of Pharmaceutical Technology
Jadavpur University
Kolkata, India

Ramesh K. Goyal
Delhi Pharmaceutical Sciences Research
    University
New Delhi, India

Leonardo Guzmán-Martínez
Laboratory of Cellular and Molecular Biology
    and Neuroscience
Faculty of Sciences International Centre for
    Biomedicine (ICC)
University of Chile
Santiago, Chile

Gunter Haesaerts
Pharmatoka SAS
Rueil-Malmaison, France

Ahmed R. Hamed
Phytochemistry Department and Biology Unit
Central Laboratory for Pharmaceutical
    and Drug Industries Research Division
National Research Centre
Giza, Egypt

Mohamed-Elamir F. Hegazy
Department of Pharmaceutical Biology
Institute of Pharmacy and Biochemistry
Johannes Gutenberg University
Mainz, Germany

and

Phytochemistry Department
National Research Centre
Giza, Egypt

Soleiman E. Helaly
Department of Microbial Drugs
Helmholtz Centre for Infection Research
Braunschweig, Germany

and

Department of Chemistry
Faculty of Science
Aswan University
Aswan, Egypt

L. Hingorani
Pharmanza Herbal Pvt. Ltd.
Gujarat, India

Nazar Ul Islam
Department of Pharmacy
Sarhad University of Science and Information
    Technology
Peshawar, Pakistan

Amit Kar
School of Natural Product Studies
Department of Pharmaceutical
    Technology
Jadavpur University
Kolkata, India

Chandra Kant Katiyar
Emami Ltd.
Kolkata, India

James Kean
Centre for Human Psychopharmacology
    Swinburne University of Technology
Melbourne, Australia

Kam Ming Ko
Division of Life Science
Hong Kong University of Science and
    Technology
Hong Kong, China

N. Lall
University of Pretoria
Pretoria, South Africa

I.A. Lambrechts
University of Pretoria
Pretoria, South Africa

Pou Kuan Leong
Division of Life Science
Hong Kong University of Science and
    Technology
Hong Kong, China

Ricardo B. Maccioni
Laboratory of Cellular and Molecular Biology
  and Neuroscience
Faculty of Sciences International Centre for
  Biomedicine (ICC)
University of Chile
Santiago, Chile

F. Mahomoodally
Department of Health Sciences
Faculty of Science
University of Mauritius
Réduit, Mauritius

Rutusmita Mishra
Molecular Endocrinology Laboratory
Department of Biotechnology
Indian Institute of Technology Roorkee
Uttarakhand, India

Tahia K. Mohamed
Natural Compounds Chemistry Department
National Research Centre
Giza, Egypt

Tarik A. Mohamed
Phytochemistry Department
National Research Centre
Giza, Egypt

Pulok K. Mukherjee
School of Natural Product Studies
Department of Pharmaceutical Technology
Jadavpur University
Kolkata, India

Isabella Muscari
Department of Surgery and Biomedical
  Sciences
University of Perugia
Perugia, Italy

D.B. Anantha Narayana
Ayurvidye Trust
Bengaluru, India

Masaaki Noji
Faculty of Pharmaceutical Sciences
Tokushima Bunri University
Tokushima, Japan

Panadda Nontahnum
Faculty of Agroindustry
King Mongkut's Institute of Technology
  Ladkrabang
Bangkok, Thailand

Paul W. Paré
Department of Chemistry and Biochemistry
Texas Tech University
Lubbock, Texas

Bhoomika M. Patel
Institute of Pharmacy
Nirma University
Ahmedabad, India

Jamuna Prakash
Department of Food Science and Nutrition
University of Mysore
Mysuru, India

and

Zhejiang Gongshang University
Hongzhou, China

and

International Academy of Food Science and
  Technology
Toronto, Canada

Hemangi Rawal
Institute of Pharmacy
Nirma University
Ahmedabad, India

Partha Roy
Molecular Endocrinology Laboratory
Department of Biotechnology
Indian Institute of Technology Roorkee
Uttarakhand, India

Mohamed E.M. Saeed
Department of Pharmaceutical Biology
Institute of Pharmacy and Biochemistry
Johannes Gutenberg University
Mainz, Germany

Romanee Sanguandeekul
Department of Food Technology
Faculty of Science
Chulalongkorn University
Bangkok, Thailand

Muhammad Shahid
Department of Pharmacy
Sarhad University of Science and Information
    Technology
Peshawar, Pakistan

Khaled A. Shams
Phytochemistry Department
National Research Centre
Giza, Egypt

R.B. Smarta
Interlink Marketing Consultancy Pvt Ltd
Mumbai, India

Pimpinan Somsong
School of Agricultural Resources
Chulalongkorn University
Bangkok, Thailand

George Srzednicki
School of Chemical Engineering
University of New South Wales
Sydney, Australia

Con Stough
Centre for Human Psychopharmacology
Swinburne University of Technology
Melbourne, Australia

Fazal Subhan
Department of Pharmacy
CECOS University
Peshawar, Pakistan

Elin Yulinah Sukandar
Bandung Institute of Technology
Bandung, Indonesia

Tran Van Sung
Institute of Chemistry
Vietnam Academy of Science and Technology
Hanoi, Vietnam

S. Suroowan
Department of Health Sciences
Faculty of Science
University of Mauritius
Réduit, Mauritius

Neeraj Tandon
Indian Council of Medical Research
New Delhi, India

Tan Tengli
Glycaemic Index Research Unit
Temasek Polytechnic
Singapore

Trinh Thi Thuy
Institute of Chemistry
Vietnam Academy of Science and
    Technology
Hanoi, Vietnam

Ong Jing Ting
Glycaemic Index Research Unit
Temasek Polytechnic
Singapore

Shobha Udipi
Medical Research Centre
Kasturba Health Society
Mumbai, India

Ihsan Ullah
Department of Pharmacy
University of Swabi
Swabi, Pakistan

Akemi Umeyama
Faculty of Pharmaceutical Sciences
Tokushima Bunri University
Tokushima, Japan

Ashok Vaidya
Medical Research Centre
Kasturba Health Society
Mumbai, India

Ajay George Varghese
Bipha Drug Laboratories Pvt Ltd
Kottayam, India

Ritu Varshney
Molecular Endocrinology Laboratory
Department of Biotechnology
Indian Institute of Technology Roorkee
Uttarakhand, India

Jayantha Wijayabandara
Faculty of Medical Sciences
University of Sri Jayewardenepura
Nugegoda, Sri Lanka

and

Bandaranaike Memorial Ayurvedic Research
    Institute
Department of Ayurveda
Maharagama, Sri Lanka

Satyapal Singh Yadav
Indian Council of Medical Research
New Delhi, India

Introduction

Globally, herbal medicine has been considered an important alternative to modern allopathic medicine. Although herbal medicines are very popular in society, only a few medicinal herbs have been scientifically evaluated for their potential in medical treatment. In most countries, herbal drugs are poorly regulated and are often neither registered nor controlled by the health authorities. The safety of herbal medicines remains a major concern. In the United States, the Food and Drug Administration (FDA) has estimated that over 50,000 adverse events are caused by botanical and other dietary supplements. In addition, for most herbal drugs, efficacy has not been proved at the clinical level and quality is not assured. The World Health Organization's (WHO) Traditional Medicine (TM) Strategy 2014–2023 focuses on promoting the safety, efficacy and quality of TM by expanding the knowledge base and providing guidance on regulatory and quality assurance standards.

The use of herbal drugs for the prevention and treatment of various health ailments has been in practice from time immemorial. Nearly one third of the world's population uses herbal medicine as the primary form of healthcare. Because of their unique effects, herbal medicines have been gaining popularity all over the world. Generally, it is believed that the risk associated with herbal drugs is significantly lower, but several reports on serious reactions are indicating the need for development of effective regulatory guidelines and quality control systems for authentication, isolation and standardisation of herbal medicine. At the same time, however, the lack of harmonised international regulatory guidelines regarding the manufacturing of herbal medicines represents a major obstacle in achieving the required quality assurance of herbal products worldwide.

Plants are producing numerous chemically and pharmacologically active, highly diverse secondary metabolites that are optimised to exert therapeutic functions, but are still far from being exhaustively investigated. Resulting from huge scientific and consumer demand for natural product–based drug discovery, new approaches for the identification, characterisation and pharmaceutical level clinical trials of natural products are being developed to address some of the challenges related with the development of plant-based therapeutics. One major asset of medicinal plant–based drug discovery is the existence of ethnopharmacological information providing hints for compounds therapeutically effective in humans. In order to harvest its full potential, of particular importance is the adoption of a broad interdisciplinary approach involving ethnopharmacological knowledge, botany, phytochemistry and more relevant pharmacological testing strategies (e.g. early *in vivo* efficacy studies and compound identification strategies including metabolism and synergistic action of the plant constituents). Resupply from the original plant species is very often unfeasible to meet market demands upon commercialisation of a natural product, and alternative resupply approaches are being developed that rely on biotechnological production or chemical synthesis. Total chemical synthesis is an effective resupply strategy in cases of natural products or natural product derivatives with simple structures, such as acetylsalicylic acid and ephedrine. For complex structures with multiple chiral centres, however, total synthesis is, at present, both difficult and economically unfeasible in most cases, requiring significant technological advances to be successfully applied. For the resupply of complex natural products, usually harvesting from plant sources and semi-synthesis from naturally occurring precursors still remain the most economically viable approaches. Although biotechnological production is currently not broadly applied for industry-scale production of plant-derived natural products, it bears potential that can be harvested in the future in alignment with the progress of the knowledge of plant biosynthetic pathways and the development of more efficient genetic engineering strategies and tools.

Natural product–based drug discovery and development represents a complex endeavour demanding a highly integrated interdisciplinary approach based on ethnopharmacological knowledge. All recent scientific developments, technologic advances and research trends clearly indicate that natural products will be among the most important sources of new drugs in the future.

The paradigm shift in natural product research has resulted in an extensive revolution in phytochemistry, which has strengthened its importance through the application of powerful new technologies in enhancing the original link between phytochemistry and traditional medicine. To establish an evidence base for traditional medicine, there are some essential requirements, including the development of guidelines for safety, efficacy and quality. To appreciate that perception, it is important to be aware of the goals for traditional medicine. One of the important goals that should be included is that it is a vital aspect of the health system and for patients to be covered by health insurance for their use of traditional medicine products. Traditional medicine for healthcare requires reproducible quality and a strong evidence base that will assure safety and efficacy for patients, as well as practitioners.

As per WHO definitions, there are three kinds of herbal medicines: raw plant material, processed plant material and medicinal herbal products. The use of herbal medicines has increased markedly in line with the global trend of people returning to natural therapies. Natural medicinal products are classified in different countries as dietary supplements, nutraceuticals, complementary medicines or health supplements. These are traditionally considered harmless and increasingly being consumed by people without prescriptions. However, some of these products can cause health problems, some are not effective, and some may interact with other drugs. Standardisation of natural medicine formulations is essential to assess the quality of drugs based on the concentration of their active principles. Quality evaluation of natural medicine preparations is a fundamental requirement of the industry and other organisations dealing with herbal products.

Considering the entire supply chain of natural medicines, this book emphasises the safety, quality and efficacy of clinically proven herbal and/or natural medicines. We have divided the book into five main categories: Quality and Chemistry; Safety; Regulation; Clinical Efficacy; and Reviews. We have tried to incorporate more industry contributions from those who are closely involved with evidence-based product development. Every effort has been made to provide maximum input for the readers to gain insight into contemporary scientific happenings in the field of natural medicine and particularly herbal drugs research, which might be effective in allowing them to forecast their own research work.

Section I

Quality and Chemistry

1 Efficacy, Quality, Safety and Toxicity of Herbal Medicine
Safeguarding Public Health

S. Suroowan and F. Mahomoodally

CONTENTS

1.1 INTRODUCTION

The relationship between humans and plants dates back to antiquity (Hakeem et al. 2019). Man has always been curious by nature and passionate about plants. Early attempts by primitive man to assuage suffering included the exploration of the medicinal virtues of plants by trial and error and employing the doctrine of signatures (Attard and Attard 2019). Indeed, traditional medicine, including herbal medicine, involves the diagnosis, prevention and elimination of physical, social or mental imbalance (Mosihuzzaman and Choudhary 2008). Successful therapeutic attempts have, since then, been transferred from one generation to the other verbally, as well as recorded in writing (Kunle et al. 2012).

Interestingly, the consumption of herbal products has become an integral part of healthcare after that several limitations of conventional medicine have been pinpointed in the West. Between the years 1999 and 2000 an increase of over 380% in sales of herbal medicine was observed due to the increasing complexity of diseases, as well as the failure of conventional medicinal approaches to address a wide array of ailments (Zhang et al. 2015). Scientists have used herbs as inspiration to discover new conventional therapeutic agents. Indeed, up to 25% of conventional medicines are derived from plants, the most obvious examples being aspirin, artemisinin, ephedrine and paclitacxel (Bent 2008).

Although mankind has employed the same plants for centuries, the regulations surrounding their contemporary use have been divided regionally, and different legal provisions prevail in diverse regions regarding the authorisation for their use (Chan et al. 2012). Currently, more than one terminology is employed to describe the medicinal use of plants, including 'herbal medicinal products', 'natural health products' and 'botanical medicines' (Chan et al. 2012; Wiesner and Knöss 2014). Different strategies have been devised to evaluate the safety profile of herbal medicines, and in some countries the classification and acceptance of herbal plants varies based on cultural habits (Wiesner and Knöss 2014).

One pertinent issue to safeguard public health includes the quality, efficacy, safety and toxicity of herbal medicine, given that there is a paucity of data surrounding these concerns. Even though there are different legislations governing the authorisation of use of herbal products, evaluation of key factors corresponding to their quality, efficacy, safety and toxicity should be regulated by scientifically validated methods. Therefore, this chapter endeavours to disseminate currently used approaches to ensure this and attempts to provide suggestions to ensure that herbal medicines of reasonable standard are marketed and thus can significantly improve public health.

1.2 HERBS AND HERBAL MEDICINE

A herb is any form of a plant or a plant product such as the flowers, leaves, stems, roots, seeds and tubers. These can either be sold raw or preparations of them can be concocted where the herb is macerated in a solvent to extract the phytoconstituents. Common solvents used for extraction include water and alcohol, among others. The phytoconstituents of a herb are also referred to as 'phytochemicals' or 'secondary metabolites' and form part of diverse classes of chemical compounds including alkaloids, fatty acids, flavonoids, glycosides and saponins and confer the therapeutic or medicinal benefits. Given the fact that diverse chemical entities occur in herbs, manufacturers of herbal products design standardised preparations of the herbs whereby a given phytochemical is present in a consistent amount (Powers 2002). Herbal medicine involves the use of herbs for their therapeutic or medicinal value. They can be concocted from any part of the plant and are administered orally or topically and must be of reasonable quality (Kunle 2012).

1.3 QUALITY OF HERBAL MEDICINE

There is no denying that the quality of herbal products is an absolute prerequisite for regulation and application. Knowledge of the quality and the chemical composition of an herbal product ensures its safe and effective use. It also allows the reproduction of clinical results. As an act of good practice, the full botanical name of the plant species must be used while performing a literature search on the plant species during information documentation. This approach ensures that even if distinct plants species share the same Latin or common English name, they can be easily distinguished from each other. In addition, this approach enables the ruling out of cultivars, subspecies and chemovarieties (Wiesner and Knöss 2014).

Several instances of inadvertent or deliberate substitutions have been recorded, as exemplified in the literature when Chinese herbal preparations containing Siberian (*Eleutherococcus senticosus* (Rupr. & Maxim.) Maxim.), American (*Panax quinquefolius* L.) and Japanese ginseng were substituted for Korean or Chinese ginseng (*Panax ginseng* C.A. Mey.). This is of particular concern when the substitutes have a greater toxicity than the actual original components. Renal fibrosis has also resulted due to the use of *Aristolochia fangchi*, Y.C. Wu ex L.D. Chow & S.M. Hwang, as well as poisoning from *Podophyllum emodi* Wall. ex Hook.f. & Thomson species, which indicates that herbal medicines need to be of reasonable quality to ensure their safe use (Mosihuzzaman and Choudhary 2008).

During the mounting of meta-analyses, due consideration must be attributed to the type of solvent used for extraction, because different phytochemicals are soluble in different solvents. Hence, the composition of distinct extracts of the same plant will evidently contrast. It is certainly an erroneous approach to compare results of the same plant from different studies while there is no standardisation of the extract being considered. Moreover, knowledge of the major constituent is imperative, but other chemicals occurring in smaller amounts should also be investigated due to impurities and adulteration of the starting plant material, which could significantly alter clinical results and the safety profile of the product. For example, this situation can be reflected in the presence of aflatoxins that can significantly lead to toxicity. Analysis of the composition and validation of the production process will improve the reproducibility of clinical and non-clinical studies (Zhang et al. 2015).

1.4 LACK OF RESEARCH ON HERBAL MEDICINE QUALITY

When compared to conventional medicines, there are limited studies conducted on the quality, efficacy, safety, herb–drug interactions and herbal side effects (particularly hepatotoxicity) of herbal medicines. In 2014, a review mentioned that a search in PubMed using the keyword herbal medicinal products (HMPs) resulted into 30,917 articles. Most of the reviews accessed highlighted as a concluding remark the lack of scientific data on HMPs to judge the efficacy or safety of the published information (Whitten et al. 2006; Posadzki et al. 2013; Teschke et al. 2013).

One relevant cause of the lack of scientific evidence surrounding HMPs could be attributed to the fact that limited funding is allocated to this area of research. Since 1999, the National Center for Complementary and Alternative Medicine at the National Institute of Health has been allocated between US$50–128.8 million every year to research complementary and alternative medicines, including herbal medicine. Poor funding hinders interdisciplinary collaboration to train people to carry out high quality research on herbal medicine, including the refinement of existing practices (Pelkonen et al. 2014).

Research on HMPs and development of this market requires strong political commitment. In China, the use of traditional Chinese medicine dates back more than 2000 years, and over 11,000 medicinal plants and 100,000 formulations have been documented. These are often used and selected for the development of novel and multi-component drug candidates. In 2008, the Chinese state invested US$124 billion in healthcare, which also aimed to diversify research on HMPs and to develop new markets for HMPs (Wang et al. 2008).

1.5 CHANGING ATTITUDES TOWARDS HMPs

In the European Union (EU), HMPs are officially recognised as medicines based on directives set out in 2001 and 2004. On the other hand, in the United States (US), HMPs are still classified as botanical products and are controlled by food legislation due to their chemical complexity. In 2008, the FDA approved its first botanical drug Veregen® (sinecatechins) derived from green tea for application on genital and perianal warts. In 2012, Crofelemer was approved for the symptomatic relief of diarrhoea in HIV/AIDs patients under antiretroviral therapy. Despite the reluctance to register HMPs as official medicine, it is widely recognised today that they can be important alternative sources of medicines for chronic diseases such as cancer and heart conditions. For example Chinese medicine–based PHY906 has passed phase I and II trials for cancer and Dantonic® underwent phase III trial for angina in the United States (Chen et al. 2008; Yen et al. 2008; Fan et al. 2012).

1.6 SAFETY OF HERBAL MEDICINE

Given their wide use by various cultures worldwide, herbal medicine is still considered safe and devoid of adverse effects in many parts of the world. Nonetheless, a number of adverse effects have been recorded from the use of herbal medicine and in some cases these have been traced back to the presence of contaminants and adulteration. Herbs may also consist of phytochemicals that are toxic. Profound phytochemical and pharmacological studies are warranted to highlight the safety of herbal products and to rule out the risk of adverse events. Potential contaminants of herbal medicinal products may include microorganisms (*Staphylococcus aureus*, *Escherichia coli*, *Salmonella*, *Shigella*), microbial toxins (bacterial endotoxins, aflatoxins), pesticides (DDT, organic phosphates, insecticides and herbicides), fumigation agents (methyl bromide, phosphine), radioactivity and metals such as lead, cadmium and mercury (Ernst 2002; Mosihuzzaman and Choudhary 2008). Toxic metals have been identified in diverse Chinese remedies, such as the presence of lead in Bal Jivan Chamcho. Several adverse effects can result due to such contamination, including lead toxicity and alopecia from thallium (Ernst 2002; Mosihuzzaman and Choudhary 2008).

1.7   EFFICACY OF HERBAL MEDICINES

The efficacy of an HMP is the extent to which it improves health and contributes to wellbeing. The most widely chosen method for evaluating the efficacy of an HMP is by conducting clinical trials whereby clinical, laboratory and/or diagnostic outcomes are used to determine efficacy. Positive clinical outcomes such as improvement in morbidity and mortality, reduced pain or discomfort and overall improvement of quality of life are good indicators of efficacy. Laboratory and other diagnostic outcomes – for example improvement in blood pressure or findings from electrocardiogram, radiology or imaging techniques – are also good evidence of efficacy (Mosihuzzaman and Choudhary 2008).

Efficacy of herbal medicines can be evaluated using the following methods (Mosihuzzaman and Choudhary 2008):

1. Anecdotal reports: Collection and organisation of anecdotal reports is considered an important component in the evaluation of efficacy of a large group of herbs, as knowledge of many herbs is unknown.
2. Case reports: These are the first clues for new diseases, interventions and unknown undocumented adverse effects. The data published in reputed clinical journals can be an important baseline in this process. These can be retrospective (data obtained from previous documentation or occurrence) or prospective in nature (in this case a baseline is used to follow-up data). Prospective case reports can be of two kinds: observational (documentation is executed through passive observation only) or interventional (the system is adjusted by standardising design).
3. Case series: These are a collection of case reports that are organised to determine any association. These can be prospective (observational or interventional) or retrospective case reports.
4. Randomised clinical trials: In conventional medicine, these are the ultimate way to investigate efficacy. However, significant resources must be allocated or made available to conduct such trials.

1.8   REQUIREMENTS OF EFFICACY OF HERBAL PRODUCTS IN THE EUROPEAN UNION

The EU requirements for efficacy of herbal medicines are mentioned in this article, as herbal medicines are most widely regulated through these legislations. These are set out in Directive (2001)/83/ EC on medicinal products used among humans and further amended to nationally register herbal medicinal products based solely on their traditional use by Directive (2004)/24/EC. This directive also constitutes a scientific committee, namely the committee on herbal medicinal products, to harmonise the herbal medicinal product market in European countries.

Prior to its launch into the market and to obtain a marketing authorisation or registration, an HMP must be approved by the national competent authorities or the European commission after the applicant has made an application through any of these three pathways (Claeson 2014):

1. Full marketing authorisation application: This refers to article 8(3) of Directive (2001)/83/ EC and it is the usual way to apply for any new medicinal product (New Chemical Entity). Evidence of pharmaceutical tests (quality documentation), non-clinical (toxicological and pharmacological) studies and clinical trials must also be submitted. The efficacy of the product should also be demonstrated by conducting clinical trials and must be relevant to the therapeutic area being investigated. Approval is based upon evidence that the benefits of the product outweigh the associated risks. This route is rarely employed and only a scarce number of HMPs have been registered in the EU using this guideline.

2. Well-established marketing authorisation application: This type of application refers to article 10a of Directive (2001)/83/EC. It specifically targets medicinal products for which evidence of long-standing and well-established use in the EU is available. Non-controlled clinical trials as well as epidemiological studies including cohort and observational studies are used as evidence in the assessment. The directive further states the following: 'The applicant shall not be required to provide the results of toxicological and pharmacological tests or the results of clinical trials if he can demonstrate that the constituent or constituents of the medicinal product have a well-established medicinal use with recognised efficacy and an acceptable level of safety, by means of a detailed scientific bibliography'. A publicly available bibliography of scientific origin may be used as evidence for long-term use of the product, and the number of indications is dictated by available literature. Other criteria for assessing the product include at least 10 years of use within the EU, quantitative aspects of the use of the product, the extent of scientific interest in the product and the consistency of scientific assessments.

3. Traditional use marketing registration: This is a simplified approach for products that do not fulfill the requirements for recognised efficacy but which have displayed potential efficacy based on long standing use and experience. This was introduced in 2004 as an amendment to the Directive (2001)/83/EC. Requirements for clinical trials were also reduced for these products. However, no exceptions were made with regard to the pharmaceutical quality of the product, and the national competent authorities (NCA) is given full authority to investigate on its safety. In addition, the following conditions also have to be satisfied to obtain marketing authorisation or registration:
   • They can be used without the supervision of a medical practitioner for diagnostic purposes or prescription or for treatment monitoring
     – Their strength and dosage are specified
     – They are intended for oral, external or inhalation use
     – The product or corresponding product has been used medicinally for at least 30 years and at least 15 years within the community

The applicant must also submit quality clinical and non-clinical data relating to the product to be registered. The documentation must be submitted in the Common Technical Document Format as per the International Conference on Harmonisation.

1.8.1 Status of Herbal Medicine in the United States

According to the Dietary Supplement Health and Education Act (DSHEA) of 1994, all herbs are considered dietary supplements in the United States. Supplements are defined in this act as anything that supplements the diet such as amino acids, concentrates, enzymes, extracts, herbs, minerals, metabolites, organ tissues and vitamins. The major difference between a dietary supplement and a drug is that it cannot be used in the diagnosis, prophylaxis and treatment of a disease. Even so, manufacturers of herbal supplements are allowed to make claims surrounding the use of their products that can be linked to health benefits, such as an Echinacea product is claimed to enhance the immune system (Institute of Medicine 2005).

In the United States, dietary supplements can be marketed and sold without providing proof of safety and efficacy. To halt the marketing of an herbal medicine, the Food and Drug Administration (FDA) must provide proof that it is unsafe for use. These regulations differ greatly from the marketing authorisation of pharmaceutical drugs, which must provide proof of safety and efficacy. The absence of strict legislation surrounding the selling of herbal supplements has led to varying and uncontrolled amounts of the active ingredients in products from different manufacturers, and this leads to doubts concerning their safety and efficacy. An investigation into the levels of active ingredients into 25 different ginseng supplements revealed a 15- to 200-fold variation in their concentration (Bent 2008).

1.8.2 TOXICITY OF HERBAL MEDICINE

Although herbs are natural, they are not devoid of adverse effects. Side effects and herb–drug interactions are common among plants. An event of particular interest occurred when 105 Belgian patients consumed the Chinese medicine *Aristolochia fangchi* Y.C. Wu ex L.D. Chow & S.M. Hwang for weight loss. Of these, 43 developed end-stage renal failure and 39 had prophylactic kidney removal, while 18 were found to develop urothelial carcinoma (Nortier and Vanherweghem 2002). Pyrrolizidine alkaloids present in various herbs are also commonly known to induce hepatotoxicity and potentially fatal veno-occlusive disease (Stickel et al. 2005). Contaminants in herbal medicine are of particular interest among products imported from Asia. Interestingly, a study examined 260 patented herbal products from Asia, out of which 26% contained high levels of heavy metals and 7% contained undeclared drugs (Anon 2003). When assessing the toxicity of herbal medicines, the dose of the herbal product is very important, and this may be achieved by any of the following methods: *in vivo* and *in vitro* techniques, cell line and microarray techniques and standardisation or other appropriate techniques.

1.8.3 STANDARDISATION OF HERBAL MEDICINE

A document produced by the International Union of Pure and Applied Chemistry (IUPAC) recommends a series of steps for the standardisation of herbal products. These include (Mosihuzzaman and Choudhary 2008):

1. Authentication: The first step is obviously the identification of the plant species by its Latin (binomial) name. Authentication is conducted by macroscopic, microscopic and taxonomic evaluation. Alongside important information related to the plant should be recorded the botanical identity, part collected, regional status and stage of collection (phytomorphology, microscopy, histology).
2. Physical parameters: Organoleptic properties are evaluated, such as appearance, ash value, disintegration time, flowability, friability, hardness, moisture, odour, pH, sedimentation, viscosity and taste.
3. Chromatographic and spectroscopic evaluation: Quantitative and semi-quantitative data on the active constituents and marker compounds present in the crude drug or herbal product are obtained through ultraviolet (UV)–vis spectrophotometry, thin-layer chromatography (TLC), high-performance thin-layer chromatography (HPTLC) and nuclear magnetic resonance (NMR) analysis. Hence, a fingerprint of the herbal product or crude drug is produced.
4. Microbiological parameters: This can be performed using as guideline standards listed in the *Romanian* or *British Pharmacopoeia*. The herbal products are tested for *Escherichia coli* and moulds, total viable count, enterobacteria and aflatoxin.
5. Pesticide residue analysis: Common harmful pesticides should be assayed for, including DDT, BHC, toxaphene and aldrin.
6. Heavy metal analysis: The presence of toxic metals such as Cu, Zn, Mn, Fe, Cd, Pb and Hg should be investigated.

1.8.4 The Need for New Approaches

Currently, there are mounting challenges in drug development and clinical treatment for various disorders. Both in developing and developed countries there is an emergence of a larger number of chronic disease cases that are a significant cause of morbidity and mortality (Schadt 2009; Barabási et al. 2011). Notably, chronic disorders are an amalgam of various etiological factors and various molecular pathways are involved. The prophylaxis and management of chronic disorders has led to the development of various drugs to address individual symptoms and hence the use of diverse drug classes has led to the arousal of various side and adverse effects, interactions (drug–drug, herb–drug, food–drug) and polypharmacy (Hopkins et al. 2006). It seems an interesting strategy to aim at different targets using diverse active constituents in a single drug, as in the case of HMPs, but in a personalised fashion for every individual patient.

New avenues in the advent of personalised HMPs involve the use of the modern omic methods such as genomics, transcriptomics, epigenomics, proteomics and metabolomics to give the use of traditional medicines a new dimension (van der Greef and McBurney 2005; van Wietmarschen et al. 2009). The use of *in silico* models has enabled the study of a wide range of HMPs on targets, but these data need to be confirmed in experiments. Following the human genome project involving billions of dollars, advanced technological tools have become more affordable. Likewise, proteomics has become more affordable and sensitive, with various enhanced techniques including shotgun, targeted and multiplexed qualitative proteomics using isobaric tags (Doerr 2010; Engmann et al. 2010; Gilmore and Washburn 2010; Yan et al. 2010).

1.8.5 Constraints and Challenges

A plethora of secondary metabolites are naturally expressed both in the raw plant and in the extract. In this endeavour, the determination of which metabolites are responsible for the pharmacological properties becomes challenging. Environmental conditions also influence the composition of secondary metabolites, among which the most important are soil, altitude, seasonal variation of temperature, atmospheric humidity, daylight and rainfall pattern. In various areas, plant species are intentionally or unintentionally substituted to become widely available and be sold at cheaper prices, as in the case of the substitution of *Illicium verum* Hook.f. (star anise) by *Illicium anisatum* (bastard anise), which contains the highly toxic constituent anisatin (Ražić et al. 2006).

1.8.6 Recommendations for Existing and Future Practice

Herbal medicine should be treated as a drug rather than food. It should be acknowledged that despite being natural, HMPs can exert plausible side and adverse effects, including herb–drug and drug–drug interactions. In addition, HMPs should not be used in large amounts and over the long term until their standard dose has been established (Zhang 2011; Zhang et al. 2015). As for conventional drugs, herbal medicine should be reserved for specific ailment conditions rather than being used continuously. For example, the toxic dose of *Radix Bupleuri Chinensis* used in Japan is 192 g/60 kg, while the clinical dose is 9 g/60 kg. However, the use of higher doses combined with long-term use undeniably causes adverse events (Zhang 2011; Zhang et al. 2015).

The toxicity of an herbal medicine can be divided into its intrinsic and extrinsic toxicity. The intrinsic toxicity is due to the herb alone, such as the adverse effects encountered from Ephedra, *Aristolochia* and *Aconitum* species while extrinsic toxicity is due to the presence of contaminants or adulteration of the herbal product (Zhang et al. 2015).

Herbal medicine should have specific indications, for example Ma Huang, which is traditionally used to treat respiratory disorders in China, is marketed as a dietary supplement in the

United States, intended to cause weight loss. The use of the herb in high doses has led to heart attacks, strokes and several cases of mortality (Lee 2000; Haller and Benowitz 2001). Herb–drug interactions arising from the use of herbal medicine and conventional drugs are a stark reality today even if few scientific investigations have been carried out to determine this (Ernst 2002). A retrospective study among patients suffering from psychosis revealed that up to 36.4% of patients employ herbs and conventional drugs concomitantly. This is associated to at least 60% of the cases of adverse events when quetiapine, olanzapine and clozapine are administered concomitantly with herbal products from any of the following plants: *Akebia caulis*, *Fructus gardenia*, *Fructus schisandrae chinensis*, *Radix bupleuri*, *Radix rehmanniae* and *Semen plantaginis* (Zhang 2011).

Currently, pharmacological data available on most herbs are limited. In addition to the mechanism of action of each of the components present in the herb, data such as minimum toxic dose, toxic target organs, safe dose range and therapeutic window are missing. Therefore, to effectively debate on the safety and efficacy of herbal medicine and hence to warrant their use among humans, these data are of prime interest (Zhang 2011; Zhang et al. 2015).

This calls for collaborative partnership among consumers to document traditional uses and provide evidence of long-standing use, scientists to evaluate the claimed effects and investigate plausible mechanisms of action and research institutions that are well equipped for investigation, as well as with industry.

Research on HMPs requires a multidisciplinary approach and the hand-in-hand collaboration of researchers, universities and industry. In various countries, the plant as a whole or herbal preparation is considered the active ingredient. Nonetheless the occurrence of different components in the plant must be evaluated, including their action. Instead of focusing on single compounds solely, standardised and refined extracts of plants can be undertaken. Both the characterised and uncharacterised portion of the herbal product should be subjected to pharmacological assays, such as varying the dose and investigating the response in a given model. In the occurrence of a therapeutic action from the characterised portion and no therapeutic or safety concern in the uncharacterised part, the therapeutic and safe action of the herbal product or plant can be confirmed. Deeper insight into the mechanism of action of the components is also warranted (Chen et al. 2008).

Communication and knowledge of different regulatory systems for the registration of herbal products can provide a baseline for the development of a common legislation in the long run, but this is still a huge challenge. Strengths and weaknesses existing in different regulatory systems can be identified. Regulations being in line with standard practices can be highlighted and proposed for mutual adoption worldwide. Different regional laws are prevalent worldwide as can be epitomised in Europe, Asia and South America. A convergent legislative regulatory approach might be valuable in the provision of herbal-based therapeutic substances of adequately tested quality, safety and efficacy geared towards promoting an enhanced level of public health (Barnes 2003).

1.9 CONCLUSION

Given the current existing legislations, herbal medicine quality, efficacy and safety are not addressed profoundly. The toxicity and herb–drug interactions arising due to herbal medicine use require urgent attention. Even if, in some countries, strict legislation exists for the marketing and use of herbal medicines among the general public, active pharmacovigilance systems need to be set up to ensure their safe use throughout their lifetime. As herbal medicines are recognised under different terms (e.g. 'herbal medicines' and 'dietary supplements'), it is important for a worldwide organisation such as the World Health Organization to set up standard guidelines for the efficacy, safety, quality and toxicity of HMPs.

REFERENCES

Anon. (2003). Herbal medicines and perioperative care. *Obstetrics & Gynecology*, **101**(1), 197.

Attard, E. and Attard, H., 2019. Hawthorn: *Crataegus oxyacantha, Crataegus monogyna* and related species. In *Nonvitamin and Nonmineral Nutritional Supplements*, 289–293, Academic Press.

Barabási, A., Gulbahce, N. and Loscalzo, J. (2011). Network medicine: A network-based approach to human disease. *Nature Reviews Genetics*, **12**(1), 56–68.

Barnes, J. (2003). Quality, efficacy and safety of complementary medicines: Fashions, facts and the future. Part I. Regulation and quality. *British Journal of Clinical Pharmacology*, **55**(3), 226–233.

Bent, S. (2008). Herbal medicine in the United States: Review of efficacy, safety, and regulation. *Journal of General Internal Medicine*, **23**(6), 854–859.

Chan, K., Shaw, D., Simmonds, M.S., Leon, C.J., Xu, Q., Lu, A., Sutherland, et al. (2012). Good practice in reviewing and publishing studies on herbal medicine, with special emphasis on traditional Chinese medicine and Chinese materia medica. *Journal of Ethnopharmacology*, **140**(3), 469–475.

Chen, S., Dou, J., Temple, R., Agarwal, R., Wu, K. and Walker, S. (2008). New therapies from old medicines. *Nature Biotechnology*, **26**(10), 1077–1083.

Claeson, P. (2014). Requirements on efficacy of herbal medicinal products. *Journal of Ethnopharmacology*, **158**, 463–466.

Directive 2004/24/EC of the European Parliament and of the Council of 31 March 2004 with regard to traditional herbal medicinal products.

Doerr, A. (2010). Targeted proteomics. *Nature Methods*, **7**(1), 34–34.

Engmann, O., Campbell, J., Ward, M., Giese, K. and Thompson, A. (2010). Comparison of a protein-level and peptide-level labeling strategy for quantitative proteomics of synaptosomes using isobaric tags. *Journal of Proteome Research*, **9**(5), 2725–2733.

Ernst, E. (2002). Herbal medicine: Advocates need to put things right. *Trends in Pharmacological Sciences*, **23**(8), 359.

The European Parliament and the Council of the European Union. (2001) Directive 2001/83/EC of the European Parliament and of the Council of 6 November 2001 on the Community code relating to medicinal products for human use. *Official Journal of the European Union*, 67–128.

Fan, T., Deal, G., Koo, H., Rees, D., Sun, H., Chen, S., Dou, J. et al. (2012). Future development of global regulations of Chinese herbal products. *Journal of Ethnopharmacology*, **140**(3), 568–586.

Gilmore, J. and Washburn, M. (2010). Advances in shotgun proteomics and the analysis of membrane proteomes. *Journal of Proteomics*, **73**(11), 2078–2091.

Hakeem, K. R., Abdul, W. M., Hussain, M. M., and Razvi, S. S. I. (2019). Traditional Information About Herbal Medicine of Oral Activity. In *Oral Health and Herbal Medicine* (pp. 17–18). Springer, Cham.

Haller, C. and Benowitz, N. (2001). Adverse cardiovascular and central nervous system events associated with dietary supplements containing ephedra alkaloids. *ACC Current Journal Review*, **10**(3), 25–26.

Hopkins, A., Mason, J. and Overington, J. (2006). Can we rationally design promiscuous drugs? *Current Opinion in Structural Biology*, **16**(1), 127–136.

Institute of Medicine, (2005). *Dietary Supplements: A Framework for Evaluating Safety*. Washington, DC: National Academies Press.

Kunle, O. F., Egharevba, H. O. and Ahmadu, P. O. (2012). Standardization of herbal medicines – A review. *International Journal of Biodiversity and Conservation*, **4**(3), 101–112.

Lee, M. (2000). Cytotoxicity assessment of Ma-Huang (Ephedra) under different conditions of preparation. *Toxicological Sciences*, **56**(2), 424–430.

Mosihuzzaman, M. and Choudhary, M. (2008). Protocols on safety, efficacy, standardization, and documentation of herbal medicine (IUPAC technical report). *Pure and Applied Chemistry*, **80**(10), 2195–2230.

Nortier, J. and Vanherweghem, J. (2002). Renal interstitial fibrosis and urothelial carcinoma associated with the use of a Chinese herb (*Aristolochia fangchi*). *Toxicology*, *181–182*, 577–580.

Pelkonen, O., Xu, Q. and Fan, T. (2014). Why is research on herbal medicinal products important and how can we improve its quality? *Journal of Traditional and Complementary Medicine*, **4**(1), 1–7.

Posadzki, P., Watson, L. and Ernst, E. (2013). Herb-drug interactions: An overview of systematic reviews. *British Journal of Clinical Pharmacology*, **75**(3), 603–618.

Powers, M. (2002). Book review: Evidence-based herbal medicine. *Annals of Pharmacotherapy*, **36**(9), 1485–1486.

Ražić, S., Đogo, S. and Slavković, L. (2006). Multivariate characterization of herbal drugs and rhizosphere soil samples according to their metallic content. *Microchemical Journal*, **84**(1–2), 93–101.

Schadt, E. (2009). Molecular networks as sensors and drivers of common human diseases. *Nature*, **461**(7261), 218–223.

Stickel, F., Patsenker, E. and Schuppan, D. (2005). Herbal hepatotoxicity. *Journal of Hepatology*, **43**(5), 901–910.

Teschke, R., Frenzel, C., Glass, X., Schulze, J. and Eickhoff, A. (2013). Herbal hepatotoxicity: A critical review. *British Journal of Clinical Pharmacology*, **75**(3), 630–636.

van der Greef, J. and McBurney, R. (2005). Rescuing drug discovery: *In vivo* systems pathology and systems pharmacology. *Nature Reviews Drug Discovery*, **4**(12), 961–967.

van Wietmarschen, H., Yuan, K., Lu, C., Gao, P., Wang, J., Xiao, C. Yan, X. et al. (2009). Systems biology guided by Chinese medicine reveals new markers for sub-typing rheumatoid arthritis patients. *Journal of Clinical Rheumatology*, **15**(7), 330–337.

Wang, L., Zhou, G., Liu, P., Song, J., Liang, Y., Yan, X., Xu, F. et al. (2008). Dissection of mechanisms of Chinese medicinal formula Realgar-Indigo naturalis as an effective treatment for promyelocytic leukemia. *Proceedings of the National Academy of Sciences*, **105**(12), 4826–4831.

Whitten, D., Myers, S., Hawrelak, J. and Wohlmuth, H. (2006). The effect of St John's Wort extracts on CYP3A: A systematic review of prospective clinical trials. *British Journal of Clinical Pharmacology*, **62**(5), 512–526.

Wiesner, J. and Knöss, W. (2014). Future visions for traditional and herbal medicinal products—A global practice for evaluation and regulation? *Journal of Ethnopharmacology*, **158**, 516–518.

Yan, W., Luo, J., Robinson, M., Eng, J., Aebersold, R. and Ranish, J. (2010). Index-ion triggered MS2 ion quantification: A novel proteomics approach for reproducible detection and quantification of targeted proteins in complex mixtures. *Molecular & Cellular Proteomics*, **10**(3), M110.005611.

Yen, Y., So, S., Rose, M., Saif, M., Chu, E., Chen, L., Liu, S., Foo, A., Tilton, R. and Cheng, Y. (2008). Phase I/II study of capecitabine and PHY906 in hepatocellular carcinoma. *Journal of Clinical Oncology*, **26**(15), 4610–4610.

Zhang, J., Onakpoya, I., Posadzki, P. and Eddouks, M. (2015). The safety of herbal medicine: From prejudice to evidence. *Evidence-Based Complementary and Alternative Medicine*, **2015**, 1–3.

Zhang, Z. (2011). P03-366 – An epidemiological study of concomitant use of herbal medicine and antipsychotics in schizophrenic patients: Implication for herb-drug interaction. *European Psychiatry*, **26**, 1536.

2 Standardisation and Quality Control of Herbal Medicines
From Raw Materials to Finished Products

Jayantha Wijayabandara

CONTENTS

2.1 INTRODUCTION

Medicinal plants have been used as sources of medicine in virtually all cultures. The recognition of their therapeutic action through a vast amount of empirical knowledge concerning the prevention and treatment of diseases is the fundamental basis of the systems of traditional medicine, including Ayurveda. Traditional systems of medicine still make a great contribution to the health of the people around the globe, and herbal medicinal products (HMPs) represent a substantial portion of the global drug market (World Health Organization 2005). Indigenous remedies have become an economic and sound approach to spread healthcare to people in many countries. Today, there is a great deal of global interest in traditional medicine mainly due to the realisation of toxicity and harmful side effects of many modern medicines and their limitation in many areas of therapy. Furthermore, the following highlight the importance of traditional medicines in healthcare management:

- Provision of essential drugs where modern drugs are not available
- Provision of drugs for primary healthcare
- Provision of household remedies for self-medication for minor ailments
- Provision of an alternative where modern drugs are inadequate
- Provision of an alternative to modern drugs for people interested in natural products or environmental-friendly products (in both developed and developing countries)
- Consumers prefer 'green' medicines instead of 'synthetic chemicals'
- Consumers perceive modern healthcare to be ineffective, expensive, impersonal and to have undesirable side effects
- No satisfactory modern drugs are available for most degenerative disorders

Due to the increasing demand for various commonly used medicinal plants in the production of traditional medicines, coupled with the problems of different vernacular names used by people in various geographical locations where these plants grow, a great deal of adulteration or substitution is encountered in the commercial markets.

The World Health Organization (WHO) encourages, recommends and promotes traditional/ herbal remedies in national healthcare programmes (World Health Organization 2014). The attention paid by health authorities to the use of herbal medicines has increased considerably because

1. They provide an economic and sound approach to spread healthcare to the poor and to those in less developed areas.
2. They are becoming popular alternative medicine in countries where modern medicine is predominant in the healthcare system.

Parallel with increasing interest in plant-based medicines all over the world, there is a serious concern about the quality and safety of these medicines due to increasing pollution in the air, water and soil. Medicinal plant materials used in the manufacture of herbal products may be contaminated with herbicides, pesticides, heavy metals, dioxin, biphenyls, and so forth. The excess of toxic heavy metals over a specified limit may lead to several health problems (Word Health Organization 2007). The use of fake herbs to prepare drugs in some instances has also contributed to a negative opinion about herbal medicines. Several forensic reports and investigations have been published against HMPs from different parts of the world, particularly concerning heavy metal toxicity (Steenkamp et al. 1999).

A more positive approach is required for the way in which modern, scientifically based HMPs can be used in current disease management, allowing them to take on a predominant role in comparison to the more expensive and toxic synthetic compounds where these are not absolutely essential or, in many cases, desirable. Herbal products are multi-component systems containing both active and inactive compounds and metallic elements (in macro and micro quantities). The quantitative composition of these constituents also depends on agro-climatic conditions and so may vary from one place to another.

Trends in returning to traditional or natural systems in healthcare demand scientific approaches to answer the questions of quality, safety and efficacy. Very limited scientific studies and data are available on herbal medicines with respect to:

- Toxicity in animals
- Efficacy in animal models
- Sensitive quality control standards for raw materials and finished products
- Dose regimen and dose frequency
- Bioavailability studies in animals
- Shelf-life studies for raw materials and finished products

- Bioavailability studies in healthy human volunteers
- Multicenter clinical trials in patients
- Pesticides and heavy metal levels and their limits
- Microbiological and radio chemical contamination

Factors restricting the growth of the traditional medicine and herbal drug industry include:

- Lack of quality products
- Lack of legal provisions for the quality of herbal medicines – no proper regulations: unsafe nature of herbal medicines
- Lack of scientifically based standards/specifications
- Lack of user-friendly products
- Difficulty in influencing customers due to no transparency/traceability and unknown composition
- Gap in knowledge that exists in traditional medicine with regard to the nature of active constituents, mechanism of action, pharmacokinetics, pharmacodynamics, so HMPs cannot compete with Western medicine, although it is not a smart approach in disease management
- Undeveloped system to complete with Western medicine
- Lack of data on medicinal plants with regard to availability, collection, demand and supply, and so forth
- Multiple stakeholders with divergent interests (forestry department, cultivators, industry, policy makers and regulatory bodies)
- Destructive harvesting of rare medicinal plants from the wild
- End users not making contribution for conservation of medicinal plants
- No proof of safety and efficacy
- Availability of substandard and fake products on the market
- Problems in labelling
- Problems of different vernacular names for medicinal plants result in great deal adulteration or substitution in the commercial market

2.2 NEED FOR SCIENTIFIC STANDARDISATION OF TRADITIONAL MEDICINES

Standardisation of traditional medicines and medicinal plant materials has become an essential activity in promoting traditional systems of medicine in any country. Many countries do not have standard identification tests or analytical procedures to maintain consistent quality. The legal provisions for the quality of herbal medicines are not as stringent as they are for modern medicines. In fact, most HMPs go to market without testing for their quality, safety and efficacy. Concern had been expressed in many situations about persistent problems in ensuring the quality of finished herbal formulations and their starting materials.

. The monographs in some herbal pharmacopoeias (e.g. Ayurveda Pharmacopoeia of Sri Lanka) describe only the physico-chemical parameters and lack adequate and sensitive analytical procedures to maintain the consistent quality of plant materials and their formulations (Anonymous 1979). Moreover, these monographs lack sophistication and can in fact be deficient in the modern sense that they cannot ensure complete analysis or establish that the drug under analysis is correctly constituted in terms of therapeutic efficacy. In the event of any problems, the health authorities have to be responsible for the unsafe nature of herbal medicines. The WHO also supports traditional medicines when they have demonstrated benefits for the patient and minimal risks (World Health Organization 2014). Governments should actively promote the rational use of herbal medicines that have been scientifically validated in order to maximise the benefits and minimise the risks of herbal medicines. Hence, it is important to ensure that herbal medicines are of acceptable quality, safety and efficacy. The quality, safety and efficacy of the medicines used in traditional medicine depend on the pharmacopoeial standards used in the drug manufacturing process. Pharmacopoeial quality specifications and requirements provide the legal basis for regulatory control of any medicines.

Herbal medicines have been used for thousands of years in many parts of the world. A question may be asked as to why all these scientific studies cited above are now required despite our traditional systems of medicine are in practice for several centuries. It is easy to answer the question of this nature. Since the use of herbal medicines is a time-tested observation with billions of people for several centuries, there had been ample opportunity to solve problems associated with toxicities and side effects and must be acceptable to all of us. In the olden days, a traditional medical practitioner would collect the raw materials, process them and dispense them to his own patients. He used to be a one-man quality assurance system. With such unique expertise, the practitioner was able to maintain certain reliable standards. His personal experience and involvement would more than compensate for the scientific studies mentioned above. However, the scenario of manufacturing and dispensing traditional medicines has undergone a sea of change in the last 40 years or so. A number of small-scale, medium-scale and large-scale manufacturers have come up in the field of herbal drugs. This transformation of traditional medicine from an individualised system to a commercial manufacturing system resulted in great deterioration in the whole procedure and process of traditional medicines. In fact, the quality of the drug became the greatest casualty in this transformation. This is mainly because the main important activity of raw material procurement, processing and dispensing did not come under the control of a single body. Instead, transformed in the hands of unqualified and unskilled persons, mass production ultimately resulted in a great deal of adulteration or substitution of plant materials in the commercial market. The use of other plants than that mentioned in ancient traditional literature can cause deterioration of the quality of the drug. Adulteration of the genuine plant is the other cause of deterioration. Adulteration is practised either deliberately or through ignorance of the collector. Because traditional physicians are quite knowledgeable and conscientious in their field, adulterants are encountered only when a drug is commercially produced. Determination of species specificity is very essential in the standardization of herbal medicines. Standardisation therefore provides solutions to these problems and also assures a better quality of drug. In a number of resolutions, the WHO has emphasised the need to ensure quality control of medicinal plants by using modern analytical techniques and applying suitable standards (World Health Organization 1998). It is therefore imperative that scientific standardisation techniques should be adopted for validation and quality control of herbal medicines.

Standardisation is a process of developing the body of information and controls that guarantee the constancy of composition – and therefore the consistency of the efficacy of an HMP. The single and most important factor that affects wider acceptance of traditional medicine is the non-availability or inadequacy of reliable and sensitive standards for checking quality. This also affects modernisation or modification of production methods.

Many of the traditional drugs currently in use do not have well-defined analytical procedures to characterise the composition and maintain consistent quality. The main reason associated with the difficulty in developing quality control standards is that most of these products contain whole plants or parts of several plants or their total extracts, and in some cases even a combination of a number of herbs. These medicines thus quite often contain a large number of chemical constituents. The activity of the plant material or finished product does not depend on a single substance, but is believed to be influenced by a large number of compounds working synergistically. Hence, it is very important to take the holistic view of herbal medicines when they are put to modern scientific scrutiny for their standardisation. All researchers involved in standardization of herbal medicines should follow a holistic approach as practiced in our traditional systems.

In addition to the problems of efficacy, safety and the wider social and political issues, there are other scientific problems related to the quality of the plant materials used and this concerns sensitive analytical standards. Directives on the analytical control of herbal medicines must take into account the fact that the material or product to be examined has a complex and 'inconstant' composition because of variations that occur in plant materials obtained from identical botanical species. Because HMPs are made directly from crude plant material, they can show substantial variation in composition, quality and therapeutic effect. The variation and diversity of life is observed even within a species. In fact, two medicinal plants of the same species may look identical, but they may be substantially different in the levels of chemical constituents that they contain. Hence, herbal medicines made from plants that differ markedly in their chemical constituents cannot produce the same therapeutic effects. Instead, they may produce different undesirable or desirable effects, because the mechanism of action is sometimes influenced by the amount or dose of the active constituents. The consequence will be inconsistent clinical results.

Hence, the standardisation of HMPs may be influenced by several factors such as soil and climate conditions in which the plants grow, age, harvesting period, methods of collection, method of drying and so on. All of these factors affect the nature and quantities of the constituents, and strict analytical control is essential to maintain the quality of raw plant materials. It is important to use cultivated rather than wild plants, which are often heterogeneous in regard to the above factors, to eliminate some of the causes of inconstancy. Cultivated plants offer several advantages over wild plants in terms of standardisation (Bonati 1991):

- The plants can be cultivated in homogeneous climatic and soil conditions.
- Plants of known age can be harvested at the right time and rapidly, consequently homogeneous in their content of active principles.
- Plants can be dried under controlled time and temperature conditions. In fact, homogeneous and correct drying is often the most delicate and essential phase in the whole process of production of raw plant materials.

Because of the complex composition of herbal drugs, the process of HMP production is crucial to quality consistency. It has to be kept constant through the standardisation of the whole manufacturing process. Although standardisation of herbal medicines is a challenging task, because analytical and bioassay techniques have advanced greatly, it is now possible to develop reliable and sensitive quality control standards to guarantee consistency in composition (Scheme 2.1). Standardisation is necessary to establish consistency and reproducibility in the manufacture of

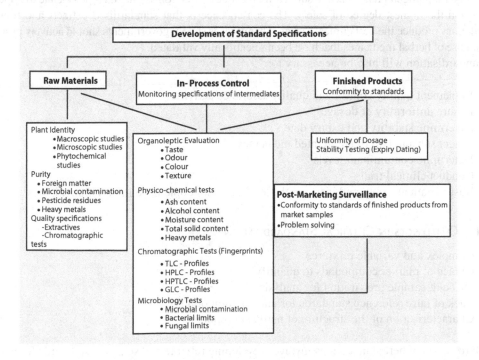

SCHEME 2.1 Summary of parameters used in the development of standard specifications.

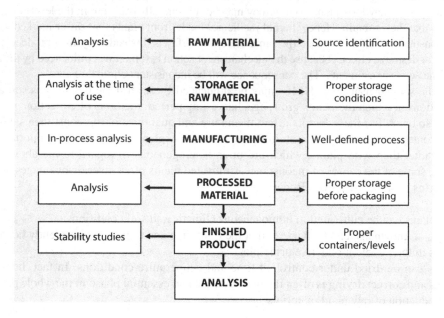

SCHEME 2.2   General protocol for standardised production of herbal medicines.

a particular HMP to ensure guaranteed potency through acceptable levels of active compounds. This process can be carried out microscopically, chemically, spectroscopically or biologically and currently involves complicated and complex procedures (Scheme 2.2).

The vast majority of clinical studies involving herbal medicines have used standardised extracts (Keller 2001). The fundamental reason is that standardised extracts offer consistent and reproducible therapeutic effects and the highest degree of safety. The consequence is that standardised extracts and finished formulations produce the best clinical results. Therefore, as stated, governments should actively promote rational use of herbal medicines that have been scientifically validated.

Standardisation will also be necessary to:

- Implement quality control and quality assurance activities
- Ensure uniformity of dosage
- Determine stability and expiry date
- Detect substandard or adulterated medicines
- Determine contaminant levels
- Conduct clinical trials
- Ensure patient safety and increase the level of trust people have in herbal medicines

2.2.1   CHALLENGES IN CHEMICAL STANDARDISATION

- Complex and variable mixtures
- Choice of marker compounds to quantify
- Difficult sample preparation for analysis
- Lack of pure reference standards for marker compounds
- Characterisation of the structure of marker compounds

Standardisation of herbal medicines involves developing reliable and sensitive standards for the following parameters (Scheme 2.3).

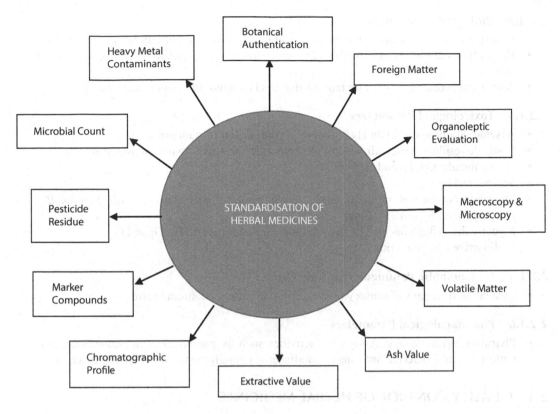

SCHEME 2.3   Standardisation of herbal medicines.

2.2.1.1   Botanical Parameters
- Visual evaluation: Includes macroscopic characteristics (external morphology)
- Foreign matter: Includes foreign plants, animals and minerals, etc.
- General microscopy: Includes histological observations and measurements
- Powder microscopy: Includes microscopic characteristics of powdered drug
- Quantitative microscopy of leaves: Includes parameters such as stomatal index, palisade ratio, vein islet number and veinlet termination number

2.2.1.2   Chemical and Physico-Chemical Parameters
- Chemical composition:
  - By chromatographic fingerprinting: TLC, HPTLC, HPLC and GC fingerprints
  - By DNA fingerprinting
  - By spectroscopic fingerprinting: UV–Vis and FTIR spectra
  - By chromatography coupled spectroscopic fingerprinting: GC-MS, LC-NMR and LC-UV fingerprints
- Ash values: Total acid-insoluble and water-soluble ash
- Extractive values: Hot water, cold water and ethanol extractives
- Moisture content and volatile matter: loss on drying, azeotropic distillation
- Volatile oils: By steam distillation
- Swelling index: In water
- Foaming index: Foam height produced under specified conditions

2.2.1.3   Biological Parameters

- Bitterness value: Unit equivalent bitterness of standard solution of quinine hydrochloride
- Haemolytic activity: On bovine blood by comparison with standard reference solution of saponin
- Astringent property: Testing on tannins that bind to standard Freiberg hide powder

2.2.1.4   Toxicological Parameters

- Arsenic: Stain produced on $HgBr_2$ paper in comparison to standard stain
- Pesticide residues: Determination of total chloride and total organic phosphates
- Heavy metals: Cd, Pb and Hg
- Solvent residues
- Microbial contamination: Total viable aerobic count of pathogens: *E. coli*, *Salmonella*, *P. aeruginosa*, *S. aureous*, fungi
- Mycotoxins: Aflatoxins by TLC using standard aflatoxins (B_1, B_2, G_1 and G_2)
- Radioactive contamination

2.2.1.5   Organoleptic Parameters for Raw Drugs

- Evaluation by means of sensory organs: Touch (texture), odour and taste

2.2.1.6   Pharmacological Parameters

- Pharmacological assays: Assays for activities such as antioxidant, immunomodulatory, anticancer, antibacterial, antifungal, antidiabetic, hypoglycaemic and hepatoprotective

2.3   QUALITY CONTROL OF HERBAL MEDICINES

While recognising the value of treatment with herbal medicines, it is important to bear in mind that improper use can cause serious adverse and side effects. Generally, people equate natural substances with safety. However, massive damage may be caused by the inappropriate use of natural products. In many countries, there is no proper quality control for the marketing of medicinal herbs and finished herbal medicines, and most herbal medicines are adulterated by contamination. Hence, quality control activities should be practised by setting high quality and safety standards for medicinal herbs and their finished products in order to safeguard the health of consumers. Consistent quality of herbal medicinal products can only be assured by the quality control of starting plant material, in-process quality controls, GMP controls, quality control of finished products and specific actions applied to them throughout development and manufacture.

Quality control should include:

1. Raw material control
2. In-process control
3. Control of manufacturing operations
4. Random checking of samples of finished products in quality control laboratories

2.3.1   Quality Control of Raw (Plant) Materials

Uniform quality of HMPs can only be achieved if the starting materials are correctly defined in an explicit and descriptive manner. Each plant used for manufacturing should be botanically authenticated and checked using its macroscopic, microscopic and taxonomic characteristics. Comparison of a sample of the raw material with a reference sample or herbarium specimen maintained in a manufacturing facility should be exercised at all times. The geographical location, season of collection, method of drying, parts of the plant used and whether it is fresh or dried should also be recorded. A general protocol followed for quality control of raw material is given in Scheme 2.4.

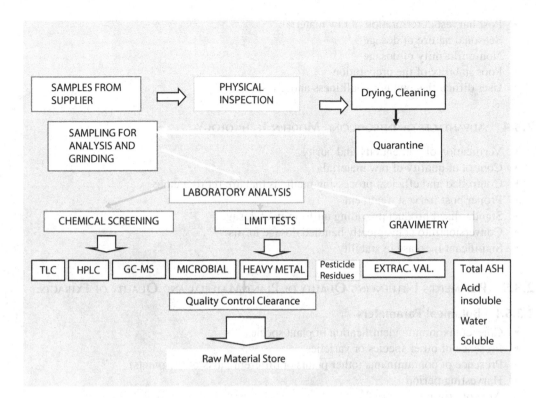

SCHEME 2.4 Quality control process for raw materials.

2.3.2 Assessment of Quality

Quality of raw materials and finished products are regulated by the relevant pharmacopoeial monographs while manufacturing operations are regulated by the code of good manufacturing practices promulgated by the World Health Organization (1998). Thus, detailed analysis of all raw materials, finished products and in-process materials should be carried out. Most of the analysis is carried out in the manufacturer's quality control laboratory using wet chemical analysis and instrumentation. This should cover all important aspects of the quality assessment of herbal medicines. It is necessary to make reference to a pharmacopoeial monograph if one exists. If such a monograph is not available, a suitable monograph must be developed and should be set out as in an official pharmacopoeia. All procedures should be in accordance with current good manufacturing practices.

In-process analysis should be adopted to ensure consistent quality of finished products rather than relying entirely on the testing of finished product prior to market release. It is important to validate manufacturing processes to control critical steps, selecting appropriate monitoring methods and periodic improvements.

There are many advances in process technology for the extraction and separation of fractions or chemical constituents from plants, as well as in pharmaceutical technology for production of new formulations and dosage forms. These advances should be applied whenever and wherever possible in the production of traditional medicines and their dosage forms (Sunil et al. 2010).

2.3.3 Disadvantages of Traditional Manufacturing Methods

- Authenticity and purity of raw materials not known
- Variability of raw material quality

- Post-harvest deterioration of raw material
- Seasonal nature of dosage
- Non-uniformity of dosage
- Poor stability of the preparation
- User difficulties owing to bulkiness and transport

2.3.4 ADVANTAGES OF INTRODUCING MODERN TECHNOLOGY

- Verification of authenticity and purity
- Control of quality of raw materials
- Controlled and efficient processing methods that are reproducible
- Proper post-harvest treatment
- Standardised product providing uniformity of dosage
- Conversion into conveniently handled dosage forms
- Significant increase in stability

2.3.5 PARAMETERS INFLUENCING QUALITY OF PLANT MATERIAL AND QUALITY OF EXTRACTS

2.3.5.1 Botanical Parameters

- Correct taxonomic identification of plant species
- Presence of other species or varieties
- Presence of contaminants (other plants or different parts of the plants)
- Harvesting period
- Area of origin
- Storage of the plant material
- Microbial counting
- Variants (ecotypic, genotypic, chemotypic variations) leading to variability in the chemical composition
- Seasonal variations
- Association patterns, including animals and insects
- Lunar period

2.3.5.2 Chemical Parameters

- Content of active principles
- Qualitative composition of the plant
- Extractive content
- Extraction procedure
- Nature of formulation
- Ratio among the various compounds
- Heave metal content
- Solvents used for extraction

2.3.6 QUALITY ASSESSMENT OF CRUDE PLANT MATERIALS

The following aspects should be considered in the quality assessment of crude plant materials:

- General description of the plant
- Part used – Fresh or dried powder
- Mode of grinding and particle size
- Production of crude drugs

- Cultivation
- Harvesting
- Post-harvest handling
- Packaging and storage

2.3.7 QUALITY SPECIFICATIONS FOR CRUDE PLANT MATERIALS

It is necessary to develop well-defined quality standards for the following parameters:

- Macroscopic and microscopic identification
- Chemical/chromatographic identification
- Foreign organic matter limit
- Ash content
- Acid-insoluble ash content
- Water-soluble extractive
- Alcohol-soluble extractive
- Moisture content
- Main/active constituent content
- Microbial limit
- Pesticide residue limit
- Heavy metal limit
- Likely contaminants
- Adulterants
- Shelf life

2.3.8 QUALITY ASSESSMENT OF FINISHED PRODUCTS

The following test parameters should be considered in the quality assessment of finished products.

- **For Tablets, Capsules and Powders**
  Weight variation, disintegration time (except for powders), content of main/active constituents, qualitative composition, microbial limit, heavy metals, determination of extractives in various solvents, moisture content, particle size (for powders).

- **For Solutions**
  pH, qualitative composition, alcohol content, content of main/active constituents, viscosity, identification of preservatives, microbial limit, heavy metals, sodium saccharin content.

- **For Creams and Lotions**
  Qualitative composition, pH, water content, peroxide value, content of main/active constituent, microbial limit, heavy metals, thermal stability.

- **For Oils and Hair Oils**
  Qualitative composition, content of main/active constituents, coloring matter, pH, acid value, peroxide value, fatty acid content.

- **For Herbal Tea**
  Qualitative composition, colouring matter, moisture content, microbial purity, heavy metals, content of main/active constituents.

REFERENCES

Anonymous. (1979). *Ayurveda Pharmacopoeia of Sri Lanka*, Vol. 2. Colombo, Sri Lanka: Department of Ayurveda.

Bonati, A. (1991). How and why should we standardize pharmaceutical drugs for clinical validation. *Journal of Ethnopharmacology*, **32**, 195–197.

Keller, K. (2001). *Herbal Medicinal Products in the EU Biopharmaceutical/Quality Issues.* London, UK: European Medicines Evaluation Agency.

Steenkamp V, Stewart, M.J, Curoswska, E, Zuckerman, M. (1999). A severe case of multiple metals poisoning in a child treated with a traditional medicine. Forensic Science International, 128: 177–183.

Sunil, K. S., Jha, S. K., Chaudhary, A., Yadava, R. D. S. and Rai, S. B. (2010). Quality control of herbal medicines using spectroscopic techniques and multivariate statistical analysis. *Pharmaceutical Biology*, **48**(2), 134–141.

World Health Organization. (1998). *Quality Control Methods for Medicinal Plant Materials.* Geneva, Switzerland: WHO.

World Health Organization. (2005). *National Policy on Traditional Medicine and Regulation of Herbal Medicines: Report of a WHO Global Survey.* Geneva, Switzerland: WHO.

World Health Organization. (2007). *WHO Guidelines on Assessing Quality of Herbal Medicines with Reference to Contaminants and Residues.* Geneva, Switzerland: WHO.

World Health Organization. (2014). *WHO Traditional Medicine Strategy: 2014–2023.* Geneva, Switzerland: WHO.

3 Structure-Function Elucidation of Flavonoids by Modern Technologies

Role in Management of Diabetes and Cancer

Ritu Varshney, Neeladrisingha Das,
Rutusmita Mishra and Partha Roy

CONTENTS

3.1 PHYTOCHEMICALS

Phytochemicals are the natural plant-derived compounds that are produced for the plant's own defense and protection against various environmental stresses such as bacteria, fungi, insects, pollution, weather change and various diseases (Romeo 2012). Although phytochemicals are considered non-essential nutrients because they are not required to sustain life, recent research has revealed that they can also protect humans against several diseases such as oxidative damage (Zhang et al. 2015; Lee et al. 2017), diabetes (Firdous 2014), cancer (Li et al. 2016), cardiovascular disorders (Vasanthi et al. 2012), neurodegenerative disorders (Vankatesan et al. 2015) and ageing (Larsson 2009) to name a few. Although there are more than a thousand known phytochemicals, the most studied include polyphenols and carotenoids. Among polyphenols, flavonoids and isoflavones are well-known subclasses found to be beneficial in combating various health conditions and disorders.

3.2 NEED OF PHYTOCHEMICALS

In the past few decades, food and nutrition have been recognised as critical factors in the management and cure of diseases. Since time immemorial, by virtue of traditional knowledge, indigenous people have utilized various herbs and medicinal plants for the treatment of disorders. Because the new generation of treatment modalities to mitigate dreadful diseases is constrained to mainly use synthetic drugs – which are costly and may cause unpredictable side effects – there is a need to identify novel phytochemicals that can modulate and maintain physiological functions with minimum side effects. Because of their lesser side effects, more reliable pharmacological action and cost-effectiveness, phytochemicals are also emerging as the new generation's therapeutic strategy to combat various diseases like cancer, diabetes, cardiovascular disease, bone disorders and neurodegeneration.

Phytochemicals are considered important nutraceuticals with health benefits described in the later part of this review. They play a role as substrates for biochemical reactions, act as cofactors/inhibitors of enzymatic reactions, ligands for surface/intracellular receptors as agonist/antagonist, scavengers of reactive or toxic substances, enhancers of the bioavailability of essential nutrients and selective growth factors for beneficial gastrointestinal microbiota or selective inhibitors of deleterious intestinal bacteria (Dillard and German 2000).

3.3 CLASSIFICATION OF PHYTOCHEMICALS

The phytochemicals can be classified based upon their chemical structures. The major classifications could be alkaloids, aromatic acids, phenolics, lactones, terpenoids, fatty acids and organosulphur compounds. The detailed classification along with examples is provided in Figure 3.1.

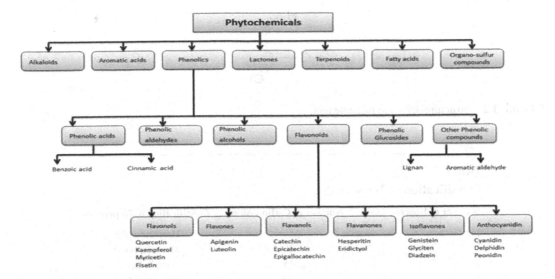

FIGURE 3.1   A brief classification of various phytochemicals.

A brief description of different types of phytochemicals is given below.

1. **Alkaloids** – Alkaloids are the cyclic organic compounds having nitrogen in a negative oxidation state. Their presence is mainly restricted to most of the Angiospermae and a few Gymnospermae (Waller 2012). They are further classified mainly based either on the similarity of the carbon skeleton (*indole-, isoquinoline-* or *pyridine*-like) or based on the biochemical precursors (tryptophan, ornithine, lysine, etc.). However, in general, we can classify alkaloids as true alkaloids, proto-alkaloids and pseudo-alkaloids.

2. **Aromatic Acids** – These phytochemicals are aromatic in nature and have organic acid functional groups.

3. **Phenolics** – Phenolic phytochemicals have a phenol ring with different functional groups attached to it. These are the largest category of phytochemicals and are distributed widely throughout the plant kingdom. Based on the functional group side chains, phenolic compounds can be further classified as phenolic acids, phenolic aldehydes, phenolic glucosides, flavonoids, lignans, and so forth. The structural diversity of this group of phytochemicals is mainly due to hydroxylation patterns, stereochemistry and different patterns of methoxylation and glycosylation (Koleckar et al. 2008).

4. **Lactones** – These are mainly sesquiterpene lactones having a lactone ring. These compounds are mainly confined to the species of the family compositeae (Rodriguez et al. 1976) and a few are also isolated from species of cactaceae and solanaceae (Canales et al. 2005). The structural modifications in the group mainly involve the incorporation of an epoxide ring, esterified hydrogen groups and a 5-carbon acid (Yoshioka et al. 1973). Some sesquiterpene lactones also possess covalently added halogen atoms (Siuda and DeBarnardis 1973).

5. **Terpenoids** – The word 'terpene' is mainly adapted from turpentine oil. It was initially used to describe the $C_{10}H_{18}$ hydrocarbons occurring in the oil. Terpenoids are further classified in terms of the isoprene units (Figure 3.2) they have. Table 3.1 shows the basic classification of terpenoids based on the number of carbon atoms.

6. **Fatty Acids** – In terms of chemistry, fatty acids are carboxylic acids having a long aliphatic chain (saturated or unsaturated). Although plants synthesize a large number of fatty acids, only a few are major and taken into account (Gunstone et al. 2007). However, a wide diversity is observed in plant fatty acids. This group of phytochemicals can be further divided into *n*-saturated fatty acids, *n*-unsaturated fatty acids, branched-chain acids and cyclic acids (Shorland 2012).

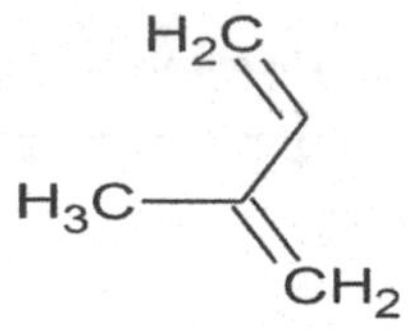

FIGURE 3.2 Structure depicting isoprene unit.

TABLE 3.1
Classification of Terpenoids

Number of Isoprene Units	Number of Carbon Atoms	Classification of Terpenoids
1	5	Hemiterpenoid
2	10	Monoterpenoid
3	15	Sesquiterpenoid
4	20	Diterpenoid
5	25	Sesterterpenoid
6	30	Triterpenoid
8	40	Tetraterpenoids
>8	>40	Polyterpenoids

7. **Organosulphur compounds** – These are the sulphur-containing organic compounds found naturally in plants. Organosulphur compounds are volatile in nature and mainly account for the odour and flavour of some plant products such as wine, nuts and coffee (Qian et al. 2011). Organosulphur compounds are currently generating tremendous interest among researchers due to their promising actions against different diseases. As far as further classification is concerned, these compounds are classified according to the sulphur-containing functional groups such as thioesters, thioethers, thioacetals, thiols, disulphides and polysulphides.

Because these phytochemicals contain a large number of entities, it is beyond the scope of this chapter to discuss all of them. Based on our literature review and data collected from various scientific search engines, flavonoids are the most widely studied phytochemicals and are being used for the management of different diseases. Hence in order to narrow down the topic of discussion, in this chapter, the major focus will be on flavonoids and their use for the management of different diseases.

3.4 FLAVONOIDS

3.4.1 BASICS OF FLAVONOIDS

The term 'flavonoid' is derived from the Latin word *flavus*, meaning yellow (Miranda et al. 2001; Procházková et al. 2011). These are ubiquitous secondary metabolites that are also responsible for red, blue and purple pigmentation in plants (Winkel-Shirley 2001). This clearly indicates that these molecules are linked to pigmentation in plants. In earlier days, flavonoids were thought to be the toxic metabolic waste of plants and therefore stored away in vacuoles. Some authors also described the same to be an evolutionary remnant having no current function. However, due to their wide range of biological activities, major research focus has shifted to decipher their medicinal properties and mode of actions in cellular level. Flavonoids have various roles in plants and some of the most important roles are discussed here. Flavonoids play an important role in the interaction between plants and the environment. Flavonoids protect plants from various biotic as well as abiotic stresses (Winkel-Shirley 2002; Treutter 2006; Pourcel et al. 2007). Flavonoids as well as other phenolic compounds are also responsible for drought resistance in certain species (Pizzi and Cameron 1986; Moore et al. 2005). Although flavonoids are not essential for plant survival, they influence/regulate the transport of the plant hormone auxin (Murphy et al. 2000; Buer et al. 2010). Another important role of flavonoids is protection of plants from solar UV radiation. Most anthocyanins absorb UV radiation between 270 and 290 nm. However, acylated anthocyanins, in particular, are strong UV absorbers (Markham 1982; Giusti et al. 1999). Apart from all these possible roles, flavonoids are also associated with protecting plants from different microbes and insects (Barry et al. 2002; Gallet et al. 2004; Griesbach 2005).

3.4.2 CLASSIFICATION OF FLAVONOIDS

Flavonoids can be mainly classified based upon their chemical structures. The basic skeleton of almost all flavonoids is the same: 2-phenylbenzopyrone (Figure 3.3). Flavonoids differ from one another in the pattern of hydroxylation or methylation, degree of unsaturation and type of sugars attached. In general, flavonoids can be classified into the following types: (a) flavonols, (b) flavones, (c) flavanols, (d) flavanones, (e) anthocyanidins and (f) isoflavones (Figure 3.1). It is beyond the scope of this review to discuss the structures of all flavonoids due to their extensive beneficial health effects, but the structures of some of the important flavonols are discussed below.

3.4.3 FLAVONOLS

Flavonols have a 3-hydroxyflavone backbone (Figure 3.4). The different positions of the −OH group in the backbone is the only reason for the chemical diversity of this group. As far as flavonols in human diets are concerned, these are mainly found in vegetables, fruits and beverages like tea and wine (Hertog et al. 1993; Crozier et al. 1997; McDonald et al. 1998). Some of the widely studied flavonols are discussed below.

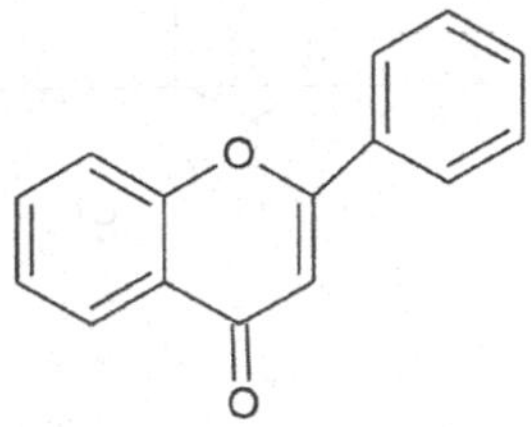

FIGURE 3.3   Structure of 2-phenylbenzopyrone.

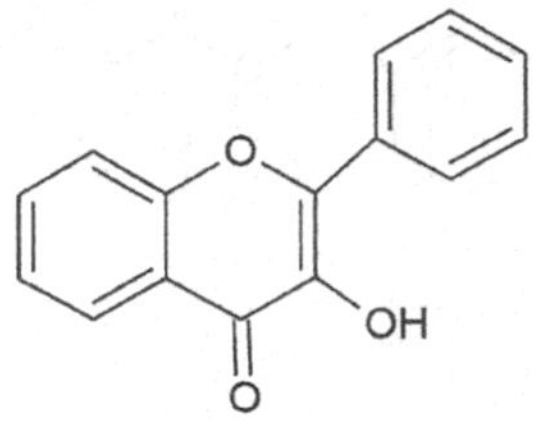

FIGURE 3.4   3-Hydroxyflavone as a basic flavone structure.

3.4.3.1 Myricetin

The IUPAC name for myricetin is 3,5,7-trihrdroxy-2-(3,4,5-trihydroxyphenyl)-4-chromenone. Myricetin is found throughout the plant kingdom, but mostly in species of the families Myricaceae (Lau-Cam and Chan 1973; Jones et al. 2010), Polygonaceae (Abd El-Kader et al. 2013) and Pinaceae (Hergert 1956). Structurally, myricetin (Figure 3.5) is closely related to kaempferol, quercetin, morin and fisetin. Due to its structural closeness with quercetin, it is also referred as hydroxyquercetin. Myricetin was first isolated from *Myricanagi* Thunb (from the family Myricaceae; Perken and Hummel 1896). These are mainly found in vegetables, berries, nuts, tea (Ross and Kasum 2002) and wine (Basli et al. 2012). This compound possesses various pharmaceutical properties, including anticancer (Sun et al. 2012; Kim et al. 2014), antidiabetic (Ong and Khoo 2000; Al-Awwadi et al. 2004), anti-inflammatory (Hiermann et al. 1998; Wang et al. 2010), antioxidant (Gordon and Roedig-Penman 1998) and hepatoprotective (Chattopadhyay and Bandyopadhyay 2005).

3.4.3.2 Kaempferol

The IUPAC name of kaempferol is 3,5,7-trihydroxy-2-(4-hydroxyphenyl)-4H-chromen-4-one. These are common in plants and are widely distributed throughout the plant kingdom. As per a review article by Calderon-Montano et al. (2011), 400 plant species from various families are listed along with the types of kaempferol isolated (Calderón-Montaño et al. 2011). Kaempferol (Figure 3.6) is found either in its native form or may be bound to glucose, galactose and rhamnose to form glycosides. As far as dietary kaempferol is concerned, it is found abundantly in tea, broccoli, apples, strawberries and beans (Somerset and Johannot 2008). Kaempferol exhibits various therapeutic effects and is supposed to be a potent drug against various ailments. The biggest advantage of this phytochemical is its selective cytotoxicity to cancerous cells (Ramos 2007; Mylonis et al. 2010;

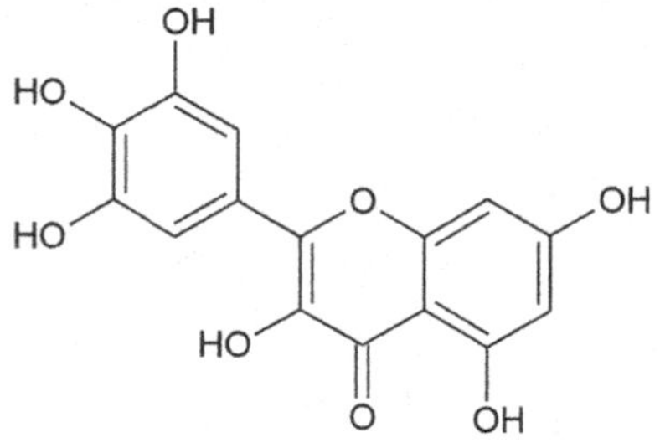

FIGURE 3.5   Structure of myricetin.

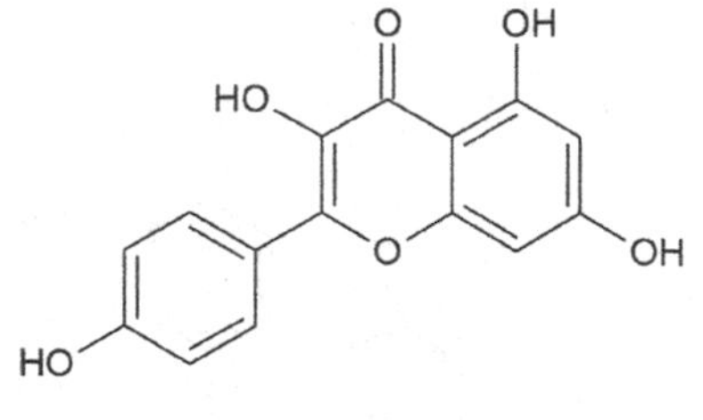

FIGURE 3.6   Structure of kaempferol.

Kim and Choi 2013) rather than normal cells (Zhang et al. 2008). Apart from this, kaempferol also has potential therapeutic activity against diabetes (de Sousa et al. 2004; Zang et al. 2011; Zhang and Liu 2011), inflammation (Rho et al. 2011; Kong et al. 2013) and cardiovascular diseases (Curin and Andriantsitohaina 2005).

3.4.3.3 Quercetin

According to the IUPAC system, quercetin is known as 2-(3,4-dihydroxyphenyl)-3,5,7-trihydroxy-4H-chromen-4-one. It is the most abundant dietary flavonoid found in fruits, green leafy vegetables, olive oil, red wine and tea. Structurally, quercetin contains five hydroxyl groups (Figure 3.7) and the position of these determines its diversity. Glycosides and ethers are the major derivatives of the compound. However, sulphate and prenyl substituents are also observed, but less frequently (Harborne and Roberts 1994; Williams and Grayer 2004). Normally, quercetin is not found in free form, but rather forms a complex with phenolic acids, sugars and alcohols. After ingestion, the derivatives of the quercetin are hydrolysed in the gastrointestinal tract and then absorbed in the body (Scalbert and Williamson 2000; Walle 2004). This group of flavonols also exhibits diverse pharmacological effects, including antiviral (Vrijsen et al. 1988; Cushnie and Lamb 2005), anti-carcinogenic (Shi et al. 2003; Zheng et al. 2012) and anti-inflammatory (Guardia et al. 2001; Rogerio et al. 2007, 2010).

3.4.3.4 Fisetin

According to the IUPAC system, fisetin is known as 2-(3,4-dihydroxyphenyl)-3,7-dihydrochromen-4-one. Fisetin (Figure 3.8) mainly acts as a coloring agent in plants. It is abundantly present in strawberries, apples, grapes, onions and cucumbers (Arai et al. 2000; Lall et al. 2015). Fisetin has been reported to have a wide variety of therapeutic activities, including antioxidant (Firuzi et al. 2005), anti-metastatic (Chien et al. 2010) and anti-inflammatory (Higa et al. 2003).

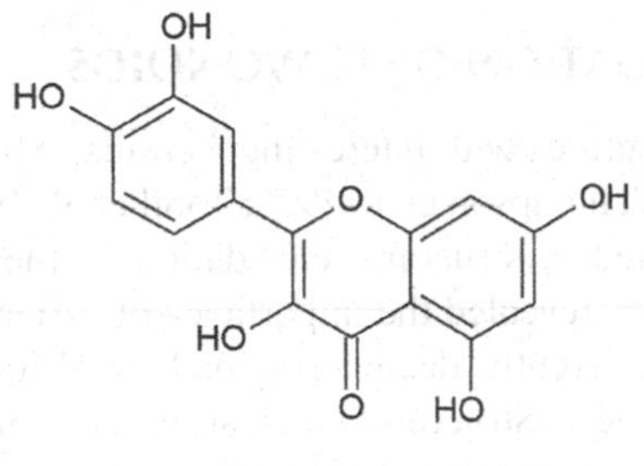

FIGURE 3.7 Structure of quercetin.

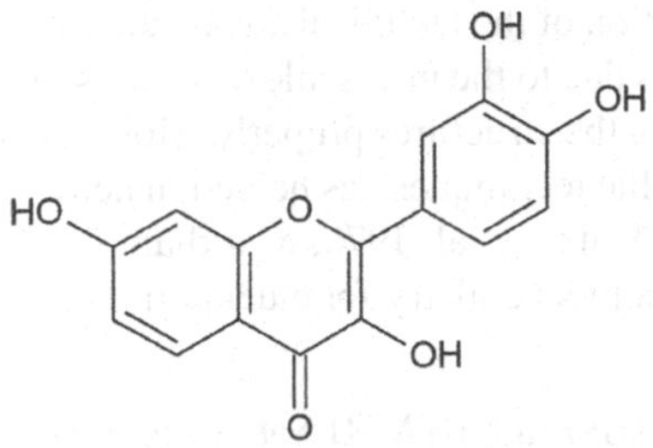

FIGURE 3.8 Structure of fisetin.

3.4.4 Dietary Flavonoids and Health

Previous epidemiological studies and associated meta-analyses strongly support that long-term consumption of dietary flavonoids offer some protection against various chronic ailments, especially cancer (Lipkin et al. 1985; Steinmetz and Potter 1991, 1996; Block et al. 1992). In cancer, uncontrolled production of free radicals is mainly observed. This led to focused attention on the possible roles of flavonoids in suppressing and scavenging free radical activities. The antioxidant property of the flavonoids helped researchers to decipher a possible link between dietary flavonoids and various other diseases. At present, more than 4000 flavonoids have been isolated (Middleton 1998) and these are the most common constituents of our daily diets. Epidemiological data also suggest that these compounds have potent activity against coronary heart diseases. According to an early study by Hertog et al. (1995), the populations with a higher intake of dietary flavonoids have better results than those who did not take the same. This study was carried out among 16 cohorts across seven countries. If we also consider the Zutphen study reports, in which the tests were conducted on an elderly population within the age group of 40–59 years, and higher intake of flavonoids was found to reduce the risk of death from coronary heart diseases (Keys et al. 1966). Although dietary flavonoids have a tremendous effect on health, their low bioavailability has always been a concern. Some studies confirm that the bioavailability of flavonoids is mainly affected by phase-2 metabolism (Manach et al. 2005). As far as flavonoid ingestion is concerned, they undergo sulphation, methylation and glucuronidation in the small intestine and liver (Mullen et al. 2006). However, studies reveal that metabolites are found in conjugated form in plasma after flavonoid ingestion (Rupasinghe et al. 2010). Despite its bioactive role at a cellular level (*in vitro* tests), bioavailability is a major challenge for these compounds, so they have comparatively reduced action in animal models. Currently efforts are being made to increase the bioavailability of these phytochemicals by adding absorption enhancers (Shen et al. 2011), novel delivery strategies (Zhang et al. 2011) and enhancing metabolic stability (Walle 2007; Cao et al. 2013).

3.5 STRUCTURAL ELUCIDATION OF FLAVONOIDS

Flavonoids have a variety of structures with interesting features. After the antioxidant properties of the flavonoids were deciphered (Thompson et al. 1976; Torel et al. 1986; Husain et al. 1987; Larson 1988), researchers were interested in structural elucidation of these phytochemicals. Structure–activity relationship (SAR) studies revealed the importance of different functional groups and their pharmacological effectiveness. Currently, deciphering biological functions from structural aspects is gaining momentum in our society. Structural elucidation, continual improvement and advancement in separation as well as spectroscopic techniques have made it easier to depict the exact structure of a flavonoid with increasing precision. As depicted by Davies et al. (2006), more than 7000 structures of various flavonoid classes are mentioned and nearly half of them were reported after 1993. This shows a clear implication of the technical advancement on structural elucidation. At later stages, lack of available materials due to the miniscule quantities of flavonoids in plant tissues posed a serious challenge for elucidating the structures properly. More recently, the availability of sensitive spectroscopic and chromatographic techniques has helped in achieving prominence for defining the structure of various flavonoids (Mabry et al. 1970; Markham 1982; Harborne 1998). A few of the major techniques used in modern biochemistry for elucidating the structures are discussed below.

3.5.1 Nuclear Magnetic Resonance (NMR) Spectroscopy

Nuclear magnetic resonance (NMR) spectroscopy is an important tool for the structural elucidation of flavonoids (Wenkert and Gottlieb 1977; Markham et al. 1982; Andersen and Fossen 2003; Agrawal 2013). It used to be quite complex to elucidate the complete structure of the flavonoids due to poor sensitivity, slow throughput and difficulties in analysing the mixtures. Recent advancement in NMR spectroscopy techniques have made it arguably the most potent technology to analyse the complete structure of flavonoids even with low sample concentration. The chemical shift and J-coupling parameters obtained from the NMR data are used for structural elucidation of the compounds. Chemical shift (δ) – expressed in parts per million (ppm) – gives a measure of the resonant frequency of a nucleus relative to that of a reference compound, such as tetramethylsilane (TMS) at a given magnetic field (Kemp 1991; Wishart et al. 1992; Balci 2005; Silverstein et al. 2014). The coupling constant (J) gives information about the bonding framework (Kessler et al. 1988; Massiot et al. 2003) because it is mediated through chemical bonds connecting the two spins (Hahn and Maxwell 1952). Although several variations are used for structural elucidation, due to the limitation of space some important NMR experiments used in evaluating flavonoid structures are described below.

3.5.1.1 ¹H-NMR and ¹³C-NMR

The main purpose of a standard ¹H-NMR is to provide information on the relative number of hydrogen atoms with a distinct chemical environment. It is mainly used to record the chemical shifts and spin–spin couplings. The H-atoms are analysed based upon four different results from ¹H-NMR: number of signals, position of signals (chemical shift), relative intensity of signals (integration) and splitting of signals (spin–spin coupling). As far as flavonoid structure is concerned, these are mainly used for analysing the aglycone and acyl groups, the anomeric configuration of and number of monosaccharides. ¹H-NMR is not sufficient to elucidate the structure of all flavonoids, so ¹³C-NMR is also used. ¹³C-NMR, also known as carbon NMR, is mainly used to detect the carbon content in the molecule. This is one of the most advanced tools for structural elucidation of organic molecules. This technique detects the ¹³C isotope of carbon. The chemical shift principle is same as that of the ¹H-NMR. However, the reference standard for ¹³C is the carbon in TMS (Wishart et al. 1995; Morcombe and Zilm 2003; Strothers 2012). A protocol having a modern NMR experimental setup has been described by Andersen and Fossen (2003).

3.5.1.2 2D-NMR- COSY/TOCSY and ¹H-¹³C Heteronuclear Experiments

One of the major drawbacks of 1D-NMR was overlapping of peaks in multi-spin systems. These overlaps made it difficult to assign the coupling constant and chemical shift to a particular nucleus (Morris 1986). To overcome such problems and to identify the structural components with precision, 2D-NMR was used. For increased sensitivity of ¹³C-NMR experiments, the results are often combined with 2D-NMR experiments, especially those using gradient techniques. The 2D-NMR techniques give data plotted in a space from two different frequency sources rather than one (as in case of 1D-NMR). The 2D-NMR consists of sequences of radio frequency (RF) pulses with delay periods in between them. All 2D-NMR experiments have four stages: preparation, evolution, mixing and detection. In the preparation period, the equilibrium magnetization is converted into a coherence signal. This signal is evolved during the evolution period, where it is frequency labelled for indirectly detected ¹³C-frequency. In the mixing period, the coherence signal obtained from the evolution period is manipulated into an observable signal that is directly detected (usually through ¹H spin; Bruch 1996; Berger and Braun 2004). The 2D-NMR spectra are mainly produced by both homonuclear as well as heteronuclear experiments. The homonuclear experiments consist of ¹H-¹H COSY (correlation spectroscopy) or ¹H-¹H DQF-COSY and ¹H-¹H TOCSY, whereas the heteronuclear experiments consist of ¹H-¹³C HSQC experiments. ¹H-¹H COSY is mainly used to determine the signals arising from the neighbouring protons (usually up to four bonds). Correlation mainly appears when there is a probability of spin–spin coupling between protons. DQF-COSY is Double Quantum Filtered–COSY, one of the advanced forms of COSY. The advantage of DQF-COSY is that it eliminates the non-coupled proton signals: that is, the strong solvent signal and the H_2O signal that may overlap with flavonoid sugar signals. TOCSY (total correlation spectroscopy) produces high-quality spectra and is used to determine the stereochemistry of compounds. It is mainly used in determining the oligosaccharides, where each sugar is an isolated spin system. As mentioned by Davies et al. (2006),

TOCSY experiments together with other NMR experiment were used to elucidate the structure of flavonoids from *Mammea longifolia* (Jagan et al. 2002), *Erythrina abyssinica* (Kamusiime et al. 1996), *Polygonum viscosum* (Datta et al. 2000) and *Centaurium spicatum* (Shahat et al. 2003).

Heteronuclear NMR experiments are mainly performed by heteronuclear single quantum coherence spectroscopy (HSQC). In this case, the resulting spectrum is a 2D spectrum having one axis designated for the proton (^{1}H) and the other axis designated for other heteronucleus, which is usually ^{13}C or ^{15}N. ^{1}H-^{13}C-HSQC is generally conducted to deduce the structural aspects of most of the organic compounds. It mainly provides the correlation between the aliphatic carbon and the associated protons. The main advantage of this experiment is increased sensitivity (<1.0 mg flavonoid sample).

3.5.2 VIBRATIONAL SPECTROSCOPY (IR AND RAMAN)

Vibrational spectroscopy is a term used collectively for two important analytical techniques: infrared (IR) and Raman spectroscopy. These two techniques are most frequently used to detect the fundamental modes of molecular vibrations (Mirabella 1998). Since its use in structure elucidation of flavonoids from 1950, its application was believed to be limited to hydroxyl and carbonyl absorption frequencies (Briggs and Colebrook 1962). However, with the advancement of technology, now vibrational analysis plays a vital role in the field of flavonoid analysis (Cornard et al. 1994; Chen et al. 2003). The fundamental principle of the working of these spectroscopies is the measurement of the vibrational energy level associated with the chemical bonds in the sample. As a result, they provide complementary information about the molecular structure. As far as IR is concerned, the sample is usually irradiated with a polychromatic light, and a photon of light is absorbed if the absorbed light (energy) matches the vibrational energy required for the vibration of a particular bond (Ferrari et al. 2004; Siesler et al. 2008). Eventually, the structure can be elucidated from the spectra formed. Unlike IR, in Raman spectroscopy, the sample is irradiated with a monochromatic light and the photons are scattered either elastically or in-elastically. The in-elastically scattered photons or Raman scatters have lost (Stokes) or gained (anti-Stokes) energy during the interaction with the emitted photon (Tu 1982). This gives information about the molecular structure of test compound. These techniques have been extensively used by Cornard, Merlin and their colleagues for the structural elucidation of many flavonoids (Cornard et al. 1995, 1997; Cornard and Merlin, 1999, 2001).

3.5.3 X-RAY CRYSTALLOGRAPHY

This technique is mainly used to determine the atomic and molecular structure of a crystalline compound. This technique is therefore used to determine only a selected class of flavonoids having only crystalline structures. The basic principle of this technique depends upon the diffraction of the X-ray beam. In this case, the crystalline atoms cause a beam of incident X-ray to diffract into various directions. This, in turn, helps in calculating the electron density distribution in the crystal. From this electron density, the mean distance of the atoms in the crystals and the chemical bonds can be deduced (Ladd and Palmer 1985; Drenth 2007). The structure of several flavanonols (Hufford et al. 1993; Selivanova et al. 1999) and flavones (Cornard et al. 1995; Cornard and Merlin 1999; Hong et al. 2001; Paula et al. 2002) were elucidated using X-ray crystallography. However, recently the molecular structures of various synthesized flavonoids were also deciphered using the same technique (Uchida et al. 1995; Artali et al. 2003; Cotelle et al. 2004).

3.5.4 OTHER METHODS

Various other methods for elucidating structures include ultraviolet–visible spectroscopy (UV–Vis spectroscopy), circular dichroism spectroscopy and colorimetric analysis. Previously, UV–Vis spectroscopy was routinely used to determine flavonoid structures for two characteristics. These polyphenolic compounds provide two characteristic peaks at 240–285 nm (arising from the A-ring) and 300–550 nm (arising from the B-ring). The use of UV–Vis spectroscopy in predicting structures has diminished after the technical advancement in NMR, along with modern spectroscopic techniques. However, it is now mostly used for quantitative analyses of the flavonoids. UV–Vis spectroscopy is also widely used in the analysis of anthocyanins, which frequently change their colour with respect to pH (Melo et al. 2000; Giusti and Wrolstad 2001; Moncada et al. 2004). As far as circular dichromism is concerned, it is mainly used to determine the optical properties of the flavonoids. The principle behind dichromism is that when a polarized light is passed through a substance containing chiral molecules, the direction of the polarization can be altered (Berova et al. 2000). This technique is mainly used to define the stereochemistry of the flavonoids having a stereogenic centre or chiral molecule.

3.6 FUNCTIONAL ELUCIDATION OF FLAVONOIDS

Flavonoids, as a vast and diverse class of polyphenols, have an inevitable role in maintaining several major physiological functions in multicellular organisms. The role of flavonoids is being elucidated in the prevention and management of various health complications, as this class of phytochemicals exerts modulatory effects on various signalling pathways at the genomic and non-genomic level. The broad therapeutic actions of flavonoids are attributed to their antioxidant, anti-inflammatory and immunomodulatory effects. The antioxidant activity of flavonoids is well recognised and documented in literature within the last 40 years, with nearly 23,000 publications including 20,000 research articles and 2600 reviews mentioned in the Scopus database (Pérez-Cano and Castell 2016). Nevertheless the biological activities of flavonoids are not confined only to their antioxidant role. Several signalling cascades are activated in response to flavonoids, giving them their protective role in metabolic disorders like diabetes, cancer, cardiovascular diseases, cognitive disorders, osteoporosis and gastrointestinal complications. Because it is beyond the scope of this chapter to include every disease condition modulated by flavonoid intake, we have focused on providing a brief outlook on the modulatory effects of flavonoids in the two most common physiological malfunctions: diabetes and cancer.

3.6.1 DIABETES

Diabetes mellitus (DM) is one of the most prevalent diseases worldwide and its incidence is progressively increasing. It is a group of metabolic ailments characterized by increased level of blood glucose due to defects in insulin secretion or insulin action or both, which is further associated with other long-term complications such as diabetic retinopathy, cardiovascular disorders, liver dysfunction, kidney dysfunction and neurovascular dysfunction (American Diabetes Association 2009).

The World Health Organization (WHO 2016) validated that the worldwide number of people with diabetes has risen to 422 million in 2014 from 108 million in 1980, with an estimated 1.5 million deaths in 2012. The global prevalence of diabetes among adults has risen to 8.5% in 2014 from 4.7% in 1980. WHO projects that by 2030, diabetes will be the world's seventh leading cause of death. Worldwide, the number of individuals with diabetes is rising due to the increasing prevalence of obesity and physical inactivity, population growth, ageing and urbanization (Wild et al. 2004; Nanditha et al. 2016).

DM is classified into two main categories: (1) insulin-dependent diabetes mellitus (IDDM)/ type 1 diabetes and (2) noninsulin-dependent diabetes mellitus (NIDDM)/type 2 diabetes. Type 2 DM is the more prevalent type of diabetes and accounts for 90–95% of all diagnosed cases (American Diabetes Association 2014). In type 1 diabetes, the body does not produce enough insulin due to the gradual destruction of insulin-secreting pancreatic β-cells by the autoimmune system which results in increased blood glucose levels, while in type 2 diabetes, the body stops responding to secreted insulin, a condition known as insulin resistance, which results in a hyperglycaemic condition. To overcome this condition, the pancreas produces a higher amount of insulin and over time, the pancreas fails to produce enough insulin to lower the elevated glucose level, which leads to pancreatic β-cell death. The foremost cause of type 2 diabetes is a combination of genetic and environmental factors such as lifestyle, poor dietary intake, physical inactivity and obesity (Cerf 2013; American Diabetes Association 2014).

With the increased incidence of diabetes, many synthetic drugs have been established to combat this disease, such as α-glucosidase inhibitors, sulfonylurea, biguanides, thiazolidinediones and meglitinide derivatives. These drugs pose several limitations, including lack of effectiveness, higher cost and various side effects, such as hypoglycaemia, weight gain, oedema, anaemia, congestive heart failure, liver dysfunction and gastrointestinal side effects including abdominal discomfort, bloating, anorexia and diarrhoea (Cheng and Fantus 2005; Gupta et al. 2016). Considering all of the disadvantages and side effects of already established drugs, there is need for more efficient compounds/drugs with lesser side effects. Traditional plant-based medicines are effective, economical and safe with no or lesser side effects. These herbal plants or active phytoconstituents are thus considered to be substitutive and outstanding candidates in combating diabetes (Amiot et al. 2016). As the occurrence of the disease is succeeding unabated, there is a critical need for finding effective natural plants/phytochemicals to develop new competent therapeutics (Sharma et al. 2008; Amiot et al. 2016).

In recent years, our group tried to elucidate the antidiabetic potential of various plants and phytoconstituents. Our group has demonstrated the hypoglycaemic and hypolipidemic potential of a flavonoid-rich extract of *Eugenia jambolana* seeds in streptozotocin-induced diabetic rats (Sharma et al. 2008). In another finding, the same group has shown the hypoglycaemic and hypolipidemic effect of guggulsterone, isolated from *Commiphora mukul* resin in high fat–diet fed diabetic rats (Sharma et al. 2009). One more report from our laboratory has shown that an alkaloid rich fraction of *Capparis deciduas* inhibited the elevated blood glucose level, triglyceride content and total cholesterol level in diabetic mice (Sharma 2010). We have recently reported that kaempferol – a well-known flavonoid present in various herbs and medicinal plants including *Eugenia jambolana*, *Ginkgo biloba*, citrus fruits, apples, grapes, onions, leeks and red wines – has been found to have antidiabetic potential and exerts a cytoprotective role on pancreatic β-cells undergoing apoptosis in a lipotoxic environment through activation of autophagy via AMPK/mTOR pathway. Kaempferol was also found to increase β-cell proliferation (Varshney et al. 2017).

Various plants and their active components have been found to have antidiabetic potential. Some of the potent plants include *Allium cepa*, *Aloe vera*, *Allium sativum*, *Aegle marmelos*, *Azadirachta indica*, *Camellia sinensis*, *Citrullus colocynthis*, *Eugenia jambolana*, *Ficus religiosa*, *Gymnema sylvestre*, *Mangifera indica*, *Momordica charantia*, *Ocimum sanctum*, *Opuntia streptacantha*, *Phyllanthus amarus*, *Silybum marianum* and *Trigonella foenum-graecum* (Patel et al. 2012; Prakash 2015).

3.6.2 ANTIDIABETIC POTENTIAL OF FLAVONOIDS AND THEIR MECHANISM OF ACTIONS

Insulin is produced from pancreatic β-cells and stored in granules that are further secreted on demand, which usually occurs just after consuming food. Insulin binds to insulin receptors present on the liver, muscle and adipose cells and in turn translocates GLUT-4 to the cell membrane to facilitate uptake of glucose inside the cells. In liver and muscle cells, glucose is further stored as glycogen. Thus, in this way, insulin lowers the postprandial blood glucose level (Arnoff et al. 2004). In diabetic conditions, either the insulin level goes down or the cells become resistant to insulin. To overcome these conditions any of the steps can be targeted as mentioned below (Kim et al. 2016; Zhou et al. 2016; Chaudhury et al. 2017; Dias et al. 2017; Gupta et al. 2017):

- Improvement of glucose uptake and utilization in muscles, adipose tissues
- Pancreatic β-cell regeneration
- Insulin sensitizer
- Insulin secretion enhancer
- Lowering glucose absorption in the intestine (α-glucosidase inhibitor, α-amylase inhibitor)
- Regulation of crucial signalling pathways to cell homeostasis

- Inhibition of gluconeogenesis and glycogenolysis in the liver
- Stimulation of glycogenesis
- Reduction of inflammation and oxidative stress

In this chapter, we focus on reviewing most significant and effective methods that can be used as tools to investigate the antidiabetic potential of any herb/phytochemical and its mechanism of action.

In vitro **analyses:** It is evident that for a phytochemical to have antidiabetic potential it must be capable of lowering the blood glucose level through a different mechanism of action, as discussed earlier. The antidiabetic potential of herbs and their active constituents can be determined using a variety of *in vitro* assays as an initial screening tool prior to *in vivo* studies (Reed and Scribner 1999; Vinayagam et al. 2017). Advantages of using *in vitro* test systems include: (1) relatively economical, (2) fast and high-throughput screening helps to eliminate non-effective compounds in initial stages and minimizes the use of animals for further testing, (3) considered significant to determine the cellular and molecular mechanisms and (4) benefits in terms of ethical considerations. Thus, *in vitro* studies are the perfect model for obtaining active principles with defined biological activities that can be further tested *in vivo* to confirm their bioactivity and mode of action (Reed and Scribner 1999; Ranganatha and Kuppast 2012; Doke and Shawale 2012; Karthikeyan 2016; Vinayagam et al. 2017).

However, *in vitro* studies also have several limitations, as cells and tissues are treated outside their natural environment without a blood supply, surrounding tissues, nutrients and hormones present inside the body. This may directly or indirectly interact with the target tissue or compound tested, thus enhancing the possibility of artefactual results. Thus it should be taken into consideration that compounds showing some effects on a cellular level are not the final confirmation about their effects under physiological conditions (Ranganatha and Kuppast 2012; Doke and Shawale 2012; Karthikeyan 2016) and must be confirmed using *in vivo* test systems.

3.6.2.1 *In Vitro* Enzymatic Assays

3.6.2.1.1 *The Alpha-Amylase Inhibition Assay*

Pancreatic alpha-amylase (α-amylase) is a key enzyme of carbohydrate metabolism. It hydrolyses dietary starch into smaller oligosaccharides – oligoglucans, maltose and maltotriose – that are further degraded into glucose by α-glucosidase. Thereafter, glucose enters into the bloodstream through intestinal absorption and results in elevated postprandial glucose levels. Targeting α-amylase can thus be an effective strategy in lowering blood glucose levels in a hyperglycaemic condition. Inhibition of the activity of α-amylase reduces the elevated glucose peaks that occur after a meal in a low insulin condition (type 1 diabetes) and insulin-resistant condition (type 2 diabetes), keeping the glucose level under control (Brayer et al. 2010). To determine the α-amylase inhibitory activity of any phytochemical, the inhibition assay can be performed using the chromogenic 3,5-dinitrosalicylic acid (DNS) method as described by Miller, which is based on detection of reducing sugar (Miller 1959). Some of the flavonoids that have been reported to have α-amylase inhibition activity are rutin (Obot et al. 2015), quercetin (Tadera et al. 2006; Oboh et al. 2015; Semaan et al. 2017), myricetin (Tadera et al. 2006), luteolin (Kim et al. 2000; Tadera et al. 2006), fisetin (Tadera et al. 2006), epigallocatechin-3-gallate (EGCG; Forester et al. 2012; Xiao et al. 2013).

3.6.2.1.2 *Alpha-Glucosidase Inhibition Assay*

Alpha-glucosidase (α-glucosidase) is an important enzyme that catalyses the final step of starch digestion in the small intestine. The α-glucosidase inhibitors help to lower the postprandial blood glucose and insulin levels in diabetic patients (van de Laar 2008). Acarbose and miglitol are extensively studied α-glucosidase inhibitors and have been found to be effective in lowering blood glucose level in type 1 and type 2 diabetic patients. In older type 2 diabetic patients, acarbose also showed increased insulin sensitivity (Sugihara et al. 2014). The α-glucosidase inhibitory activity of phytochemicals can be determined as illustrated by Walker et al. (1993). Some examples of the flavonoids already known for their α-glucosidase inhibition activity are rutin (Li et al. 2009; Oboh et al. 2015), quercetin (Tadera et al. 2006; Li et al. 2009; Oboh et al. 2015; Semaan et al. 2017), myricetin (Tadera et al. 2006; Kang et al. 2015), kaempferol (Peng et al. 2016), luteolin (Kim et al. 2000; Tadera et al. 2006), fisetin (Tadera et al. 2006), isoquercetin (Li et al. 2009), naringenin (Tadera et al. 2006; Priscilla et al. 2014) and epigallocatechin-3-gallate (EGCG; Tadera et al. 2006).

3.6.2.1.3   *Protein Tyrosine Phosphatase 1B (PTP1B) Inhibitory Assay*

Insulin activates insulin receptor upon binding, which in turn autophosphorylates at tyrosine residues. Further, the immediate effectors – insulin receptor substrates-1 (IRS-1) and insulin receptor substrates-2 (IRS-2) – are recruited to the receptor and activated to transmit intracellular signalling. PTP1B dephosphorylates tyrosine residues at the insulin receptor and its substrate (IRS-1) constraining insulin signalling, resulting in insulin sensitivity (Vieira et al. 2017). PTP1B inhibition was found to improve insulin signalling and prevent type 2 diabetes (Tamrakar et al. 2014). Increased PTP1B activity, meanwhile, led to insulin resistance and type 2 diabetes (González-Rodríguez et al. 2010). Thus, inhibitors of PTP1B can be a promising candidate for type 2 diabetic patients. For determining the PTP1B inhibitory activity of any phytochemical, the inhibition assay can be performed as mentioned elsewhere (Na et al. 2006). Flavonoids that have recently been found to be effective in inhibiting PTP1B activity include quercetin (Chen et al. 2002; Semaan et al. 2017), uralenol (Chen et al. 2002), broussochalcone (Na et al. 2006), glycyrrhisoflavone, glisoflavone, licoflavone (Li et al. 2010), pongamol, karanjin and licochalcone (Jiang et al. 2012).

3.6.2.1.4   *Dipeptidyl Peptidase IV (DPP IV) Inhibition Assay*

Dipeptidyl peptidase IV (DPP IV) is an enzyme that cleaves *N*-terminal dipeptides from incretin hormones like glucagon-like peptide-1 (GLP-1) and glucose-dependent insulinotropic polypeptide (GIP; Juillerat-Jeanneret 2013). The incretin hormones help in insulin secretion and inhibit glucagon secretion, consequently lowering postprandial blood glucose. Preventing the degradation of incretin hormones by DPP IV enzyme has thus become an effective strategy for diabetes without causing hypoglycaemia or weight gain (Matheeussen et al. 2012; Juillerat-Jeanneret 2013; Arulmozhiraja et al. 2016). *In vitro* assessment for DPP IV inhibitory activity by various phytochemicals has been described earlier by Matheeussen et al. (2012). Various reports have established the DPP IV inhibition activity of certain phytochemicals like quercetin (Semaan et al. 2017) and anthocyanins (Fan et al. 2013).

3.6.2.2   *In Vitro* **Cell Culture-Based Assays**

In vitro cell and tissue culture is the reliable model to test effects of different types of compounds on specific cell/tissue types. These cultures are used to study physiological and pathophysiological processes of cells without using animal models. The main advantage of using cell/tissue culture as *in vitro* model is that the results obtained are more reliable and reproducible from a batch of clonal cell lines (Doke and Dhawale 2015). The cells/tissue from various organs can be isolated and grown outside the body in suitable growth medium and environment for several days to months or even few years. On the contrary, a major disadvantage of using established immortalized cell lines are their characteristic features that keeps changing with increasing passage number which could be linked with abnormal behaviour, abnormal gene or protein expression or various genetic mutations (Ranganatha and Kuppast 2012; Doke and Dhawale 2015). Although a precise alternative to immortalised cell lines is primary cell/tissue culture, it also has some limitations such as the primary culture can be grown for a limited period only. Overall, the *in vitro* cell or tissue culture-based methods are potential alternatives over animal models in terms of being less laborious, expensive and time-consuming; they can also be routinely used for preliminary screening of potential target molecules for their cytocompatibility and efficacy. In the following section, we have summarised the methods that can be used to determine the antidiabetic property of any phytochemical by using cell and tissue culture as a model.

3.6.2.2.1 Glucose Uptake Assay and Glucose Transporter Assay

Glucose uptake is an important and widely used biological assay to study glucose metabolism in muscles, adipose and liver cells (Yamamoto et al. 2011). Insulin stimulates glucose uptake by activating phosphorylation of insulin receptor substrate (IRS) which in turn instigates PI3 kinase, protein kinase B and protein kinase C isoforms. Subsequently, protein kinase B activates glucose transporter 4 (GLUT-4) translocation to the cell surface and stimulates glucose uptake in the cell (Chang et al. 2004). Various natural phytochemicals are found to be insulin mimetic and effective in increasing glucose uptake. Some of these phytochemicals reported are epigallocatechin (Daisy et al. 2010) and myricetin (Kandasamy and Ashokkumar 2014). Apart from this, AMPK-mediated translocation of GLUT-4 is another alternative mechanism by which various phytochemicals such as kaempferol (Alkhalidy et al. 2015), quercetin (Alam et al. 2014), and naringin (Jung et al. 2004; Pu et al. 2012) along with some other phytochemicals are found to be effective in increasing glucose transport into cells (Huang and Czech 2007). Thus, improved glucose uptake is one of the efficient ways that can help in improving hyperglycaemia in diabetic condition (Boucher et al. 2014). To elucidate the glucose uptake stimulatory activity of phytochemicals, the cells are incubated with test compounds in presence or absence of insulin.

There are several methods to quantify cellular glucose uptake and these differ mainly in terms of the substrate for glucose transport. Upon transport glucose is shuttled to various pathways, so non-metabolizable analogues are used in these assays. These methods can be divided into two categories: (1) detection of accumulated intracellular 2-[3H] deoxy-D-glucose-6-phosphate (^{3}H-2DG6P) by radioactive method and (2) enzymatic detection of 2-deoxy-D-glucose-6-phosphate (2DG6P) by colorimetric/fluorometric/luminometric methods (Saito et al. 2011; Fan et al. 2013; Boucher et al. 2014). Of these methods, the non-radioactive enzymatic detection of 2DG6P has been widely used because of its simplicity and the lack of any need to handle or dispose of radioactive materials. In this method, 2-deoxy-D-glucose (the glucose analogue), is added to cells and taken up by glucose transporters, which is then further phosphorylated to 2DG6P by hexokinase. However, 2DG6P cannot be metabolized further and thus accumulates in the cells, which is directly proportional to 2-deoxy-D-glucose taken up by cells. The accumulated 2-deoxy-D-glucose can be further detected by colorimetric/fluorometric/luminometric enzymatic assay methods (Saito et al. 2011; Fan et al. 2013; Valley et al. 2016).

3.6.2.2.2 Pancreatic β-Cell Proliferation Assay

Pancreatic β-cells are located in the islets of Langerhans and produce and store insulin, which helps in glucose homeostasis. Loss of β-cell mass and function is one of the major causes of type 1 and type 2 diabetes. Importantly, recent research has focused mainly on improving hyperglycaemia by regenerating β-cells. Thus compounds that can protect and regenerate β-cells in diabetic conditions are of great importance (Wu and Mahato 2013; Liu and Wu 2014; Chala and Ali 2016). Some of the flavonoids recently found to be effective in β-cell regeneration are kaempferol (Zhang and Liu 2011; Alkhalidy et al. 2015; Varshney et al. 2017), genistein (Fu et al. 2010; Kim et al. 2007), quercetin (Dai et al. 2013), anthocyanins (Zhang et al. 2010), epigallocatechin-3-gallate (Cai and Lin 2009) and baicalein (Oh 2015). In vitro assays that can be performed to identify β-cell proliferative activity are BrdU uptake studies, clonogenic assay, scratch assay and cell counting, as described earlier (Fu et al. 2014; Varshney et al. 2017). Also, the cell models widely used for β-cell regeneration studies are the RIN-m5F, RIN-5F, MIN6, HIT-T15, INS-1 and β-TC-6 cell lines and isolated mice/rat/human pancreatic islets (Labriola et al. 2009).

3.6.2.2.3 Insulin Biosynthesis and Secretion Assay

Pancreatic β-cell degeneration and dysfunction plays an important role in the pathogenesis of type 1 and type 2 diabetes. Insulin, which is secreted from β-cells, is a key mediator of glucose metabolism. Thus, deficiency of insulin synthesis and secretion or lack of insulin sensitivity leads to decreased glucose tolerance which results in diabetes. Insulin is synthesized from preproinsulin which is further processed to proinsulin. Proinsulin is then processed to insulin and C-peptide and stored in secretory granules until release on stimulation. Insulin biosynthesis is regulated at both transcriptional as well as translation level. Thus, flavonoids can play a role in increasing insulin synthesis or secretion or both the activities, which can be tested using suitable assays. Some of the phytochemicals such as genistein (Skelin et al. 2010; Fu and Liu 2009), quercetin (Youl et al. 2010), berberine, ginsenoside, curcumin (Dai et al. 2013), and epigallocatechin-3-gallate (Youl et al. 2010) have been reported to be effective in augmenting insulin secretory activity of pancreatic β-cells. To elucidate the insulin synthesis activity of any phytochemical, insulin promoter activity assay can also be performed over and above transcriptional analysis of insulin gene, while for insulin secretion assay, the secreted insulin level in cell cultures can be quantified by insulin ELISA (enzyme-linked immunosorbent assay; Jang et al. 2013). For *in vitro* insulin synthesis and secretory assays, the most widely used pancreatic β-cell lines are RIN-m5F, RIN-5F, MIN6, HIT-T15, INS-1 and β-TC-6 (Labriola et al. 2009).

3.6.2.2.4 *Peroxisome Proliferator-Activated Receptor-γ Promoter Assay*

Peroxisome proliferator-activated receptor-γ (PPAR-γ) is a nuclear receptor that plays a key role in insulin sensitivity and glucose uptake (Liao et al. 2007; Fu et al. 2013). PPAR-γ agonists enhance glucose disposal in insulin-resistant animals and humans. Thiazolidinediones (TZDs), the PPAR-γ agonists improve plasma and insulin levels in diabetic and obese conditions. This class of drug is also associated with severe weight gain, which may lead to obesity and associated diseases (Fu et al. 2013). Recently, there has been an extensive search for partial agonists of PPAR-γ, the target drugs that may improve insulin sensitivity without promoting fat deposition (Larsen et al. 2003). Recently, the plant molecule nymphayol was found to be a partial agonist of PPAR-γ. It has been shown to increase insulin sensitization and decrease body weight in diabetic mice (Wang et al. 2014). Thus, PPAR-γ could be a good target for developing anti-hyperglycaemic drugs with special reference to obesity-linked type 2 diabetes. To elucidate this activity, PPAR-γ reporter gene assay can be performed as described elsewhere (Sharma et al. 2008; Choi et al. 2010). Some flavonoids, such as quercetin and kaempferol, have been reported as partial agonists of PPAR-γ and stimulated glucose uptake in mature adipocytes without any significant adipogenic activity (Fang et al. 2008).

3.6.2.2.5 *Glucagon-Like Peptide 1 Receptor Agonists Activity*

Glucagon-like peptide 1 (GLP-1) is an incretin hormone that stimulates insulin secretion and inhibits glucagon secretion, consequently lowering postprandial blood glucose (Gupta 2013; Tölle 2014; Tomlinson et al. 2016). Thus, a phytochemical agonist of GLP-1 receptor could be very effective in type 1 as well as type 2 diabetes (Kalra et al. 2016; Tomlinson et al. 2016; Lovshin 2017; Tran et al. 2017). This class of anti-hyperglycaemic agent reduces both fasting and postprandial blood glucose level in a glucose-dependent manner. Interestingly, GLP-1 receptor agonists – when adminsitered along with metformin – do not pose the increased risk of weight gain and hypoglycaemia typically observed with most other classes of anti-hyperglycaemic agents. These receptor agonists have even been found to be associated with weight loss in most of the patients (Kalra et al. 2016; Lovshin 2017; Tran et al. 2017). The GLP-1 receptor agonist also exerts cytoprotective and cell proliferative effect on β-cells, thus inducing insulin synthesis and secretion (Tran et al. 2017). Functional elucidation of GLP-1 receptor agonist activity of various phytochemicals can be performed by a GLP-1 reporter luciferase assay, as has been reported earlier (Sloop et al. 2010). This assay indicates the role of these phytochemicals in regulating the transactivation of GLP-1 gene. Some of the recently reported flavonoids containing GLP-1 agonist activity are quercetin (Wootten et al. 2011) and myricetin (Li et al. 2017).

3.6.3 Flavonoids as Antidiabetic Agents

Various *in vitro* and *in vivo* findings have proven the antidiabetic activity of some dietary flavonoids. The following table summarizes the detailed mechanism of action and antidiabetic potentials of some common flavonoids (Table 3.2).

TABLE 3.2

Mechanism of Action of Some Selected Flavonoids Demonstrating Antidiabetic Activities

Flavonoid	Mechanism of Action	Experimental Model	References
Genistein	Reduces pancreatic inflammation and tissue damage via SIRT1 activation	STZ and high-fat diet induced diabetic mice	Yousefi et al. (2017)
	Exerts protective effect on pancreatic β-cells damages regenerates β-cells and improves serum levels of insulin and glucose	STZ-induced diabetic rat	El-Kordy and Alshahranni (2015)
	Attenuates kidney oxidative stress and decreases inflammatory markers	Alloxan-induced diabetic neuropathy mice model	Kim and Lim (2013)
	Increases serum insulin and decreases β-cell apoptosis	STZ-induced C57BL/6 mice	Fu and Liu (2009)
	Decreases fasting blood glucose, increases serum insulin, improves glucose tolerance, increases β-cell mass and decreases apoptosis	STZ-induced C57BL/6 mice	Fu et al. (2010)
	Increases glucose uptake, AMPK phosphorylation; increases GLUT-1 and GLUT-4 mRNA expressions and PTP1B inhibition	L6 myotubes	Lee et al. (2009)
Quercetin	Ameliorates oxidative stress and inflammation	STZ-nicotinamide induced diabetic rats	Roslan et al. (2017)
	Decreases blood glucose and serum triglycerides and ameliorates diabetic neuropathy condition	C57BL/6J model of diabetic neuropathy	Gomes et al. (2015)
	Increases in GLUT-4 expression and exerts antioxidant activity	Alloxan-induced diabetic mice	Alam et al. (2014)
	Protects β-cell mass and function under high-fructose induction by reducing serum insulin and leptin via Akt/FoxO1 activation	Fructose-treated rats and INS-1β cells	Li et al. (2013)
	Protects against cytokine-induced β-cell death via the mitochondrial pathway and NF-κB signalling	RINm5F β-cells	Dai et al. (2013)
	Ameliorates hyperglycaemia and dyslipidaemia; increased activity of superoxide dismutase, catalase, glutathione peroxidase and HDL-cholesterol	Diet-C57BL/KsJ-db/db mice	Jeong et al. (2012)

(Continued)

TABLE 3.2 (*Continued*)

Mechanism of Action of Some Selected Flavonoids Demonstrating Antidiabetic Activities

Flavonoid	Mechanism of Action	Experimental Model	References
Myricetin	GLP-1R agonist and increases insulin secretion	Isolated islets and Wistar rats	Li et al. (2017)
	Inhibits α-glucosidase enzyme	STZ-induced diabetic rats	Kang et al. (2015)
	Improves carbohydrate metabolism; increases GLUT-2, GLUT-4, IRS-1, IRS-2 and ultimately enhances glucose utilization and renal function	STZ-(Cd) induced diabetic nephrotoxic rats	Kandasamy and Ashokkumar (2014)
	Alleviates insulin resistance; improves obesity and reduces serum pro-inflammatory cytokine levels	High-fat, high-sucrose diet-induced mice	Choi et al. (2014)
	Exerts antioxidant activity with increased glutathione peroxidase, superoxide dismutase and catalase activity	*db/db* mice	Choi et al. (2013)
EGCG	Attenuates insulin secretion; activates AMPK through the inhibition of glutamate dehydrogenase	Pancreatic β-cells and muscle cells	Pournourmohammadi et al. (2017)
	Improves insulin resistance and increases glucagon-like peptide 1 expression	Double-blinded, randomised and placebo-controlled clinical trial	C.Y. Liu et al. (2014)
	Improves glucose tolerance, insulin sensitivity and endothelial function	High-fat diet-induced C57BL/6J mice	Youl et al. (2010)
	Improves glucose tolerance; increases glucose-stimulated insulin secretion and increasing number and size of islets	*db/db* mice	Ortsäter et al. (2012)
	Exerts antioxidant activity; causes AT_1 receptor upregulation	Streptozotocin-induced diabetic rats	Thomson et al. (2012)
Kaempferol	Rescues pancreatic β-cells from palmitic acid-induced apoptosis; modulates autophagy regulation via AMPK/mTOR pathway	RIN-5F cells and primary islets	Varshney et al. (2017)
	Improves fasting blood glucose levels; glucose intolerance; insulin sensitivity and suppress blood glucose production	STZ induced mice, primary human skeletal muscles and HepG2 cells	Moore et al. (2017)
	Inhibits α-glucosidase enzyme	Enzymatic activity	Peng et al. (2016)
	Improves hyperglycaemia; glucose tolerance; increase blood insulin levels and islet β-cell mass via increased GLUT-4 and AMPK expression	High-fat diet-induced diabetic mice	Alkhalidy et al. (2015)
	Increases antioxidant activity and decreases lipid peroxidation markers	STZ-induced diabetic rats	Al-Numair et al. (2015)
	Ameliorates hypertlipidaemia and diabetes by increasing lipid metabolism; downregulates PPAR-γ and SREBP-1c activities	High-fat diet obese C57BL/6J mice	Zang et al. (2015)

3.6.4 ANTICANCER POTENTIAL OF FLAVONOIDS AND THEIR MECHANISM OF ACTIONS

As far as the pharmacological effects of dietary flavonoids are concerned, they are found to be potent in various disorders such as diabetes (Y.-J. Liu et al. 2014; Chen, Mangelinckx et al. 2015), cancer (Androutsopoulos et al. 2010; Yao et al. 2011; Park and Pezzuto 2012), cardiovascular diseases (Muldoon and Kritchevsky 1996; Gross 2004) and microbial diseases (Cushnie and Lamb 2005, 2011). Considered the second deadliest disease in the world, cancer is being widely studied across the globe. Modification of present drugs and discovery of new molecular entities are presently being carried out by various research communities. Scientific discoveries and technological advancement from the last 5 decades – including modern molecular biology techniques, high-throughput screening and structure-based drug designing – have helped in knowing the mechanisms of the disease better, as well as developing new drug candidates against cancer. Currently, nature-based molecules or their modified versions are considered to be a priority area of research due to their high pharmacological effectiveness and fewer side effects. Many new plant-based molecules have been considered as prototypes or leads of series, and their structural modification has led to pharmacologically active compounds (Lee 2004; Koehn and Carter 2005; Paterson and Anderson 2005; Butler 2008). In this chapter, we focused on diabetes in the first part, in the second part we briefly discuss cancer as the disease target. First, we discuss some commonly used cell-based assays to assess the anticancer activities of various phytochemical entities with special emphasis on flavonoids. It is to be noted that there are a large number of assays available, but we focus only on some of the major ones considering the limited scope of this chapter.

3.6.4.1 Cytotoxicity Assay

This is a simple and rapid colorimetric-based assay for analysing the cytotoxicity of drugs (Mosmann 1983; Denizot and Lang 1986). MTT or 3-(4,5-dimethylthiazol-2-yl)-2,5-diphenyltetrazolium bromide is a tetrazolium dye used in this assay. The basic principle behind the assay is that the viable cells have active mitochondria, which in turn produce NA(D)PH-dependent oxidoreductase enzymes (Slater et al. 1963). The yellow-coloured tetrazolium MTT or 3-(4,5-dimethylthiazol-2-yl)-2,5-diphenyltetrazolium bromide is reduced to violet-coloured formazan crystals when it comes in contact with the oxidoreductase enzymes. These intracellular formazan crystals can be solubilized and quantified using a spectrophotometer (usually between 550 and 600 nm). However, some other related dyes can also be used in place of MTT to determine viability. For example, XTT (2,3-bis-(2-methoxy-4-nitro-5-sulfophenyl)-2H-tetrazolium-5-carboxanilide) and MTS (3-(4,5-dimethylthiazol-2-yl)-5-(3-carboxymethoxyphenyl)-2-(4-sulfophenyl)-2H-tetrazolium) are also sometimes used as an alternative to MTT dye. This type of assay provides a first-hand reference about the cytotoxic nature of the test chemicals.

3.6.4.2 Clonogenic Assay

Another cell-based assay frequently used for evaluating the anticancer activity of any drug is the clonogenic assay. This is mainly used to evaluate the loss of reproductive integrity or death of the cells after treatment of the same with any radiation or any chemotherapeutic agents. The basic principle of this assay lies in the fact that the ability of a single cell to grow into a large colony can be visualized by the naked eye/microscopically. This gives a clear cut implication that these cells have retained their reproductive integrity. Loss of this ability as a function of radiation and chemotherapy can be deduced by the dose-survival curve. Although the assay produces accurate results, the only drawback is that the process is quite time consuming. Eventually, the percentage of cells that survive the drug treatment is measured and analysed further. Normally in this type of assay, limited numbers of cells are seeded initially and on completion of the incubation, the cells are fixed and stained to draw a conclusion. As far as the functional activity of the flavonoids are concerned, different dosages of the flavonoids can be used to determine the dose-survival curve and related cytotoxicity. The detailed protocol for this assay has been described elsewhere (Munshi et al. 2005).

3.6.4.3 Nuclear Staining of Cells

DAPI or 4′,6-diamidino-2-phenylindole is a florescent dye used to stain the nucleus of a cell. This stain has the property of binding to the A-T rich regions in the DNA (Eriksson et al. 1993) and the DAPI-DNA complex emits fluorescence. Most of the modern anticancer drugs focus on DNA damage, as it leads to apoptosis and other forms of cell death (Kawanishi and Kiraku 2004; Havelka et al. 2007; Cheung-Ong et al. 2013). This method is mainly used for deducing the DNA damage inside the cells by microscopic visualization. The main principle behind this assay is that the binding of DAPI to the ds-DNA produces a ~20-fold fluorescence enhancement (Barcellona et al. 1990). This is observed due to displacement of water molecules from both DNA as well as DAPI. DAPI also binds to RNA at selective A-U intercalation (Tanious et al. 1992) but the intensity of fluorescence is comparatively low compared to that of DNA. The cells treated with cytotoxic drugs will have nuclear damage (Cheung-Ong et al. 2013), and the fragmented DNA will have clusters of DAPI-DNA complexes that can be distinguished morphologically under a microscopic. Based upon the image, the quantification and a relative dosage-survival analysis can be carried out. As far as the fluorescence characteristic is concerned, the excitation and emission maximum of DAPI (bound to ds-DNA) is 358 and 461 nm, respectively. DAPI is usually excited by a UV lamp, but xenon and mercury-arc lamps can also be used for the excitation.

3.6.4.4 COMET Assay or Single Cell Gel Electrophoresis (SCGE)

COMET assay is one of the standard methods for assessing DNA damage. Cook et al. (1976) first studied the nuclear structure based on the lysis of the cells using non-ionic detergent and sodium chloride. Based upon their study, Ostling and Johanson (1984) modified the technique and described the tails in terms of DNA supercoiling. However the term "COMET" is used due to pattern of migration of the DNA fragments through the electrophoresis gel (Tice et al. 2000). The basic principle of the assay is that the cells are first encapsulated in agarose and then lysed with detergents and high salts so that nucleoids having supercoiled DNA will be formed. The cells having damaged DNA will have many more short fragments in comparison to those having intact DNA. These cells, when electrophoresed, will have a larger tail-like stretch than normal cells. This is because the nucleoids, having breaks, will lose their supercoiling and tends to move towards anode. Later any dye intercalating or binding DNA can be used to detect the pattern of migration, which in turn can be visualized in a florescent microscope. The DNA damage is then quantified based upon the migration scores either performed manually or by software (Klaude et al. 1996; Collins et al. 1997). Currently there are different variants of the COMET assays. Some important variants include alkaline single cell gel electrophoresis (Singh et al. 1988; Olive et al. 1990), neutral single cell gel electrophoresis (Collins 1999), fluorescent in situ hybridization comet assay (Santos et al. 1997; Rapp et al. 1999; Mladinic et al. 2012) and bromodeoxyuridine labelled detection (McGlynn et al. 1999). Tice et al. (2000) provided a detailed protocol for the COMET assay.

3.6.4.5 Cell Cycle Analysis with Flow Cytometry

The flow cytometer is an important tool having enormous potential for studying various aspects of cells, including cell counting, sorting and biomarker detection. The most important applications of flow cytometry are measurement of cellular DNA content and cell cycle analysis. Proliferating cells undergo five phases of the cell cycle: G_0, G_1, S, G_2 and M. Different phases of the cell cycle have different quantities of DNA content. However, the M phase is indistinguishable from the G_2 phase and G_0 from G_1. Hence, when cell cycle analysis is carried out on the basis of DNA content alone, the cell cycle is commonly described as G_0/G_1, S and G_2/M phases. DNA content or ploidy represents the total number of chromosomes in a cell. Any abnormality (e.g. cancer cells) in the variation in ploidy is observed and this can be detected by flow cytometry. Many modern anticancer drugs act on DNA topoisomerases, which in turn affects DNA replication (Sorenson et al. 1990; Buolamwini 2000; Gamet-Payrastre et al. 2000). These drugs also help in cell cycle arrest and all these phenomena can be confirmed by flow cytometry. The main detection in this system is performed by fluorescence from DNA binding dyes used in the assay. Some important DNA binding dyes usually used for cytometric analysis are propidium iodide, 7-aminoactinomycin-D, Hoechst 33342, 33258 and S769121, TO-PRO-3 and 4'6'-diamidino-2-phenylindole. The advantage of modern flow cytometers is that they can analyse more than a thousand samples per second and, if associated with cell sorters, can then separate and isolate the cells at the same rate.

3.6.5 FLAVONOIDS AS ANTICANCER AGENTS

Various *in vitro*, *in vivo* and epidemiological evidence has established the anticancer activities of dietary flavonoids. Some flavonoids are found to induce apoptosis (Wang et al. 1999; Q. Zhang et al. 2008), necrosis (Habtemariam 1997) and senescence (Zamin et al. 2009) or inhibit angiogenesis (Fotsis et al. 1997; Kim 2003) and metastasis (Caltagirone et al. 2000; Ni et al. 2012) of cancerous cells. Because describing the mechanism of action of each and every flavonoid is beyond the scope of this review, we represent the mechanisms of action of some major flavonoids that have been reported recently for their anticancer properties in Table 3.3.

TABLE 3.3

Mechanism of Action of Some Selected Flavonoids Demonstrating Anticancer Activities

Compounds	Mechanism of Action	Experimental Model	Reference
Quercetin	Induction of apoptosis by inhibition of HSP70 synthesis	K562, Molt-4, Raji and MCAS tumour cell lines	Wei et al. (1994)
	Induction of apoptosis via ROS mediated ERK activation	Acute myeloid leukaemia (AML) cells	Lee et al. (2015)
	Induction of mitochondrial-mediated apoptosis by downregulation of IL6/STAT3	A549 cells	Mukherjee and Khuda-Bukhsh (2015)
	Inhibition of metastasis by regulation of mir21 in prostate cancer cells	PC3 cells	Yang et al. (2015)
	Inhibits the migration of triple negative breast cancer cells by regulating β-catenin signalling pathway	MDA-MB-231 and MDA-MB-468 cells	Srinivasan et al. (2016)
Kaempferol	Induction of apoptosis by ER-stress and mitochondria-dependent pathways in bone cells	BALB/c (nu/nu) mice and U-2 OS, HOB and 143B cells	Huang et al. (2010)
	Induction of caspase-3 dependent apoptosis in oral cavity cancer cells	SCC-1483, SCC-25 and SCC-QLL1 cells	Kang et al. (2010)
	Suppression of transforming growth factor β-1-induced epithelial-mesenchymal transition (EMT) and cell migration	A549 lung cancer cells	Jo et al. (2015)
	Induction of TRAIL-induced apoptosis in colon cancer cells	SW480 cells	Yoshida et al. (2008)

(Continued)

TABLE 3.3 (*Continued*)

Mechanism of Action of Some Selected Flavonoids Demonstrating Anticancer Activities

Compounds	Mechanism of Action	Experimental Model	Reference
Quercetin	Induction of apoptosis by inhibiting the expression of MMP-9 and fibronectin involving ERK and AKT pathways in glioblastoma cells	U87-MG glioblastoma U251 and SHG44 glioma cell lines	Pan et al. (2015)
	Induction of apoptosis in human colon cancer cells by inhibiting NF-kappa B pathway	CaCO-2 and SW-620 cells	X.-A. Zhang et al. (2015)
	Suppression of hepatocyte growth factor (HGF)-stimulated melanoma cell migration and invasion by inhibiting HGF/c-Met/HGF-receptor signalling	A2058 and A375 cells	Cao et al. (2015)
	Suppression of metastatic activity of lung cancer cells by inhibiting Snail-dependent Akt activation	A549, H1975 and HCC827 and female SCID mice	Chang et al. (2017)
Genistein	Induction of apoptosis by inactivation of IGF-1R/p-Akt signalling pathway in breast cancer cells	MCF-7 cells	Chen, Duan et al. (2015)
	Inhibition of hepatocellular cell migration by reversing the epithelial-mesenchymal transition	HepG2, SMMC-7721 and Bel-7402 cells	Dai et al. (2015)
	Inhibition of human colorectal cancer metastasis by suppressing Fms-Related Tyrosine Kinase 4 (FLT4)	HCT116, HT29 and SW620 cells	Xiao et al. (2015)
Diadzein	Exhibition of anti-tumour activity in bladder cancer cells by inhibition of fibroblast growth factor receptors 3 pathway	RT112, RT4 and SW780 cells and female nude mice	He et al. (2015)
Catechin	Induction of apoptosis by cell cycle arrest and potential synergism with cisplatin in bilary tract cancer cells	CCSW-1, BDC, EGI-1, SkChA-1, TFK-1 (bile duct carcinoma cell lines) and MzChA-1, MzChA-2, GBC (gallbladder cancer cell lines)	Mayr et al. (2015)
Epigallocatechingallate (EGCG)	Suppression of osteosarcoma cell growth by upregulation of miR-1	MG-63 and U-2OS cells	Zhu and Wang (2016)
	Induction of apoptosis in human prostate cancer cells by inhibiting HSP90	BCaPT1 (early tumorigenic), BCaPT10 (late tumorigenic) and BCaPM-T10 (metastatic) human PRCA cells	Moses et al. (2015)
	Suppression of melanoma cell growth and metastasis by targeting TNF-α receptor-associated factor 6 (TRAF6)	Male Balb/c and SK-MEL-5, SK-MEL-28, A375, and G361 cells	Zhang et al. (2016)

(*Continued*)

TABLE 3.3 (*Continued*)

Mechanism of Action of Some Selected Flavonoids Demonstrating Anticancer Activities

Compounds	Mechanism of Action	Experimental Model	Reference
Hesperetin	Induction of apoptosis in breast carcinoma by accumulation of ROS and activation of apoptosis signal-regulating kinase 1 and c-Jun n-terminal kinases pathway	MCF-7 cells	Palit et al. (2015)
	Induction of apoptosis in gastric cancer cells by activating mitochondrial pathways and by increasing ROS	Male BALB/c-nu/nu nude mice and SGC-7901, MGC-803, and HGC-27 cells	J. Zhang et al. (2015)
	Induction of cell death in HER2 positive breast cancer cells by inhibiting HER2 tyrosine kinase activity	SKBR3 and MDA-MB-231 cells	Chandrika et al. (2016)
Naringenin	Induction of apoptosis in human colorectal cells by p38-dependant downregulation of cyclin D1	HCT116 and SW480 cells	Song et al. (2015)
	Induction of apoptosis and inhibition of proliferation, migration and invasion of gastric cancer cells by downregulating AKT pathway	SGC-7901 cells	Bao et al. (2016)
Apigenin	Induction of apoptosis in choriocarcinoma cells via PI3K/AKT and ERK1/2 MAPK pathways	JAR and JEG3 cells	Lim et al. (2016)
	Inhibition of metastasis in melanoma cells by inhibition of STAT-3 signalling pathway	C57BL/6 mice injected with B16F10 melanoma cells	Cao et al. (2016)
	Inhibition of metastasis by downregulating neural precursor cell expressed developmentally down-regulated protein 9 (NEDD9) in colorectal cancer cells	Female athymic nude mice and DLD1 and SW480 cells	Dai et al. (2017)
Luteolin	Inhibition of IL-6 induced epithelial-mesenchymal transition and matrix metaloproteases (MMPs) secretion of pancreatic cells by deactivating STAT signalling	PANC-1 and SW1990 cells	Huang et al. (2015)
	Induction of apoptosis in brain tumour cells (neuroblastoma) by G0/G1 cell cycle growth arrest and mitochondrial membrane potential loss in brain tumour cells	SH-SY5Y cells	Wang et al. (2015)

3.7 CURRENT RESEARCH GAPS AND FUTURE PROSPECTS

Over the past few decades, flavonoids have been among some of the most studied phytochemicals for drug discovery research due to their potential health beneficiary effects. Although several research groups globally are aiming to elucidate the mechanistic actions of these phytochemicals for the maintenance of physiological processes, there are certain limitations or gaps in the research that have to be considered for the establishment of phyto-therapeutics in the treatment of several ailments in future. The structural heterogeneity and scarcity of data on solubilisation, matrix release through digestion (bioaccessibility), cellular uptake of the bioactive form (bioavailability) and bio-transformation of phytochemicals are month the reasons for the lag of achievement in therapeutic interventions (Nijveldt et al. 2001). There is a need to analyse the long-term consequences of chronic flavonoid ingestion and more data should be collected on absorption and excretion, including stability. The *in vitro* and *in silico* studies have elucidated many significant pathways involved in the maintenance of physiological functions and homeostasis. Therefore, detailed *in vivo* and preclinical studies are expected to be performed in the coming years for the elucidation of the functional attribution of flavonoids in the improvement of human health conditions. Moreover, research gaps should be mitigated by exploring the interactions of flavonoids with receptor molecules at the time of acute and chronic diseases that may pave the path for the discovery of new flavonoids from nature's bounty so as to curtail the use of synthetic drugs. The use of certain strategies – (i) innovative processing techniques for abating bioavailability issues; (ii) explicit knowledge on wholesome and synergistic effects of mixed diets; (iii) understanding the constituents influencing influx and efflux by transporter systems or altering phase I/II metabolism; (iv) innovation of improved cell models of absorption and metabolism (mucus producing, liver cells, 3D models); and (v) knockout variants of certain transporters in animal models to study pathways of bioabsorption and bioactivity of metabolites (Bohn et al. 2015) – will aid our future with the possible novel, effective, affordable and easily accessible phyto-therapeutics for the improvement of the healthcare system. Therefore, a comprehensive analysis of these phytochemicals is the need of the hour.

ACKNOWLEDGEMENTS

This study was supported by research grants from the Department of Science and Technology (File no. SR/SO/HS-39/2009), Department of Biotechnology (File no. BT/PR12138/MED/30/1471/2014), Government of India and Uttarakhand State Council for Science and Technology (No. UCS&T/R&D/LS-10/11-12/4224), Government of Uttarakhand as funded projects to PR. The authors would like to thank Dr Sulakshana P. Mukherjee, Department of Biotechnology, Indian Institute of Technology, Roorkee, India, for critical review of the chapter, especially the NMR part.

REFERENCES

Abd El-kader, A. M., El-Readi, M. Z., Ahmed, A. S., Nafady, A. M., Wink, M. and Ibraheim, Z. Z. (2013). Polyphenols from aerial parts of *Polygonum bellardii* and their biological activities. *Pharmaceutical Biology*, 51(8), 1026–1034.

Agrawal, P. K., ed. (2013). *Carbon-13 NMR of Flavonoids*. Vol. 39. Amsterdam, the Netherlands, Elsevier.

Alam, M. M., Meerza, D. and Naseem, I. (2014). Protective effect of quercetin on hyperglycemia, oxidative stress and DNA damage in alloxan induced type 2 diabetic mice. *Life Sciences*, 109(1), 8–14.

Al-Awwadi, N., Azay, J., Poucheret, P., Cassanas, G., Krosniak, M., Auger, C., Gasc, F., Rouanet, J.-M., Cros, G., and Teissèdre, P.-L. (2004). Antidiabetic activity of red wine polyphenolic extract, ethanol, or both in streptozotocin-treated rats. *Journal of Agricultural and Food Chemistry*, 52(4), 1008–1016.

Alkhalidy, H., Moore, W., Zhang, Y., McMillan, R., Wang, A., Ali, M., Suh, J.-S., et al. (2015). Small molecule kaempferol promotes insulin sensitivity and preserved pancreatic β-cell mass in middle-aged obese diabetic mice. *Journal of Diabetes Research*, 2015, 532984.

Al-Numair, K. S., Chandramohan, G., Veeramani, C., and Alsaif, M. A. (2015). Ameliorative effect of kaempferol, a flavonoid, on oxidative stress in streptozotocin-induced diabetic rats. *Redox Report*, 20(5), 198–209.

American Diabetes Association. (2009). Standards of medical care in diabetes—2009. *Diabetes Care*, 32(Suppl 1), S13.

American Diabetes Association. (2014). Diagnosis and classification of diabetes mellitus. *Diabetes Care*, 37(1), S81–S90.

Amiot, M. J., Riva, C. and Vinet, A. (2016). Effects of dietary polyphenols on metabolic syndrome features in humans: A systematic review. *Obesity Reviews*, 17(7), 573–586.

Andersen, Ø. M. and Fossen, T. (2003). Characterization of anthocyanins by NMR. *Current Protocols in Food Analytical Chemistry*, **9**(1), F1.4.1–F1.4.23.

Androutsopoulos, V. P., Papakyriakou, A., Vourloumis, D., Tsatsakis, A. M. and Spandidos, D. M. (2010). Dietary flavonoids in cancer therapy and prevention: Substrates and inhibitors of cytochrome P450 CYP1 enzymes. *Pharmacology & Therapeutics*, **126**(1), 9–20.

Arai, Yi, Watanabe, S., Kimira, M., Shimoi, K., Mochizuki, R., and Kinae, N. (2000). Dietary intakes of flavonols, flavones and isoflavones by Japanese women and the inverse correlation between quercetin intake and plasma LDL cholesterol concentration. *Journal of Nutrition*, **130**(9), 2243–2250.

Aronoff, S. L., Berkowitz, K., Shreiner, B. and Want, L. (2004). Glucose metabolism and regulation: Beyond insulin and glucagon. *Diabetes Spectrum*, **17**(3), 183–190.

Artali, R., Barili, P. L., Bombieri, G., Da Re, P., Marchini, N., Meneghetti, F., and Valenti, P. (2003). Synthesis, X-ray crystal structure and biological properties of acetylenic flavone derivatives. *Il Farmaco*, **58**(9), 875–881.

Arulmozhiraja, S., Matsuo, N., Ishitsubo, E., Okazaki, S., Shimano, H. and Tokiwa, H. (2016). Comparative binding analysis of dipeptidyl peptidase IV (DPP-4) with antidiabetic drugs–an Ab initio fragment molecular orbital study. *PLoS One*, **11**(11), e0166275.

Balci, M. (2005). *Basic 1H-and 13C-NMR spectroscopy*. Amsterdam, the Netherlands: Elsevier.

Bao, L., Liu, F., Guo, H.-B., Li, Y., Tan, B.-B., Zhang, W.-X. and Peng, Y.-H. (2016). Naringenin inhibits proliferation, migration, and invasion as well as induces apoptosis of gastric cancer SGC7901 cell line by downregulation of AKT pathway. *Tumor Biology*, **37**(8), 11365–11374.

Barcellona, M. L., Cardiel, G. and Gratton, E. (1990). Time-resolved fluorescence of DAPI in solution and bound to polydeoxynucleotides. *Biochemical and Biophysical Research Communications*, **170**(1), 270–280.

Barry, K. M., Davies, N. W. and Mohammed, C. L. (2002). Effect of season and different fungi on phenolics in response to xylem wounding and inoculation in *Eucalyptus nitens*. *Forest Pathology*, **32**(3), 163–178.

Basli, A., Soulet, S., Chaher, N., Mérillon, J.-M., Chibane, M., Monti, J.-P. and Richard, T. (2012). Wine polyphenols: Potential agents in neuroprotection. *Oxidative Medicine and Cellular Longevity*, **2012**, 805762.

Berger, S. and Braun, S. (2004). *200 and More NMR Experiments: A Practical Course*. Weinheim, Germany: Wiley-VCH.

Berova, N., Nakanishi, K. and Woody, R., eds. (2000). *Circular Dichroism: Principles and Applications*. New York: John Wiley & Sons.

Block, G., Patterson, B. and Subar, A. (1992). Fruit, vegetables, and cancer prevention: A review of the epidemiological evidence. *Nutrition and Cancer*, **18**(1), 1–29.

Bohn, T., McDougall, G. J., Alegría, A., Alminger, M., Arrigoni, E., Aura, A.-M., Brito, C., et al. (2015). Mind the gap—Deficits in our knowledge of aspects impacting the bioavailability of phytochemicals and their metabolites—A position paper focusing on carotenoids and polyphenols. *Molecular Nutrition & Food Research*, **59**(7), 1307–1323.

Boucher, J., Kleinridders, A. and Kahn, C. R. (2014). Insulin receptor signaling in normal and insulin-resistant states. *Cold Spring Harbor Perspectives in Biology*, **6**(1), a009191.

Brayer, G.D., Williams, L. K., Tarling, C. A., Woods, K., Li, C., Zhang, R., Mahpour, A. A., Andersen, R. J. and Withers, S. G. (2010). The search for human alpha-amylase inhibitors as therapeutics for diabetes and obesity. *The FASEB Journal*, **24**(1), 681–684.

Briggs, L. H. and Colebrook, L. D. (1962). Infra-red spectra of flavanones and flavones: Carbonyl and hydroxyl stretching and CH out-of-plane bending absorption. *Spectrochimica Acta*, **18**(7), 939–957.

Bruch, M. (1996). *NMR Spectroscopy Techniques*. Boca Raton, FL: CRC Press.

Buer, C. S., Imin, N. and. Djordjevic, M. A. (2010). Flavonoids: New roles for old molecules. *Journal of Integrative Plant Biology*, **52**(1), 98–111.

Buolamwini, J. K. (2000). Cell cycle molecular targets in novel anticancer drug discovery. *Current Pharmaceutical Design*, **6**(4), 379–392.

Butler, M. S. (2008). Natural products to drugs: Natural product-derived compounds in clinical trials. *Natural Product Reports*, **25**(3), 475–516.

Cai, E. P. and Lin, J.-K. (2009). Epigallocatechin gallate (EGCG) and rutin suppress the glucotoxicity through activating IRS2 and AMPK signaling in rat pancreatic β cells. *Journal of Agricultural and Food Chemistry*, **57**(20), 9817–9827.

Calderón-Montaño, J. M., Burgos-Morón, E., Pérez-Guerrero, C. and López-Lázaro, M. (2011). A review on the dietary flavonoid kaempferol. *Mini Reviews in Medicinal Chemistry*, **11**(4), 298–344.

Caltagirone, S., Rossi, C., Poggi, A., Ranelletti, F. O., Natali, P. G., Brunetti, M., Aiello, F. B. and Piantelli, M. (2000). Flavonoids apigenin and quercetin inhibit melanoma growth and metastatic potential. *International Journal of Cancer*, **87**(4), 595–600.

Canales, M., Hernández, T., Caballero, J., Romo De Vivar, A., Avila, G., Duran, A. and Lira, R. (2005). Informant consensus factor and antibacterial activity of the medicinal plants used by the people of San Rafael Coxcatlán, Puebla, México. *Journal of Ethnopharmacology*, **97**(3), 429–439.

Cao, H., Jing, X., Wu, D. and Shi, Y. (2013). Methylation of genistein and kaempferol improves their affinities for proteins. *International Journal of Food Sciences and Nutrition*, **64**(4), 437–443.

Cao, H.-H., Cheng, C.-Y., Su, T., Fu, X.-Q., Guo, H., Li, T., Tse, A. K.-W., Kwan, H.-Y., Yu, H.and Yu, Z-L. (2015). Quercetin inhibits HGF/c-Met signaling and HGF-stimulated melanoma cell migration and invasion. *Molecular Cancer*, **14**(1), 103.

Cao, H.-H., Chu, J.-H., Kwan, H.-Y., Su, T., Yu, H., Cheng, C.-Y., Fu, X.-Q. et al. (2016). Inhibition of the STAT3 signaling pathway contributes to apigenin-mediated anti-metastatic effect in melanoma. *Scientific Reports*, **6**, 21731.

Cerf, M. E. (2013). Beta cell dysfunction and insulin resistance. *Frontiers in Endocrinology*, **4**, 37.

Chala, T. S. and Ali, G. Y. (2016). Recent advance in diabetes therapy: Pancreatic beta cell regeneration approaches. *Diabetes Management*, **6**(6), 108–118.

Chandrika, B. B., Steephan, M., Santhosh Kumar, T. R. S., Sabu, A. and Haridas, M. (2016). Hesperetin and naringenin sensitize HER2 positive cancer cells to death by serving as HER2 tyrosine kinase inhibitors. *Life Sciences*, **160**, 47–56.

Chang L., Chiang S-H. and Saltiel A.R. (2004). Insulin signaling and the regulation of glucose transport. *Molecular Medicine*, **10**(7–12), 65–71.

Chang, J.-H., Lai, S.-L., Chen, W.-S., Hung, W.-Y., Chow, J.-M., Hsiao, M., Lee, W.-J. and Chien, M.-H. (2017). Quercetin suppresses the metastatic ability of lung cancer through inhibiting Snail-dependent Akt activation and Snail-independent ADAM9 expression pathways. *Biochimica et Biophysica Acta (BBA)-Molecular Cell Research*, **1864**(10), 1746–1758.

Chattopadhyay, R. R. and Bandyopadhyay, M. (2005). Possible mechanism of hepatoprotective activity of *Azadirachta indica* leaf extract against paracetamol-induced hepatic damage in rats: Part III. *Indian Journal of Pharmacology*, **37**(3), 184.

Chaudhury, A., Duvoor, C., Dendi, V. S. R., Kraleti, S., Chada, A., Ravilla, R., Marco, A., et al. (2017). Clinical review of antidiabetic drugs: Implications for type 2 diabetes mellitus management. *Frontiers in Endocrinology*, **8**, 6.

Chen, J., Duan, Y., Zhang, X., Ye, Y., Ge, B. and Chen, J. (2015). Genistein induces apoptosis by the inactivation of the IGF-1R/p-Akt signaling pathway in MCF-7 human breast cancer cells. *Food & Function*, **6**(3), 995–1000.

Chen, J., Mangelinckx, S., Adams, A., Wang, Z. T., Li, W. L. and De Kimpe, N. (2015). Natural flavonoids as potential herbal medication for the treatment of diabetes mellitus and its complications. *Natural Product Communications*, **10**(1), 187–200.

Chen, L.-J., Games, D. E., Jones, J. and Kidwell, H. (2003). Separation and identification of flavonoids in an extract from the seeds of *Oroxylum indicum* by CCC. *Journal of Liquid Chromatography & Related Technologies*, **26**(9–10), 1623–1636.

Chen, R. M., Hu, L. H., An, T. Y., Li, J. and Shen, Q. (2002). Natural PTP1B inhibitors from *Broussonetia papyrifera*. *Bioorganic & Medicinal Chemistry Letters*, **12**(23), 3387–3390.

Cheng, A. Y. Y. and Fantus, I. G. (2005). Oral antihyperglycemic therapy for type 2 diabetes mellitus. *Canadian Medical Association Journal*, **172**(2), 213–226.

Cheung-Ong, K., Giaever, G. and Nislow, C. (2013). DNA-damaging agents in cancer chemotherapy: Serendipity and chemical biology. *Chemistry & Biology*, **20**(5), 648–659.

Chien, C.-S., Shen, K.-H., Huang, J.-S., Ko, S.-C. and Shih, Y.-W. (2010). Antimetastatic potential of fisetin involves inactivation of the PI3K/Akt and JNK signaling pathways with downregulation of MMP-2/9 expressions in prostate cancer PC-3 cells. *Molecular and Cellular Biochemistry*, **333**(1–2), 169.

Choi, H.-N., Kang, M.-J., and Kim, J.-I. (2013). Antioxidant effect of myricetin in animal model of type 2 diabetes. *The FASEB Journal*, **27**(1), 855–854.

Choi, H.-N., Kang, M.-J., Lee, S.-J. and Kim, J.-I. (2014). Ameliorative effect of myricetin on insulin resistance in mice fed a high-fat, high-sucrose diet. *Nutrition Research and Practice*, **8**(5), 544–549.

Choi, J. H., Banks, A. S., Estall, J. L., Kajimura, S., PBoström, P., Laznik, D., Ruas, J. L., et al. (2010). Anti-diabetic drugs inhibit obesity-linked phosphorylation of PPAR [ggr] by Cdk5. *Nature*, **466**(7305), 451–456.

Collins, A. R. (1999). Single cell gel electrophoresis: Detection of DNA damage at different levels of sensitivity. *Electrophoresis*, **20**, 2133–2138.

Collins, A. R., Dobson, V. L., Dušinská, M., Kennedy, G. and Štětina, R. (1997). The comet assay: What can it really tell us?. *Mutation Research/Fundamental and Molecular Mechanisms of Mutagenesis*, **375**(2), 183–193.

Cook, P. R., Brazell, I. A. and Jost, E. (1976). Characterization of nuclear structures containing superhelical DNA. *Journal of Cell Science*, **22**(2), 303–324.

Cornard, J. P. and Merlin, J. C. (1999). Structural and spectroscopic investigation of 2′-methoxyflavone. *Asian Journal of Spectroscopy*, **3**(3), 97–104.

Cornard, J. P. and Merlin, J. C. (2001). Structural and spectroscopic investigation of 5-hydroxyflavone and its complex with aluminium. *Journal of Molecular Structure*, **569**(1), 129–138.

Cornard, J. P., Barbillat, J. and Merlin, J. C. (1994). Performance of a versatile multichannel microprobein Raman, fluorescence, and absorption measurements. *Microbeam Analysis*, **3**, 13.

Cornard, J. P., Merlin, J. C., Boudet, A. C. and Vrielynck, L. (1997). Structural study of quercetin by vibrational and electronic spectroscopies combined with semiempirical calculations. *Biospectroscopy*, **3**(3), 183–193.

Cornard, J. P., Vrielynck, L., Merlin, J. C. and Wallet, J. C. (1995). Structural and vibrational study of 3-hydroxyflavone and 3-methoxyflavone. *Spectrochimica Acta Part A: Molecular and Biomolecular Spectroscopy*, **51**(5), 913–923.

Cotelle, N., Vrielynck, L., Nowogrocki, G., Cotelle, P. and Vezin, H. (2004). Synthesis, X-ray structure and spectroscopic and electronic properties of two new synthesized flavones. *Journal of Physical Organic Chemistry*, **17**(3), 226–232.

Crozier, A., Lean, M. E. J., McDonald, M. S. and Black, C. (1997). Quantitative analysis of the flavonoid content of commercial tomatoes, onions, lettuce, and celery. *Journal of Agricultural and Food Chemistry*, **45**(3) 590–595.

Curin, Y., and Andriantsitohaina, R. (2005). Polyphenols as potential therapeutical agents against cardiovascular diseases. *Pharmacological Reports*, **57**, 97.

Cushnie, T. P. and Lamb, A. J. (2005). Antimicrobial activity of flavonoids. *International Journal of Antimicrobial Agents*, **26**(5), 343–356.

Cushnie, T. P. and Lamb, A. J. (2011). Recent advances in understanding the antibacterial properties of flavonoids. *International Journal of Antimicrobial Agents*.**38**(2), 99–107.

Dai, J., Van Wie, P. G., Fai, L. Y., Kim, D., Wang, L., Poyil, P., Luo, J. and Zhang, Z. (2016). Downregulation of NEDD9 by apigenin suppresses migration, invasion, and metastasis of colorectal cancer cells. *Toxicology and Applied Pharmacology*, **311**, 106–112.

Dai, W., Wang, F., He, L., Lin, C., Wu, S., Chen, P., Zhang, Y., et al. (2015). Genistein inhibits hepatocellular carcinoma cell migration by reversing the epithelial–mesenchymal transition: Partial mediation by the transcription factor NFAT1. *Molecular Carcinogenesis*, **54**(4), 301–311.

Dai, X., Ding, Y., Zhang, Z., Cai, X. and Li, Y. (2013). Quercetin and quercitrin protect against cytokine-induced injuries in RINm5F β-cells via the mitochondrial pathway and NF-κB signaling. *International Journal of Molecular Medicine*, **31**(1), 265–271.

Daisy, P., Balasubramanian K., Rajalakshmi M., Eliza J. and Selvaraj J. (2010). Insulin mimetic impact of Catechin isolated from *Cassia fistula* on the glucose oxidation and molecular mechanisms of glucose uptake on Streptozotocin-induced diabetic Wistar rats. *Phytomedicine*, **17**(1), 28–36.

Datta, B. K., Datta, S. K., Rashid, M. A., Nash, R. J. and Sarker, S. D. (2000). A sesquiterpene acid and flavonoids from *Polygonum viscosum*. *Phytochemistry*, **54**(2), 201–205.

Davies, K. M. and Schwinn, K. E. (2006). Molecular biology and biotechnology of flavonoid biosynthesis. In Ø. M. Andersen and K. R. Markham, eds., *Flavonoids: Chemistry, Biochemistry and Applications*. Boca Raton, FL: CRC Press. pp. 143–218.

de Sousa, E., Zanatta, L. Seifriz, I., Creczynski-Pasa, T. B., Pizzolatti, M. G., Szpoganicz, B. and Silva, F. R. (2004). Hypoglycemic effect and antioxidant potential of kaempferol-3, 7-O-(α)-dirhamnoside from *Bauhinia f orficata* leaves. *Journal of Natural Products*, **67**(5), 829–832.

Denizot, F. and Lang, R. (1986). Rapid colorimetric assay for cell growth and survival: Modifications to the tetrazolium dye procedure giving improved sensitivity and reliability. *Journal of Immunological Methods*, **89**(2), 271–277.

Dias, T. R., Alves, M. G., Casal, S., Oliveira, P. F., and Silva, B. M. (2017). Promising potential of dietary (Poly) phenolic compounds in the prevention and treatment of diabetes mellitus. *Current Medicinal Chemistry*, **24**(4), 334–354.

Dillard, C. J. and German, J. B. (2000). Phytochemicals: Nutraceuticals and human health. *Journal of the Science of Food and Agriculture*, **80**(12), 1744–1756.

Doke, S. K. and Dhawale, S. C. (2015). Alternatives to animal testing: A review. *Saudi Pharmaceutical Journal*, **23**(3), 223–229.

Drenth, J. (2007). *Principles of Protein X-Ray Crystallography*. New York: Springer Science & Business Media.

El-Kordy, E. A., and Alshahrani, A. M. (2015). Effect of genistein, a natural soy isoflavone, on pancreatic β-Cells of streptozotocin-induced diabetic rats: Histological and immunohistochemical study. *Journal of Microscopy and Ultrastructure*, **3**(3), 108–119.

Eriksson, S., Kim, S. K., Kubista, M. and Norden, B. (1993). Binding of 4′, 6-diamidino-2-phenylindole (DAPI) to AT regions of DNA: Evidence for an allosteric conformational change. *Biochemistry*, **32**(12), 2987–2998.

Fan, J., Johnson, M. H., Lila, M. A., Yousef, G., and Gonzalez de Mejia, E. (2013). Berry and citrus phenolic compounds inhibit dipeptidyl peptidase IV: Implications in diabetes management. *Evidence-Based Complementary and Alternative Medicine*, **2013**, 479505.

Fang, X.-K., Gao, J. and Zhu, D.-N. (2008). Kaempferol and quercetin isolated from *Euonymus alatus* improve glucose uptake of 3T3-L1 cells without adipogenesis activity. *Life Sciences*, **82**(11), 615–622.

Ferrari, M., Mottola, L. and Quaresima, V. (2004). Principles, techniques, and limitations of near infrared spectroscopy. *Canadian Journal of Applied Physiology*, **29**(4), 463–487.

Firdous, S. M. (2014). Phytochemicals for treatment of diabetes. *EXCLI Journal*, **13**, 451.

Firuzi, O., Lacanna, A., Petrucci, R., Marrosu, G. and Saso, L. (2005). Evaluation of the antioxidant activity of flavonoids by "ferric reducing antioxidant power" assay and cyclic voltammetry. *Biochimica et Biophysica Acta (BBA)-General Subjects*, **1721**(1), 174–184.

Forester, S. C., Gu, Y. and Lambert, J. D. (2012). Inhibition of starch digestion by the green tea polyphenol, (−)-epigallocatechin-3-gallate. *Molecular Nutrition & Food Research*, **56**(11), 1647–1654.

Fotsis, T., Pepper, M. S., Aktas, E., Breit, S., Rasku, S., Adlercreutz, H., Wähälä, K., Montesano, R. and Schweigerer, L. (1997). Flavonoids, dietary-derived inhibitors of cell proliferation and in vitro angiogenesis. *Cancer Research*, **57**(14), 2916–2921.

Fu, Y., Luo, J., Jia, Z., Zhen, W., Zhou, K., Gilbert, E. and Liu, D. (2014). Baicalein protects against type 2 diabetes via promoting islet β-cell function in obese diabetic mice. *International Journal of Endocrinology*, **2014**, 846742.

Fu, Z. and Liu, D. (2009). Long-term exposure to genistein improves insulin secretory function of pancreatic β-cells. *European Journal of Pharmacology*, **616**(1), 321–327.

Fu, Z., Gilbert, E. R. and Liu, D. (2013). Regulation of insulin synthesis and secretion and pancreatic Beta-cell dysfunction in diabetes. *Current Diabetes Reviews*, **9**(1), 25–53.

Fu, Z., Gilbert, E. R., Pfeiffer, L., Zhang, Y., Fu, Y. and Liu, D. (2012). Genistein ameliorates hyperglycemia in a mouse model of nongenetic type 2 diabetes. *Applied Physiology, Nutrition, and Metabolism*, **37**(3), 480–488.

Fu, Z., Zhang, W., Zhen, W., Lum, H., J Nadler, J., Bassaganya-Riera, J., Jia, Z., Wang, Y., Misra, H. and Liu, D. (2010). Genistein induces pancreatic β-cell proliferation through activation of multiple signaling pathways and prevents insulin-deficient diabetes in mice. *Endocrinology*, **151**(7), 3026–3037.

Gallet, C., Després, L. and Tollenaere, C. (2004). Phenolic response of *Trollius europaeus* to *Chiastocheta* invasion. *Polyphenol Communication*, **2004**, 759–760.

Gamet-Payrastre, L., Li, P., Lumeau, S., Cassar, G., Dupont, M.-A., Chevolleau, S., Nicole Gasc, Tulliez, J. and Tercé, F. (2000). Sulforaphane, a naturally occurring isothiocyanate, induces cell cycle arrest and apoptosis in HT29 human colon cancer cells. *Cancer Research*, **60**(5), 1426–1433.

Giusti, M. M., and Wrolstad, R. E. (2001). Characterization and measurement of anthocyanins by UV-visible spectroscopy. *Current Protocols in Food Analytical Chemistry*, **0**(1), F1.2.1–F1.2.13.

Giusti, M. M., Rodríguez-Saona, L. E. and Wrolstad, R. E. (1999). Molar absorptivity and color characteristics of acylated and non-acylated pelargonidin-based anthocyanins. *Journal of Agricultural and Food Chemistry*, **47**(11), 4631–4637.

Gomes, I. B. S., Porto, M. L., Santos, M., Campagnaro, B. P., Gava, A. L., Meyrelles, S. S., Pereira, T. M., and Vasquez, E. C. (2015). The protective effects of oral low-dose quercetin on diabetic nephropathy in hypercholesterolemic mice. *Frontiers in Physiology*, **6**, doi:10.3389/fphys.2015.00247.

González-Rodríguez, Á., Mas Gutierrez, J. A., Sanz-González, Manuel Ros, M., Burks, D. J. and Valverde, Á. M. (2010). Inhibition of PTP1B restores IRS1-mediated hepatic insulin signaling in IRS2-deficient mice. *Diabetes*, **59**(3), 588–599.

Gordon, M. H., and Roedig-Penman, A. (1998). Antioxidant activity of quercetin and myricetin in liposomes. *Chemistry and Physics of Lipids*, **97**(1), 79–85.

Griesbach, R. J. (2005). Biochemistry and genetics of flower color. *Plant Breeding Reviews*, **25**, 89–114.

Gross, M. (2004). Flavonoids and cardiovascular disease. *Pharmaceutical Biology*, **42**, 21–35.

Guardia, T., Rotelli, A. E., Juarez, A. O. and Pelzer, L. E. (2001). Anti-inflammatory properties of plant flavonoids. Effects of rutin, quercetin and hesperidin on adjuvant arthritis in rat. *Il Farmaco*, **56**(9), 683–687.

Gunstone, F. D., Harwood, J. L. and Dijkstra, A. J. (2007). *The Lipid Handbook with CD-ROM*. Boca Raton, FL: CRC Press.

Gupta, P., Bala, M., Gupta, S., Dua, A., Dabur, R., Injeti, E. and Mittal, A. (2016). Efficacy and risk profile of anti-diabetic therapies: Conventional versus traditional drugs—A mechanistic revisit to understand their mode of action. *Pharmacological Research*, **113**, 636–674.

Gupta, R. C., Chang, D., Nammi, S., Bensoussan, A., Bilinski, K. and Roufogalis, B. D. (2017). Interactions between antidiabetic drugs and herbs: An overview of mechanisms of action and clinical implications. *Diabetology & Metabolic Syndrome*, **9**(1), 59.

Gupta, V. (2013). Glucagon-like peptide-1 analogues: An overview. *Indian Journal of Endocrinology and Metabolism*, **17**(3), 413.

Habtemariam, S. (1997). Flavonoids as inhibitors or enhancers of the cytotoxicity of tumor necrosis factor-α in L-929 tumor cells. *Journal of Natural Products*, **60**(8), 775–778.

Hahn, E. L. and Maxwell, D. E. (1952). Spin echo measurements of nuclear spin coupling in molecules. *Physical Review*, **88**(5), 1070.

Harborne, A. J. (1998). *Phytochemical Methods a Guide to Modern Techniques of Plant Analysis*. New Delhi, India: Springer Science & Business Media.

Harborne, J. B. and Roberts, M. F. (1994). The flavonoids, advances in research since 1986. *Phytochemistry*, **37**(3), 913.

Havelka, A. M., Berndtsson, M., Olofsson, M. H., Shoshan, M. C. and Linder, S. (2007). Mechanisms of action of DNA-damaging anticancer drugs in treatment of carcinomas: Is acute apoptosis an off-target effect? *Mini Reviews in Medicinal Chemistry*, **7**(10), 1035–1039.

He, Y., X. Wu, Y. Cao, Y. Hou, H. Chen, L. Wu, L. Lu, W. Zhu, and Y. Gu. (2015). Daidzein exerts anti-tumor activity against bladder cancer cells via inhibition of FGFR3 pathway. *Neoplasma*, **63**(4), 523–531.

Hergert, H. L. (1956). The flavonoids of lodgepole pine bark. *The Journal of Organic Chemistry*, **21**(5), 534–537.

Hertog, M. G. L., Hollman, P. C. H. and Van de Putte, B. (1993). Content of potentially anticarcinogenic flavonoids of tea infusions, wines, and fruit juices. *Journal of Agricultural and Food Chemistry*, **41**(8), 1242–1246.

Hertog, M. G. L., Kromhout, D., Aravanis, C., Blackburn, H., Buzina, R., Fidanza, F., Giampaoli, S., et al. (1995). Flavonoid intake and long-term risk of coronary heart disease and cancer in the seven countries study. *Archives of Internal Medicine*, **155**(4), 381–386.

Hiermann, A., Schramm, H. W. and Laufer, S. (1998). Anti-inflammatory activity of myricetin-3-O-ß-D-glucuronide and related compounds. *Inflammation Research*, **47**(11), 421–427.

Higa, S., Hirano, T., Kotani, K., Matsumoto, M., Fujita, A., Suemura, M., Kawase, I. and Tanaka, T. (2003). Fisetin, a flavonol, inhibits T H 2-type cytokine production by activated human basophils. *Journal of Allergy and Clinical Immunology*, **111**(6), 1299–1306.

Huang, S. and Czech., M. P. (2007). The GLUT4 glucose transporter. *Cell Metabolism*, **5**(4), 237–252.

Huang, W.-W., Chiu, Y.-J., Fan, M.-J., Lu, H.-F., Yeh, H.-F., Li, K.-H., Chen, P.-Y., Chung, J.-G. and Yang, J.-S. (2010). Kaempferol induced apoptosis via endoplasmic reticulum stress and mitochondria-dependent pathway in human osteosarcoma U-2 OS cells. *Molecular Nutrition & Food Research*, **54**(11), 1585–1595.

Huang, X., Dai, S., Dai, J., Xiao, Y., Bai, Y., Chen, B. and Zhou, M. (2015). Luteolin decreases invasiveness, deactivates STAT3 signaling, and reverses interleukin-6 induced epithelial–mesenchymal transition and matrix metalloproteinase secretion of pancreatic cancer cells. *OncoTargets and Therapy*, **8**, 2989.

Hufford, C. D., Jia, Y., Croom, E. M. Jr., Muhammed, I., Okunade, A. L., Clark, A. M. and Rogers, R. D. (1993). Antimicrobial compounds from *Petalostemum purpureum*. *Journal of Natural Products*, **56**(11), 1878–1889.

Husain, S. R., Cillard, J. and Cillard, P. (1987). Hydroxyl radical scavenging activity of flavonoids. *Phytochemistry*, **26**(9), 2489–2491.

Jagan, M., Rao, L., Yada, H., Ono, H. and Yoshida, M. (2002). Acylated and non-acylated flavonol monoglycosides from the Indian minor spice nagkesar (*Mammea longifolia*). *Journal of Agricultural and Food Chemistry*, **50**(11), 3143–3153.

Jang, H.-J., Ridgeway, S. D. and Kim, J.-A. (2013). Effects of the green tea polyphenol epigallocatechin-3-gallate on high-fat diet-induced insulin resistance and endothelial dysfunction. *American Journal of Physiology-Endocrinology and Metabolism*, **305**(12), E1444–E1451.

Jeong, S.-M., Kang, M.-J., Choi, H.-N., Kim, J.-H. and Kim, J.-I. (2012). Quercetin ameliorates hyperglycemia and dyslipidemia and improves antioxidant status in type 2 diabetic db/db mice. *Nutrition Research and Practice*, **6**(3), 201–207.

Jiang, C.-S., Liang, L.-F. and Guo, Y.-W. (2012). Natural products possessing protein tyrosine phosphatase 1B (PTP1B) inhibitory activity found in the last decades. *Acta Pharmacologica Sinica*, **33**(10), 1217.

Jianhong, W. U., Shi Long, M. A. O., Shi Xuan, L. I. A. O., Yang Hua, Y. I., Chuan Qing, L. A. N. and Zhong Wu, S. U. (2001). Desmosdumotin B: A new special flavone from desmos dumosus. *Chinese Chemical Letters*, **12**(1), 49–50.

Jo, E., Park, S. J., Choi, Y. S., Jeon, W.-K. and Kim, B.-C. (2015). Kaempferol suppresses transforming growth factor-β1–induced epithelial-to-mesenchymal transition and migration of A549 lung cancer cells by inhibiting Akt1-mediated phosphorylation of Smad3 at threonine-179. *Neoplasia*, **17**(7), 525–537.

Jones, J. R., Lebar, M. D., Jinwal, U. K., Abisambra, J. F., Koren, J. III, Blair, L.,,. O'Leary, J. C., et al. (2010). The diarylheptanoid (+)-a R, 11 S-myricanol and two flavones from bayberry (Myrica cerifera) destabilize the microtubule-associated protein Tau. *Journal of Natural Products*, **74**(1), 38–44.

Juillerat-Jeanneret, L. (2013). Dipeptidyl peptidase IV and its inhibitors: Therapeutics for type 2 diabetes and what else?. *Journal of Medicinal Chemistry*, **57**(6), 2197–2212.

Jung, U. J., Lee, M.-K., Jeong, K.-S. and Choi, M.-S. (2004). The hypoglycemic effects of hesperidin and naringin are partly mediated by hepatic glucose-regulating enzymes in C57BL/KsJ-db/db mice. *Journal of Nutrition*, **134**(10), 2499–2503.

Kalra, S., Baruah, M. P., Sahay, R. K., Unnikrishnan, A. G., Uppal, S. and Adetunji, O. (2016). Glucagon-like peptide-1 receptor agonists in the treatment of type 2 diabetes: Past, present, and future. *Indian Journal of Endocrinology and Metabolism*, **20**(2), 254.

Kamusiime, H., Pedersen, A. T., Andersen, Ø. M. and Kiremire, B. (1996). Kaempferol 3-O-(2-O-ß-D-glucopyranosyl-6-OaL-rhamnopyranosyl-ß-D-glucopyranoside) from the African plant *Erythrina abyssinica*. *International Journal of Pharmacognosy*, **34**(5), 370–373.

Kandasamy N. and Ashokkumar N. (2014). Protective effect of bioflavonoid myricetin enhances carbohydrate metabolic enzymes and insulin signaling molecules in streptozotocin–cadmium induced diabetic nephrotoxic rats. *Toxicology and Applied Pharmacology*, **279**(2), 173–185.

Kang, J. W, Kim, J. H., Song, K., Kim, S. H., Yoon, J.-H. and Kim, K.-S. (2010). Kaempferol and quercetin, components of *Ginkgo biloba* extract (EGb 761), induce caspase-3-dependent apoptosis in oral cavity cancer cells. *Phytotherapy Research*, **24**(S1).

Kang, S.-J., Yoon Park, J.-H., Choi, H.-N. and Kim, J.-I. (2015). α-Glucosidase inhibitory activities of myricetin in animal models of diabetes mellitus. *Food Science and Biotechnology*, **24**(5), 1897–1900.

Karthikeyan, M. (2016). *In-vivo* animal models and *in-vitro* techniques for screening antidiabetic activity. *Journal of Developing Drugs*, **5**, 153.

Kawanishi, S. and Hiraku, Y. (2004). Amplification of anticancer drug-induced DNA damage and apoptosis by DNA-binding compounds. *Current Medicinal Chemistry—Anti-Cancer Agents*, **4**(5), 415–419.

Kemp, W. (1991). Organic spectroscopy. *Molecules*, **7**(1), 11.

Kessler, H., Griesinger, C., Lautz, J., Mueller, A., Van Gunsteren, W. F. and Berendsen, H. J. C. (1988). Conformational dynamics detected by nuclear magnetic resonance NOE values and J coupling constants. *Journal of the American Chemical Society*, **110**(11), 3393–3396.

Keys, A., Aravanis, C., Blackburn, H. W., Van Buchem, F. S., Buzina, R., Djordjevic, B. D., Dontas, A. S. et al. (1966). *Epidemiological Studies Related to Coronary Heart Disease: Characteristics of Men Aged 40–59 in Seven Countries*. Tampere, Finland: Kirjapaino.

Kim, E.-K., Kwon, K.-B., Song, M.-Y., Seo, S.-W., Park, S.- J., Ka, S.-O., Na, L. et al. (2007). Genistein protects pancreatic β cells against cytokine-mediated toxicity. *Molecular and Cellular Endocrinology*, **278**(1), 18–28.

Kim, J.-S., Kwon, C.-S. and Son, K. H. (2000). Inhibition of alpha-glucosidase and amylase by luteolin, a flavonoid. *Bioscience, Biotechnology, and Biochemistry*, **64**(11), 2458–2461.

Kim, M. E., Ha, T. K., Yoon, J. H. and Lee, J. S. (2014). Myricetin induces cell death of human colon cancer cells via BAX/BCL2-dependent pathway. *Anticancer Research*, **34**(2), 701–706.

Kim, M. H. (2003). Flavonoids inhibit VEGF/bFGF-induced angiogenesis *in vitro* by inhibiting the matrix-degrading proteases. *Journal of Cellular Biochemistry*, **89**(3), 529–538.

Kim, M. J. and Lim, Y. (2013). Protective effect of short-term genistein supplementation on the early stage in diabetes-induced renal damage. *Mediators of Inflammation*, **2013**, 510212.

Kim, S.-H., and Choi, K.-C. (2013). Anti-cancer effect and underlying mechanism(s) of kaempferol, a phytoestrogen, on the regulation of apoptosis in diverse cancer cell models. *Toxicological Research*, 29(4), 229.

Kim, Y., Keogh, J. B. and Clifton, P. M. (2016). Polyphenols and glycemic control. *Nutrients*, 8(1), 17.

Klaude, M., Eriksson, S., Nygren, J. and Ahnström, G. (1996). The comet assay: Mechanisms and technical considerations. *Mutation Research/DNA Repair*, 363(2), 89–96.

Koehn, F. E. and Carter, G. T. (2005). The evolving role of natural products in drug discovery. *Nature Reviews: Drug Discovery*, 4(3), 206.

Koleckar, V., Kubikova, K., Rehakova, Z., Kuca, K., Jun, D., Jahodar, L. and Opletal, L. (2008). Condensed and hydrolysable tannins as antioxidants influencing the health. *Mini Reviews in Medicinal Chemistry*, 8(5), 436–447.

Kong, L., Luo, C., Li, X., Zhou, Y. and He, H. (2013). The anti-inflammatory effect of kaempferol on early atherosclerosis in high cholesterol fed rabbits. *Lipids in Health and Disease*, 12(1), 115.

Labriola, L., Peters, M. G., Krogh, K., Stigliano, I., Terra, L. F., Buchanan, C., Machado, M. Cc., Joffé, E., Puricelli, L. and Sogayar, M. C. (2009). Generation and characterization of human insulin-releasing cell lines. *BMC Cell Biology*, 10(1), 49.

Ladd, M. F. C. and Palmer, R. A. (1985). *Structure Determination by X-ray Crystallography*. New York: Plenum Press.

Lall, R. K., Syed, D. N., Adhami, V. M., Khan, M. I. and Mukhtar, H. (2015). Dietary polyphenols in prevention and treatment of prostate cancer. *International Journal of Molecular Sciences*, 16(2), 3350–3376.

Larsen, T. M., Toubro, S., and Astrup, A. (2003). PPARgamma agonists in the treatment of type II diabetes: Is increased fatness commensurate with long-term efficacy? *International Journal of Obesity*, 27(2), 147.

Larson, R. A. (1988). The antioxidants of higher plants. *Phytochemistry*, 27(4), 969–978.

Larsson, S. (2009). Phytochemicals: Aging and health. *Annals of Botany*, 104(7), ix.

Lau-Cam, C. A. and Chan, H. H. (1973). Flavonoids from *Comptonia peregrina*. *Phytochemistry*, 12(7), 1829.

Lee, K.-H. (2004). Current developments in the discovery and design of new drug candidates from plant natural product leads. *Journal of Natural Products*, 67(2), 273–283.

Lee, M. S., Kim, C. H., Hoang, D. M., Kim, B. Y., Sohn, C. B., Kim, M. R. and Ahn, J. S. (2009). Genistein-derivatives from *Tetracera scandens* stimulate glucose-uptake in L6 myotubes. *Biological and Pharmaceutical Bulletin*, 32(3), 504–508.

Lee, M. T., Lin, W. C., Yu, B. and Lee, T. T. (2017). Antioxidant capacity of phytochemicals and their potential effects on oxidative status in animals—A review. *Asian-Australasian Journal of Animal Sciences*, 30(3), 299.

Lee, W.-J., Hsiao, M., Chang, J.-L., Yang, S.-F., Tseng, T.-H., Cheng, C.-W., Chow, J.-M., et al. (2015). Quercetin induces mitochondrial-derived apoptosis via reactive oxygen species-mediated ERK activation in HL-60 leukemia cells and xenograft. *Archives of Toxicology*, 89(7), 1103–1117.

Li, J.-M., Wang, W., Fan, C.-Y., Wang, M.-X., Zhang, X., Hu, Q.-H. and Kong, L.-D. (2013). Quercetin preserves β-cell mass and function in fructose-induced hyperinsulinemia through modulating pancreatic Akt/FoxO1 activation. *Evidence-Based Complementary and Alternative Medicine*, 2013, 303902.

Li, S., Li, W., Wang, Y., Asada, Y. and Koike, K. (2010). Prenylflavonoids from *Glycyrrhiza uralensis* and their protein tyrosine phosphatase-1B inhibitory activities. *Bioorganic & Medicinal Chemistry Letters*, 20(18), 5398–5401.

Li, W., Guo, Y., Zhang, C., Wu, R., Yang, A. Y., Gaspar, J. and Kong, A. T. (2016). Dietary phytochemicals and cancer chemoprevention: A perspective on oxidative stress, inflammation, and epigenetics. *Chemical Research in Toxicology*, 29(12), 2071–2095.

Li, Y. Q., Zhou, F. C., Gao, F., Bian, J. S. and Shan, F. (2009). Comparative evaluation of quercetin, isoquercetin and rutin as inhibitors of α-glucosidase. *Journal of Agricultural and Food Chemistry*, 57(24), 11463–11468.

Li, Y., Zheng, X., Yi, X., Liu, C., Kong, D., Zhang, J. and Gong, M. (2017). Myricetin: A potent approach for the treatment of type 2 diabetes as a natural class B GPCR agonist. *The FASEB Journal*, 31(6), 2603–2611

Liao, W., Nguyen, M. T. A., Yoshizaki, T., Favelyukis, S., David Patsouris, D., Imamura, T., Verma, I. M. and Olefsky, J. M. (2007). Suppression of PPAR-γ attenuates insulin-stimulated glucose uptake by affecting both GLUT1 and GLUT4 in 3T3-L1 adipocytes. *American Journal of Physiology-Endocrinology and Metabolism*, 293(1), E219–E227.

Lim, W., Park, S., Bazer, F. W. and Song, G. (2016). Apigenin reduces survival of choriocarcinoma cells by inducing apoptosis via the PI3K/AKT and ERK1/2 MAPK pathways. *Journal of Cellular Physiology*, 231(12), 2690–2699.

Lipkin, M., Uehara, K., Winawer, S., Sanchez, A., Bauer, C., Phillips, R., Lynch, H. T., Blattner, W. A. and Fraumeni, J. F. (1985). Seventh-Day Adventist vegetarians have a quiescent proliferative activity in colonic mucosa. *Cancer Letters*, **26**(2), 139–144.

Liu, C. and Wu, H. (2014). From beta cell replacement to beta cell regeneration: Implications for antidiabetic therapy. *Journal of Diabetes Science and Technology*, **8**(6), 1221–1226.

Liu, C.-Y., Huang, C.-J., Huang, L.-H., Chen, I.-J., Chiu, J.-P. and Hsu, C.-H. (2014). Effects of green tea extract on insulin resistance and glucagon-like peptide 1 in patients with type 2 diabetes and lipid abnormalities: a randomized, double-blinded, and placebo-controlled trial. *PLoS One*, **9**(3), e91163.

Liu, Y.-J., Zhan, J., Liu, X.-L., Wang, Y., Ji, J. and He, Q.-Q. (2014). Dietary flavonoids intake and risk of type 2 diabetes: A meta-analysis of prospective cohort studies. *Clinical Nutrition* 33(1), 59–63.

Lovshin, J. A. (2017). Glucagon-like peptide-1 receptor agonists: A class update for treating type 2 diabetes. *Canadian Journal of Diabetes*, **41**(5), 524–535.

Mabry, T. J., Markham, K. R. and Thomas, M. B. (1970). The ultraviolet spectra of flavones and flavonols. In *The Systematic Identification of Flavonoids*. Berlin, Germany: Springer. pp. 41–164.

Manach, C., Williamson, G., Morand, C., Scalbert, A. and Rémésy, C. (2005). Bioavailability and bioefficacy of polyphenols in humans. I. Review of 97 bioavailability studies. *The American Journal of Clinical Nutrition*, **81**(1), 230S–242S.

Markham, K. R. (1982). *Techniques of Flavonoid Identification*. Vol. 31. London, UK: Academic Press.

Markham, K. R. and Chari, V. M. (1982). Carbon-13 NMR spectroscopy of flavonoids. In: J. B. Harborne and T. J. Mabry, eds., *The Flavonoids*. Boston, MA: Springer. pp. 19–134.

Massiot, D., Fayon, F., Alonso, B., Trebosc, J. and Amoureux, J.-P. (2003). Chemical bonding differences evidenced from J-coupling in solid state NMR experiments involving quadrupolar nuclei. *Journal of Magnetic Resonance*, **164**(1), 160–164.

Matheeussen, V., Lambeir, A. M., Jungraithmayr, W., Gomez, N., Mc Entee, K., Van der Veken, P., Scharpé, S.,and De Meester, I. (2012). Method comparison of dipeptidyl peptidase IV activity assays and their application in biological samples containing reversible inhibitors. *Clinica Chimica Acta*, **413**(3), 456–462.

Mayr, C., Wagner, A., Neureiter, D., Pichler, M., Jakab, M., Illig, R., Berr, F. and Kiesslich, T. (2015). The green tea catechin epigallocatechin gallate induces cell cycle arrest and shows potential synergism with cisplatin in biliary tract cancer cells. *BMC Complementary and Alternative Medicine*, **15**(1), 194.

McDonald, M. S., Hughes, M., Burns, J., Lean, M. E. J. Matthews, D. and Crozier, A. (1998). Survey of the free and conjugated myricetin and quercetin content of red wines of different geographical origins. *Journal of Agricultural and Food Chemistry*, **46**(2), 368–375.

McGlynn, A. P., Wasson, G., O'Connor, J., McKelvey-Martin, V. J. and Downes, C. S. (1999). The bromodeoxyuridine comet assay. *Cancer Research*, **59**(23), 5912–5916.

Melo, M. J., Moura, S., Roque, A., Maestri, M. and Pina, F. (2000). Photochemistry of luteolinidin: "Write-lock-read-unlock-erase" with a natural compound. *Journal of Photochemistry and Photobiology A: Chemistry*, **135**(1), 33–39.

Middleton, E. (1998). Effect of plant flavonoids on immune and inflammatory cell function. In J. Manthey and B. Buslig, eds., *Flavonoids in the Living System*. Boston, MA: Springer. pp. 175–182.

Miller, G. L. (1959). Use of dinitrosalicylic acid reagent for determination of reducing sugar. *Analytical Chemistry*, **31**(3), 426–428.

Mirabella, F. M., ed. (1998). *Modern Techniques in Applied Molecular Spectroscopy*. Vol. 14. New York: John Wiley & Sons.

Miranda, C. L., Maier, C. S. and Stevens, J. F. (2001). *Flavonoids*. In eLS (Ed.). doi:10.1002/9780470015902. a0003068.pub2.

Mladinic, M., Zeljezic, D., Shaposhnikov, S. A. and Collins, A. R. (2012). The use of FISH-comet to detect c-Myc and TP 53 damage in extended-term lymphocyte cultures treated with terbuthylazine and carbofuran. *Toxicology Letters*, **211**(1), 62–69.

Moncada, M. C., Fernández, D., Lima, J. C., Parola, A. J., Lodeiro, C., Folgosa, F., Melo, M. J. and Pina, F. (2004). Multistate properties of 7-(*N*, *N*-diethylamino)-4′-hydroxyflavylium: An example of an unidirectional reaction cycle driven by pH. *Organic & Biomolecular Chemistry*, **2**(19), 2802–2808.

Moore, J. P., Westall, K. L., Ravenscroft, N., Farrant, J. M., Lindsey, G. G. and Brandt, W. F. (2005). The predominant polyphenol in the leaves of the resurrection plant Myrothamnus flabellifolius, 3, 4, 5 tri-O-galloylquinic acid, protects membranes against desiccation and free radical-induced oxidation. *Biochemical Journal*, **385**(1), 301–308.

Moore, W., Alkhalidy, H. Zhou, K. and Liu, D. (2017). Flavonol kaempferol improves glucose homeostasis via suppressing hepatic glucose production and enhancing insulin sensitivity in diabetic mice. *The FASEB Journal*, **31**(1), 646–652.

Morcombe, C. R. and Zilm, K. W. (2003). Chemical shift referencing in MAS solid state NMR. *Journal of Magnetic Resonance*, **162**(2), 479–486.

Morris, G. A. (1987). Book Review: Atta-Ur Rahman, A.U. *Nuclear Magnetic Resonance: Basic Principles.* Springer-Verlag, Berlin, Germany, 1986, 358 p. *Magnetic Resonance in Chemistry*, **25**(4), 375–375.

Moses, M. A., Henry, E. C., Ricke, W. A. and Gasiewicz, T. A. (2015). The heat shock protein 90 inhibitor, (–)-epigallocatechin gallate, has anticancer activity in a novel human prostate cancer progression model. *Cancer Prevention Research*, **8**(3), 249–257.

Mosmann, T. (1983). Rapid colorimetric assay for cellular growth and survival: Application to proliferation and cytotoxicity assays. *Journal of Immunological Methods*, **65**(1–2) 55–63.

Mukherjee, A. and Khuda-Bukhsh, A. R. (2015). Quercetin down-regulates IL-6/STAT-3 signals to induce mitochondrial-mediated apoptosis in a nonsmall-cell lung-cancer cell line, A549. *Journal of Pharmacopuncture*, **18**(1), 19.

Muldoon, M. F. and Kritchevsky, S. B. (1996). Flavonoids and heart disease. *British Medical Journal*, **312**(7029), 458.

Mullen, W., Edwards, C. A. and Crozier, A. (2006). Absorption, excretion and metabolite profiling of methyl-, glucuronyl-, glucosyl-and sulpho-conjugates of quercetin in human plasma and urine after ingestion of onions. *British Journal of Nutrition*, **96**(1), 107–116.

Munshi A., Hobbs M., Meyn R. E. (2005). Clonogenic cell survival assay. In R. D. Blumenthal, ed., *Chemosensitivity: Volume 1 In Vitro Assays*, 1st ed. New York: Humana Press. pp. 21–28.

Murphy, A., Peer, W. A. and Taiz, L. (2000). Regulation of auxin transport by aminopeptidases and endogenous flavonoids. *Planta*, **211**(3), 315–324.

Mylonis, I., Lakka, A., Tsakalof, A., and Simos, G. (2010). The dietary flavonoid kaempferol effectively inhibits HIF-1 activity and hepatoma cancer cell viability under hypoxic conditions. *Biochemical and Biophysical Research Communications*, **398**(1), 74–78.

Na, M.-K., Jang, J.-P., Njamen, D., Mbafor, J. T., Fomum, Z. T., Kim, B. Y., Oh, W. K. and Ahn, J. S. (2006). Protein tyrosine phosphatase-1B inhibitory activity of isoprenylated flavonoids isolated from erythrina mildbraedii. *Journal of Natural Products*, **69**(11), 1572–1576.

Nanditha, A., Ma, R. C. W., Ramachandran, A., Snehalatha, C., Chan, J. C. N., Chia, K. S., Shaw, J. E. and Zimmet, P. Z. (2016). Diabetes in Asia and the Pacific: Implications for the global epidemic. *Diabetes Care*, **39**(3), 472–485.

Ni, F., Gong, Y., Li, L., Abdolmaleky, H. M. and Zhou, J.-R. (2012). Flavonoid ampelopsin inhibits the growth and metastasis of prostate cancer *in vitro* and in mice. *PLoS One*, **7**(6), e38802.

Nijveldt, R. J., Van Nood, E. L. S., Van Hoorn, D. E., Boelens, P. G., Van Norren, K. and Van Leeuwen, P. A. (2001). Flavonoids: A review of probable mechanisms of action and potential applications. *The American Journal of Clinical Nutrition*, **74**(4), 418–425.

Oboh, G., Ademosun, A. O., Ayeni, P. O.,. Omojokun, O. S. and Bello, F. (2015). Comparative effect of quercetin and rutin on α-amylase, α-glucosidase, and some pro-oxidant-induced lipid peroxidation in rat pancreas. *Comparative Clinical Pathology*, **24**(5), 1103–1110.

Oh, Y. S. (2015). Plant-derived compounds targeting pancreatic beta cells for the treatment of diabetes. *Evidence-Based Complementary and Alternative Medicine*, **2015**, 629863.

Olive, P. L., Banáth, J. P. and Durand, R. E. (1990). Heterogeneity in radiation-induced DNA damage and repair in tumor and normal cells measured using the comet assay. *Radiation Research*, **122**(1), 86–94.

Ong, K. C. and Khoo, H.-E. (2000). Effects of myricetin on glycemia and glycogen metabolism in diabetic rats. *Life Sciences*, **67**(14), 1695–1705.

Ortsäter, H., Grankvist, N., Wolfram, S., Kuehn, N. and Sjöholm, Å. (2012). Diet supplementation with green tea extract epigallocatechin gallate prevents progression to glucose intolerance in db/db mice. *Nutrition & Metabolism*, **9**(1), 11.

Ostling, O. and Johanson, K. J. (1984). Microelectrophoretic study of radiation-induced DNA damages in individual mammalian cells. *Biochemical and Biophysical Research Communications*, **123**(1), 291–298.

Palit, S., Kar, S., Sharma, G. and Das, P. K. (2015). Hesperetin induces apoptosis in breast carcinoma by triggering accumulation of ROS and activation of ASK1/JNK pathway. *Journal of Cellular Physiology*, **230**(8), 1729–1739.

Pan, H.-C., Jiang, Q., Yu, Y., Mei, J.-P., Cui, Y.-K. and Zhao, W.-J. (2015). Quercetin promotes cell apoptosis and inhibits the expression of MMP-9 and fibronectin via the AKT and ERK signalling pathways in human glioma cells. *Neurochemistry International*, **80**, 60–71.

Park, E.-J. and Pezzuto, J. M. (2012). Flavonoids in cancer prevention. *Anti-Cancer Agents in Medicinal Chemistry (Formerly Current Medicinal Chemistry-Anti-Cancer Agents)*, **12**(8), 836–851.

Patel, D. K., Prasad, S. K., Kumar, R. and Hemalatha, S. (2012). An overview on antidiabetic medicinal plants having insulin mimetic property. *Asian Pacific Journal of Tropical Biomedicine*, **2**(4), 320–330.

Paterson, I. and Anderson, E. A. (2005). The renaissance of natural products as drug candidates. *Science*, **310**(5747), 451–453.

Paula, V. F., Barbosa, L., Errington, W., Howarth, O. W. and Cruz, M. P. (2002). Chemical constituents from bombacopsis glabra (Pasq.) A. Robyns: Complete ^{1}H and 13C NMR assignments and X-ray structure of 5-Hydroxy-3, 6, 7, 8, 4′-pentamethoxyflavone. *Journal of the Brazilian Chemical Society*, **13**(2), 276–280.

Peng, X., Zhang, G., Liao, Y. and Gong, D. (2016). Inhibitory kinetics and mechanism of kaempferol on α-glucosidase. *Food Chemistry*, **190**, 207–215.

Pérez-Cano, F. J. and Castell, M. (2016). Flavonoids, inflammation and immune system. *Nutrients*, **8**(10), 659.

Perkin, A. G., and Hummel, J. J. (1896). LXXVI.—The colouring principle contained in the bark of Myrica nagi. Part I. *Journal of the Chemical Society Transactions*, **69**, 1287–1294.

Pizzi, A. and Cameron, F. A. (1986). Flavonoid tannins—Structural wood components for drought-resistance mechanisms of plants. *Wood Science and Technology*, **20**(2), 119–124.

Pourcel, L., Routaboul, J.-M., Cheynier, V., Lepiniec, L. and Debeaujon, I. (2007). Flavonoid oxidation in plants: From biochemical properties to physiological functions. *Trends in Plant Science*, **12**(1), 29–36.

Pournourmohammadi. S., Grimaldi, M., Stridh, M. H., Lavallard, V., Waagepetersen, H. S., Wollheim, C. B. and Maechler, P. (2017). Epigallocatechin-3-gallate (EGCG) activates AMPK through the inhibition of glutamate dehydrogenase in muscle and pancreatic ß-cells: A potential beneficial effect in the pre-diabetic state? *The International Journal of Biochemistry & Cell Biology*, **88**, 220–225.

Prakash, O., Kumar, R., Srivastava, R., Tripathi, P. and Mishra, S. (2015). Plants explored with anti-diabetic properties: A review. *American Journal of Pharmacological Sciences*, **3**(3), 55–66.

Priscilla, D. H., Roy, D., Suresh, A., Kumar, V. and Thirumurugan, K. (2014). Naringenin inhibits α-glucosidase activity: A promising strategy for the regulation of postprandial hyperglycemia in high fat diet fed strep-tozotocin induced diabetic rats. *Chemico-Biological Interactions*, **210**, 77–85.

Procházková, D., Boušová, I. and Wilhelmová, N. (2011). Antioxidant and prooxidant properties of flavonoids. *Fitoterapia*, **82**(4), 513–523.

Pu, P., Gao, D.-M., Mohamed, S., Chen, J., Zhang, J., Zhou, X.-Y., Zhou, N.- J., JXie, J. and Jiang, H. (2012). Naringin ameliorates metabolic syndrome by activating AMP-activated protein kinase in mice fed a high-fat diet. *Archives of Biochemistry and Biophysics*, **518**(1), 61–70.

Qian, M. C., Fan, X. and Mahattanatawee, K., eds. (2011). *Volatile Sulfur Compounds in Food*. Washington, DC: American Chemical Society.

Ramos, S. (2007). Effects of dietary flavonoids on apoptotic pathways related to cancer chemoprevention. *Journal of Nutritional Biochemistry*, **18**(7), 427–442.

Ranganatha, N. and Kuppast, I. J. (2012). A review on alternatives to animal testing methods in drug develop-ment. *International Journal of Pharmacy and Pharmaceutical Sciences*, **4**(5), 28–32.

Rapp, A., Bock, C., Dittmar, H. and Greulich, K. O. (1999). COMET-FISH used to detect UV-A sensitive regions in the whole human genome and on chromosome 8. *Neoplasma*, **46**, 99–101.

Reed, M. J. and Scribner, K. A. (1999). *In-vivo* and *in-vitro* models of type 2 diabetes in pharmaceutical drug discovery. *Diabetes, Obesity and Metabolism*, **1**(2), 75–86.

Rho, H. S., Ghimeray, A. K., Yoo, D. S., Ahn, S. M., Kwon, S. S., Lee, K. H., Cho, D. H. and Cho, J. Y. (2011). Kaempferol and kaempferol rhamnosides with depigmenting and anti-inflammatory properties. *Molecules*, **16**(4), 3338–3344.

Rodriguez, E., Towers, G. H. N. and Mitchell, J. C. (1976). Biological activities of sesquiterpene lactones. *Phytochemistry*, **15**(11), 1573–1580.

Rogerio, A. P., Dora, C. L., Andrade, E. L., Chaves, J. S., Silva, L., Lemos-Senna, E. and Calixto, J. B. (2010). Anti-inflammatory effect of quercetin-loaded microemulsion in the airways allergic inflamma-tory model in mice. *Pharmacological Research*, **61**(4), 288–297.

Rogerio, A. P., Kanashiro, A., Fontanari, C., Da Silva, E. V. G., Lucisano-Valim, Y. M., Soares, E. G. and Faccioli, L. H. (2007). Anti-inflammatory activity of quercetin and isoquercitrin in experimental murine allergic asthma. *Inflammation Research*, **56**(10), 402–408.

Romeo, J. T., ed. (2012). *Phytochemicals in Human Health Protection, Nutrition, and Plant Defense.* Vol. 33. Pullman, WA: Springer Science & Business Media.

Roslan, J., Giribabu, N. Karim, K. and Salleh, N. (2017). Quercetin ameliorates oxidative stress, inflammation and apoptosis in the heart of streptozotocin-nicotinamide-induced adult male diabetic rats. *Biomedicine & Pharmacotherapy*, **86**, 570–582.

Ross, J. A., and Kasum, C. M. (2002). Dietary flavonoids: Bioavailability, metabolic effects, and safety. *Annual Review of Nutrition*, **22**(1), 19–34.

Rupasinghe, H. P., Ronalds, C. M., Rathgeber, B. and Robinson, R. A. (2010). Absorption and tissue distribution of dietary quercetin and quercetin glycosides of apple skin in broiler chickens. *Journal of the Science of Food and Agriculture*, **90**(7), 1172–1178.

Saito, K., Lee, S., Shiuchi, T., Toda, C., Kamijo, M., Inagaki-Ohara, K., Okamoto, S. and Yasuhiko Minokoshi, Y. (2011). An enzymatic photometric assay for 2-deoxyglucose uptake in insulin-responsive tissues and 3T3-L1 adipocytes. *Analytical Biochemistry*, **412**(1), 9–17.

Santos, S. J., Singh, N. P. and Natarajan, A. T. (1997). Fluorescence in situ Hybridization with Comets. *Experimental Cell Research*, **232**(2), 407–411.

Scalbert, A. and Williamson, G. (2000). Dietary intake and bioavailability of polyphenols. *Journal of Nutrition*, **130**(8), 2073S–2085S.

Selivanova, I. A., Tyukavkina, N. A., Kolesnik, Y. A., Nesterov, V. N., Kuleshova, L. N., Khutoryanskii, V. A., Bazhenov, B. N. and Saibotalov, M. Y. (1999). Study of the crystalline structure of dihydroquercetin. *Pharmaceutical Chemistry Journal*, **33**(4), 2.

Semaan, D. G., Igoli, J. O., Young, L., Marrero, E., Gray, A. I. and Rowan, E. G. (2017). In vitro anti-diabetic activity of flavonoids and pheophytins from *Allophylus cominia* Sw. on PTP1B, DPPIV, alpha-glucosidase and alpha-amylase enzymes. *Journal of Ethnopharmacology*, **203**, 39–46.

Shahat, A. A., Cos, P., Hermans, N., Apers, S., De Bruyne, T., Pieters, L., Vanden Berghe, D. and Vlietinck, A. J. (2003). Anticomplement and antioxidant activities of new acetylated flavonoid glycosides from Centaurium spicatum. *Planta Medica*, **69**(12), 1153–1156.

Sharma, B., Balomajumder, C. and Roy, P. (2008). Hypoglycemic and hypolipidemic effects of flavonoid rich extract from *Eugenia jambolana* seeds on streptozotocin induced diabetic rats. *Food and Chemical Toxicology*, **46**(7), 2376–2383.

Sharma, B., Salunke, R., Balomajumder, C., Daniel, S. and Roy, P. (2010). Anti-diabetic potential of alkaloid rich fraction from *Capparis decidua* on diabetic mice. *Journal of Ethnopharmacology*, **127**(2), 457–462.

Sharma, B., Salunke, R., Srivastava, S., Majumder, C. and Roy, P. (2009). Effects of guggulsterone isolated from *Commiphora mukul* in high fat diet induced diabetic rats. *Food and Chemical Toxicology*, **47**(10), 2631–2639.

Shen, Q., Li, X., Li, W. and Zhao, X. (2011). Enhanced intestinal absorption of daidzein by borneol/menthol eutectic mixture and microemulsion. *American Association of Pharmaceutical Scientists Technology*, **12**(4), 1044–1049.

Shi, M., Wang, F.-S., and Wu, Z.-Z. (2003). Synergetic anticancer effect of combined quercetin and recombinant adenoviral vector expressing human wild-type p53, GM-CSF and B7-1 genes on hepatocellular carcinoma cells *in vitro*. *World Journal of Gastroenterology*, **9**(1), 73.

Shorland, F. B. (2012). The comparative aspects of fatty acid occurrence and distribution. *Comparative Biochemistry*, **3**, 1.

Siesler, H. W., Ozaki, Y., Kawata, S. and Heise, H. M., eds. (2008). *Near-Infrared Spectroscopy: Principles, Instruments, Applications.* New York: John Wiley & Sons.

Silverstein, R. M., Webster, F. X., Kiemle, D. J. and Bryce, D. L. (2014). *Spectrometric Identification of Organic Compounds.* Hoboken, NJ: John Wiley & Sons.

Singh, N. P., McCoy, M. T., Tice, R. R. and Schneider, E. L. (1988). A simple technique for quantitation of low levels of DNA damage in individual cells. *Experimental Cell Research*, **175**(1), 184–191.

Siuda, J. F. and DeBernardis, J. F. (1973). Naturally occurring halogenated organic compounds. *Lloydia*, **36**(2), 107–143.

Skelin, M., Rupnik, M. and Cencic, A. (2010). Pancreatic beta cell lines and their applications in diabetes mellitus research. *ALTEX*, **27**(2), 105–113.

Slater, T. F., Sawyer, B. and Sträuli, U. (1963). Studies on succinate-tetrazolium reductase systems: III. Points of coupling of four different tetrazolium salts III. Points of coupling of four different tetrazolium salts. *Biochimica et Biophysica Acta*, **77**, 383–393.

Sloop, K. W., Willard, S. W., Brenner, M. B., Ficorilli, J., Valasek, K., Showalter, A. D., Farb, T. B., et al. (2010). Novel small molecule glucagon-like peptide-1 receptor agonist stimulates insulin secretion in rodents and from human islets. *Diabetes*, **59**(12), 3099–3107.

Somerset, S. M., and Johannot, L. (2008). Dietary flavonoid sources in Australian adults. *Nutrition and Cancer*, **60**(4), 442–449.

Song, H. M., Park, G. H., Eo, H. J., Lee, J. W., Kim, M. K., Lee, J. R., Lee, M. H., Koo, J. S. and Jeong, J. B. (2015). Anti-proliferative effect of naringenin through p38-dependent downregulation of cyclin D1 in human colorectal cancer cells. *Biomolecules & Therapeutics*, **23**(4), 339.

Sorenson, C. M., Barry, M. A. and Eastman, A. (1990). Analysis of events associated with cell cycle arrest at G2 phase and cell death induced by cisplatin. *Journal of the National Cancer Institute*, **82**(9), 749–755.

Srinivasan, A., Thangavel, C., Liu, Y., Shoyele, S., Den, R. B., Selvakumar, P., and Lakshmikuttyamma, A. (2016). Quercetin regulates β-catenin signaling and reduces the migration of triple negative breast cancer. *Molecular Carcinogenesis*, **55**(5), 743–756.

Stalin, A., Irudayaraj, S. S., Kumar, D. R., Balakrishna, K., Ignacimuthu, S., Al-Dhabi, N. A. and Veeramuthu Duraipandiyan, V. (2016). Identifying potential PPARγ agonist/partial agonist from plant molecules to control type 2 diabetes using *in silico* and *in vivo* models. *Medicinal Chemistry Research*, **25**(9), 1980–1992.

Steinmetz, K. A. and Potter, J. D. (1991). Vegetables, fruit, and cancer. I. Epidemiology. *Cancer Causes & Control*, **2**(5), 325–357.

Steinmetz, K. A. and Potter, J. D. (1996). Vegetables, fruit, and cancer prevention: A review. *Journal of the American Dietetic Association*, **96**(10), 1027–1039.

Stothers, J. B. (2012). *Carbon-13 NMR Spectroscopy: Organic Chemistry, A Series of Monographs*. Vol. 24. St. Louis, MO: Elsevier.

Sugihara, H., Nagao, M., Harada, T., Nakajima, Y., Tanimura-Inagaki, K., Okajima, K., Tamura, H., et al. (2014). Comparison of three α-glucosidase inhibitors for glycemic control and bodyweight reduction in Japanese patients with obese type 2 diabetes. *Journal of Diabetes Investigation*, **5**(2), 206–212.

Sun, F., Zheng, X. Y., Ye, J., Wu, T. T., Wang, J. L. and Chen, W. (2012). Potential anticancer activity of myricetin in human T24 bladder cancer cells both *in vitro* and *in vivo*. *Nutrition and Cancer*, **64**(4), 599–606.

Tadera, K., Minami, Y., Takamatsu, K. and Matsuoka, T. (2006). Inhibition of α-glucosidase and α-amylase by flavonoids. *Journal of Nutritional Science and Vitaminology*, **52**(2), 149–153.

Tamrakar, A. K., Maurya, C. K. and Rai, A. K. (2014). PTP1B inhibitors for type 2 diabetes treatment: A patent review (2011–2014). *Expert Opinion on Therapeutic Patents*, **24**(10), 1101–1115.

Tanious, F. A., Veal, J. M., Buczak, H., Ratmeyer, L. S. and Wilson, W. D. (1992). DAPI (4′, 6-diamidino-2-phenylindole) binds differently to DNA and RNA: Minor-groove binding at AT sites and intercalation at AU sites. *Biochemistry*, **31**(12), 3103–3112.

Thompson, M., Williams, C. R. and Elliot, G. E. P. (1976). Stability of flavonoid complexes of copper (II) and flavonoid antioxidant activity. *Analytica Chimica Acta*, **85**(2), 375–381.

Thomson, M., Al-Qattan, K., Mohamed H. M. H. and Ali, M. (2012). Green tea attenuates oxidative stress and downregulates the expression of angiotensin ii AT1 receptor in renal and hepatic tissues of streptozotocin-induced diabetic rats. *Evidence-Based Complementary and Alternative Medicine*, **2012**, 409047.

Tice, Raymond R., E. Agurell, D. Anderson, B. Burlinson, A. Hartmann, H. Kobayashi, Y. Miyamae, E. Rojas, J-C. Ryu, and Y. F. Sasaki. (2000). Single cell gel/comet assay: Guidelines for *in vitro* and *in vivo* genetic toxicology testing. *Environmental and Molecular Mutagenesis*, **35**(3) 206–221.

Tölle, S. (2014). GLP-1 analogues in treatment of type 1 diabetes mellitus. *Deutsche Medizinische Wochenschrift*, **139**(42), 2123–2126.

Tomlinson, B., Hu, M., Zhang, Y., Chan, P. and Liu, Z.-M. (2016). An overview of new GLP-1 receptor agonists for type 2 diabetes. *Expert Opinion on Investigational Drugs*, **25**(2), 145–158.

Torel, J., Cillard, J. and Cillard, P. (1986). Antioxidant activity of flavonoids and reactivity with peroxy radical. *Phytochemistry*, **25**(2), 383–385.

Tran, K. L., Park, Y. I., Pandya, S., Muliyil, N. J., Jensen, B. D., Huynh, K. and Nguyen, Q. T. (2017). Overview of glucagon-like peptide-1 receptor agonists for the treatment of patients with type 2 diabetes. *American Health & Drug Benefits*, **10**(4), 178.

Treutter, D. (2006). Significance of flavonoids in plant resistance: A review. *Environmental Chemistry Letters*, **4**(3), 147.

Tu, A. T. (1982). *Raman Spectroscopy in Biology: Principles and Applications*. New York: John Wiley & Sons.

Uchida, T., Kozawa, K., Kimura, Y. and Goto, Y. (1995). Structural study on chalcone derivatives. *Synthetic Metals*, **71**(1), 1705–1706.

Valley, M. P., Karassina, N., Aoyama, N., Carlson, C., Cali, J. J. and Vidugiriene, J. (2016). A bioluminescent assay for measuring glucose uptake. *Analytical Biochemistry*, **505**, 43–50.

van de Laar, F. A. (2008). Alpha-glucosidase inhibitors in the early treatment of type 2 diabetes. *Vascular Health and Risk Management*, **4**(6), 1189.

Varshney, R., Gupta, S. and Roy, P. (2017). Cytoprotective effect of kaempferol against palmitic acid-induced pancreatic β-cell death through modulation of autophagy via AMPK/mTOR signaling pathway.*Molecular and Cellular Endocrinology*, **448**, 1–20.

Vasanthi, H. R., ShriShriMal, N. and Das, D. K. (2012). Phytochemicals from plants to combat cardiovascular disease. *Current Medicinal Chemistry*, **19**(14), 2242–2251.

Venkatesan, R., Ji, E. and Kim, S. Y. (2015). Phytochemicals that regulate neurodegenerative disease by targeting neurotrophins: A comprehensive review. *BioMed Research International*, **2015**, 814068.

Vieira, M., Lyra e Silva, N. M., Ferreira, S. T., and. De Felice, F. G. (2017). Protein tyrosine phosphatase 1B (PTP1B). A potential target for Alzheimer's therapy? *Frontiers in Aging Neuroscience*, **9**, 7.

Vinayagam, R., Xiao, J. and Xu, B. (2017). An insight into anti-diabetic properties of dietary phytochemicals. *Phytochemistry Reviews*, **16**(3), 535–553.

Vrijsen, R., Everaert, L. and Boeyé, A. (1988). Antiviral activity of flavones and potentiation by ascorbate. *Journal of General Virology*, **69**(7), 1749–1751.

Walker, J. M., Winder, J. S. and Kellam, S. J. (1993). High-throughput microtiter plate-based chromogenic assays for glycosidase inhibitors. *Applied Biochemistry and Biotechnology*, **38**(1–2), 141–146.

Walle, T. (2004). Absorption and metabolism of flavonoids. *Free Radical Biology and Medicine*, **36**(7), 829–837.

Walle, T. (2007). Methylation of dietary flavones greatly improves their hepatic metabolic stability and intestinal absorption. *Molecular Pharmaceutics*, **4**(6), 826–832.

Waller, G. R. (2012). *Alkaloid Biology and Metabolism in Plants*. New York: Springer Science & Business Media.

Wang, F., Gao, F., Pan, S., Zhao, S. and Xue, Y. (2015). Luteolin induces apoptosis, G0/G1 cell cycle growth arrest and mitochondrial membrane potential loss in neuroblastoma brain tumor cells. *Drug Research*, **65**(02) 91–95.

Wang, I.-K., Lin-Shiau, S-Y.and Lin, J-K. (1999). Induction of apoptosis by apigenin and related flavonoids through cytochrome c release and activation of caspase-9 and caspase-3 in leukaemia HL-60 cells. *European Journal of Cancer*, **35**(10), 1517–1525.

Wang, L., Waltenberger, B., Pferschy-Wenzig, E.-M., Blunder, M., Liu, X., Malainer, C., Blazevic, T. et al. (2014). Natural product agonists of peroxisome proliferator-activated receptor gamma (PPARγ). A review. *Biochemical Pharmacology*, **92**(1), 73–89.

Wang, S.-J., Tong, Y., Lu, S., Yang, R., Liao, X., Xu, Y.-F. and Li, X. (2010). Anti-inflammatory activity of myricetin isolated from *Myrica rubra Sieb. et Zucc.* leaves. *Planta Medica*, **76**(14), 1492–1496.

Wei, Y.-Q., Zhao, X., Y Kariya, Y., Fukata, H., Keisuke Teshigawara, K. and Uchida, A. (1994). Induction of apoptosis by quercetin: Involvement of heat shock protein. *Cancer Research*, **54**(18), 4952–4957.

Wenkert, E. and Gottlieb, H. E. (1977). Carbon-13 nuclear magnetic resonance spectroscopy of flavonoid and isoflavonoid compounds. *Phytochemistry*, **16**(11), 1811–1816.

Wild, S. H., Roglic, G., Green, A., Sicree, R. and King, H. (2004). Global prevalence of diabetes: Estimates for the year 2000 and projections for 2030: Response to Rathman and Giani. *Diabetes Care*, **27**(10), 2569–2569.

Williams, C. A. and Grayer, R. J. (2004).Anthocyanins and other flavonoids. *Natural Product Reports*, **21**(4), 539–573.

Winkel-Shirley, B. (2001). Flavonoid biosynthesis. A colorful model for genetics, biochemistry, cell biology, and biotechnology. *Plant Physiology*, **126**(2), 485–493.

Winkel-Shirley, B. (2002). Biosynthesis of flavonoids and effects of stress. *Current Opinion in Plant Biology*, **5**(3), 218–223.

Wishart, D. S., Bigam, C. G., Yao, J., Abildgaard, F., Dyson, H. J., Oldfield, E., Markley, J. L. and Sykes, B. D. (1995). 1 H, 13 C and 15 N chemical shift referencing in biomolecular NMR. *Journal of Biomolecular NMR*, **6**(2), 135–140.

Wishart, D. S., Sykes, B. D. and Richards, F. M. (1992). The chemical shift index: A fast and simple method for the assignment of protein secondary structure through NMR spectroscopy. *Biochemistry*, **31**(6), 1647–1651.

Wootten, D., Simms, J., Koole, C., Woodman, O. L., Summers, R. J., Christopoulos, A. and Sexton, P. M. (2011). Modulation of the glucagon-like peptide-1 receptor signaling by naturally occurring and synthetic flavonoids. *Journal of Pharmacology and Experimental Therapeutics*, **336**(2), 540–550.

World Health Organization. (2016). *Global Report on Diabetes.* Geneva, Switzerland: World Health Organization.

Wu, H. and Mahato, R. I. (2013). Beta cell regeneration: A novel strategy for treating type 1 diabetes. *Gene Technology*, **2**, e106.

Xiao, J., Ni, X., Kai, G. and Chen, X. (2013). A review on structure–activity relationship of dietary polyphenols inhibiting α-amylase. *Critical Reviews in Food Science and Nutrition*, **53**(5), 497–506.

Xiao, X., Liu, Z., Wang, R., Wang, J., Zhang, S., Cai, X., Wu, K., Bergan, R. C., Xu, L. and Fan, D. (2015). Genistein suppresses FLT4 and inhibits human colorectal cancer metastasis. *Oncotarget*, **6**(5), 3225.

Yamamoto N., Ueda-Wakagi M., Sato T., Kawasaki K., Sawada K., Kawabata K., Akagawa M. and Ashida H. (2011). Measurement of glucose uptake in cultured cells. *Current Protocols in Pharmacology*, **71**(12.14), 1–26.

Yang, F.-Q., Liu, M., Li, W., Che, J.-P., Wang, G.-C. and Zheng, J.-H. (2015). Combination of quercetin and hyperoside inhibits prostate cancer cell growth and metastasis via regulation of microRNA-21. *Molecular Medicine Reports*, **11**(2), 1085–1092.

Yao, H., Xu, W., Shi, X. and Zhang, Z. (2011). Dietary flavonoids as cancer prevention agents. *Journal of Environmental Science and Health, Part C*, **29**(1), 1–31.

Yoshida, T., Konishi, M., Horinaka, M., Yasuda, T., Goda, A. E., Taniguchi, H., Yano, K., Wakada, M., and Sakai, T. (2008) Kaempferol sensitizes colon cancer cells to TRAIL-induced apoptosis. *Biochemical and Biophysical Research Communications*, **375**(1), 129–133.

Yoshioka, H., Mabry, T. J. and Timmermann, B. N. (1973). *Sesquiterpene Lactones: Chemistry, NMR and Plant Distribution.* Tokyo, Japan: University of Tokyo Press.

Youl, E., G. Bardy, R. Magous, G. Cros, F. Sejalon, A. Virsolvy, S. Richard et al. (2010). Quercetin potentiates insulin secretion and protects INS-1 pancreatic β-cells against oxidative damage via the ERK1/2 pathway. *British Journal of Pharmacology*, **161**(4), 799–814.

Yousefi, H., Alihemmati, A., Karimi, P., Alipour, M. R., Habibi, P. and Ahmadiasl, N. (2017). Effect of genistein on expression of pancreatic SIRT1, inflammatory cytokines and histological changes in ovariectomized diabetic rat. *Iranian Journal of Basic Medical Sciences*, **20**(4), 423–429.

Zamin, L. L., Filippi-Chiela, E. C., PDillenburg-Pilla, P., Horn, F., Salbego, C. and Lenz, G. (2009). Resveratrol and quercetin cooperate to induce senescence-like growth arrest in C6 rat glioma cells. *Cancer Science*, **100**(9), 1655–1662.

Zang, Y., Sato, H. and Igarashi, K. (2011). Anti-diabetic effects of a kaempferol glycoside-rich fraction from unripe soybean (Edamame, Glycine max L. Merrill.'Jindai') leaves on KK-Ay mice. *Bioscience, Biotechnology, and Biochemistry*, **75**(9), 1677–1684.

Zang, Y., Zhang, L., Igarashi, K., and Yu, C. (2015). The anti-obesity and anti-diabetic effects of kaempferol glycosides from unripe soybean leaves in high-fat-diet mice. *Food & Function*, **6**(3), 834–841.

Zhang, B., Kang, M., Xie, Q., Xu, B., Sun, C., Chen, K. and Wu, Y. (2010). Anthocyanins from Chinese bayberry extract protect β cells from oxidative stress-mediated injury via HO-1 upregulation. *Journal of Agricultural and Food Chemistry*, **59**(2), 537–545.

Zhang, J., Lei, Z., Huang, Z., Zhang, X., Zhou, Y., Luo, Z., Zeng, W., Su, J., Peng, C. and Chen, X. (2016). Epigallocatechin-3-gallate (EGCG) suppresses melanoma cell growth and metastasis by targeting TRAF6 activity. *Oncotarget*, **7**(48), 79557.

Zhang, J., Wu, D., Song, J., Wang, J., Yi, J. and Dong, W. (2015). Hesperetin induces the apoptosis of gastric cancer cells via activating mitochondrial pathway by increasing reactive oxygen species. *Digestive Diseases and Sciences*, **60**(10), 2985–2995.

Zhang, Q., Zhao, X.-H. and Wang, Z.-J. (2008). Flavones and flavonols exert cytotoxic effects on a human oesophageal adenocarcinoma cell line (OE33) by causing G2/M arrest and inducing apoptosis. *Food and Chemical Toxicology*, **46**(6), 2042–2053.

Zhang, X.-A., Zhang, S., Yin, Q. and Zhang, J. (2015). Quercetin induces human colon cancer cells apoptosis by inhibiting the nuclear factor-kappa B Pathway. *Pharmacognosy Magazine*, **11**(42), 404.

Zhang, Y., Chen, A. Y., Li, M., Chen, C. and Yao, Q. (2008). Ginkgo biloba extract kaempferol inhibits cell proliferation and induces apoptosis in pancreatic cancer cells. *Journal of Surgical Research*, **148**(1), 17–23.

Zhang, Y.-J., Gan, R.-Y., Li, S., Zhou, Y. Li, A.-N., Xu, D.-P. and Li. H.-B. (2015). Antioxidant phytochemicals for the prevention and treatment of chronic diseases. *Molecules*, **20**(12), 21138–21156.

Zhang, Y. and Liu, D. (2011). Flavonol kaempferol improves chronic hyperglycemia-impaired pancreatic beta-cell viability and insulin secretory function. *European Journal of Pharmacology*, **670**(1), 325–332.

Zhang, Z., Huang, Y., Gao, F., Gao, Z., Bu, H., Gu, W. and Li, Y. (2011). A self-assembled nanodelivery system enhances the oral bioavailability of daidzein: *In vitro* characteristics and *in vivo* performance. *Nanomedicine*, **6**(8), 136.

Zheng, S.-Y., Li, Y., Jiang, D., Zhao, J. and Ge, J.-F. (2012). Anticancer effect and apoptosis induction by quercetin in the human lung cancer cell line A-549. *Molecular Medicine Reports*, **5**(3), 822–826.

Zhou, K., Pedersen, H. K., Dawed, A. Y. and Pearson, E. R. (2016). Pharmacogenomics in diabetes mellitus: Insights into drug action and drug discovery. *Nature Reviews Endocrinology*, **12**(6), 337.

Zhu, K. and Wang, W. (2016). Green tea polyphenol EGCG suppresses osteosarcoma cell growth through upregulating miR-1. *Tumor Biology*, **37**(4), 4373–4382.

4 Tanshinone Diterpenes
Chemistry and Multifunctional Biological Activities

*Mohamed-Elamir F. Hegazy, Tarik A. Mohamed,
Abdelsamed I. Elshamy, Ahmed R. Hamed,
Sara Abdelfatah, Soleiman E. Helaly, Nahla S. Abdel-Azim,
Khaled A. Shams, Abdel-Razik H. Farrag,
Abdessamad Debbab, Tahia K. Mohamed,
Hesham R. El-Seedi, Mohamed E.M. Saeed, Masaaki Noji,
Akemi Umeyama, Paul W. Paré and Thomas Efferth*

CONTENTS

4.1   NATURAL PRODUCTS AND MODERN DRUGS

In a recent study by the World Health Organization (WHO), it is stated that about 80% of the world population depends on traditional medicines (WHO 2002). In the United States alone, 121 drugs are derived from natural sources and 85% of these compounds either directly or indirectly originate from plants (Benowitz 1996). Of the anticancer drugs on the market, around 47% are derived from natural materials (Newman and Cragg 2007). The contribution of natural product drug discovery from select countries is presented in Figure 4.1 (Newman et al. 2003).

Natural products are derived from several biological sources, including microorganisms (soil/aquatic bacteria and fungi), plants, soft and hard coral, sponges and animals (Figure 4.2).

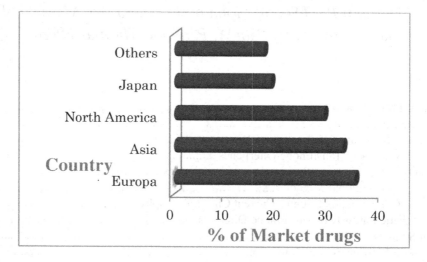

FIGURE 4.1   The percentage of the global market of naturally derived medications developed from a given region.

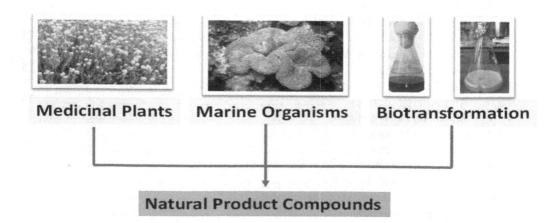

FIGURE 4.2   Examples of natural product sources.

4.2 TANSHINONES

Tanshinones are classified as abietane-type diterpenoids originally isolated from the Chinese plant *Salvia miltiorrhiza* (*Danshen* or *Tanshen* in Chinese). The first identified tanshinone metabolite was reported by Nakao and Fukushima in 1934. Since then, more than 40 lipophilic tanshinones have been isolated and chemically identified (Wang et al. 2007a,b; Dong et al. 2011; Zhang et al. 2012). Recently, several studies have been published concerning the isolation, identification, synthesis and biological activity of tanshinone metabolites. These compounds have been reported to exhibit significant *in vitro* and *in vivo* pharmacological activity, especially as cardiovascular (Gao et al. 2012; Zeng et al. 2012) and anticancer agents. Indeed, biological activity has been observed against several human cancer cell lines (Nizamutdinova et al. 2008a,b; Su et al. 2008; Zhou et al. 2011; Gong et al. 2012).

4.3 THE BASIC STRUCTURES OF TANSHINONE DITERPENES

Tanshinones are a class of compounds belonging to the abietane diterpenoid structure type (Figure 4.3). Known tanshinone compounds are: tanshinone I (TI), tanshinone IIA (TIIA), cryptotanshinone, dihydrotanshinone I (DH-TI), tanshinlactone and neo-tanshinlactone (Figure 4.3) as well as isotanshinone I, tanshinone IIB, methyltanshinone, isocryptotanshinone I, and isocryptotanshinone II (Gu et al. 2004; Don et al. 2006; Yang et al. 2006; Wang et al. 2007; Wei et al. 2007; Dong et al. 2011; Zhang et al. 2012).

Up to now, more than 90 tanshinone metabolites have been identified, which can be classified into two major groups: (1) lipophilic abietane diterpene constituents such as tanshinones derivatives (Wang et al. 2007; Dong et al. 2011), and (2) hydrophilic compounds including salvianic acid A and B, protocatechuic acid, protocatechuic aldehyde, rosmarinic acid, salvianolic acid A–C, which are also known as lithospermic acids A–C, or magnesium lithospermates A–C or tanshinoates A–C (Zhou et al. 2005; Liu et al. 2006; Ma et al. 2006; Bi et al. 2008). In addition to these two major classes, baicalin, 5,3′-dihydroxy-7,4′-dimethoxy flavanone, ursolic acid, β-sitosterol, daucosterol, vitamin E and tannin have been identified from *Danshen* (Kong 1989). Twelve natural tanshinones isolated from *Salvia miltiorrhiza* bunge (Lamiaceae) (Figure 4.4), deoxyneocryptotanshinone (VII), grandifolia F (VIII), ferruginol (IX), cryptotanshinone (III), tanshinone IIA (II), tanshinol B (X),

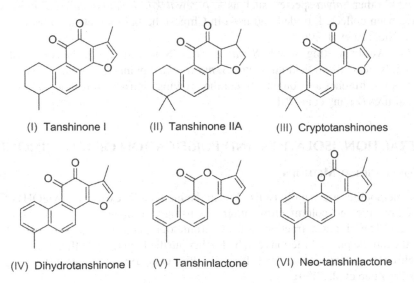

(I) Tanshinone I   (II) Tanshinone IIA   (III) Cryptotanshinones

(IV) Dihydrotanshinone I   (V) Tanshinlactone   (VI) Neo-tanshinlactone

FIGURE 4.3 The chemical structure of some tanshinone skeletons.

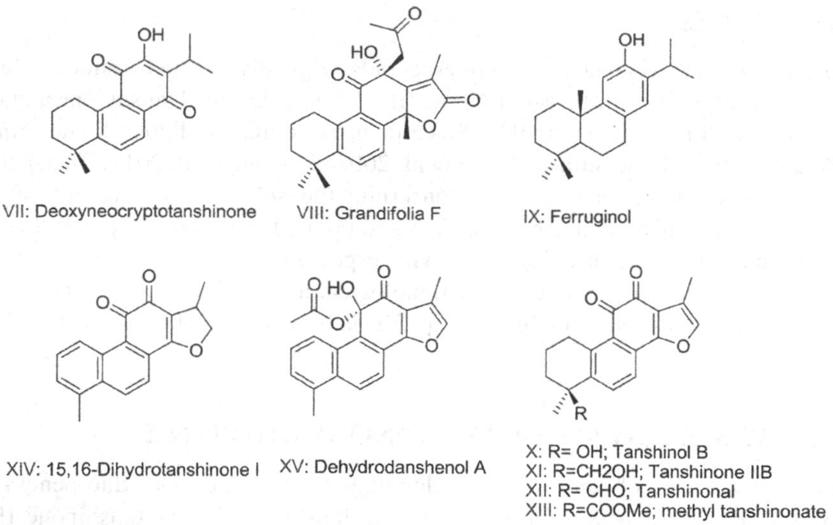

VII: Deoxyneocryptotanshinone   VIII: Grandifolia F   IX: Ferruginol

XIV: 15,16-Dihydrotanshinone I   XV: Dehydrodanshenol A

X: R= OH; Tanshinol B
XI: R=CH2OH; Tanshinone IIB
XII: R= CHO; Tanshinonal
XIII: R=COOMe; methyl tanshinonate

FIGURE 4.4 Structures of selected tanshinones.

tanshinone IIB (XI), tanshinonal (XII), methyl tanshinonate (XIII), 15,16-dihydrotanshinone I (XIV), tanshinone I (I) and dehydrodanshenol A (XV) (Kim et al. 2017).

4.4 NATURAL SOURCES OF TANSHINONE DITERPENES

Tanshinone was first isolated from the rhizomes of *S. miltiorrhiza* present in the hilly areas of China, Korea, Mongolia and Japan.

Most of the identified compounds from *S. miltiorrhiza* have also been identified from other *Salvia* species (Romanova et al. 1972; Lee et al. 1987; Wang et al. 1988; Chang et al. 1990a, 1990b; Li et al. 1991; Kasimu et al. 1998; Tezuka et al. 1998; Yang et al. 2003; Adams et al. 2005; Matkowski et al. 2008; Qiao et al. 2009; Li et al. 2010a). Although *S. miltiorrhiza* is the only official source of *Danshen*, 17 other *Salvia* species, such as *S. przewalskii*, *S. yunnanensis*, *S. bowleyana* and *S. trijuga*, have been collected, traded and used in Chinese herbal markets as substitutes (Skała and Wysokińska 2005; Li et al. 2008).

Because of over-harvesting of wild *S. miltiorrhiza* (Sun et al. 2012), the source of commercial *Danshen* mainly depends on field-cultivated *S. miltiorrhiza* plants (Lin et al. 2008). Other alternative sources of tanshinones are sought to meet the growing pharmaceutical demand involving plant cell/organ cultures (Zhang et al. 2012).

4.5 EXTRACTION, ISOLATION AND PURIFICATION OF TANSHINONES

4.5.1 CONVENTIONAL METHODS

Tanshinone metabolites are usually isolated from the methanolic extraction (MeOH) of *Salvia* species followed by silica gel column chromatography using a gradient CH_2Cl_2-MeOH mixture as the elution solvent. The obtained fractions are re-chromatographed using a gradient of C_6H_6-MeOH mixture as the mobile phase. Fractions can be further purified via recrystallization or by preparative thin-layer chromatography (Honda et al. 1988; Ikeshiro et al. 1991; Li et al. 1993; Yang et al. 1996; Gu et al. 2006; Zhao et al. 2006).

Reversed HPLC (high-performance liquid chromatography) separation has also been performed using a gradient profile with methanol (solvent A) and water (solvent B): starting with 70% A to 100% A over 20 min and then holding for 8 min with a constant flow rate of 1 mL/min; injection volume is 20 µL using a 230 nm wavelength of the diode array detector for monitoring compound elution (Dittmann et al. 2004).

4.5.2 Conical Coils Counter-Current Chromatography

Modern conical coil counter-current chromatography (CCC) has been reported for tanshinone isolation and is an advancement for natural products isolation (Figure 4.5; Liang et al. 2013). A solvent system of hexane–ethyl acetate–methanol–water (HEMWat) showed higher efficiency with a volume ratio of 5:5:7:3.

Six diterpenoids including dihydrotanshinone I (88.1%), cryptotanshinone (98.8%), methylene-tanshiquinone (97.6%), tanshinone I (93.5%), tanshinone IIA (96.8%) and danshenxinkun B (94.3%) have been successfully isolated from 300 mg of a crude extract in a single run via high-speed counter-current chromatography (HSCCC) with a two-phase solvent systems composed of n-hexane–ethanol–water (10:5.5:4.5, v/v) and n-hexane–ethanol–water (10:7:3, v/v) (Li and Chen 2001).

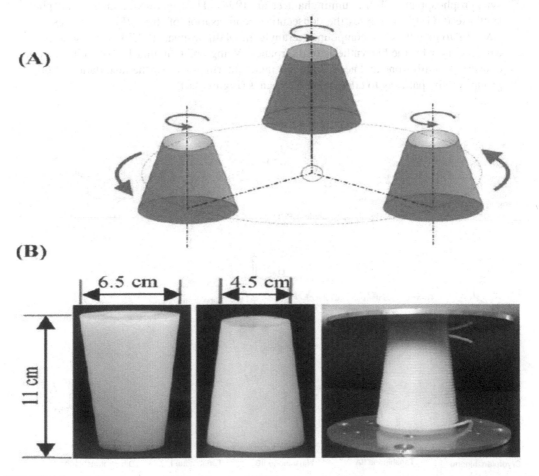

FIGURE 4.5 (A) The design principle of tapered CCC apparatus with three upright conical coils connected in series and (B) the photographs of holder and a part of coils.

4.6 BIOSYNTHETIC PATHWAY OF TANSHINONE DITERPENES

The biosynthesis of the terpenoids in higher plants occurs through two distinct pathways as outlined below.

1. The mevalonic acid (MVA) pathway occurs in the cytosol (Seto et al. 1996) and is responsible for the synthesis of sterols, certain sesquiterpenes and the side chain of ubiquinone (Arigoni et al. 1997; Wang et al. 2010). The MVA pathway plays a role in tanshinone synthesis with extensive crosstalk between the two pathways.

2. The 2-C-methyl-D-erythritol-4-phosphate (MEP) or non-MVA pathway occurs in plastids (Seto et al. 1996) and is responsible for tanshinone biosynthesis. In MEP pathways, 1-deoxy-D-xylulose-5-phosphate synthase (DXS) catalysed the coupling of pyruvate and glyceraldehyde-3-phosphate (GA-3P) into 1-deoxy-D-xylulose-5-phosphate (DXP), which is consecutively converted into MEP through the action of 1-deoxy-D-xylulose-5-phosphate reductoisomerase (DXR). Through a series of enzymatic conversions MEP is converted to the universal precursors isopentenyl-diphosphate (IPP) and dimethylallyl diphosphate (DMAPP) for terpene formation (Rohmer 1999). In the reacting of IPP or DMAPP with carbonium ion, IPP leads to the production of geranyl diphosphate (GPP). GPP, with an active allylic phosphate group reversely reacts with IPP to produce farnesyl pyrophosphate (FPP) (Cunningham et al. 1994). Then, geranylgeranyl diphosphate synthase (GGPPS) catalyses the consecutive condensation of three IPP molecules with DMAPP to give the C-20 compound, geranylgeranyl diphosphate (GGPP), an essential linear precursor for the biosynthesis of diterpenes (Wang and Ohnuma 1999). GGPP can be converted to miltirone and neocryptotanshinone intermediates by the installation of other groups on the pathway to tanshinone diterpenes (Figure 4.6).

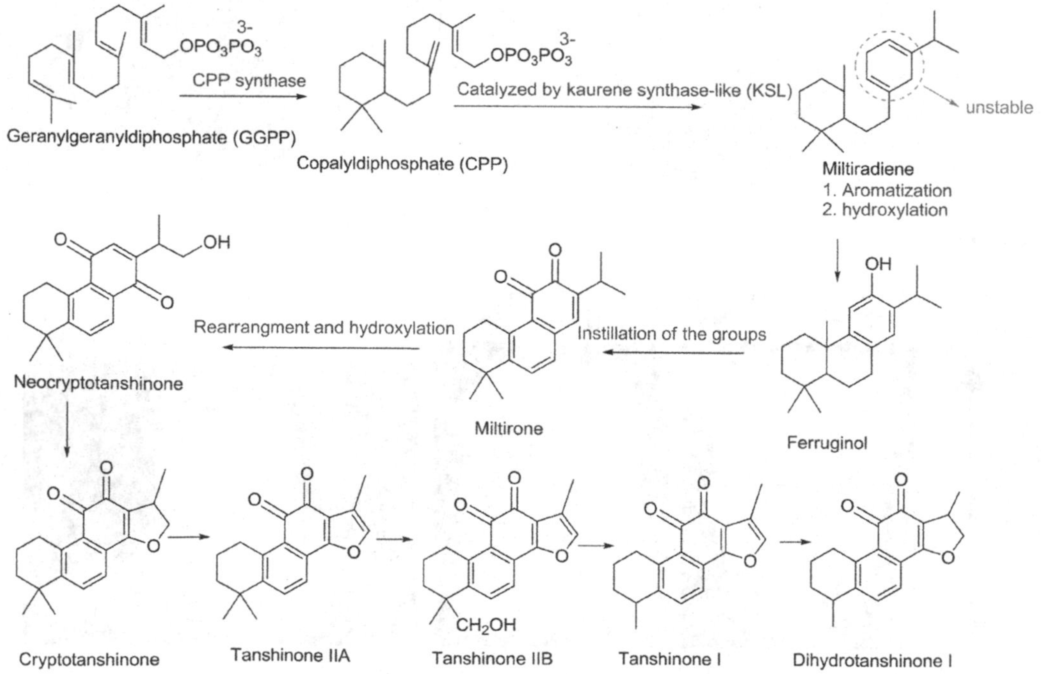

FIGURE 4.6 Plausible biosynthetic pathways of tanshinones in *S. miltiorrhiza*. (From Wang, J.W. and Wu, J.Y., *Appl. Microbiol. Biotechnol.*, 88, 437–449, 2010.)

4.7 TOTAL SYNTHESIS OF TANSHINONE

Tanshinone diterpenoids have significant bioactivity such antibacterial, antidermatophytic, antioxidant, anticancer and cardiovascular. Therefore, researchers focus on the systematic isolation and identification of its biological activities, especially the interactions with central benzodiazepine receptors. In one of several total synthesis trials of these compounds, Chang et al. (1990a, 1990b) reported the total synthesis of several tanshinones via anisole as a starting compound as described in Figure 4.7 as examples.

Recently, a novel total synthesis of tanshinone I via the intermediate 3-hydroxy-8-methyl-1,4-phenanthrenedione has been described (Wu et al. 2017). The low overall yield and the use of expensive reagents in the synthesis process were minimized by the use of the Diels–Alder reaction to directly construct the 1,4-phenanthrenedione scaffold, generating tanshinone I in only three steps. The synthesis of tanshinone I started by the reaction of 2-methylstyrene and 2-methoxy-1,4-benzoquinone. The non-catalysed Diels–Alder reaction between these two starting compounds in toluene afforded 3-methoxy-8-methyl-1,4-phenanthrenedione in 52% yield. Subsequent demethylation of this unstable intermediate with NaOH in aqueous EtOH afforded 3-hydroxy-8-methyl-1,4-phenanthrenedione with a 79% yield. In the final step, the Feist–Benary reaction of compound 3-hydroxy-8-methyl-1,4-phenanthrenedione with chloroacetone in HOAc–NH$_4$OAc gave the target tanshinone I in 45% yield. The overall yield for the three-step synthesis was approximately 18.5% (Figure 4.8).

4.8 STRUCTURAL MODIFICATION OF TANSHINONES

Due to the high hydrophobicity of tanshinones, structural modifications have been made to increase absorption when given orally or intraperitoneally (Zhang et al. 2006). Sodium tanshinone IIA sulphonate (STS), a water-soluble derivative of tanshinone IIA, has been widely used to treat patients with cardiovascular diseases for more than 30 years and as an antioxidant agent (Lee et al. 1999; Nizamutdinova et al. 2008b; Chen et al. 2009). STS has been proposed to possess a broad range of pharmacological activities (Zhang et al. 1990; Kang et al. 2000; Tan et al. 2011).

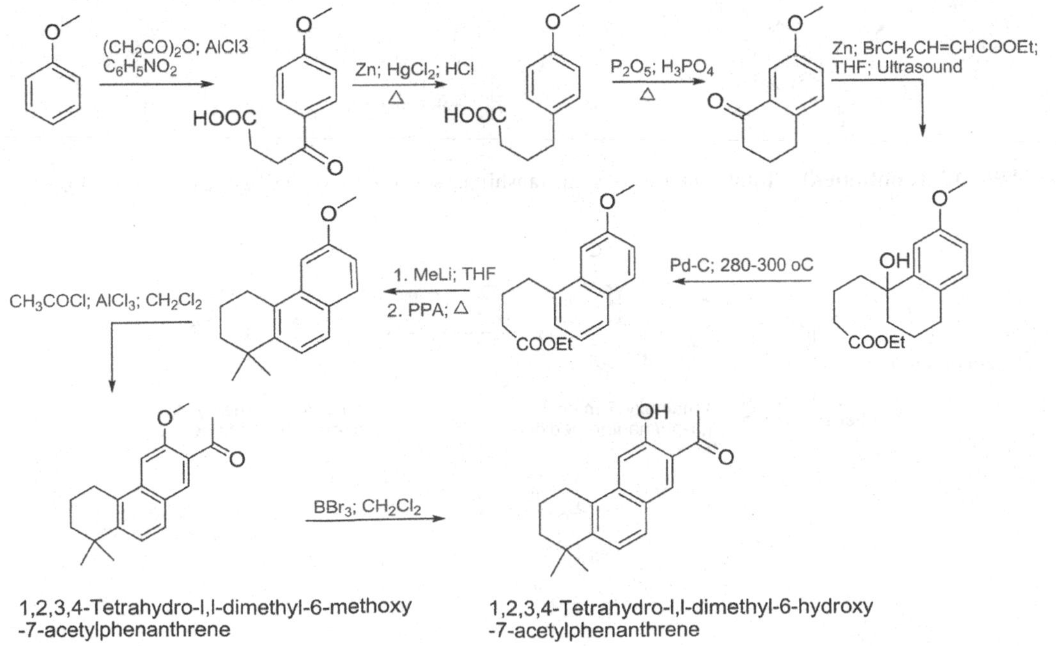

1,2,3,4-Tetrahydro-l,l-dimethyl-6-methoxy
-7-acetylphenanthrene

1,2,3,4-Tetrahydro-l,l-dimethyl-6-hydroxy
-7-acetylphenanthrene

FIGURE 4.7 Total synthesis of some tanshinones as reported by Chang et al. (1990a,b).

(Continued)

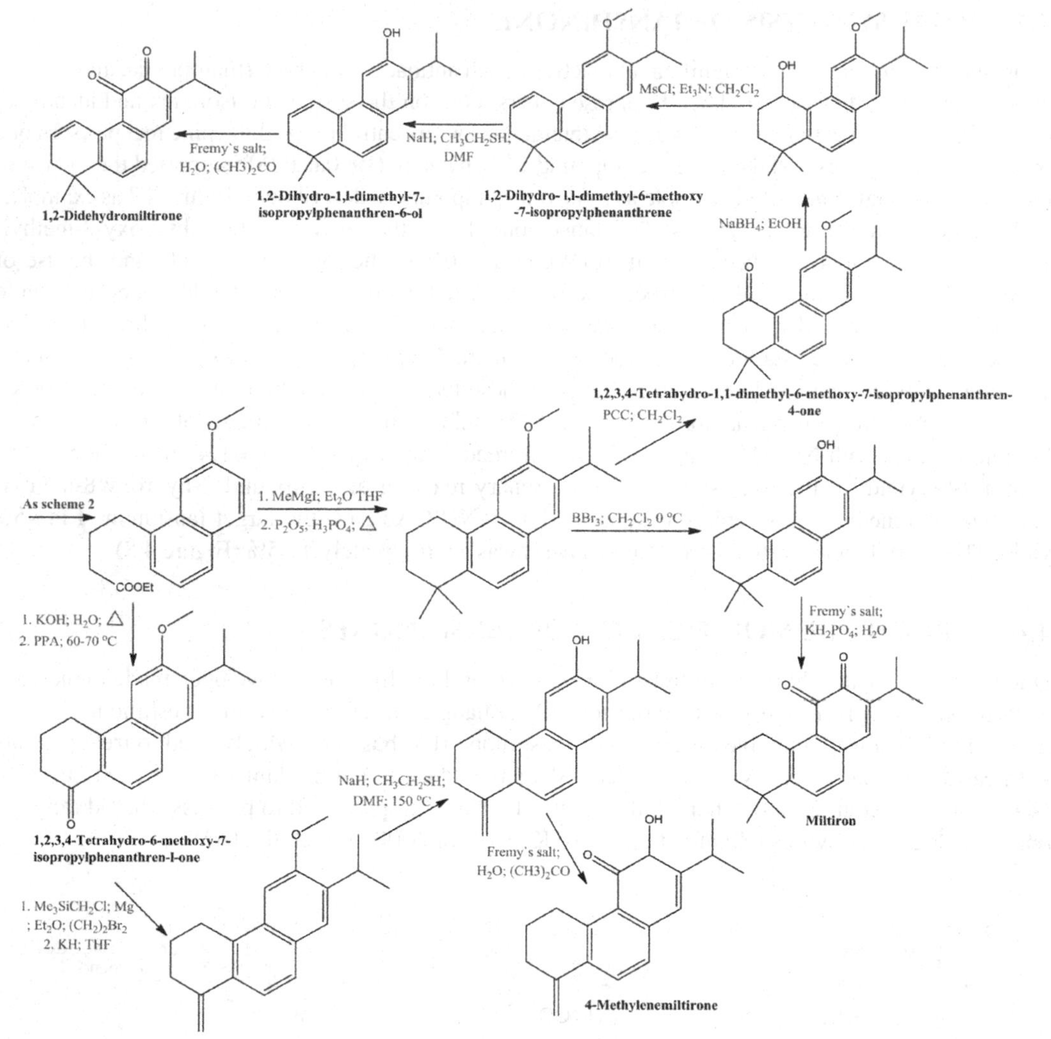

FIGURE 4.7 (Continued) Total synthesis of some tanshinones as reported by Chang et al. (1990a,b).

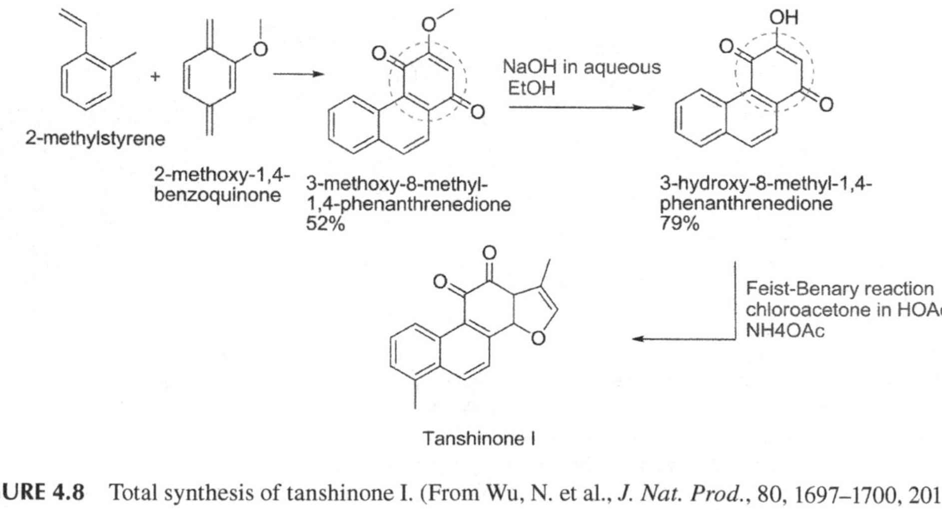

FIGURE 4.8 Total synthesis of tanshinone I. (From Wu, N. et al., *J. Nat. Prod.*, 80, 1697–1700, 2017.)

4.9 MULTIFUNCTIONAL BIOLOGICAL ACTIVITY OF TANSHINONE DITERPENES

Tanshinones are abietane diterpenes, isolated mainly from *S. miltiorrhiza* (Lamiaceae), a plant largely used in traditional Chinese medicine for the treatment of cardiovascular and inflammatory diseases. *Danshen*, a crude herbal drug isolated from the dried root or rhizome of *S. miltiorrhiza*, has long been traditionally used in Asian countries for multiple therapeutic remedies, including myocardial infarction, angina pectoris, stroke and atherosclerosis (Wang et al. 2007; Han et al. 2008). The protective effects of *Danshen* are listed (Figure 4.9).

4.9.1 Anticancer Activity

Tanshinones exhibit cytotoxicity activity against all tested cell lines (IC_{50}: 2.4–39.6 µM), with comparable or higher potencies compared to cisplatin (IC_{50}: 1.6–11.8 µM) but lower potencies compared to paclitaxel (IC_{50}: < 0.008–0.2 µM; Xu et al. 2010a,b).

Tanshinones and/or tanshinone-containing herbal formulae exhibit broad anticancer properties in cell culture models, which have been discussed in several reviews (Yuan et al. 2003; Wang et al. 2007; Dong et al. 2011). Tanshinlactone and neo-tanshinlactone derivatives (Figure 4.4) are potent metabolites for anticancer activities (Dong et al. 2011). These results suggest that the presence of the lipophilic group in most of diterpenoid tanshinones support the prominent anticancer potential, along with anti-inflammatory and antioxidant activity (Zhang et al. 2012). Cryptotanshinone, tanshinone I and tanshinone IIA are the three major elements of the lipophilic group (Figures 4.4 and 4.5) and numerous

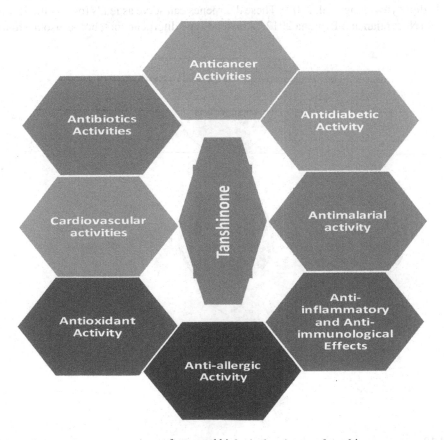

FIGURE 4.9 Schematic representations of reported biological activates of tanshinones.

in vitro and *in vivo* studies have revealed the anticancer actions as well as the underlying mechanisms of these tanshinone components (Figure 4.11; Ho and Chang 2015).

Tanshinone IIA possesses anticancer activity against several human cancer cells, including solid tumours and haematological malignancies. Tanshinone IIA also showed anticancer activity *in vivo* in mouse xenograft models (Sung et al. 1999; Lu et al. 2009; Chen et al. 2012; Liu et al. 2012). Tanshinone IIA showed the best synergistic effect with doxorubicin in the same cells (Lee et al. 2010).

The tanshinone-related compounds cryptotanshinone, dihydrotanshinone, tanshinone I and tanshinone IIA isolated from *S. miltiorrhiza* also exerted anticancer properties against hepatocellular carcinoma cell lines, HepG2, Hep3B and PLC/PRF/5. Cryptotanshinone suppressed doxorubicin efflux, a process mediated by P-glycoprotein in HepG2 cells. In another study, cryptotanshinone caused apoptosis in HL-60 cells via the mitochondrial pathway (Ni and Qian 2014). Tanshinone I also induced apoptosis in the breast cancer cell lines MCF-7 and MDA-MB-231 (Nizamutdinova et al. 2008a). Dihydroneotanshinlactone and neotanshinlactone showed selective cytotoxic activity towards SK-BR-3, breast adenocarcinoma cells, with a higher potency compared to cisplatin, but lower than paclitaxel.

Neotanshinlactone and methyl tanshinonate showed considerable cytotoxicity against SMMC-7721, A-549, MCF-7 and SW480 (Pan et al. 2012). A schematic summary of the cellular and molecular activities of tanshinones is provided in Figure 4.10.

4.9.2 ANTIDIABETIC ACTIVITY

Tanshinone was tested for tyrosine phosphorylation activity with the insulin receptor (IR) β-subunit and in 3T3-L1 adipocytes (Jung et al. 2009). These diterpenes can serve as leads for specific IR activators for diabetes (Nagarajan and Brindha 2012). Abietane-type diterpene metabolites isotanshinone IIA,

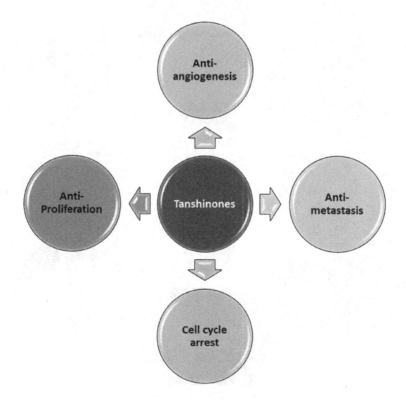

FIGURE 4.10   Anticancer tanshinone mechanisms.

dihydro-isotanshinone I and isocryptotanshinone obtained through bioassay guided fractionation exerted non-competitive PTP1B inhibition (Han et al. 2005). Different mechanisms of action for isotanshinone antidiabetic activity were evaluated by Nagarajan and Brindha (2012).

Recently, Kim et al. (2017) investigated the antidiabetic potential of 12 natural tanshinones isolated from *S. miltiorrhiza* and evaluated their inhibitory activity against PTP1B. Cryptotanshinone, tanshinol B and dehydrodanshenol A exhibited potent PTP1B inhibitory activity with IC_{50} values of 5.5 ± 0.9, 4.7 ± 0.4 and 8.5 ± 0.5 µM, respectively. Enzyme kinetic analysis of PTP1B inhibition revealed that cryptotanshinone and tanshinol B were mixed non-competitive type inhibitors, whereas dehydrodanshenol A was a classical non-competitive type inhibitor confirmed by molecular docking simulations.

A total plant extract of *S. miltiorrhiza* as well as the isolated compounds tanshinone I, IIA and 15,16-dihydrotanshinone I enhanced the activity of insulin (1 nM) on the tyrosine phosphorylation of the IR as well as the activation of the downstream kinases Akt, ERK1/2 and GSK3b. In adipocytes, the same insulin receptor (IR) downstream signalling and the translocation of glucose transporter 4 were demonstrated by the three tanshinones in the presence of insulin. These insulin-sensitizing activities of tanshinones may be useful for developing a new class of specific IR activators as antidiabetic agents (Jung et al. 2009).

4.9.3 ANTIBIOTIC ACTIVITIES

4.9.3.1 Antimicrobial Activity

Tanshinone IIA and tanshinone I showed the potent antimicrobial activity of *S. miltiorrhiza* hairy roots, which can be used for large-scale production of antimicrobial agents (Zhao et al. 2011).

4.9.3.2 Antibacterial Activity

Cryptotanshinone and dihydrotanshinone I, two nor abietane-type diterpenes (tanshinone) derived from the roots of *S. miltiorrhiza* possess antibacterial activity against a broad range of Gram-positive bacteria including the *B. subtilis* strain KCTC 3069 both with low MICs; 3.1 L g/mL (Lee et al. 1999).

4.9.3.3 Antifungal Activity

Tanshinone IIA, cryptotanshinone and dihydrotanshinone I exhibit antifungal activity against *Candida albicans* at a concentration of 100 µg/mL (Yongmoon and Lnkyung 2013).

4.9.4 ANTIMALARIAL ACTIVITY

Tanshinone IIA, tanshinone I, 1,2-dihydrotanshinquinone, methylene tanshinquinone and methyl tanshinonate were the most active antiplasmodial agents with IC_{50}s of 1–10 µM. The presence of the furan ring and/or double bond of the heterocycle in the diterpenoid structure, can affect the antiplasmodial activity (Lusarczyk et al. 2011).

4.9.5 ANTI-INFLAMMATORY AND ANTI-IMMUNOLOGICAL EFFECTS

Tanshinone's anti-inflammatory effect led to the speculation that some tanshinones might be used in the treatment of immunological diseases (Kang et al. 2000). Tanshinone I, cryptotanshinone and dihydrotanshinone significantly inhibited interleukin-12 (IL-12) and interferon-gamma (IFN-γ) production (Kang et al. 2000). Furthermore, tanshinones inhibited the expression of IL-12 p40 gene at the mRNA level and negatively regulated IL-12 production at the transcription level. Tanshinone IIA also strongly inhibited the production of inflammatory mediators such as IL-1β, IL-6 and TNF-α (Jang et al. 2003). Phospholipase A2 (PLA2) plays an important role in inflammatory and/or immunoregulatory responses. The *in vivo* anti-inflammatory activity of tanshinone I has been mechanistically linked to PLA2 inhibition. These results validated the traditional use of *S. miltiorrhiza* as part of anti-inflammatory regimens (Gao 1983; Kim et al. 2002; Jang et al. 2003; Wang et al. 2007).

4.9.6   ANTI-ALLERGIC ACTIVITY

Dihydrotanshinone I and cryptotanshinone revealed significant activity with IC_{50} values of 16 and 36 mM, respectively, with IgE receptor-mediated tyrosine phosphorylation of PLCg2 and MAPK, suggesting that the dihydrofuran ring may be important for biological activity (Ryu et al. 1999; Choi and Kim 2004; Wang et al. 2007).

4.9.7   EFFECTS ON HEART DISEASE

Tanshinone I, tanshinone IIA, cryptotanshinone, 1,2-dihydro tanshinquinone and danshenxinkun A were effective coronary artery dilators (Chen et al. 1986). A water-soluble derivative, sodium tanshinonate IIA sulphonate, has been clinically tested in coronary heart disease patients with biological efficacy (Chen 1984; Chang et al. 1990). Sodium tanshinonate IIA sulphonate attenuated hypertrophy induced by angiotensin II (Takahashi et al. 2002). Tanshinone VI also attenuated the humoral-induced hypertrophy of cardiac myocytes and fibrosis of cardiac fibroblasts to protect against hypoxia/reoxygenation injury and improved post-hypoxic cardiac function in the heart (Takeo et al. 1990; Maki et al. 2002; Yagi and Takeo 2003). Moreover, tanshinone I, tanshinone IIA, cryptotanshinone and dihydrotanshinone I protected from myocardial ischaemia (Yagi et al. 1994; Wang et al. 2007).

Tanshinone IIA is one of the tanshinones with well-documented anti-atherosclerotic effects. The excellent anti-atherosclerotic profile of TSN has inspired the synthesis, chemical modification and *in vitro* biological evaluation of novel substituted tanshinone derivatives as potent anti-atherosclerotic agents. Structurally, tanshinone IIA is made up of four rings (I–IV, Figure 4.4; Fang et al. 2018).

4.9.8   EFFECTS ON HEPATIC FIBROSIS

Tanshen can be used to treat hepatitis and hepatic fibrosis. Tanshinone I showed activity against hepatic stellate cells (HSCs), which play a central role in hepatic fibrosis (Kim et al. 2003). Tanshinone IIA had protective effects on injured primary cultured rat hepatocytes induced by carbon tetrachloride (CCl_4; Liu et al. 2003; Wang et al. 2007).

4.9.9   ANTIOXIDANT ACTIVITY

Tanshinone I, tanshinone IIB, cryptotanshinone, dihydrotanshinone I, methylenetanshinquinone and danshenxinkun B have demonstrated antioxidant activity (Zhang et al. 1990; Weng and Gordon 1992). Tanshinone IIA inhibited the association of lipid peroxidation products with DNA (Cao et al. 1996). Additionally, it was an effective antioxidant against LDL oxidation *in vitro*, and the mechanism appears to be related to its peroxyl radical scavenging and LDL binding activity. Tanshinone IIA's inhibition of LDL oxidation was beneficial in preventing development of atherosclerosis (Niu et al. 2000; Wang et al. 2007).

4.9.10   CARDIOVASCULAR ACTIVITY

Tanshinones and hydrophilic derivatives from *Danshen* have been extensively studied for cardiovascular activity (Ho and Hong 2011; Gao et al. 2012; Jia et al. 2012; Zeng et al. 2012).

4.9.11 OTHER BIOLOGICAL ACTIVITIES

Methyl tanshinonate, hydroxytanshinone, tanshinone IIA, and tanshinone IIB showed anti-platelet aggregation activity (Lee et al. 1987; Chang et al. 1990) and potential neuroprotective effects (Lam et al. 2003). Tanshinone IIA has the potential to ameliorate bone resorption diseases *in vivo* by reducing both the number and activity of osteoclasts (Kim et al. 2004). Cholinesterase is one of the targets for the treatment of Alzheimer's disease (AD), while cryptotanshinone and dihydrotanshinone I revealed anti-cholinesterase activity (Ren et al. 2004).

4.10 STRUCTURE–ACTIVITY RELATIONSHIP OF TANSHINONES

Tanshinone IIA has a drug-like steroid structural skeleton. The structure–activity relationship (SAR) of tanshinones and analogues included: (i) C15-addition of –SO_3Na group (sodium tanshinone IIA sulphonate) increasing water solubility; (ii) C4-$(CH_3)_2$ change to a double bond CH_2 increased anti-inflammatory effects; (iii) one C4-CH_3 change to –CH_2OH increased anti-inflammatory activity; (iv) C15 = C16 saturation (cryptotanshinone) maintained inhibitory effects on monocyte adhesion to endothelial cells, increased anti-inflammatory effects in LPS-stimulated macrophages, but lost inhibitory effects on foam cell formation; (v) C11-C12 substitution by nicotinic anhydride led to increased potency to decrease foam cell formation; (vi) C11-C12 insertion of oxygen (change to anhydrides) maintained inhibitory effects against foam cell formation, also increased anti-inflammatory effects; and (vii) C1-addition of acetoxyl group in sodium tanshinone IIA sulphonate exhibited potent anti-inflammatory effects (Figure 4.11; Fang et al. 2018).

4.11 *IN VIVO* STUDY OF TANSHINONES

It was stated that treatment with an herbal preparation containing *Danshen* (cardiotonic pills) causes inhibition of atherogenesis in the model of ApoE deficient mice (Ling et al. 2008). However, the role of the phytochemical constituents underlying this athero-protective effect remains obscure. Tang et al. (2007) and Chen et al. (2008) reported that tanshinone IIA decreased the atherosclerosis in hypercholesterolaemic rats and rabbits. In 2011, Tang et al. demonstrated that the oral administration of a tanshinone IIA preparation decreased the size of atherosclerotic plaques in chow-fed and high-cholesterol diet fed ApoE-deficient mice (Gao et al. 2012). Fang et al. (2007, 2008) also

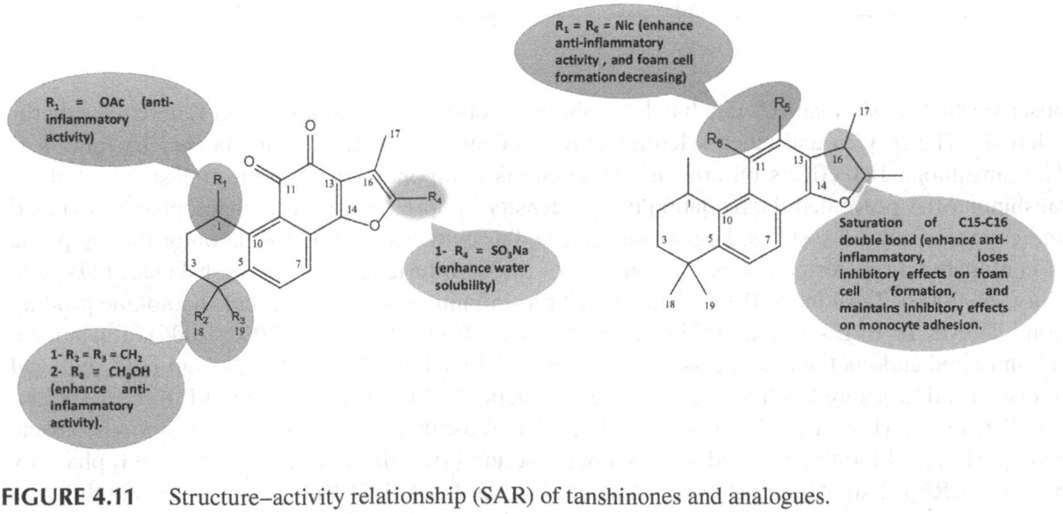

FIGURE 4.11 Structure–activity relationship (SAR) of tanshinones and analogues.

TABLE 4.1

In Vivo **Anti-Atherosclerotic Effects of** *Danshen*

Dosage (mg/kg/day)	Animal Model	Anti-Atherosclerotic Effects	References
35/70	Rat atherosclerotic calcification	↓ Vascular lipid and calcium; —Serum lipid; ↓ Serum oxLDL, ↓ superoxide anion; ↓ MDA; ↑ Cu/Zn-SOD mRNA and protein	Tang et al. (2007)
3/10/30	High-fat diet fed rabbit	—Serum lipid; ↓ Plaque burden improves pathological changes in coronary artery	Chen et al. (2008)
10/30/90	ApoE–/– mice	↓ Aortic sinus cross section lesion area; ↓ Lesion in aortic root ↓ PPAR-γ, CD36, LOX-1 mRNA expression	Tang et al. (2011)
6.25/15/37.5	High-fat diet fed rabbit	↓ Intimal lesion area; ↓ Pro-inflammatory cytokine (IL-1β, VCAM-1) ↓ MMP-2, MMP-9 expression and gelatinolytic activities	Fang et al. (2007)
6.25/15/37.5	High-fat diet fed rabbit	↑ SOD activity; ↓ MDA level, CD40 expression, MMP-2 activity	Fang et al. (2008)
13.3/40/120	Rat model of carotid artery	↓ Intima hyperplasia; Balloon injury ↓ PCNA expression in neointima ↓ FBS induced VSMC proliferation, BrdU incorporation cell cycle arrest at G0/G1 phase; ↓ ERK1/2 phosphorylation, c-fos expression	Li et al. (2010b)
300/600	Mouse carotid artery ligation model	↓ Intima hyperplasia; ↓ Intima/media ratio; ↓ PCNA expression in neointima	Du et al. (2005)
35	High-fat induced obesity in mice	↓ Obesity, ↓weight gain; ↑ Glucose tolerance; ↓ Lipid accumulation,; ↓LDL-C/HDL-C	Gong et al. (2009)

Source: Gao, S. et al., *Atherosclerosis*, 220, 3–10, 2012.

Note: ApoE–/–, ApoE deficient; ERK, extracellular signal-regulated kinases; FBS, fetal bovine serum; HDL, high-density lipoprotein; IL, interleukin; LDL, low-density lipoprotein; LOX-1, lectin-like oxidized LDL receptor-1; MDA, malondialdehyde; MMP, matrix metalloproteinase; oxLDL, oxidized LDL; PCNA, proliferating cell nuclear antigen; PPAR-γ, peroxisome proliferator-activated receptor gamma; SOD, superoxide dismutase; VCAM-1, vascular cellular adhesion molecule-1; VSMC, vascular smooth muscle cell.

observed that tanshinone IIA exhibited an inhibitory effect in high-fat diet fed rabbits on atherosclerosis. The *in vivo* anti-atherosclerotic activity of tanshinone IIA is summarized in Table 4.1. The tanshinone IIA effects on critical atherogenesis components have been intensively studied: tanshinone IIA prevented the oxidation of low-density lipoprotein (LDL) in macrophage-mediated and copper-catalysed systems. Its role was detected as evidenced by prolongation of the lag phase of conjugated diene formation and a reduction of thiobarbituric acid-reactive substances (TBARS; Niu et al. 2000). Tanshinone IIA downregulated pro-inflammatory cytokine and chemokine production (TNF-α, IL-6, IL-1β and iNOS) by inactivating NF-*k*B (Jang et al. 2003, 2006). Tanshinone IIA inhibited endothelial dysfunction by protecting endothelial cells (HUVEC) from H_2O_2-induced injury with decreasing CD40 expression and enhancing NO production *via* the PI3K-Akt-AMPK-eNOS pathway (Lin et al. 2006; Pan et al. 2011). Tanshinone IIA inhibited rat smooth muscle cells (SMC) proliferation induced by fetal bovine serum (via cell cycle arrest at the G_0/G_1 phase by blocking ERK1/2 signalling pathway; Wang et al. 2005; Li et al. 2010b) and Ang-II (via inhibition of calcineurin activity; Pan et al. 2009); and tanshinone IIA also prevented TNF-α-induced migration of human SMC through inhibition of the Akt-NF-kB-MMP-9 and ERK1/2 pathways (Jin et al. 2008). These *in vitro* data were confirmed by recent *in vivo* studies that tanshinone IIA prevents the formation of balloon injury-induced neointima (Du et al. 2005; Li et al. 2010b). Tanshinone IIA inhibited the formation of macrophage-derived foam cells by suppressing the expression of receptors of scavenger (CD36, SR-A, LOX-1) and resultant oxLDL uptake (Xu et al. 2010; Tang et al. 2011). Furthermore, tanshinone IIA caused the downregulation of MMP expression/activity and favourably modified plaque composition that increase stabilization of plaques (Gao et al. 2012).

4.12 CLINICAL TRIALS WITH *DANSHEN*

Danshen or Tanshen (Figure 4.12), the dried root or rhizomes of *S. miltiorrhiza* Bunge, has been and is used in traditional Chinese medicine throughout many Asian countries as a preventive or therapeutic remedy for coronary heart diseases, vascular diseases, stroke, hyperlipidaemia, endangiitis, arthritis and hepatitis (Zhou et al. 2005; Dong et al. 2011). Fufang *Danshen*, a composite multi-herbal formula containing *Danshen* as the major ingredient, is officially listed in the Chinese Pharmacopoeia for many health ailments. The Fufang *Danshen* dripping pill (one of the commercial forms of Fufang *Danshen*) has completed Phase II clinical trials for evaluating the efficacy and safety in patients with chronic stable angina pectoris in the United States (No. NCT00797953; Gao et al. 2012). Since the first isolation from *Danshen* by Nakao and Fukushima (1934) in the 1930s, tanshinones have been recognised for their potent biological activity.

4.13 CONCLUSION AND PERSPECTIVES

The potent biological activity of tanshinones such as their antibacterial, antioxidant, anti-inflammatory, antineoplastic and cardio-cerebrovascular protection effects make them attractive lead compounds. Further chemical and biological investigations are needed to enhance their solubility as well as biological activity. The cellular and molecular modes of action are still incompletely understood. Only cryptotanshinone, tanshinone I and tanshinone IIA are validated as TRAIL sensitizers to date, because of the lack of *in vivo* studies of tanshinone metabolites.

Sustainable sources for such compounds through synthetic and/or semi-synthetic routes as well as enzymatic transformation are important large-scale production.

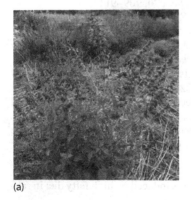 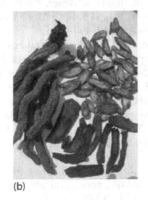 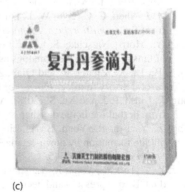

(a)   (b)   (c)

FIGURE 4.12 **(See color insert.)** (a) *Salvia miltiorrhiza* (*Danshen* or *Tanshen*), (b) root or rhizomes and (c) manufactured by Tasly Pharmaceuticals (http://www.tasly.com/) has completed phase II clinical trials in the United States (No. NCT00797953).

ACKNOWLEDGEMENT

Prof. Mohamed Hegazy gratefully acknowledges the financial support from the Alexander von Humboldt Foundation for the 'Georg Foster Research Fellowship for Experienced Researcher'.

REFERENCES

Adams, J. D., Wall, M. and Garcia, C. (2005). *Salvia columbariae* contains tanshinones. *Evidence-Based Complementary Alternative Medicine*, **2**, 107–110.

Arigoni, D., Sagner, S., Latzel, C., Eisenreich, W., Bacher, A. and Zenk, M. H. (1997). Terpenoid biosynthesis from 1-deoxy-D-xylulose in higher plants by intramolecular skeletal rearrangement. *Proceedings of the National Academy of Sciences of the USA*, **94**, 10600–10605.

Benowitz, S. (1996). As war on cancer hits 25-year mark, scientists see progress, challenges. *Scientist*, **10**, 1–7.

Bi, H. C., Zuo, Z., Chen, X., Xu, C. S., Wen, Y. Y., Sun, H. Y., Zhao, L. Z. et al. (2008). Preclinical factors affecting the pharmacokinetic behaviour of tanshinone IIA, an investigational new drug isolated from *Salvia miltiorrhiza* for the treatment of ischaemic heart diseases. *Xenobiotica*, **38**, 185–222.

Cao, E. H., Liu, X. Q., Wang, J. J. and Xu, N.F. (1996). Effect of natural antioxidant tanshinone II-A on DNA damage by lipid peroxidation in liver cells. *Free Radical Biology and Medicine*, **20**, 801–806.

Chang, H. M., Cheng, K. P., Choang, T. F., Chow, H. F., Chui, K. Y., Hon, P. M., Tan, F. W., Yang, Y. and Zhong, Z. P. (1990a). Structure elucidation and total synthesis of new tanshinones isolated from *Salvia miltiorrhiza* Bunge (Danshen). *Journal of Organic Chemistry*, **55**, 3537–3543.

Chang, W. L., Wu, W. L., Chen, Y. C. and Lin, H. C. (1990b). Biological activity of tanshinones. *Zhonghua Yaoxue Zazhi*, **42**, 183–185.

Chen, C. C., Chen, H. T., Chen, Y. P., Hsu, H. Y. and Hsieh, T. C. (1986). Isolation of the components of *Salviae miltiorrhizae* radix and their coronary dilator activities. *Taiwan Yaoxue Zazhi*, **38**, 226–230.

Chen, J., Shi, D. Y., Liu, S. L. and Zhong, L. (2012). Tanshinone IIA induces growth inhibition and apoptosis in gastric cancer in vitro and in vivo. *Oncology Reports*, **27**(2), 523–528.

Chen, W. Z. (1983). Pharmacology of *Salvia miltiorrhiza*. *Yaoxue Xuebao*, **19**, 876–880.

Chen, W. Y., Tang, F. T., Chen, S. R. and Liu, P. Q. (2008). Phylactic effect of tanshinone II-A on atherogenesis. *Zhong Guo Yao Fang*, **19**, 884–887.

Chen, Y., Tu, J. H., He, Y. J., Zhang, W., Wang, G., Tan, Z. R., Zhou, G., Fan, L. and Zhou, H. H. (2009). Effect of sodium tanshinone II A sulfonate on the activity of CYP1A2 in healthy volunteers. *Xenobiotica*, **39**, 508–513.

Choi, H. S. and Kim, K. M. (2004). Tanshinones inhibit mast cell degranulation by interfering with IgE receptor-mediated tyrosine phosphorylation of PLCg2 and MAPK. *Planta Medica*, **70**, 178–180.

Cunningham, F. X., Sun, Z., Chamovitz, D., Hirschberg, J. and Gantt, E. (1994). Molecular structure and enzymatic function of lycopene cyclase from the cyanobacterium *Synechococcus* sp. Strain PCC7942. *Plant Cell*, **6**, 1107–1121.

Dittmann, K., Gerhaeuser, C., Klimo, K. and Hamburger, M. (2004). HPLC-based activity profiling of *Salvia miltiorrhiza* for MAO A and iNOS inhibitory activities. *Planta Medica*, **70**, 909–913.

Don, M. J., Shen, C. C., Syu, W. J., Ding, Y. H. and Sun, C. M. (2006). Cytotoxic and aromatic constituents from *Salvia miltiorrhiza*. *Phytochemistry*, **67**, 497–503.

Dong, Y., Morris-Natschke, S. L. and Lee, K. H. (2011). Biosynthesis, total syntheses, and antitumor activity of tanshinones and their analogs as potential therapeutic agents. *Natural Product Reports*, **28**, 529–542.

Du, J. R., Li, X., Zhang, R. and Qian, Z. M. (2005). Tanshinone inhibits intimal hyperplasia in the ligated carotid artery in mice. *Journal of Ethnopharmacology*, **98**, 319–322.

Fang, J., Little, P. J. and Xu, S. (2018). Atheroprotective effects and molecular targets of tanshinones derived from herbal medicine danshen. *Medicinal Research Reviews*, **38**(1), 201–228.

Fang, Z. Y., Lin, R., Yuan, B. X., Liu, Y. and Zhang, H. (2007). Tanshinone IIA inhibits atherosclerotic plaque formation by down-regulating MMP-2 and MMP-9 expression in rabbits fed a high-fat diet. *Life Sciences*, **81**, 1339–1345.

Fang, Z. Y., Lin, R., Yuan, B. X., Yang, G. D., Liu, Y. and Zhang, H. (2008). Tanshinone IIA downregulates the CD40 expression and decreases MMP-2 activity on atherosclerosis induced by high fatty diet in rabbit. *Journal of Ethnopharmacology*, **115**, 217–222.

Gao, S., Liu, Z., Li, H., Little, P. J., Liu, P. and Xu, S. (2012). Cardiovascular actions and therapeutic potential of tanshinone IIA. *Atherosclerosis*, **220**, 3–10.

Gao, Y. G. (1983). Anti-inflammatory actions of tanshinone. *Zhong Xi Yi Jie He Za Zhi*, **3**, 300–301.

Gong, Y., Li, Y., Abdolmaleky, H. M., Li, L. and Zhou, J. R. (2012). Tanshinones inhibit the growth of breast cancer cells through epigenetic modification of Aurora A expression and function. *PLoS One*, **2012**, 7.

Gong, Z., Huang, C., Sheng, X., Zhang, Y., Li, Q., Wang, M. W., Peng, L. and Zang, Y. Q. (2009). The role of tanshinone IIA in the treatment of obesity through peroxisome proliferator-activated receptor gamma antagonism. *Endocrinology*, **150**, 104–113.

Gu, M., Su, Z. and Ouyang, F. (2006). Fingerprinting of *Salvia miltiorrhiza* Bunge by thin-layer chromatography scan compared with high speed countercurrent chromatography. *Journal of Liquid Chromatography & Related Technologies*, **29**, 1503–1514.

Gu, M., Zhang, G., Su, Z. and Ouyang, F. (2004). Identification of major active constituents in the fingerprint of *Salvia miltiorrhiza* Bunge developed by high-speed counter-current chromatography. *Journal of Chromatography A*, **1041**(1–2), 239–243.

Han, J. Y., Fan, J. Y., Horie, Y., Miura, S., Cui, D. H., Ishii, H., Hibi, T., Tsuneki, H. and Kimura, I. (2008). Ameliorating effects of compounds derived from *Salviamiltiorrhiza* root extract on microcirculatory disturbance and target organ injury by ischemia and reperfusion. *Pharmacology & Therapeutics*, **117**, 280–295.

Han, Y. M., Oh, H., Na, M., Kim, B. S., Oh, W. K., Kim, B. Y., Jeong, D. G., Ryu, S. E., Sok, D. E. and Ahn, J. S. (2005). PTP1B inhibitory effect of abietane Diterpenes isolated from *Salvia miltiorrhiza*. *Biological and Pharmaceutical Bulletin*, **28**(9), 1795–1797.

Ho, J. H. and Hong, C. Y. (2011). Salvianolic acids: Small compounds with multiple mechanisms for cardiovascular protection. *Journal of Biomedical Science*, **18**. doi:10.1186/1423-0127-18.

Ho, T. F. and Chang, C. C. (2015). A promising "TRAIL" of tanshinones for cancer therapy. *BioMedicine*, **5**(4), 29–35.

Honda, G., Koezuka, Y. and Tabata, M. (1988). Isolation of an antidermatophytic substance from the root of *Salvia miltiorrhiza*. *Chemical and Pharmaceutical Bulletin*, **36**, 408–411.

Ikeshiro, Y., Hashimoto, I., Iwamoto, Y., Mase, I. and Tomita, Y. (1991). Diterpenoids from *Salvia miltiorrhiza*. *Phytochemistry*, **30**, 2791–2792.

Jang, S. I., Jeong, S. I., Kim, K. J., Kim, H. J., Yu, H. H., Park, R., Kim, H. M. and You, Y. O. (2003). Tanshinone IIA from *Salvia miltiorrhiza* inhibits inducible nitric oxide synthase expression and production of TNF-α, IL-1beta and IL-6 in activated RAW 264.7 cells. *Planta Medica*, **69**, 1057–1059.

Jang, S. I., Kim, H. J., Kim, Y. J., Jeong, S. I. and You, Y. O. (2006). Tanshinone IIA inhibits LPS-induced NF-kappa B activation in RAW 264.7 cells: Possible involvement of the NIK-IKK, ERK1/2, p38 and JNK pathways. *European Journal of Pharmacology*, **542**, 1–7.

Jia, Y., Huang, F., Zhang, S. and Leung, S. W. (2012). Is danshen (*Salvia miltiorrhiza*) dripping pill more effective than isosorbide dinitrate in treating angina pectoris? A systematic review of randomized controlled trials. *International Journal of Cardiology*, **157**, 330–340.

Jin, U. H., Suh, S. J., Chang, H. W., Son, J. K., Lee, S. H., Son, K. H., Chang, Y. C. and Kim, C. H. (2008). Tanshinone IIA from *Salvia miltiorrhiza* BUNGE inhibits human aortic smooth muscle cell migration and MMP-9 activity through AKT signaling pathway. *Journal of Cellular Biochemistry*, **104**, 15–26.

Jung, S. H., Seol, H. J., Jeon, S. J., Son, K. H. and Lee, Y. R. (2009). Insulin-sensitizing activities of tanshinones, diterpene compounds of the root of *Salvia miltiorrhiza* Bunge. *Phytomedicine*, **6**(4), 327–335.

Kang, B. Y., Chung, S. W., Kim, S. H., Ryu, S. Y. and Kim, T. S. (2000). Inhibition of interleukin-12 and interferon-g production in immune cells by tanshinones from *Salvia miltiorrhiza*. *Immunopharmacology*, **49**, 355–361.

Kasimu, R., Tanaka, K., Tezuka, Y., Gong, Z. N., Li, J. X., Basnet, P., Namba, T. and Katota, S. (1998). Comparative study of seventeen *Salvia* plants: Aldose reductase inhibitory activity of water and MeOH extracts and liquid chromatography-mass spectrometry (LC-MS) analysis of water extracts. *Chemical and Pharmaceutical Bulletin*, **46**, 500–504.

Kim, D. H., Paude, P., Yu, T., Ngo, T. M., Kim, J. A., Jung, H. A., Yokozawa, T. and Choi, J. S. (2017). Characterization of the inhibitory activity of natural tanshinones from *Salvia miltiorrhiza* roots on protein tyrosine phosphatase 1B. *Chemico-Biological Interactions*, **278**, 65–73.

Kim, H. H., Kim, J. H., Kwak, H. B., Huang, H., Han, S. H., Ha, H., Lee, S. W., Woo, E. R. and Lee, Z. H. (2004). Inhibition of osteoclast differentiation and bone resorption by tanshinone IIA isolated from *Salvia miltiorrhiza* Bunge. *Biochemical Pharmacology*, **67**, 1647–1656.

Kim, J. Y., Kim, K. M., Nan, J. X., Zhao, Y. Z., Park, P. H., Lee, S. J. and Sohn, D. H. (2003). Induction of apoptosis by tanshinone I via cytochrome c release in activated hepatic stellate cells. *Pharmacology & Toxicology*, **92**, 195–200.

Kim, S. Y., Moon, T. C., Chang, H. W., Son, K. H., Kang, S. S. and Kim, H. P. (2002). Effects of tanshinone I isolated from *Salvia miltiorrhiza* Bunge on arachidonic acid metabolism and *in vivo* inflammatory responses. *Phytotherapy Research*, **16**, 616–620.

Kong, D. Y. (1989). Chemical constituents of *Salvia miltiorrhiza* (Danshen). *Zhongguo Yiyao Gongye Zazhi*, **20**, 279–285.

Lam, B. Y. H., Lo, A. C. Y., Sun, X., Luo, H.W., Chung, S. K. and Sucher, N. J. (2003). Neuroprotective effects of tanshinones in transient focal cerebral ischemia in mice. *Phytomedicine*, **10**, 286–291.

Lee, A. R., Wu, W. L., Chang, W. L., Lin, H. C. and King, M. L. (1987). Isolation and bioactivity of new tanshinones. *Journal of Natural Products*, **50**, 157–160.

Lee, D. S., Lee, S. H., Noh, J. G. and Hong, S. D. (1999). Antibacterial activities of cryptotanshinone and dihydrotanshinone I from a medicinal herb, *Salvia miltiorrhiza* Bunge. *Bioscience, Biotechnology, and Biochemistry*, **63**, 2236–2239.

Lee, W. Y. W., Cheung, C. C. M., Liu, K. W., Fung, K. P., Wong, J., Lai, P. B. and Yeung, J. H. (2010). Cytotoxic effects of tanshinones from *Salvia miltiorrhiza* on doxorubicin-resistant human liver cancer cells. *Journal of Natural Products*, **73**(5), 854–859.

Li, B., Niu, F. D., Li, Z. W., Zhang, H. J., Wang, D. Z. and Sun, H. D. (1991). Diterpenoids from the roots of *Salvia przewalskii*. *Phytochemistry*, **30**, 3815–3817.

Li, H. and Chen F. (2001). Preparative isolation and purification of six diterpenoids from the Chinese medicinal plant *Salvia miltiorrhiza* by high-speed counter-current chromatography. *Journal of Chromatography A*, **925**, 109–114.

Li, J., He, L. Y. and Song, W. Z. (1993). Separation and quantitative determination of seven aqueous depsides in *Salvia miltiorrhiza* by HPTLC scanning. *Yaoxue Xuebao*, **28**, 543–547.

Li, M. H., Chen, J. M., Peng, Y., Wu, Q. and Xiao, P. G. (2008). Investigation of Danshen and related medicinal plants in China. *Journal of Ethnopharmacology*, **120**, 419–426.

Li, M. H., Peng, Y. and Xiao, P. G. (2010a). Distribution of tanshinones in the genus *Salvia* (family Lamiaceae) from China and its systematic significance. *International Journal of Systematic and Evolutionary Microbiology*, **48**, 118–122.

Li, X., Du, J. R., Yu, Y., Bai, B. and Zheng, X. Y. (2010b). Tanshinone IIA inhibits smooth muscle proliferation and intimal hyperplasia in the rat carotid balloon-injured model through inhibition of MAPK signaling pathway. *Journal of Ethnopharmacology*, **129**, 273–279.

Liang, J., Meng, J., Guo, M., Yang, Z. and Wu, S. (2013). Conical coils counter-current chromatography for preparative isolation and purification of tanshinones from *Salvia miltiorrhiza* Bunge. *Journal of Chromatography A*, **1288**, 35–39.

Lin, R., Wang, W. R., Liu, J. T., Yang, G. D. and Han, C. J. (2006). Protective effect of tanshinone IIA on human umbilical vein endothelial cell injured by hydrogen peroxide and its mechanism. *Journal of Ethnopharmacology*, **108**, 217–222.

Lin, W., Deng, J., Lu, M., Ou, X., Lin, N., Yang, G. and Liang, H. (2008). The research in production of Danshen in three main cultivations in China. *Journal of Chinese Medicinal Materials*, **31**, 338–340.

Ling, S., Dai, A., Guo, Z. and Paul, A. (2008). A preparation of herbal medicine *Salvia miltiorrhiza* reduces expression of intercellular adhesion molecule-1 and development of atherosclerosis in apolipoprotein E-deficient mice. *Journal of Cardiovascular Pharmacology and Therapeutics*, **51**, 38–44.

Liu, A. H., Li, L., Xu, M., Lin, Y. H., Guo, H. Z. and Guo, D. A. (2006). Simultaneous quantification of six major phenolic acids in the roots of *Salvia miltiorrhiza* and four related traditional Chinese medicinal preparations by HPLC–DAD method. *Journal of Pharmaceutical and Biomedical Analysis*, **41**, 48–56.

Liu, C., Li, J., Wang, L., Wu, F., Huang, L., Xu, Y., Ye, J., Xiao, B., Meng, F., Chen, S. and Yang, M. (2012). Analysis of tanshinone IIA induced cellular apoptosis in leukemia cells by genomewide expression profiling. *BMC Complementary and Alternative Medicine*, **12**(5), 1–10.

Liu, Y., Wang, X. and Liu, Y. (2003). Protective effects of tanshinone IIA on injured primary cultured rat hepatocytes induced by CCl4. *Zhong Yao Cai*, **26**, 415–417.

Lu, Q., Zhang, P., Zhang, X. and Chen, J. (2009). Experimental study of the anti-cancer mechanism of tanshinone IIA against human breast cancer. *International Journal of Molecular Medicine*, **24**(6), 773–780.

Lusarczyk, S., Zimmermann, S., Kaiser, M., Matkowki, A., Hamburger, M. and Adams, M. (2011). Antiplasmodial and antitrypanosomal activity of tanshinone-type diterpenoids from *Salvia miltiorrhiza*. *Planta Medica*, **77**(14), 1594–1596.

Ma, L., Zhang, X., Guo, H. and Gan, Y. (2006). Determination of four water-soluble compounds in *Salvia miltiorrhiza* Bunge by high-performance liquid chromatography with a coulometric electrode array system. *Journal of Chromatography B*, **833**, 260–263.

Maki, T., Kawahara, Y., Tanonaka, K., Yagi, A. and Takeo, S. (2002). Effects of tanshinone VI on the hypertrophy of cardiac myocytes and fibrosis of cardiac fibroblasts of neonatal rats. *Planta Medica*, **68**, 1103–1107.

Matkowski, A., Zielińska, S., Oszmiański, J. and Lamer-Zarawska, E. (2008). Antioxidant activity of extracts from leaves and roots of *Salvia miltiorrhiza* Bunge, *S. przewalskii* Maxim., and *S. verticillata* L. *Bioresource Technology*, **99**, 7892–7896.

Nagarajan, A. and Brindha, P. (2012). Diterpenes–A review on therapeutic uses with special emphasis on antidiabetic activity. *Journal of Pharmacy Research*, **5**(8), 4530–4540.

Nakao, M. and Fukushima, T. (1934). On the chemical composition of *Salvia miltiorrhiza* (Chinese drug Tanshen). *Yakugaku Zasshi*, **54**, 844–858.

Newman, D. J. and Cragg, G. M. (2007). Natural products as sources of new drugs over the last 25 years. *Journal of Natural Products*, **70**, 461–477.

Newman, D. J., Cragg, G. M. and Snader, K. M. (2003). Natural products as sources of new drugs over the period 1981–2002. *Journal of Natural Products*, **66**, 1022–1037.

Ni, W., Qian, W. and Tong, X. (2014). Cryptotanshinone induces apoptosis of HL-60 cells via mitochondrial pathway. *Tropical Journal of Pharmacy Research*, **13**(4), 545–551.

Niu, X. L., Ichimori, K., Yang, X., Hirota, Y., Hoshiai, K., Li, M. and Nakazawa, H. (2000). Tanshinone II-A inhibits lowdensity lipoprotein oxidation in vitro. *Free Radical Research*, **33**, 305–312.

Nizamutdinova, I. T., Lee, G. W., Son, K. H., Jeon, S. J., Kang, S. S., Kim, Y. S., Lee, J. H., Seo, H. G., Chang, K. C. and Kim, H. J. (2008a). Tanshinone I effectively induces apoptosis in estrogen receptor-positive (MCF-7) and estrogen receptor-negative (MDA-MB-231) breast cancer cells. *International Journal of Oncology*, **33**(3), 485–491.

Nizamutdinova, I. T., Lee, G. W., Lee, J. S., Cho, M. K., Son, K. H., Jeon, S. J., Kang, S. S. et al. (2008b). Tanshinone I suppresses growth and invasion of humanbreast cancer cells, MDA-MB-231, through regulation of adhesion molecules. *Carcinogenesis*, **29**, 1885–1892.

Pan, C., Lou, L., Huo, Y., Singh, G., Chen, M., Zhang, D., Wu, A., Zhao, M., Wang, S. and Li, J. (2011). Salvianolic acid B and tanshinone IIA attenuate myocardial ischemia injury in mice by NO production through multiple pathways. *Therapeutic Advances in Cardiovascular Disease*, **5**, 99–111.

Pan, Y. J., Li, X. Y. and Yang, G. T. (2009). Effect of tanshinone II A on the calcineurin activity in proliferating vascular smooth muscle cells of rats. *Chinese Journal of Integrative Medicine*, **29**, 133–135.

Pan, Z. H., Li, Y., Wu, X. D., He, J., Chen, X. Q., Xu, G., Peng, L. Y. and Zhao, Q. S. (2012). Norditerpenoids from *Salvia castanea* Diels f. pubescens. *Fitoterapia*, **83**(6), 1072–1075.

Qiao, X., Zhang, Y. T., Ye, M., Wang, B. R., Han, J. and Guo, D. (2009). Analysis of chemical constituents and taxonomic similarity of *Salvia* species in China using LC/MS. *Planta Medica*, **75**, 1613–1617.

Ren, Y., Houghton, P. J., Hider, R. C. and Howes, M. J. R. (2004). Novel diterpenoid acetylcholinesterase inhibitors from *Salvia miltiorrhiza*. *Planta Medica*, **70**, 201–204.

Rohmer, M. (1999). The discovery of a mevalonate-independent pathway for isoprenoid biosynthesis in bacteria, algae and higher plants. *Natural Product Reports*, **16**, 565–574.

Romanova, A., Pribylova, G., Patudin, A., Leskova, E., Pakaln, D. and Ban'kovskii, A. (1972). The quinones of some species of sage. *Chemistry of Natural Compounds*, **8**, 231–232.

Ryu, S. Y., Oak, M. H. and Kim, K. M. (1999). Inhibition of mast cell degranulation by tanshinones from the roots of *Salvia miltiorrhiza*. *Planta Medica*, **65**, 654–655.

Seto, H., Watanabe, H. and Furihata, K. (1996). Simultaneous operation of the mevalonate and non-mevalonate pathways in the biosynthesis of isopentenyl diphosphate in *Streptomyces aeriouvifer*. *Tetrahedron Letters*, **37**, 7979–7982.

Skała, E. and Wysokińska, H. (2005). Tanshinone production in roots of micropropagated *Salvia przewalskii* Maxim. *Zeitschrift für Naturforschung C*, **60**, 583–586.

Su, C. C., Chen, G. W. and Lin, J. G. (2008). Growth inhibition and apoptosis induction by tanshinone I in human colon cancer Colo 205 cells. *International Journal of Molecular Medicine*, **22**, 613–618.

Sun, P., He, Y. L., Zhou, L. L., Qi, J. J., Rui, Y. and Li, X. E. (2012). Effects of genotype and environment on active components of *Salviae miltiorrhizae* by HPLC. *Asian Journal of Chemistry*, **24**, 2146–2150.

Sung, H. J., Choi S. M., Yoon, Y. and An, K. S. (1999). Tanshinone IIA, an ingredient of *Salvia miltiorrhiza* BUNGE, induces apoptosis in human leukemia cell lines through the activation of caspase-3. *Experimental and Molecular Medicine*, **31**(4), 174–178.

Takahashi, K., Ouyang, X., Komatsu, K., Nakamura, N., Hattori, M., Baba, A. and Azuma, J. (2002). Sodium tanshinone IIA sulfonate derived from Danshen (*Salvia miltiorrhiza*) attenuates hypertrophy induced by angiotensin II in cultured neonatal rat cardiac cells. *Biochemical Pharmacology*, **64**, 745–750.

Takeo, S., Tanonaka, K., Hirai, K., Kawaguchi, K., Ogawa, M., Yagi, A. and Fujimoto, K. (1990). Beneficial effect of Tan-Shen, an extract from the root of *Salvia*, on post-hypoxic recovery of cardiac contractile force. *Biochemical Pharmacology*, **40**, 1137–1143.

Tan, X., Yang, Y., Cheng, J., Li, P., Inoue, I. and Zeng, X. (2011). Unique action of sodium tanshinone II-A sulfonate (DS-201) on the Ca^{2+} dependent BK_{Ca} activation in mouse cerebral arterial smooth muscle cells. *European Journal of Pharmacology*, **656**, 27–32.

Tang, F., Wu, X., Wang, T., Wang, L. J., Guo, J., Zhou, X. S., Xu, S. W., Liu, W. H., Liu, P. Q. and Huang, H. Q. (2007). Tanshinone II A attenuates atherosclerotic calcification in rat model by inhibition of oxidative stress. *Vascular Pharmacology*, **46**, 427–438.

Tang, F. T., Cao, Y., Wang, T. Q., Wang, L. J., Guo, J., Zhou, X. S., Xu, S. W., Liu, W. H., Liu, P. Q. and Huang, H.Q. (2011). Tanshinone IIA attenuates atherosclerosis in ApoE(–/–) mice through down-regulation of scavenger receptor expression. *European Journal of Pharmacology*, **650**, 275–284.

Tezuka, Y., Kasimu, R., Li, J. X., Basnet, P., Tanaka, K., Namba, T. and Kadota, S. (1998). ChemInform abstract: Constituents of roots of *Salvia deserta* SCHANG. (Xinjiang-Danshen). *ChemInform*, **29**. doi:10.1002/chin.199828287.

Wang, H., Gao, X. and Zhang, B. (2005). Tanshinone: An inhibitor of proliferation of vascular smooth muscle cells. *Journal of Ethnopharmacology*, **99**, 93–98.

Wang, J. W. and Wu, J. Y. (2010). Tanshinone biosynthesis in *Salvia miltiorrhiza* and production in plant tissue cultures. *Applied Microbiology and Biotechnology*, **88**, 437–449.

Wang, K. and Ohnuma, S. (1999). Chain-length determination mechanism of isoprenyl diphosphate synthases and implications for molecular evolution. *Trends in Biochemical Sciences*, **24**, 445–451.

Wang, N., Niwa, M. and Luo, H. W. (1988). Triterpenoids from *Salvia przewalskii*. *Phytochemistry*, **27**, 299–301.

Wang, X., Cui, G., Huang, L. and Qiu, D. (2007a). Effects of methyl jasmonate on accumulation and release of tanshinones in suspension cultures of *Salvia miltiorrhiza* hairy root. *Zhongguo Zhongyao Zazhi*, **32**, 300–302.

Wang, X., Morris-Natschke, S. L. and Lee, K. H. (2007b). New developments in the chemistry and biology of the bioactive constituents of Tanshen. *Medicinal Research Reviews*, **27**(1), 133–148.

Wei, Y. J., Li, S. L. and Li, P. (2007). Simultaneous determination of seven active components of Fufang Danshen tablet by high-performance liquid chromatography. *Biomedical Chromatography*, **21**, 1–9.

Weng, X. C. and Gordon, M. H. (1992). Antioxidant activity of quinones extracted from tanshen (*Salvia miltiorrhiza* Bunge). *Journal of Agricultural and Food Chemistry*, **40**, 1331–1336.

Wu, N., Ma, W. C., Mao, S. J., Wu, Y. and Jin, H. (2017). Total synthesis of tanshinone I. *Journal of Natural Products*, **80**(5), 1697–1700.

Xu, G., Yang, J., Wang, Y. Y., Peng, L. Y., Yang, X. W., Pan, Z. H., Liu, E. D., Li, Y. and Zhao, Q. S. (2010a). Diterpenoid constituents of the roots of *Salvia digitaloides*. *Journal of Agricultural and Food Chemistry*, **58**(23), 12157–12161.

Xu, S. W., Tang, F. T., Le, K., Lan, T., Shen, X. Y., Huang H. Q. and Liu P. Q. (2010b). Tanshinone IIA inhibits oxidized low-density lipoprotein induced LOX-1 expression in murine macrophages by reduction of intracellular reactive oxygen species and NF-kappa B activation (Abstract). *Circulation*, **122**, 292.

Yagi, A., Okamura, N., Tanonaka, K. and Takeo, S. (1994). Effects of tanshinone VI derivatives on post-hypoxic contractile dysfunction of perfused rat hearts. *Planta Medica*, **60**, 405–409.

Yagi, A. and Takeo, S. (2003). Anti-inflammatory constituents, aloesin and aloemannan in Aloe species and effects of tanshinone VI in *Salvia miltiorrhiza* on heart. *Yakugaku Zasshi*, **123**, 517–532.

Yang, H., Ip, S. P., Sun, H. D. and Che, C. T. (2003). Constituents of *Salvia trijuga*. *Pharmaceutical Biology*, **41**, 375–378.

Yang, M., Liu, A., Guan, S., Sun, J., Xu, M. and Guo, D. (2006). Characterization of tanshinones in the roots of *Salvia miltiorrhiza* (Dan-shen) by high-performance liquid chromatography with electrospray ionization tandem mass spectrometry. *Rapid Communications in Mass Spectrometry*, **20**, 1266–1280.

Yang, M. H., Blunden, G., Xu, Y. X., Nagy, G. and MáThé, I. (1996). Diterpenoids from *Salvia* species. *Pharmacy and Pharmacology Communications*, **2**, 69–71.

Yongmoon, H. and Lnkyung, J. (2013). Antifungal effect of tanshinone from *Salvia miltiorrhiza* against disseminated candidiasis. *Yakhak Hoeji*, **57**(2), 119–124.

Yuan, S. L., Wang, X. J. and Wei, Y. Q. (2003). Anticancer effect of tanshinone and its mechanisms. *Ai Zheng*, **22**, 1363–1366.

Zeng, Y., Song, J. X. and Shen, X. C. (2012). Herbal remedies supply a novel prospect for the treatment of atherosclerosis: A review of current mechanism studies. *Phytotherapy Research*, **26**, 159–167.

Zhang, J., Huang, M., Guan, S., Bi, H. C., Pan, Y., Duan, W., Chan, S. Y. et al. (2006). A mechanistic study of the intestinal absorption of cryptotanshinone, the major active constituent of *Salvia miltiorrhiza*. *Journal of Pharmacology and Experimental Therapeutics*, **317**, 1285–1294.

Zhang, K. Q., Bao, Y., Wu, P., Rosen, R. T. and Ho, C. T. (1990). Antioxidative components of tanshen (*Salvia miltiorhiza* Bung). *Journal of Agricultural and Food Chemistry*, **38**, 1194–1197.

Zhang, Y., Jiang, P., Ye, M., Kim, S. H., Jiang, C. and Lu, J. (2012). Tanshinones: Sources, pharmacokinetics and anti-cancer activities. *International Journal of Molecular Sciences*, **13**(10), 13621–13666.

Zhao, J., Lou, J., Mou, Y., Li, P., Wu, J. and Zhou, L. (2011). Diterpenoid tanshinones and phenolic acids from cultured hairy roots of *Salvia miltiorrhiza* Bunge and their antimicrobial activities. *Molecules*, **16**, 2259–2267.

Zhao, R. N., Xie, P. S., Yin, W. P., Lu, P. H., Yan, Y. Z. and Wang, Z. D. (2006). Quality analysis of "whitish" radix *Salvia mltiorrhiza* in Luanchuan region of Henan province by TLC and HPLC. *Chinese Traditional Herbal Drugs*, **37**, 119–122.

Zhou, L., Zuo, Z. and Chow, M. S. (2005). Danshen: An overview of its chemistry, pharmacology, pharmacokinetics, and clinical use. *Journal of Clinical Pharmacology*, **45**(12), 1345–1359.

Zhou, X., Jia, M. and Zhang, Y. (2011). The effect of Tanshinone I on proliferation and apoptosis of human gastric adenocarcinoma cell line SGC-7901. *Journal of Modern Oncology*, **19**, 23–27.

5 Bacognize
A Standardised Extract of *Bacopa monnieri*

L. Hingorani

CONTENTS

5.1 INTRODUCTION

Bacopa monnieri, known as Brahmi in Ayurveda, has been used in India since antiquity. This herb grows in wet and damp areas. Its habitat is throughout India, Nepal, Sri Lanka, China, Taiwan, Vietnam, Florida, Hawaii and some southern states of the United States. Brahmi is a small, creeping, succulent herb with short, petiolate, oblong leaves, rooting at the nodes. The stem is 10–30 cm long, 1–2 mm thick, with soft, glabrous ascending branches. Leaves are 0.6–2.5 cm long and 3–8 mm wide. Flowers are white or purple and have four to five petals. Brahmi has no distinct odour, but it tastes bitter. It is mentioned in *Charaka Samhita*, which calls it Madhya rasayan, meaning it has cognitive and memory-improving properties with neuronal protective and regenerative capabilities. *Charaka* also mentioned this herb under Prajasthapan (herbs that stabilise pregnancy) and Balya (herbs that improve strength and immunity). Traditionally, juice of Brahmi leaves is used to treat dementia, insomnia, epilepsy and insanity. It is also a well-known brain tonic recommended for memory and cognitive improvement in children. It is also used in the treatment of anaemia, bronchitis, asthma and diabetes.

According to Ayurveda, Brahmi balances Pitta, rejuvenates Sadhaka pitta – which has influence on Dhi (power of learning), Dhruti (power of retention) and Smriti (power of recall) – hence it is used for memory and cognitive improvement. Brahmi reduces Kapha dosha and controls aggravation of Vata dosha. It replenishes deficient Majja Dhatu (nervous system) and that is the reason it is used in Alzheimer's disease, Parkinson's disease, attention-deficit/hyperactivity disorder, insomnia and depression.

Kapodvadk, Somvalli and Saraswati are the synonyms of Brahmi. Manduki, Twastri, Divya and Mahaushadhi are the synonyms of Mandukaparni. Charaka, Sushruta and Vagbhata have mentioned Brahmi (*Bacopa monnieri*) and Mandukaparni (*Centella asiatica*) as two herbs, but due to the similarity of properties Bhavprakash and Hemadri treated both as same.

Over the last few decades, research interest in Brahmi has grown to evaluate its efficacy in brain health, particularly in mood regulation, memory improvement, age-related cognitive decline (senile dementia) and Alzheimer's disease.

Bacopa has been widely studied for its activity in enhancing memory. Most of the studies have been done on its alcoholic or hydro-alcoholic extracts. Earlier studies referred to Bacoside A and B being its active components, which have now been found to be a mixture of phytochemicals. In the search for studies with the standardised product of Bacopa, we found that like any other herbal product, the studies lacked standardisation of the product used in those studies. Bacognize® is the standardised extract of *Bacopa monnieri* used in our studies.

5.2 PHYTOCHEMISTRY

Due to the pharmacological importance of *Bacopa monnieri*, chemical examinations of the plant have been carried out by various groups of researchers globally. Detailed investigations were first documented as early as 1931, when Bose and Bose reported the isolation of the 'brahmine' (alkaloid) from *B. monnieri* followed by identification of other alkaloids like nicotine and herpestine (Chopra et al. 1956), D-mannitol, saponin, hersaponin and potassium salts (Sastri et al. 1959).

During the isolation of Bacoside A, an artefact Bacoside B usually co-occurs. Bacoside A was found to be levorotary and Bacoside B as dextrorotatory due to differences in their carbohydrate chain configuration (Gohil and Patel 2010).

The major chemical constituents isolated and characterised using various major spectral, 2D NMR and chemical studies by various research groups from the alcoholic extract of the herb are dammarane-type triterpenoid saponins with jujubogenin and pseudojujubogenin as aglycones. The chemical composition of bacosides contained in the polar fraction has also been established on the basis of chemical and physical degradation studies. On acid hydrolysis, bacosides yield a mixture of aglycones, bacogenin A1, A2, A3 and A4 (Kulshreshtha and Rastogi 1973, 1974; Chandel et al. 1977; Rastogi et al. 1994), among which the major component was ebelin lactone pseudojujubogenin (bacogenin A4). In view of the increasing interest in this herbal drug, Chakravarty et al. (2002) isolated three phenylethanoid glycosides: monnierasides I–III along with the known analogue plantainoside B from the glycosidic fraction of *B. monnieri*. The composition of bacoside A was established as a mixture of four triglycosidic saponins: Bacoside A3, Bacopaside II, 3-*O*-[α-L-arabinofuranosyl-(1→2)-{β-D-glucopyranosyl-(1→3)-}-α-L-arabinopyranosyl] jujubogenin and Bacopasaponin C (Deepak et al. 2005). Impugned bacoside B has also been reported as a mixture of four diglycosidic saponins – Bacopaside N1, Bacopaside N2, Bacopaside-IV and Bacopaside-V (Sivaramakrishna et al. 2005) – and their identity needs further establishment (Mundkinajeddu and Agarwal 2013). Pawar and Bhutani (2006) isolated two dammarane glycosides from aqueous extracts of the plant. The chemical structure of these compounds have been established as 20-*O*-α-L-arabinopyranosyl jujubogenin and 3-*O*-α-L-arabinopyranosyl jujubogenin on the basis of LC-MS, IR,1D- and 2D-NMR studies.

A new sterol glycoside, bacosterol-3-O-β-D-glucopyranoside along with bacopasaponin C, baco-paside I, bacopaside II, bacosterol, bacosine, luteolin-7-O-β-glucopyranoside and four cucurbitacins, bacobitacin A (I)-D, a known cytotoxic, cucurbitacin E, together with three known phenylethanoid glycosides – monnieraside I, III and plantioside B – were also isolated from *B. monnieri* (Bhandari et al. 2006, 2007). Zhou et al. (2007) isolated three new triterpene glycosides, bacopasides VI–VIII, together with three known analogues from the whole plant: bacopaside I, bacopaside II, and baco-pasaponin C. Suresh et al. (2010) also extracted using ethyl acetate a chalcone-type compound 2,4,6-trihydroxy-5-(3,3-di-Me propenyl)-3-(4-hydroxyphenyl) propiophenone from *B. monnieri*. Other major compounds reported from this plant include phenylethanoid glycosides, flavonoids, amino acids such as alpha-alanine, aspartic acid, glutamic acid, and betulinic acid, stigmasterol, b-sitosterol and stigmastanol (Chatterji et al. 1963; Jain and Kulshreshtha 1993; Russo and Borrelli 2005) (Table 5.1).

TABLE 5.1
Saponins Characterised in *B. monnieri* Using Different Spectroscopic and Chemical Transformation Methods

Name	Derivative	References
Jujubogenin Derivatives		
Bacoside A$_1$	3-O-[α-L-arabinofuranosyl(1→3)]-α-L-arabinopyranoside	Jain and Kulshreshtha (1993)
Bacoside A3	3-O-α-L-arabinofuranosyl-(1→2)-[β-D-glucopyranosyl-(1→3)]-β-D-glucopyranoside	Rastogi et al. (1994)
Bacopasaponin A	3,20-di-O-α-L-arabinopyranoside	Garai et al. (1996a)
Bacopasaponin E	3-O-α-L-arabinofuranosyl-(1→2)-[β-D-glucopyranosyl-(1→3)]-α-L-arabinopyranoside, 20-O-α-L-arabinopyranoside	Mahato et al. (2000)
Bacopasaponin F	3-O-α-L-arabinofuranosyl-(1→2)-[β-D-glucopyranosyl-(1→3)]-β-D-glucopyranoside, 20-O-α-L-arabinopyranoside	
Bacopasaponin G	3-O-[α-L-arabinofuranosyl-(1→2)]-α-L-arabinopyranoside	Hou et al. (2002)
Bacopaside III	3-O-α-L-arabinofuranosyl-(1→2)-ß-D-glucopyranosyl	Chakravarty et al. (2003)
Bacopaside IV	3-O-ß-D-glucopyranosyl-(1→3)-α-L-arabinopyranosyl	
Bacopaside IX	3-O-{ß-D-glucopyranosyl(1→4)[α-L-arabinofuranosyl-(1→2)]-ß-D-glucopyranosyl}-20-O-α-L-arabinopyranosyl	Zhou et al. (2009)
Pseudojujubogenin Derivatives		
Bacopasaponin B	3-O-[α-L-arabinofuranosyl-(1→2)]-α-L-arabinopyranoside	Garai et al. (1996a, 1996b)
Bacopasaponin C	3-O-α-L-arabinofuranosyl-(1→2)-[β-D-glucopyranosyl-(1→3)]-α-L-arabinopyranoside	
Bacopasaponin D	3-O-[α-L-arabinofuranosyl-(1→2)]-β-D-glucopyranoside	
Bacoside A$_2$	3-O-α-L-arabinopyranosyl-(1→5)-[α-L-arabinofuranosyl-(1→6)]-α-D-glucofuranoside	Rastogi and Kulshreshtha (1999)
Bacopaside III	3-O-[6-O-sulfonyl-β-D-glucopyranosyl-(1→3)]-α-L-arabinopyranoside	Hou et al. (2002)
Bacopaside I, Bacopaside V	3-O-α-L-arabinofuranosyl-(1→2)-[6-O-sulfonyl-β-D-glucopyranosyl-(1→3)]-α-L-arabinopyranoside, 3-O-ß-D-glucopyranosyl-(1→3)-α-L-arabinofuranosyl	Chakravarty et al. (2001, 2003)
Bacopaside II	3-O-α-L-arabinofuranosyl-(1→2)-[β-D-glucopyranosyl-(1→3)]-β-D-glucopyranoside	
Bacopasaponin H	3-O-[α-L-arabinopyranosyl]	Mandal and Mukhopadhyay (2004)
Bacopaside XI	3-O-[ß-D-arabinofuranosyl (1→3)]-6-O-sulfonyl-ß-D-glucopyranosyl	Bhandari et al. (2009)
Bacopaside XII	3-O-{ß-D-glucopyranosyl(1→3)[ß-D-arabinofuranosyl(1→2)]-ß-D-glucopyranosyl}-20-O-ß-D-arabinopyranosyl	

5.3 QUANTIFICATION METHODS

Some methods have been reported in the literature for the quantification of bacosides in plant extracts and formulations. In accordance with the method elaborated by Pal and co-workers, Bacoside A, a triterpenoid glycoside, was primarily hydrolysed to release aglycone which was then quantified by UV spectrophotometry. As far as TLC is concerned 'Bacoside A', despite being a mixture of saponins, gives single spot on normal phase TLC and this behaviour has been utilised for HPTLC based estimations. Due to this reason, the HPTLC method has an inherent limitation of not estimating the individual saponins of 'Bacoside A'. The major limitation of this method is that it lacks specificity and has interference from other hydrolysed compounds.

Over the years, HPLC methods were also developed for the quantification of bacosides in *Bacopa monnieri* extracts and formulations. Ganzera et al. (2004) reported the method for quantification of six saponins using gradient HPLC with PDA detector, but one of the major peaks was not completely characterised.

Deepak et al. determined bacoside A, which contains 4 compounds by HPLC, but did not consider bacoside B. In another report, bacosides were estimated by HPLC, coupled NMR and MS, and the bioassay methods were described.

As the number of aged people suffering from cognitive problems increases, memory boosters have gained immense importance and there is an urgent need to develop sensitive and reliable quality control techniques to establish the authenticity and purity of memory boosting formulations. The value of the method increases with the estimation of all the characteristic compounds present in the extracts, because the major components could be present in several closely related species.

Later in another publication, 12 different saponins were determined by HPLC in the dried herb samples of *B. monnieri*. As per the findings of this paper, a set of five saponins – the four saponins of 'bacoside A' as Bacoside A3 (1), Bacopaside II (2), Bacopasaponin C (3), jujubogenin isomer of bacopasaponin C (4) and another saponin bacopaside I (5) – constituted more than 96% w/w of the total saponins of *B. monnieri*. Interestingly, these five saponins are now required to be measured to study the compliance to analytical monographs on *B. monnieri* published in the United States Pharmacopoeia. The Indian Pharmacopoeia and the Ayurvedic Pharmacopoeia of India have monographs based on the estimation of the four saponins (1–4) of 'bacoside A', while the British Pharmacopoeia monograph on *B. monnieri* has a procedure for the estimation of total content of Bacopa saponins calculated using compound 2 as the reference standard. Many chromatographic methods based on HPLC and HPTLC have been published for determination of saponins of 'bacoside A' in the literature (Shrikumar et al. 2004; Agrawal et al. 2006; Phrompittayarat et al. 2007; Bhandari et al. 2009; Shinde et al. 2011; Tothiam et al. 2011; Srivastava et al. 2012). Most of the reported HPLC methods utilised classical reverse phase HPLC columns (based on C18) using gradient elution with acetonitrile and water mixtures.

Strangely, no major scientific studies have been published on 'bacoside B'. The only available paper, to the best of our knowledge, indicated that 'bacoside B' is a mixture of four saponins: bacopaside N1 (6), bacopaside N2 (7), bacopaside IV (8) and bacopaside V (9). Although the authors provided data to support the given chemical structures of 6–9 in the paper, they did not provide the basis to call the mixture 'bacoside B'. The details given by Sivaramakrishna et al. (2005) contradicts the original papers which described the structural features and chromatographic behaviour of 'bacoside B'.

As per the report of Deepak and Agarwal (2013), it can be concluded that the identity of 'bacoside B' does not seem to have been clearly established in the literature and the proposed identity of 'bacoside B' appears ambiguous. In addition, the 'impugned bacoside B' can potentially be formed during extraction of the herb via hydrolysis of saponins of 'bacoside A', the major saponin mixture present in the plant material. These observations, along with the fact that saponins of 'impugned bacoside B' form less than 3% w/w of the total saponins of dried plant material of *B. monnieri*, make a strong case for developing a negative limit for the content of saponins of 'impugned bacoside B' in the analytical monographs on the plant in various Pharmacopoeia.

5.4   BACOGNIZE®: A STANDARDISED EXTRACT WITH CLINICAL EFFICACY AND SAFETY

Botanical Description

Bacopa: *Bacopa monnieri*, well known as 'Brahmi' has been identified botanically as:

Botanical Name: *Bacopa monnieri* (Linn.) Wettst.

Family: Scrophulariaceae

Other Names

> English – Thyme-leaved gratiola or water hyssop
>
> Sanskrit – Saraswati
>
> Gujarati – Neerbrahmi
>
> Hindi – Mandukaparni
>
> Tamil – Nirabrahmi
>
> Urdu – Brahmi
>
> Telugu – Sambarenu

Morphological/Macroscopic Characters

> Root – Thin, wiry, small, branched creamy yellow
>
> Stem – Thin, green or purplish green, about 1–2 mm thick, soft, nodes and internodes prominent, glabrous; taste: slightly bitter
>
> Leaf – Simple, opposite, decussate, green sessile, 1–2 cm long, obovate – oblong; taste – slightly bitter. Flower – small, axillary and solitary, pedicels 6–30 mm long, bracteoles shorter than pedicle. Fruit – capsules up to 5 mm long, ovoid and glabrous

Distribution

It is distributed throughout India in all plain districts, ascending to an altitude of 1320 m

5.5   MICROSCOPY AND POWDER DRUG CHARACTERISTICS

5.5.1   Microscopic Characters

T.S. of Leaf

Figure 5.1 shows the T.S. of the leaf as done in the laboratory of Pharmanza Herbal Pvt. Ltd. For comparison and authentication of the species.

T.S. of Stem

Figure 5.2 shows the T.S. of the stem of *Bacopa monnieri* (Linn.) Wettst. as done in the laboratory of Pharmanza Herbal Pvt. Ltd. For comparison and authentication of the species.

T.S. of Root

Figure 5.3 shows the T.S. of root of *Bacopa monnieri* (Linn.) Wettst. as done in the laboratory of Pharmanza Herbal Pvt. Ltd. For comparison and authentication of the species.

5.5.2   Powdered Drug Analysis

> **Leaf**: Powder has greenish tinge, characteristic smell and slightly astringent taste. Microscopic examination of the leaf powder shows stomata, spiral vessel, xylem vessel, calcium oxalate crystal, crystal and starch grains mostly round, rarely oval and irregular (Figure 5.4).
>
> **Stem**: Powder is light brown in colour with characteristic smell and slightly bitter and astringent taste. Microscopic examination of the stem powder shows annular xylem vessel, pitted xylem vessel, spirals mostly round, rarely oval and irregular (Figure 5.5).

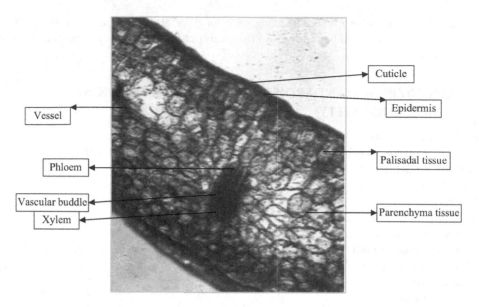

FIGURE 5.1   The cross section of leaf shows a single layer of upper and lower epidermis covered with thin cuticle; glandular hairs sessile, subsidiary cells present on both surface; few prismatic crystals calcium oxalate occasionally found distributed in mesophyll cells; mesophyll traversed by small veins surrounded by bundle sheath; no distinct midrib present.

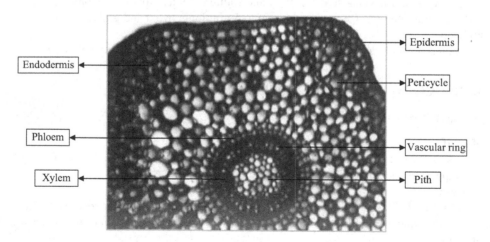

FIGURE 5.2   The cross section of stem shows single layer of epidermis followed by a wide cortex of thin-walled cells with very large intercellular spaces; endodermis single layered; pericycle 3 consisting of 1–2 layers; vascular ring continuous, composed of a narrow zone of phloem towards periphery and a wide ring of xylem towards centre; centre occupied by a small pith with distinct intercellular spaces; starch grain simple; round to oval, present in a few cells of cortex and endodermis.

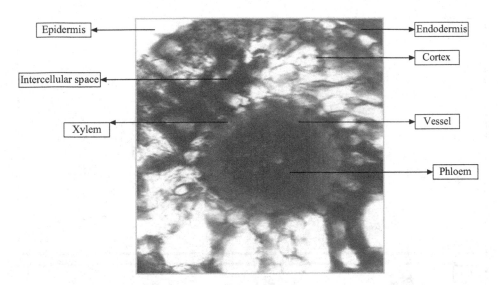

FIGURE 5.3 The cross section of stem shows a single layer of epidermis, cortex having large air cavities; endodermis single layered; pericycle not distinct; stele consists of a thin layer of phloem with a few sieve elements and isolated material from xylem shows vessels with reticulate thinking.

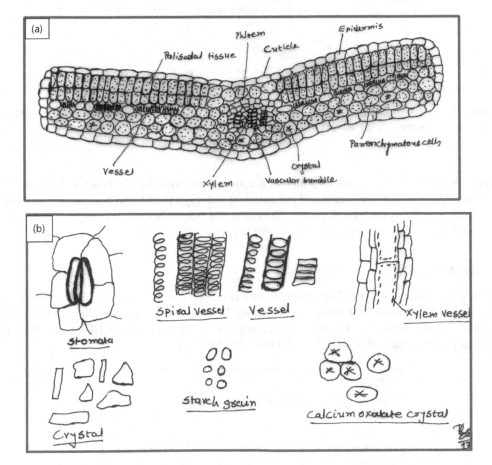

FIGURE 5.4 (a) T.S. of leaf of *Bacopa monnieri* (Linn.) Wettst and (b) powder drug of the leaf of *Bacopa monnieri* (Linn.) Wettst (Lucida sketch).

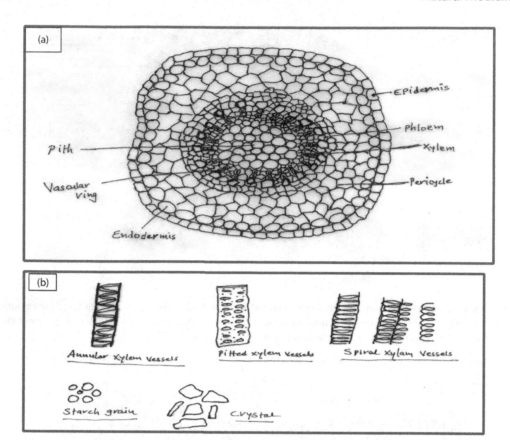

FIGURE 5.5   (a) T.S. of stem of *Bacopa monnieri* (Linn.) Wettst and (b) powder drug of the stem of *Bacopa monnieri* (Linn.) Wettst (Lucida sketch).

Root: Powder is brown in colour with characteristic smell and slightly bitter and astringent taste. Microscopic examination of the xylem vessel, crystal and starch grain root powder shows annular xylem vessel, pitted xylem vessel, crock cells (brown colour), crystal and starch grains mostly round, rarely oval and irregular (Figure 5.6).

5.6   DNA TESTING

Molecular diagnostic test: The DNA concentration is assessed using a Qubit Fluorometer in addition to the TRU-ID DNA authentication test using TRU-ID mini-sequence analysis technology. Molecular diagnostics in this test uses Sanger sequencing of standardised DNA sequences of a plant. Samples are analysed against TRU-ID Plant DNA library.

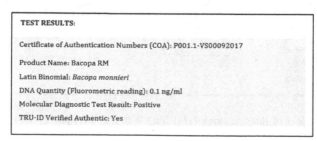

TEST RESULTS:

Certificate of Authentication Numbers (COA): P001.1-VS00092017

Product Name: Bacopa RM

Latin Binomial: *Bacopa monnieri*

DNA Quantity (Fluorometric reading): 0.1 ng/ml

Molecular Diagnostic Test Result: Positive

TRU-ID Verified Authentic: Yes

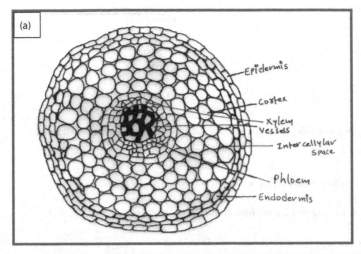

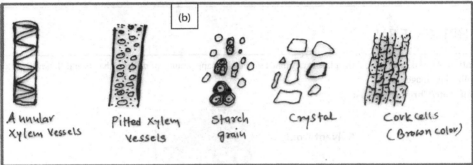

FIGURE 5.6 (a) T.S. of root of *Bacopa monnieri* (Linn.) Wettst and (b) powder drug of the root of *Bacopa monnieri* (Linn.) Wettst (Lucida sketch).

5.7 THE BACOPA RM SPECIFICATION

Physical Characteristics	Specification	Test Method
Identification	Positive	TLC
Description	*Bacopa monnieri* is a small, creeping herb with numerous branches, succulent, rooting at the nodes, with numerous prostrate branches, each 10–30 cm long. Brahmi leaves are petiole, oblong, sessile, and dried. Flowers are purple brown in colour, axillary, solitary with peduncles.	Visual
Colour	Greenish brown	Visual
Odour	Slightly mucilaginous, bitter and acrid.	Organoleptic
Taste	Bitter	Organoleptic
Foreign Matter	NMT 2%	In-house specification
Chemical Analysis	**Specification**	**Test Method**
Assay for Actives:		
Total Bacosides	NLT 10%	UV Spectrophotometer
Total Ash Content	NMT 18%	USP <281>
Ash Content (Acid Insoluble)	NMT 6%	USP <281>
Alcohol Soluble Extractives	NLT 6%	Indian Pharmacopoeia
Water Soluble Extractives	NLT 15%	Indian Pharmacopoeia

(Continued)

Impurities	Specification	Test Method
Total Heavy Metals	<10 ppm	USP <231>
Lead	<0.5 ppm	AAS
Mercury	<1 ppm	AAS
Cadmium	<1 ppm	AAS
Arsenic	<1 ppm	AAS

References

Ayurvedic Pharmacopoeia of India and In-house specifications of M/s Pharmanza Herbal Pvt. Ltd.

Packaging Details:

Packaging:

Raw material packed in fresh gunny bag/pp woven bag.

Retesting frequency:

Unused material to be retested after 2 years from the date of material received.

Storage:

Store at room temperature, away from moisture, sunlight and heat

5.8   HPTLC OF RM

Observation: After derivatisation, the plate is examined visually for appearance of different bands at different Rf. Please refer following image:

Images of Plate/Chromatograms:

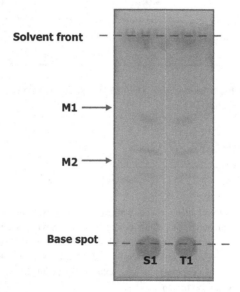

Where:

S1 = *Bacopa monnieri* (L.) Pennell (Brahmi) raw material Powder PHPL secondary standard raw material RM Batch no. RMBM277 T1, = *Bacopa monnieri* (L.) Pennell (Brahmi) raw material (RMBM277). M1 = Marker Compound 1, M2 = Marker Compound 2.

Evaluation of Results: The test reference solution of *Bacopa monnieri* (L.) Pennell (Brahmi) raw material Powder PHPL secondary standard raw material (RMBM277). Track (1) shows two bands, one is Purple blue band at approximate Rf value of M1 = 0.65. Second is brown colour band at approximate Rf value M2 = 0.32. The major zone in the samples (T1) corresponds in colour and position to that of two markers of test reference solution.

Comments and Conclusions: Blue line = Base Spot at 10 mm, Red line = solvent front at 90 mm, Track 1 is the test reference solution of *Bacopa monnieri* PHPL secondary standard raw material (RMBM277). Track 2 is *Bacopa monnieri* (L.) Pennell (Brahmi) raw material Powder of Batch no. (RMBM277) respectively. The correspondence in colour and position of band confirms presence of *Bacopa monnieri* raw material.

5.9   SUPPLY CHAIN CHALLENGES FROM FARM TO PRODUCT

Bacopa is a creeper that usually grows in waste water, therefore in the resultant in the muddy land. Therefore, the problems of contaminants and microbes are always identified with it.

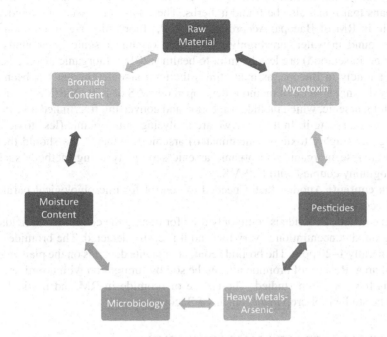

1. **Mycotoxins:** Currently, the concern in dietary herbals is the presence of Mycotoxins. These are toxic secondary metabolites of fungi belonging, essentially, to the Aspergillus, Penicillium and Fusarium genera. Mycotoxins are chemical compounds that can be produced on herbs and agricultural material. The Food and Agriculture Organization (FAO) of the United Nations estimates that 25% of agricultural crops are contaminated by mycotoxins.

    The accumulation of mycotoxins in foods and feeds is a major threat to human and animal health, as these are responsible for toxicities including carcinogenicity, mutagenicity and estrogenic, gastrointestinal, urogenital, vascular, kidney and nervous disorders. Some mycotoxins are also immuno-compromising and can thus reduce resistance to infectious diseases. Significant economic losses are associated with their impact on human health, animal productivity and domestic and international trade.

    There is need to protect the health of humans and susceptible animals by limiting their exposure to mycotoxins. Despite many years of research and the introduction of good practices in the food production, storage and distribution chain, mycotoxins continue to be a problem. Many countries regulate for, or suggest permissible levels of, mycotoxins in foods and feed because of their public health significance and commercial impact.

2. **Pesticide content:** Most herbal material grows in rice fields, from which it is harvested. Whatever pesticides are used in rice crop are therefore found in herbals growing in the same field. There is a very small amount of material that grows in the forest. Exclusive cultivation of the herbal is a difficult and costly affair. A few companies, including our Pharmanza Herbal Pvt. Ltd., have started cultivation of herbs and are successful. This will take care of pesticide residues.

3. **Microbiological infestation:** The usual control parameter for safe *B. monnieri* extract is control of microbiological contamination. As discussed earlier, crop management is also one of the major contributing factors, along with location and harvesting, that contribute to the increase in total platelet counts, yeast and mould contents in *B. monnieri*.

4. **Arsenic content:** It has been always challenging to address heavy metals issues and specifically arsenic. Arsenic is found in the Earth's crust. It is everywhere in the environment and can be found in water, air and soil, in both organic and inorganic forms. The main concern will be the human activities also can introduce arsenic into the environment. That means that it can also be found in herbs. There has been issue of extended amount of arsenic in RM of Bacopa. According to WHO, 'Inorganic arsenic compounds (such as those found in water) are highly toxic while organic arsenic compounds (such as those found in seafood) are less harmful to health' (2018). Inorganic arsenic needs to be tested separately in Bacopa, as many times the total arsenic amount has been reported. Currently the major share of methods developed on AAS or ICP-OES/MS are designed to analyse total arsenic, which includes digestion and converting free/linked arsenic into free arsenic and analysing it. In this way we are analysing both organic (less toxic – natural) and inorganic (highly toxic – contaminated) arsenic together. Care should therefore be taken to analyse inorganic and organic arsenic separately using methods such as Ion-chromatography coupled with ICP-MS.

5. **Moisture content:** Another factor needed to control for microbiological parameters, as well as Bacoside stability.

6. **Bromide content:** Bromide is commonly used for tracing the conditions of fields, because its background concentration is very low and it is easily detected. The bromide content in soil is generally 1–20 ppm. The bromide content in plants depends on the plant and the geographical area. Release of bromide ions in the soil by fumigation with bromine-containing fumigants has also been studied. The uptake of bromide in RM and pesticide methods needs to be studied for crop management of Bacopa.

5.10   BOTANICAL EXTRACT STANDARDISATION

1. **Total Bacoside content by UV spectrophotometer:** Bacosides are reported to be ebelin lactones, which can be further formed leading to acidic hydrolysis of various triterpenoids. The latter method can be established via UV analysis to determine the presence of chromophore during UV-spectroscopy.

2. **Total Bacoside content by HPLC:** The HPLC method was developed and identified for the standardisation of Bacopa. The British Pharmacopoeia (BP) included this method of estimation of bacosides (Murthy et al. 2006). Later, the United States Pharmacopoeia (USP) included monographs for *Bacopa monnieri*. The HPLC method (Deepak 2005) currently focuses on Bacoside A, which has been found as a mixture of saponins with bacoside A3, bacopaside I, bacopaside II, jujubogenin isomer of bacopasaponin C and bacopasaponin C is analysed as a major constituent.

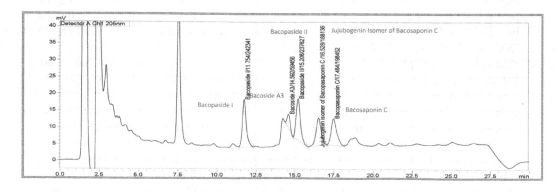

TABLE 5.2

Quantification of Markers in Bacognize

Analytes	Result (%w/w)
Bacoside A3	4.57
Bacopaside II	2.13
Bacopaside X	1.70
Bacopasaponin C	2.98
Total Bacopasaponin (Identified)	11.38
Total Bacopasaponin (Identified + Unidentified)	15.57

As mentioned in Kumar et al. (2016), Bacognize was standardised to have a concentration of a total of four bacosides as 11.38% by HPLC (Table 5.2).

Bacopa monnieri extract has been standardised per USP method using five saponins. The standardised extract has been reported to have NLT 45% saponin by UV spectrophotometry and NLT 12% by HPLC.

5.11 MANUFACTURING OF BACOGNIZE EXTRACT

Process flow for *Bacopa monnieri* extract (Ethanol Extract)

Raw material receipt

Approval of raw material

Approved material storage

Extraction (Ethanol)

Filtration

Distillation (CCP#1)

Sterilization (if required) (CCP# 2&3)

Drying (CCP#4)

Sifting

Blending

For granulated product

Granulation

Milling (CCP#5)

Sifting

Blending

Metal & Magnet Detection (CCP#6)

Final Sifting

5.12   FORMULATION

5.12.1   STANDARDISATION

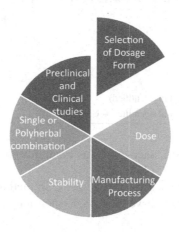

5.13   SPECIFICATION OF TABLET

Bacognize Tablet: The standardised formulation manufactured at PHPL after careful observation of *B. monnieri* and its nature. The general dosage form was finalised from clinical trials conducted on 'Bacognize'. The film coating technique as adapted to protect it from moisture and other parameters. Bacognize was further tested according to in-house parameters for standardisation.

Physical Characteristics	Specification	Test Method	Result
Identification	Positive	TLC	Confirms
Appearance	Round shape	Visual	Confirms
Colour	Sky blue	Visual	Confirms
Hardness	NLT 3.0 kg/cm^2	In-house specification	3.0 kg/cm^2
Thickness	5.2–5.7 mm	In-house specification	5.3 mm
Disintegration test	NMT 60 min	In-house specification	32 min
Average weight	522.5–577.5 mg	In-house specification	550 mg
Uniformity of weight	Average weight ± 7.5%	USP 30 NF <905>	Confirms
Chemical Analysis	**Specification**	**Test Method**	**Result**
Assay for actives			
Total Bacopa glycosides (Bacosides)	NLT 27%	UV spectrophotometer	28.32%
pH	5–8	USP 29 NF <791>	6.70
LOD	NMT 6%	USP 29 NF <731> (vacuum oven)	2.65%
Moisture	NMT 8%	USP 29 NF <921>(KF)	3.90%
Carrier	None	In-house specification	Confirms
Excipients	NMT 40% starch, talc, magnesium stearate, polyvinylpyrrolidone, crospovidone	In-house specification	Confirms
Impurities	**Specification**	**Test Method**	**Result**
Total heavy metals	<10 ppm	USP 29 NF <231>	Complies
Lead	<0.5 ppm	By AAS	0.32 ppm
Mercury	<0.1 ppm	By AAS	Absent
Cadmium	<1 ppm	By AAS	Absent
Arsenic	<1 ppm	By AAS	Absent

(Continued)

Microbiology	Specification	Test Method	Result
Total plate count	<5000 Cfu/g	USP 30 NF 25 <2021>	3000 Cfu/g
Yeast and mould	<200 Cfu/g	USP 30 NF 25 <2021>	90 Cfu/g
Coliforms	<10 Cfu/g	USP 30 NF 25 <2021>	Absent
Enterobacteriaceae	<100 Cfu/g	USP 30 NF 25 <2021>	<1 Cfu/g
Escherichia coli	Absent	USP 30 NF 25 <2021>	Absent
Salmonella	Absent	USP 30 NF 25 <2021>	Absent
S. aureus	Absent	USP 30 NF 25 <2021>	Absent

Bacognize Tablet

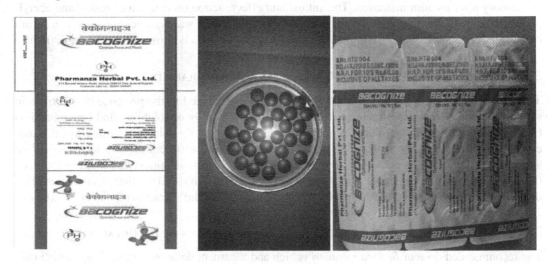

5.14 CLINICAL TRIALS AND PHARMACOKINETICS

5.14.1 ALZHEIMER'S DISEASE

Alzheimer's disease is a degenerative condition mainly affecting the elderly population. The cause and pathogenesis of this disease is still uncertain. It significantly affects the quality of life of patients suffering from this disease. So far there is no proven effective therapeutic intervention available for this disease. *Bacopa monnieri* has an inhibitory effect on the enzyme cholinesterase, which can result in a decrease in the breakdown of acetylcholine, an important neurotransmitter whose decreased levels are seen in Alzheimer's disease. An open label, prospective, uncontrolled, non-randomised trial was conducted. The study population included all newly diagnosed patients with Alzheimer's disease in the Psychiatry Out-Patient Department between 60 and 65 years of age. Baseline scores on the Mini Mental State Examination Scale (MMSES) were recorded for all patients. Subsequently all patients took 300 mg of Bacognize (*Bacopa monnieri* standardised extract) orally twice a day for 6 months. MMSES scores were recorded again after the completion of the study drug. Out of the 60 patients enrolled, 39 completed the study, 2 patients died during course of study and 9 patients were lost. Consumption of Bacognize® (*Bacopa monnieri* standardised extract) 300 mg twice a day orally for 6 months resulted in improvement in some aspects of cognitive functions in geriatric patients suffering from Alzheimer's disease. Significant improvement was seen in orientation of time, place and person and attention. Language showed improvement in terms of reading, writing and comprehension (Goswami et al. 2011).

5.14.2 PLACEBO-CONTROLLED TRIAL OF BACOGNIZE
BACOPA MONNIERI ON INTELLECT FOR MEMORY

This study was planned to evaluate the effect of Bacognize on the memory of medical students for 6 weeks. This was a randomised double blind placebo-controlled, non-crossover parallel trial. Sixty medical students of either gender from the second year of medical school, third term, regular batch, were enrolled from the Government Medical College, Nagpur, India. Baseline biochemical and memory tests were done. The participants were randomly divided in two groups to receive either 150 mg of standardised extract of *Bacopa monnieri* (Bacognize) or matching placebo twice daily for 6 weeks. All baseline investigations were repeated at the end of the trial. Students were followed up for 15 days after the intervention.

The administration of the standardised extract produced a significant effect on some components of memory after its administration. The antioxidant effect, action on calcium channels and acetylcholine level have been credited for the action of *Bacopa*. There was significant increase in serum calcium levels (in normal range) in medical students after *Bacopa* administration (Kumar 2016).

5.14.3 FORMULATIONS TO INCREASE COMPLIANCE AND BIOAVAILABILITY

The memory-enhancing effects of *Bacopa monnieri* are attributed to the presence of triterpenoid saponins called 'Bacosides'. Bacopa extract has the problem of poor solubility and hence has less bioavailability. To enhance solubility and bioavailability of poorly soluble bacoside a self nano-emulsifying drug delivery system (SNEDDS) was tried using different oils, surfactants and co surfactants. This formula could help in reducing dose of *Bacopa monnieri* and making the drug thermodynamically more stable with high-solubilisation capacity and so that it could be filled directly into soft or hard gelatine capsules for convenient oral administration (Gohel et al. 2016).

5.14.4 PHARMACOKINETIC STUDY WITH LIPOPHILIC FORMULATION OF *BACOPA MONNIERI*

The recommended dose of *Bacopa monnieri* is high and treatment duration is rather long, which may cause gastric irritation. A new lipophilic formulation of *Bacopa monnieri* with phosphatidylcholine was therefore prepared. The new lipophilic formulation was evaluated for its penetration in the brain and pharmacokinetic profile in rats. Analysis of the plasma and brain samples of rats was done after 24 h of dosing, which revealed the high concentration of bacosides. This indicates the better penetration of bacosides and their metabolites into the brain. The lipophilic formulation had more permeability to cross the blood–brain barrier and its duration of action was longer. Such lipophilic formulation can increase compliance and quality of life in patients suffering from dementia and Alzheimer's disease (Parihar et al. 2016).

5.14.5 DISPERSIBLE TABLET AND TASTE MASKING

Poor solubility, patient compliance and bitterness were a major driving forces to develop taste masked β-cyclodextrin complexed Bacognize, which disperses very quickly. The product was converted to tablets and stability studies were conducted (Thakkar 2016).

5.14.6 MECHANISM OF ACTION

The 5-hydroxytryptophan (5-HTP), also known as serotonin, is a neurotransmitter responsible for learning ability, mood regulation and sleep cycles. Serotonin works by fitting into 5-HTP receptors, which are membrane bound proteins. These receptor proteins affect a variety of brain functions like learning, mood and sleep. Bacognize® acts as 5-HTP receptor agonist and thereby improves the memory, learning ability, sleep and mood. (On file research performed by the Department of Biomedical and Pharmaceutical Sciences and the COBRE Center for Structural and Functional Neuroscience at the University of Montana, April 2004.)

REFERENCES

Achaliya, G. S., Wododkar, S. G. and Dorle, A. K. (2005). Evaluation of CNS activity of *Brahmi ghirta*. *Indian Journal of Pharmacology*, **37**, 33–36.

Agrawal, H., Kaul, N., Paradkar, A. R. and Mahadik, K. R. (2006). Separation of bacoside A3 and bacopaside II, major triterpenoid saponins in *Bacopa monnieri*, by HPTLC and SFC. Application of SFC in implementation of uniform design for herbal drug standardization, with thermodynamic study. *Acta Chromatographica*, **17**, 125–50.

Aithal, H. N. and Sirsi, M. (1961). Pharmacological investigation on *Herpestis monniera*. *Indian Journal of Pharmaceutical Sciences*, **23**, 2–5.

Alan, K., Parvey, N., Yadav, S., Molvi, K., Hwisa, N., Al Sharif, S. M., Pathak, D. et al. (2011). Anti microbial activity of leaf callus of *Bacopa monnieri* L. *Der Pharmacia Lettre*, **3**(7), 287–291.

Aloe, A., Alleve, E. and Fiore, M. (2002). Stress and growth factor findings in animal models. *Pharmacology Biochemistry and Behavior*, **73**, 159–166.

Bafna, P. A. and Balaraman, R. (2005). Antioxidant activity of DHC-I, an herbal formulation in experimentally induced cardiac and rental damage. *Phytotherapy Research*, **19**, 216–221.

Bhakuni, D. S., Dhar, M. L., Dhar, M. M., Dhawan, B. N. and Mehrotra, B. N. (1969). Screening of Indian plants for biological activity- II. *Indian Journal of Experimental Biology*, **7**(4), 250–262.

Bhandari, P., Kumar, N., Singh, B. and Kaul, V. K. (2006). Bacosterol Glycoside, a New 13,14-Seco-steroid Glycoside from *Bacopa monnieri* (L.). *Chemical and Pharmaceutical Bulletin*, **54**(2), 240–241.

Bhandari, P., Kumar, N., Singh, B. and Kaul, V. K. (2007). Cucurbitacins from *Bacopa monnieri*. *Phytochemistry*, **68**(9), 1248–1254.

Bhandari, P., Kumar N., Singh, B. and Kaur, I. (2009a). Dammarane triterpenoid saponins from *Bacopa monnieri*. *Canadian Journal of Chemistry*, **87**(9), 1230–1234.

Bhandari, P., Kumar, N., Singh, B., Singh, V. and Kaur, I. (2009b). Silica-based monolithic column with evaporative light scattering detector for HPLC analysis of bacosides and apigenin in *Bacopa monnieri*. *Journal of Separation Science*, **32**, 2812–2818.

Bhaskar, M. and Jagtap, A. G. (2011). Exploring the possible mechanism of action behind antinoceptive activity of *Bacopa monnieri*. *International Journal of Ayurveda Research*, **2**, 2–7.

Bhattacharya, S. K., Bhattacharya, A., Kumar, A. and Ghosal, S. (2000). Antioxidant activity of *Bacopa monniera* in rat frontal cortex, Striatum and hippocampus. *Phytotherapy Research*, **14**(3), 174–179.

Bhattacharya, S. K., Bhattacharya, A., Kumar, A. and Ghosal, S. (2001). Effect of *Bacopa monnieri* on animal models of Alzheimer's disease and perturbed central cholinergic markers of cognition in rats. In A. Mori and T. Satoh, eds. *Emerging Drugs, Vol. 1 (Molecular Aspects of Asian Medicines)*. Westbury, NY: PJD Publications, pp. 21–32.

Bhattacharya, S. K. and Ghosal, S. (1998). Anxiolytic activity of a standardized extract of *Bacopa monnieri*: An experimental study. *Phytomedicine*, **5**, 77–82.

Bose, K. C. and Bose, N. K. (1931). Observations on the actions and uses of *Herpestis monniera*. *Journal of the Indian Medical Association*, **1**, 60.

Chakravarty, A. K., Garai, S., Masuda, K., Nakane, T. and Kawahara, N. (2003). Bacopasides III–V: Three new triterpenoid glycosides from *Bacopa monniera*. *Chemical and Pharmaceutical Bulletin*, **51**, 215–217.

Chakravarty, A. K., Sarkar, T., Masuda K., Shiojima, K., Nakane, T. and Kawahara, N. (2001). Bacopaside I and II: Two pseudojujubogenin glycosides from *Bacopa monniera*. *Phytochemistry*, **58**, 553–556.

Chandel, R. S., Kulshreshtha, D. K. and Rastogi, R. P. (1977). Bacogenin A$_3$ – A new sapogenin from *Bacopa monniera*. *Phytochemistry*, **16**, 141–143.

Chatterji, N., Rastogi, R. P. and Dhar, M. L. (1963). Chemical examination of *Bacopa monnieri* West. Part I: Isolation of chemical constituents. *Indian Journal of Chemistry*, **1**, 212–215.

Chaudhuri, P. K., Srivastava, R., Kumar, S. and Kumar, S. (2004). Phytotoxic and antimicrobial constituents of *Bacopa monnieri* and Holmskioldia sanguinea. *Phytotherapy Research*, **18**(2), 114–117.

Chopra, R. N., Nayar, L. and Chopra, I. C. (1956). *Glossary of Indian Medicinal Plants*, Vol. 32. New Delhi, India: Council of Scientific and Industrial Research.

Cook, N. C. and Samman, S. (1996). Flavonoids – Chemistry metabolism, cardioprotective effects and dietary sources. *Journal of Nutritional Biochemistry*, **7**, 66–76.

D'Souza, P., Deepak, M., Rani, P. and Kadamboor, S. (2002). Brine shrimp lethality assay of *Bacopa monnieri*. *Phytotherapy Research*, **16**(2), 197–198.

Dar, A. and Channa, S. (1997). Relaxant effect of ethanol extract of *Bacopa monniera* on trachea, pulmonary artery and aorta from rabbit and guinea-pig. *Phytotherapy Research*, **11**, 323–325.

Dar, A. and Channa, S. (1999). Calcium antagonistic activity of *Bacopa monniera* on vascular and intestinal smooth muscles of rabbit and guinea-pig. *Journal of Ethnopharmacology*, **66**, 167–174.

Das, A., Shanker, G., Nath, C., Pal, R., Singh, S. and Singh, H. A. (2002). Comparative study in rodents of standardized extracts of *Bacopa monniera* and Ginkgo biloba: Anticholinesterase and cognitive enhancing activities. *Pharmacology Biochemistry and Behavior*, **73**(4), 893–900.

Deepak, M. and Agarwal, A. (2013). 'Bacoside B' – The need remains for establishing identity. *Fitoterapia*, **87**, 7–10.

Deepak, M., Sangli, C. K., Arun, P. C. and Agarwal, A. (2005). Quantitative determination of the major saponin mixture bacoside A in *Bacopa monnieri* by HPLC. *Phytochemical Analysis*, **16**, 24–29.

Deepak, R., Gitika, B., Gautam, P. and Raghwendra, P. (2003). Adaptogenic effect of *Bacopa monniera* (Brahmi). *Pharmacology Biochemistry and Behavior*, **75**(4), 823–830.

Dhanasekaran, M., Tharakan, B., Holcomb, L. A., Hitt, A. R., Young, K. A. and Manyam, B. V. (2007). Neuroprotective mechanisms of ayurvedic antidementia botanical *Bacopa monniera*. *Phytotherapy Research*, **21**(10), 965–969.

Dharmani, P. and Palit, G. (2006). Exploring Indian medicinal plants for antiulcer activity. *Indian Journal of Pharmacology*, **38**, 95–99.

Dorababu, M., Prabha, T., Priyambaba, S., Agarwal, V. K., Aryya, N. C. and Goel, R. K. (2004). Effect of *Bacopa monnieri* and *Azadiracta indica* on gastric ulceration and healing in experimental NIDDM rats. *Indian Journal of Experimental Biology*, **42**, 389–397.

Elangovan, V., Govindasamy, S., Ramamoorthy, N. and Balasubramanian, K. (1995). In vitro studies on the anticancer activity of *Bacopa monnieri*. *Fitoterapia*, **66**, 211–215.

Ganzera, M., Gampenrieder, J., Pawar, R. S., Khan, I. A. and Stuppner, H. (2004). Separation of the major triterpenoid saponins in *Bacopa monnieri* by high-performance liquid chromatography. *Analytica Chimia Acta*, **516**, 149–154.

Garai, S., Mahato, S. B., Ohtani, K. and Yamasaki, K. (1996a). Dammarane type triterpenoid saponins from *Bacopa monniera*. *Phytochemistry*, **42**, 815–820.

Garai, S., Mahato, S. B., Ohtani, K. and Yamasaki, K. (1996b). Bacopasaponin D – A pseudojujubogenin glycoside from *Bacopa monniera*. *Phytochemistry*, **43**, 447–449.

Ghosh, T., Maity, T. K. and Singh, J. (2011). Antihyperglycemic activity of bacosine, a triterpene from *Bacopa monnieri* in alloxan induced diabetic rats. *Planta Medica*, **77**(8), 804–808.

Goel, R. K., Sairam, K., Babu, M. D. and Tavares, I. A. (2003). In vitro evaluation of *Bacopa monniera* on anti-Helicobacter pylori activity and accumulation of prostaglandins. *Phytomedicine*, **10**(6–7), 523–527.

Gohel, M., Purohit, A., Patel, A. and Hingorani, L. (2016). Optimization of bacoside A loaded SNEEDS using S-optimal mixture design for enhancement of solubility and bioavailability. *International Journal of Pharmacy and Pharmaceutical Sciences*, **8**(12), 213–220.

Gohil, K. J. and Patel, J. A. (2010). A review on *Bacopa monnieri*: Current research and future prospects. *International Journal of Green Pharmacy*, **4**(1), 1–9.

Gold, P. W., Goodwin, F. K. and Chrousus, G. P. (1998). Clinical and biochemical manifestation of depression in relation to neurobiology of stress: Part 1. *New England Journal of Medicine*, **319**, 348–353.

Goswami, S., Saoji, A., Kumar, N., Thawani, V., Tiwari, M. and Thawani, M. (2011). Development and optimization of dispersible tablet of *Bacopa monnieri* with improved functionality for memory enhancement. *Journal of Pharmacy and Bioallied Sciences*, **3**(4), 208–215.

Govindarajan, R., Vijayakumar, M. and Pushpangadan, P. (2005). Antioxidant approach to disease management and the role of Rasayana' herbs of Ayurveda. *Journal of Ethnopharmacology*, **99**, 165–178.

Hema, T. A., Arya, A. S., Suseelan, S., Celestinal, J. R. K. and Divya, P. V. (2013). Anti microbial activity of five medicinal plants against clinical pathogens. *International Journal of Pharma and Bio Sciences*, **4**(1), 70–80.

Holocomb, L. A., Dhanasekaran, M., Hitt, A. R., Young, K. A., Riggs, M. and Manyam, B. V. (2006). *Bacopa monnieri* extract residues amyloid levels in PSAPP mice. *Journal of Alzheimer's Disease*, **9**, 243–251.

Hou, C. C., Lin, S. J., Cheng, J. T. and Hsu, F. L. (2002). Bacopaside III, Bacopasaponin G and bacopasides A, B and C from *Bacopa monniera*. *Journal of Natural Products*, **65**, 1759–1763.

Jain, P., Khanna, N. K., Trehan, T., Pendse, V. K. and Godhwani, J. L. (1994). Anti-inflammatory effects of an Ayurvedic preparation, Brahmi Rasayan, in rodents. *Indian Journal of Experimental Biology*, **32**, 633–636.

Jain, P. and Kulshreshtha, D. K. (1993). Bacoside A_1 – A minor saponin from *Bacopa monniera*. *Phytochemistry*, **33**, 449–451.

Janani, P., Sivakumari, K. and Parthasarathy, C. (2008). Hepatoprotective activity of bacoside A against *N*-nitrosodiethylamine-induced liver toxicity in adult rats. *Cell Biology and Toxicology*, **25**(5), 425–434.

Kikuzaki, H. and Nakatani, N. (1993). Antioxidant effects of some ginger constituents. *Journal of Food Science*, **58**, 1407–1410.

Kulshreshtha, D. K. and Rastogi, R. P. (1973). Bacogenin A_1 – A novel dammerane triterpene sapogenin from *Bacopa monniera*. *Phytochemistry*, **12**, 887–892.

Kumar, N., Abhichandani, L. G., Thawani, V., Gharpure, K. J., Naidu, M. U. R. and Venkataramana, G. (2016). Efficacy of standardized extract of *Bacopa monnieri* (Bagognize) on cognitive functions of medical students: A six week randomized placebo-controlled trial. *Evidence-Based Complementary and Alternative Medicine*, 2016.

Limpeanchob, N., Jaipan, S., Rattanakaruna, S., Phrompittayarat, W. and Ingkaninan, K. (2008). The Neuroprotective effect of *Bacopa monnieri* on beta-amyloid-induced cell death on primary cortical culture. *Journal of Ethnopharmacology*, **120**(1), 112–117.

Mahato, S. B., Garai, S. and Chakravarty, A. K. (2000). Bacopasaponins E and F: Two jujubogenin bisdesmosides from *Bacopa monniera*. *Phytochemistry*, **53**, 711–714.

Maher, B. F. G., Stough, C., Shelmerdine, A., Wesnes, K. and Nathan, P. J. (2002). The acute effects of combined administration of Ginkgo biloba and *Bacopa monnieri* on cognitive function in humans. *Human Psychopharmacology: Clinical and Experimental*, **17**, 163–164.

Malhotra, C. K. and Das, P. K. (1959). Pharmacological studies of *Herpestis monniera* Linn (Brahmi). *Indian Journal of Medical Research*, **47**, 294–305.

Mandal, S. and Mukhopadhyay, S. (2004). Bacopasaponin H: A pseudojujubogenin glycoside from *Bacopa monniera*. *Indian Journal of Chemistry*, **43**(8), 1802–1804.

McLaughlin, J. L., Rogers, L. L. and Anderson, J. E. (1998). The use of biological assays to evaluate botanicals. *Drug Information Journal*, **32**, 513–524.

Mishra, M. (1998). Memory Plus Works, claim clinical studies. *The Times of India*, 29 March 1998.

Mundkinajeddu, D. and Agarwal, A. (2013). 'Bacoside B' – The need remains for establishing identity. *Fitoterapia*, **87**, 7–10.

Murthy, P. B. S., Raju, V. R., Ramakrisana, T., Chakravarthy, M. S., Kumar, K. V., Kannababu, S. and Subbaraju, G. V. (2006). Estimation of twelve bacopa saponins in *Bacopa monnieri* extracts and formulations by high-performance liquid chromatography. *Chemical and Pharmaceutical Bulletin*, **54**(6), 907–911.

Nathan, P. J., Clarke, J., Lloyd, J., Hutchison, C. W., Downey, L. and Sough, C. (2001). The acute effects of an extract of *Bacopa monnieri* (Brahmi) on cognitive function in healthy normal subjects. *Human Psychopharmacology: Clinical and Experimental*, **16**, 345–351.

Parihar, D., Kumar, S. and Thawani, V. (2016). Development of new formulation of *Bacopa monnieri* to improve its pharmacokinetic properties. *Indian Medical Gazette*, January 2016.

Paulose, C. S., Chathu, F., Khan, S. R. and Krishnakumar, A. (2008). Neuroprotective role of *Bacopa monnieri* extract in epilepsy and effect of glucose supplementation during hypoxia: Glutamate receptor gene expression. *Neurochemical Research*, **33**(9), 1663–1671.

Pawar, R., Gopalakrishnaa, C. and Bhutani, K. K. (2001). Dammarane triterpene saponin from *Bacopa monnieri* as the inhibitor in polymorphonuclear cells. *Plant Medica*, **7**, 752–754.

Pawar, R. S. and Bhutani, K. K. (2006). New dammarane triterpenoidal saponins from *Bacopa monniera*. *Indian Journal of Chemistry*, **45B**, 1511–1514.

Phrompittayarat, W., Wittaya-Areekul, S., Jetiyanon, K., Putalun, W., Tanaka, H. and Ingkaninan, K. (2007). Determination of saponin glycosides in *Bacopa monnieri* by reversed phase high-performance liquid chromatography. *Thai Pharmaceutical and Health Science Journal*, **2**, 26–32.

Prakash, J. C. and Sirsi, M. (1962). Comparative study of the effects of brahmi (*Bacopa monniera*) and chlorpromazine on learning in rats. *Journal of Scientific and Industrial Research*, **21**, 93–96.

Rakesh, A. K., Gulecha, U. S., Mahajan, M. S., Mundada, A. S. and Gangurde, H. H. (2009). Evaluation of antiulcer activity of poly herbal formulation. *International Journal of Pharmaceutical Research and Development*, **10**, 1–6.

Rao, C. H., Sairam, K. and Goel, R. K. (2000). Experimental evaluation on gastric ulceration and secretion. *Indian Journal of Physiology and Pharmacology*, **44**, 435–444.

Rashid, S., Lodhi, F., Ahmad, M. and Usmanghani, K. (1990). Cardiovascular effects of *Bacopa monnieri* (L.) pennel extract in rabbits. *Pakistan Journal of Pharmaceutical Sciences*, **3**(2), 57–62.

Rastogi, S. and Kulshreshtha, D. K. (1999). Bacoside A_2 – A triterpenoid saponin from *Bacopa monniera*. *Indian Journal of Chemistry*, **38B**, 353–356.

Rastogi, S., Pal, R. and Kulshreshtha, D. K. (1994). Bacoside A3 – A triterpenoid saponin from *Bacopa monniera*. *Phytochemistry*, **36**, 133–137.

Roodenrys, S., Booth, D., Bulzomi, S., Phipps, A., Micallef, C. and Smoker, J. (2002). Chronic effects of Brahmi (*Bacopa monnieri*) on human memory. *Neuropsychopharmacology*, **27**(2), 279–281.

Russo, A. and Borrelli, F. (2005). *Bacopa monnieri*, a reputed nootropic plant: An overview. *Phytomedicine*, **12**, 305–317.

Russo, A., Borrelli, F., Campisi, A. and Acquaviva, R. (2003). Nitric oxide-related toxicity in cultured astrocytes: Effect of *Bacopa monnieri*. *Life Sciences*, **73**(12), 1517–1526.

Saba, H., Vibhash, D., Manish, M., Prashant, K. S., Farhan, H. and Tauseef, A. (2012). Anti epileptic activity of some medicinal plants. *International Journal of Medicinal and Aromatic Plants*, **2**(2), 354–360.

Sairam, K., Dorababu, M., Goel, R. K. and Bhattacharya, S. K. (2002). Antidepressant activity of standardized extract of Bacopa monniera in experimental models of depression in rats. *Phytomedicine*, **9**, 207–211.

Sairam, K., Rao, C. V., Babu, M. D. and Goel, R. K. (2001). Prophylactic and curative effects of *Bacopa monniera* in gastric ulcer models. *Phytomedicine*, **8**, 423–430.

Sastri, M. S., Dhalla, N. S. and Malhotra, C. L. (1959). Chemical investigation of *Herpestis monniera* Linn (Brahmi). *Indian Journal of Pharmacology*, **21**, 303–304.

Shah, M., Behara, Y. R. and Jagadeesh, B. (2012). Phytochemical screening and in vitro antioxidant activity of aqueous and hydroalcoholic extract of *Bacopa monnieri* Linn. *International Journal of Pharmaceutical Sciences and Research*, **3**(9), 3418–3424.

Sharan, S. V., Rao, S. B., Chippada, S. C. and Vangalapati, M. (2011). In vitro antioxidant activity and estimation of total phenolic content in methanolic extract of *Bacopa monniera*. *Rasayan Journal of Chemistry*, **4**(2), 381–386.

Sharma, D. (2006). Neuroprotective role of *Bacopa monnieri* extract against aluminium induced oxidative stress in the hippocampus of rat brain. *Neurotoxicology*, **27**, 451–457.

Shinde, P. B., Aragade, P. D., Agrawal, M. R., Deokate, U. A. and Khadabadi, S. S. (2011). Simultaneous determination of withanolide A and bacoside A in spansules by high-performance thin-layer chromatography. *Indian Journal of Pharmaceutical Sciences*, **73**, 240–243.

Singh, H. K. and Dhawan, B. N. (1997). Neuropsychopharmacological effects of the Ayurvedic nootropic *Bacopa monniera* Linn (Brahmi). *Indian Journal of Pharmacology*, **29**, S359–S365.

Singh, R. H. and Singh, L. (1980). Studies on the anti-anxiety effect of the medhya rasayana drug Brahmi (*Bacopa monniera* Wettst.). *Journal of Research in Ayurveda and Siddha*, **1**, 133–148.

Singh, S., Eapan, S. and D'Souza, S. F. (2006). Cadmium accumulation and antioxidative system in an aquatic plant, *Bacopa monnieri* L. *Chemosphere*, **62**, 233–246.

Shrikumar, S., Sandeep, S., Ravi, T. K. and Umamaheswari, M. (2004). A HPTLC determination and fingerprinting of bacoside A in *Bacopa monnieri* and its formulation. *Indian Journal of Pharmaceutical Sciences*, **66**, 132–135.

Sivaramakrishna, C., Rao, C. V., Trimurtulu, G., Vanisree, M. and Subbaraju, G. V. (2005). Triterpenoid glycosides from *Bacopa monnieri*. *Phytochemistry*, **66**, 2719–2728.

Srivastava, P., Raut, H. N., Puntambekar, H. M. and Desai, A. C. (2012). Stability studies of crude plant material of *Bacopa monnieri* and quantitative determination of bacopaside I and bacoside A by HPLC. *Phytochemical Analysis*, **23**, 502–507.

Stough, C., Lloyd, J., Clarke, J., Downey, L. A., Hutchison, C. W., Rodgers, T. and Nathan, P. J. (2001). The chronic effects of an extract of *Bacopa monniera* (Brahmi) on cognitive function in healthy human subjects. *Psychopharmacology*, **156**, 481–484.

Subhan, F., Abbas, M., Rauf, K. and Baser, A. (2010). Anti gut motility, Toxicological and pharmacological studies on *Bacopa monnieri*. *Pharmocology Online*, **3**, 903–914.

Sudharani, D., Krishna, K. L., Deval, K., Safia, A. K. and Priya. (2011). Pharmacological profiles of *Bacopa monnieri* – A review. *International Journal of Pharmacy*, **1**(1), 15–23.

Sumathy, T., Govindasamy, S., Balakrishna, K. and Veluchamy, G. (2002). Protective role of *Bacopa monniera* on morphine-induced brain mitochondrial enzyme activity in rats. *Fitoterapia*, **73**(5), 381–385.

Sumathy, T., Subramanian, S., Govindasamy, S. and Balakrishna, K. (2001). Protective role of *Bacopa monniera* on morphine induced hepatotoxicity in rats. *Phytotherapy Research*, **15**(7), 643–645.

Suresh, A., Sheela, X., Rosary, Q., Kanmani, R., Mani, C., Easwaran, L., Stanley, A. L. et al. (2010). Isolation and identification of a chalcone from *Bacopa monnieri*. *Asian Journal of Chemistry*, **22**(2), 965–970.

Thakkar, V. T., Deshmukh, A., Hingorani, L., Juneja, P., Baldaniya, L., Patel, A., Pandya, T. and Gohel, M. (2017). Development and optimization of dispersible tablet of *Bacopa monnieri* with improved functionality for memory enhancement. *Journal of Pharmacy and Bioallied Sciences*, **9**, 208–215.

Tothiam, C., Phrompittayarat, W., Putalun, W., Tanaka, H., Sakamoto, S., Khan, I. A. et al. (2011). An enzyme-linked immunosorbant assay using monoclonal antibody against bacoside A3 for determination of jujubogenin glycosides in *Bacopa monnieri* (L.) Wettst. *Phytochemical Analysis*, **22**, 385–391.

Tripathi, Y. B., Chaurasia, S., Tripathi, E., Upadhaya, A. and Dubey, G. P. (1996). *Bacopa monnieri* Linn as an antioxidant: Mechanism of action. *Indian Journal of Experimental Biology*, **34**, 521–526.

Uabundit, N., Wattanathorn, J., Mucimapura, S. and Ingkaninan, K. (2010). Cognitive enhancement and neuroprotective effects of *Bacopa monnieri* in Alzheimer's disease model. *Journal of Ethnopharmacology*, **127**(1), 26–31.

World Health Organization (WHO). (February 2018). *Arsenic Fact Sheet*. Available from: https://www.who.int/news-room/fact-sheets/detail/arsenic.

Zhou, Y., Peng, L., Zhang, W. D. and Kong, D. Y. (2009). Effect of triterpenoid saponins from *Bacopa monniera* on scopolamine-induced memory impairment in mice. *Planta Medica*, **75**(6), 568–574.

Zhou, Y., Shen, Y. H., Zhang, C., Su, J., Liu, R. H. and Zhang, W. D. (2007). Triterpene saponins from *Bacopa monniera* and their antidepressant effects in two mice models. *Journal of Natural Products*, **70**, 652–655.

6 Role of Process Standardisation in Development of Natural Products

Arunporn Etherat, Romanee Sanguandeekul, Panadda Nontahnum, Pimpinan Somsong and George Srzednicki

CONTENTS

6.1   INTRODUCTION

Food is an essential factor for the survival of humans. Food that we are consuming provides metabolic energy that the human organism can process. Its main constituents are the nutrients and also bioactive compounds that have potential to produce various health benefits. Due to the variety of foods produced in different climates, we are all affected by the food that we consume.

Initially, the food chain consisted of only a few staples that were sufficient to sustain the life of humans. Over time, the food chain became much richer and included a number of food items that became known for particular benefits to human health. Such foods are often produced in areas with particular flora, including many medicinal plants. They were well known for generations for their health benefits but often only consumed locally.

In recent times, however, the scientific research in the area of food science, nutrition and medicine has contributed to a better understanding of the relationship between food and health. Vitamins and other essential nutrients were identified during the last century, and appropriate technologies have been developed to modify foods in order to better fulfil the specific needs of the consumer. Among these technologies we should mention food fortification that provides the required nutrients in quantities that are necessary to obtain the expected health benefits. The scientific research related to food is interdisciplinary. It includes such disciplines as agriculture, plant physiology, dietetics, clinical nutrition, epidemiology and food processing.

Food contains six essential nutrients, that is those nutrients the body cannot synthesise by itself, or not in sufficient amounts for the needs of the organism. These nutrients have to be provided by the diet. They include carbohydrates, proteins, fat, minerals, vitamins and water.

In addition to the essential nutrients that are consumed in order to satisfy the metabolic requirements of the human organism, diet can also improve human health. This occurs through the action of compounds with bioactive properties. There is so far no single definition of bioactive compounds. Guaadaoui et al. (2014) attempted to reconcile various existing definitions and eventually described them as: 'a compound which has the capability and the ability to interact with one or more component(s) of the living tissue by presenting a wide range of probable effects'. The term bioactive food (bioactive dietary) compound or components is usually associated with only positive effects on the organism (Biesalski et al. 2009). Such effects are generally the main objective of the research from the food science perspective. However, some compounds may also have negative effects such as toxicity, allergenicity or mutagenicity. Hence, the potential negative effects should also be included in the research.

Bioactive compounds may be of different origin: terrestrial or aquatic; plant, animal or other sources (e.g. microorganisms). However, given the large amount of bioactive compounds in plants, particularly in vegetables, fruits and medicinal plants, the bulk of research is focusing on them as part of the human diet. Vegetables and fruits are a major supplier of vitamins such as vitamin C and provitamin A (β-carotene) and also of polyphenols (e.g. anthocyanins) that act as antioxidants and thus protect the consumer from cancer or cardiovascular diseases. This chapter will present some selected types of bioactive compounds from these sources, the way of incorporating them in foods and examples of testing their effects on human health.

6.2 MAIN BIOACTIVE COMPOUNDS IN HONEY AND BEE PRODUCTS

Among foods that are characterised as functional foods, honey and other products originating from the beehives (i.e. propolis, royal jelly and bee pollen) take a prominent place.

6.2.1 COMPOSITION OF HONEY AND OTHER BEE PRODUCTS

Honey has been used as a stable sweetener and energy source for humans for a long time. It is a supersaturated solution of sugars, mainly fructose (38%), glucose (31%) and maltose-like sugars, with traces of sucrose (Gheldof et al. 2002). The moisture content is about 17.7%. It also contains acids, minerals, vitamins, amino acids, flavonoids and other phenolic compounds and aromatic substances. The composition is variable, depending on the botanical composition and geographical region (Nagai et al. 2006).

Propolis is a sticky resinous substance that bees collect from tree buds and the gummy exudates of plants, mainly poplar (*Populus* sp.), willow, cypress, pines and other conifer trees. Other sources include the peach, eucalyptus and rubber plant. The honey bees mix these resinous substances with beeswax and other secretions (Marcucci et al. 2001; Chen et al. 2009). Propolis is mainly composed of resin (50%), wax (30%), essential oils (10%), pollen (5%) and other organic compounds (5%; Bankova 2005).

Propolis contains at least 300 compounds. The main chemical compounds of propolis are flavonoids (flavones, flavanones, dihydro flavonols and chalcones), phenolic compounds and esters. Other compounds are terpenes, aromatic aldehydes and alcohols. Caffeic acid phenyl ester (CAPE) is also found (Aga et al. 1994).

Royal jelly is a white viscous secretion from the hypopharyngeal and mandibular glands of worker bees. It is solely consumed by the queen bee. Royal jelly is composed of water (50%–60%), proteins (18%), carbohydrate (15%), lipids (3%–6%), mineral salts (1.5%) and vitamins (Nagai and Inoue 2004) along with a large number of bioactive substances in the lipid part such as 10-hydroxy-2-decenoic acid (Caparica-Santos and Marcucci 2007).

Honey, propolis and royal jelly contain phenolic compounds because the honey bees collect nectar from the plants. In honey, propolis and royal jelly most of the phenolic compounds are in the form of flavonoids. The main flavonoids are flavonols (quercetin, kaempferol, galangin and fisetin), flavanones (pinocembrin, naringin and hesperidin) and flavones (apigenin, acacetin, chrysin and luteolin; Cushnie and Lamb 2005; Fiorani et al. 2006). The type and concentration of these flavonoids depend on various factors, such as plant species or flower source of nectar, geographical area, season and other environmental factors. Other bioactive compounds in bee products beside phenolic compounds are proteins (enzymes), peptides and amino acids. Important bioactive compounds in royal jelly are also found in lipid fraction, namely 10-hydroxy-2-decenoic acid.

6.2.2 EXTRACTION OF THE ACTIVE INGREDIENTS

Honey can be used externally for wound healing and cosmetics or internally as a sweetener providing energy or as functional food. So, it is recognised as a medicine as well as an energy-providing food due to its functional properties and nutritional value. Normally, honey is used as a functional food in the form that is obtained from nature with minimal processing.

Royal jelly is normally consumed as a fresh product. Due to its nourishing composition, it is easily degraded. Fresh royal jelly can be stored in a refrigerator (4°C) for a few days and can be kept frozen at the temperature of at least −18°C for a year. For longer shelf life, it should be freeze-dried.

Unlike honey and royal jelly, raw propolis is a resinous substance that cannot be used directly; it should be processed before use. Several extraction methods have been used to separate out the bioactive compounds and formulate products. The most common method for extracting propolis is ethanol extraction. Extraction with ethanol is suitable to obtain de-waxed propolis extracts rich in polyphenolic compounds (Pietta 2000). A 95% ethanol extraction yields the highest concentration of flavonoids and the lowest amount of beeswax (Ahn et al. 2004). Other extraction methods such as aqueous, methanol, hexane, acetone and chloroform have also been used (Pietta et al. 2002).

6.2.3 POTENTIAL APPLICATION OF BIOACTIVE COMPOUNDS FROM HONEY AND BEE PRODUCTS

Functional properties that provide health benefits and applications of honey, propolis and royal jelly are extensively reviewed in several articles (Viuda-Martos et al. 2008; Pasupuleti et al. 2017).

6.2.3.1 Antioxidant

Honey, propolis and royal jelly may be used as functional foods because they have high antioxidant potential. Phenolics are the main contributors to the antioxidant capacity of honey and propolis, which can increase the shelf life of the product, minimise or prolong the occurrence of unpleasant odours and flavours in food, colour loss and loss of nutritional value (Fernandez-Lopez et al. 2007).

In royal jelly, the small peptides (2–4 amino acids) have been shown to possess strong antioxidant activity (Guo et al. 2009).

6.2.3.2 Antimicrobial Agent

Antimicrobial properties can be divided into antibacterial, antifungal, anti-protozoa and antiviral properties. Both honey and propolis have antibacterial properties. Pure honey has bactericidal properties against pathogenic bacteria including *Salmonella* spp., *Escherichia coli*, *Shigella* spp. and many Gram-negative species (Adebolu 2005). Propolis has anti-inflammatory and anti-*Helicobacter pylori* activities, which can be used to treat gastric ulcer (Paulino et al. 2015). The application of a 5% aqueous propolis solution results in an improvement in vaginal infection from yeast-like fungi *Candida albicans*. The oral cavity has significant bacterial microflora and excessive bacterial growth may lead to oral diseases. Propolis may inhibit bacterial plaque development and bring benefits to health (Pereira et al. 2011).

Propolis is capable of inhibiting virus propagation. Amoros et al. (1992) revealed that propolis inhibited propagation of several viruses, including herpes simplex type 1 and 2, adenovirus type 2 and poliovirus type 2. Flavonoids, quercetin and rutin, which are found in both honey and propolis, show antiviral activities (Selway 1986).

Peptides and carboxylic acids in royal jelly have been shown to have antimicrobial properties. Royalisin (51 amino acids) has been reported to have antifungal activity against *Botrytis cinerea* (Fujiwara et al. 1990). The carboxylic acid, 10-HAD in royal jelly, has strong antibacterial properties against *Bacillus subtilis*, *Staphylococcus aureus* and *E. coli* (Alreshoodi and Sultanbawa 2015).

6.2.3.3 Inhibitor of Enzymatic Browning

Furthermore, honey can be used in food processing as a food protector (Osztmianski and Lee 1990; Chen et al. 2000). It can be used as an inhibitor of enzymatic browning in fruits and vegetables. So, honey is a natural alternative to sulphite for controlling the enzymatic browning reaction.

6.2.3.4 Anti-Inflammatory Agent

Honey and propolis also act as anti-inflammatory agents due to the presence of bioactive compounds such as chrysin and galangin (Mirzoeva and Calder 1996; Viuda-Martos et al. 2008).

Besides the functional properties mentioned above, other functional properties of the bioactive compounds present in honey, propolis and royal jelly have been studied. Some of them are antitumour, anticancer, wound healing, anti-ageing and neuroprotective properties (Pasupuleti et al. 2017).

From the functional properties of honey, propolis and royal jelly, it can be seen that the bee products mentioned have a high potential to develop into apitherapeutic agents for humans and animals. However, some considerations should be borne in mind. The first consideration is the form of honey, propolis and royal jelly that would be used and whether to use it in its natural form or to use only the isolated bioactive compounds for a certain purpose, as well as whether the formulation used should contain only one bioactive compound or combination of the compounds for synergistic effect. Second, the effective dose or the right intake dosage for a certain function should be considered. Beside these, we should be aware of the problem of allergens in persons who suffer from allergic reaction to bee-related allergens and impurities that the product extract might contain (e.g. heavy metals in propolis).

6.3 FRUITS AND VEGETABLES AS A SOURCE OF LUTEIN

6.3.1 Main Sources of Lutein in Fruit and Vegetables

Lutein, a yellow plant pigment that is a naturally occurring carotenoid, belongs to the xanthophyll family, one of two major carotenoid families. Among more than 700 carotenoids already isolated (Britton et al. 2004), lutein and zeaxanthin stereoisomers are the major carotenoid pigments that accumulate in human macula lutea, the area responsible for high-resolution vision (Landrum and Bone 2001; Alves-Rodrigues and Shao 2004). Possibly as a result of their action in filtering blue light and deactivating reactive oxygen species, these xanthophylls play an important protective role in maintaining ocular health (Li et al. 2010). Decreasing risk of developing early age-related macular degeneration (AMD), which may lead to the irreversible blindness in the elderly, is related to the consumption of approximately 10 mg/day of lutein, (Huang et al. 2015). There are not only eye health benefits from lutein, but the consumption of lutein may well help maintain heart health by reducing the risk of atherosclerosis, as suggested by various studies (Dwyer et al. 2001; Mares-Perlman et al. 2001). Furthermore, as an antioxidant, lutein may also be essential for skin health since the presence of lutein in skin results in the reduction of UV-induced damage (Roberts et al. 2009).

Humans cannot produce lutein by themselves; therefore, they can only obtain lutein by consuming foods that contain this compound. Although lutein can be found in most fruits and vegetables, the amount of lutein present in plants varies. The main sources of lutein are generally dark, leafy greens such as spinach, kale and parsley (Perry et al. 2009). Table 6.1 shows the sources of lutein in selected fruits and vegetables with high concentrations of lutein.

The daily consumption of 6 mg lutein was recommended in order to reduce the risk of AMD by 57% (Seddon et al. 1994), so the recommendation for adequate lutein intake is to consume 100–500 g/day of leafy green vegetables (Kaczor and Pacia 2016). Nevertheless, the amount of lutein consumption in both United States and Europe is far below this recommendation (Alves-Rodrigues and Shao 2004). Therefore, food products and dietary supplements fortified with lutein may help improve lutein intake to achieve sufficient levels, because usual dietary intake of lutein falls short of the levels associated with many of its benefits.

6.3.2 EXTRACTION OF LUTEIN

Lutein can generally be extracted from natural plants using a solvent following the saponification extraction method, which is widely used in the extraction of carotenoids (Larsen and Christensen 2005). Organic solvents such as hexane, acetone and ethanol are commonly used for the extraction of lutein, a highly lipophilic substance, from plants. The saponification process involves hydrolysing the ester linkages of the lipids to breakdown the matrix for the release of free lutein (Crombie 2004; Yue et al. 2006). Many plant sources of lutein were used in order to study the extraction of lutein, for example, cabbage and spinach as vegetable sources, grapes and oranges as fruit sources and marigold as a flower source. Marigold petals are rich in lutein and are commonly used as raw materials for the extraction of lutein. Because dried marigold flowers contain 0.1%–0.2% dry matter of carotenoids, out of which 80% are lutein diesters, the extraction of lutein from marigold is carried out for commercial purposes in many countries, including Mexico, Peru, Ecuador, Spain, India and China (Šivel et al. 2014). Due to the sensitivity of lutein in alkaline condition, other extraction methods such as using an ultrasound-assisted solvent method have also been investigated for the extraction of lutein.

TABLE 6.1
Lutein Content (mg/100 g Wet Basis) in Selected Fruits and Vegetables

Food	Treatment	Content	Sources
Kale	Fresh	18.63	Müller (1997)
	Canned	49	de Sá and Rodriguez-Amaya (2003)
Water cress	Fresh	7.54	Kimura and Rodriguez-Amaya (2003)
Spinach	Raw	6.60	Perry et al. (2009)
	Cooked	12.64	Perry et al. (2009)
Grapes (*Vitis vinifera*)	Fresh	6.60	Guedes de Pinho et al. (2001)
Parsley	Raw	4.32	Perry et al. (2009)
Broccoli	Fresh	2.83	Khachik et al. (1992)
	Steamed (5 min)	3.25	Khachik et al. (1992)

The lutein content extracted from egg yolk with the ultrasound-assisted solvent method was higher than that extracted with the alkaline solvent. This is probably because the sonication could extensively break down the egg yolk matrix to release lutein (Yue et al. 2006). In order to reduce the extraction time and decrease the amount of solvent used, the supercritical carbon dioxide has been studied for the extraction of lutein from plants as well. The level of pressure, temperature, CO_2 flow rate and co-solvent used in processing have a direct effect on the efficiency of this technique (Ma et al. 2008; Palumpitag et al. 2011). The manufacture of dietary supplements or the enrichment of foods and drinks with carotenoids use free lutein and ester lutein extracted from plants in the form of powder, oil or beadlets (Šivel et al. 2014).

6.3.3 Applications/Uses of Lutein in Food Products and Factors Affecting Its Stability

Lutein, with the levels of usage ranging from 2.0 to 330 mg/kg on fresh weight basis for foods, is generally used as a colouring agent in food products such as chewing gum, processed fruits, fruit juices, breakfast cereals and baked goods (Cantrill et al. 2016). Increasing the consumption level of lutein by increasing the amount of lutein in food products has been widely studied. When adding FloraGLO Lutein 20% in corn oil into fat-free strawberry yogurt, the physicochemical and sensory characteristics of strawberry-flavoured yogurts were not affected by the addition of lutein. However, there was a relatively small decline in lutein content of yogurts over the 5 weeks of storage, with the pH of yogurt decreasing from 4.4 to 3.9 upon storage for this period. There was no major change in yogurt characteristics when adding up to 3 mg of lutein per 170 g of yogurt (Aryana et al. 2006).

Lutein is sensitive to light, heat and oxygen (Boon et al. 2010). The degradation of lutein was observed when lutein-fortified wholegrain flours were used to produce bakery products including pan bread, flat bread, biscuits and muffins. The eminent vulnerability to heat of lutein is related to the degradation of carotenoids. Compared to bread, fortified biscuits and muffins showed greater lutein reduction. Nonetheless, the fortified bakery products still contained sufficient amounts of lutein per serving (up to 1.0 mg/serving) and would hold promise for the development of high-lutein functional foods (Abdel-Aal et al. 2010).

To produce lutein-enriched frankfurter products, lutein was added to sausages. The bioaccessibility of lutein in frankfurters fortified with lutein exceeded 30% of the amount initially present (Granado-Lorencio et al. 2010). This percentage was higher than the bioavailability of lutein detected from raw fruits and vegetables, which showed the values of bioavailability of lutein of approximately 1%–15% (Fernández-Sevilla et al. 2010).

Despite the amount of lutein present in foods, the real benefit of consuming lutein depends on its bioavailability. Zaripheh and Erdman (2002) reported that the molecular structure and physical disposition of xanthophylls in the food network and the interactions of xanthophylls with other compounds were the major factors limiting their bioavailability. Dietary lipids are important cofactors for carotenoid bioavailability (Parada and Aguilera 2007). The absorption of lutein could be enhanced by the addition of dietary fat to lutein-enriched products or lutein supplements. The presence of dietary fat was thought to be important to stimulate the gallbladder to release bile acids and digestive enzyme, and also for micelle formation for absorption in the small intestine. Therefore, plant sources that have high amounts of lutein but low lipid content are less bioavailable unless processed to destroy the food matrix to release lutein or consumed with a minimum amount of fat in the food system. Nano-scale products would also increase the bioavailability of lutein. Arunkumar et al. (2013) revealed that lutein nanoparticles entrapped in chitosan had higher lutein bioavailability in mice than lutein in mixed micelles. The bioavailability of a nano-emulsion of lutein was also reported to be greater than that of lutein supplement pills (Vishwanathan et al. 2009). When smaller nanoparticle sizes lutein were produced, the bioavailability of lutein showed a tendency to increase; however, the stability of lutein upon storage decreased due to the relatively higher surface area to volume ratio of particles exposed to environment. The stability of lutein as a function of temperature and UV exposure have been extensively studied, and it has been concluded that lutein is easily degraded by heat and susceptible to UV light. The degradation rate constant of lutein nano-emulsions stabilised by whey protein isolate when kept for 28 days at 40°C was approximately 8 times higher than that kept at 5°C (Teo et al. 2017). When exposed to UV light for only 48 h, the lutein remaining in emulsified lutein esters with oil ranged between approximately 15%–60%, depending on the types of oils used in the emulsion systems (Khalil et al. 2012). Therefore, the proper storage conditions for lutein products are at a low temperature in the absence of UV light.

6.4 ANTHOCYANINS IN BERRIES

6.4.1 REVIEW OF BERRY TYPES KNOWN AS AN IMPORTANT SOURCE OF ANTHOCYANINS

According to the common usage of the term, a berry is a small, fleshy fruit. They are often brightly coloured, juicy, with a sweet or sour taste. Berries do not have a stone or pit, but may have many pips or seeds. Some of them are produced from the ovary of a single flower in which the outer layer of the ovary wall develops into an edible fleshy portion (pericarp), as per strictly scientific definition of a berry. Others are aggregate or multiple fruits. Among the most common berries are strawberries, raspberries, blueberries, but also grapes, which are normally not considered berries. Most berries are edible, but some are toxic (e.g. *Atropa belladonna*, called 'belladonna') or toxic when unripe (e.g. white mulberry, red mulberry and elderberry) but edible when they are ripe.

Berries are not only appreciated as being very tasty and having low energy but also increasingly because of their bioactive compounds. Therefore they are often used as ingredients in functional foods. The species with a high content of bioactive compounds belong to various families, especially Rosaceae (strawberry, raspberry, blackberry), and Ericaceae (blueberry, cranberry). Among the bioactive compounds are antioxidants such as phenolic compounds and fruit colourants (anthocyanins and carotenoids). The phenolics in berries include phenolic acids, such as hydroxybenzoic and hydroxycinnamic acid conjugates, as well as further flavonoids, such as flavonols, flavanols and particularly anthocyanins. As for tannins, they are divided into condensed tannins (proanthocyanidins) and hydrolysable tannins, which have been found to be important bioactive compounds. Moreover, bioactive compounds include other antioxidants such as vitamins (ascorbic acid) and minerals with antioxidant properties. Among the cultivated berries, blueberries, cranberries, blackberries, raspberries and strawberries are a major source of anthocyanins, see Table 6.2 (Skrovankova et al. 2015).

6.4.2 EXTRACTION OF ANTHOCYANINS

Anthocyanins in plants occur as glycosides of six common anthocyanidins including cyanidin, delphinidin, petunidin, peonidin, pelargonidin and malvidin, which give a different colour spectrum of anthocyanins ranging from red to purple (Figure 6.1). The structure of anthocyanins is polar, so they can be extracted using various organic polar solvents. The common solvents used for anthocyanin extraction are methanol, ethanol, acetone, water or a mixture of these solvents. Methanol is efficient in terms of anthocyanin extraction, but its toxicity limits its use, especially when the anthocyanins are meant to be used in foods. Acetone is less toxic than many other solvents and allows an efficient and more reproducible extraction. Using acetone to extract plant anthocyanins can avoid the interference from pectin that is generally dissolved in alcohol or water. Acetone requires lower temperature for evaporation after extraction. Acid is added into the extraction solvent to keep anthocyanin in its stable flavylium cation form at an acidic pH that is generally lower than pH 2. Still, highly acidic solution may cause partial hydrolysis of acyl moieties in acylated anthocyanins. Hydrochloric acid was widely used in the past, but more recently weaker acids such as formic acid, tartaric acid or citric acid have become more commonly used. After solvent extraction, solid phase purification is used to purify anthocyanin from other compounds such as organic acids that are co-present in the crude extract.

Other techniques concerning extraction of anthocyanins have been developed including, for example, the use of ultrasonic-assisted systems to aid in plant cell disruption. Supercritical fluid

TABLE 6.2
Anthocyanin Composition in the Main Cultivated Berries

Berry	Anthocyanins
Blueberry	Cyanidin glycosides
(*Vaccinium ashei; V. angustifolium; V. corymbosum*)	Delphinidin glycosides
	Malvidin glycosides
	Petunidin glycosides
	Peonidin glycosides
Cranberry	Cyanidin glycosides
(*V. macrocarpon*)	Peonidin glycosides
	Pelargonidin glycosides
	Malvidin glycosides
	Delphinidin glycosides
	Petunidin glycosides
Red raspberry	Cyanidin glycosides
(*Rubus idaeus*)	Pelargonidin glycosides
Blackberries	Cyanidin glycosides
(*Rubus fruticosus*)	Pelargonidin glycosides
	Peonidin glycosides
Strawberry	Cyanidin glycosides
(*Fragaria ananassa*)	Pelargonidin glycosides
	Peonidin glycosides

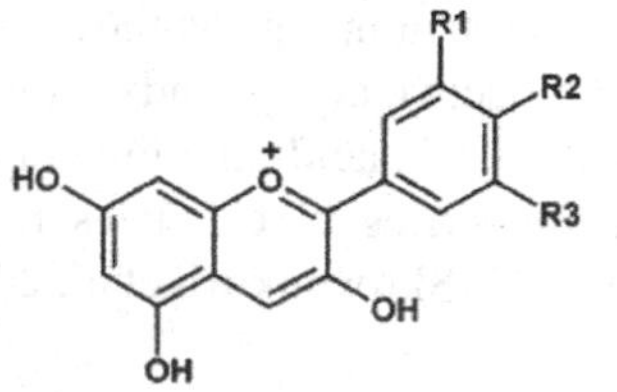

Anthocyanidins	R1	R2	R3	MW	Colour
Pelargonidin (Pg)	H	OH	H	271	Orange
Cyanidin (Cy)	OH	OH	H	287	Orange red
Peonidin (Pn)	OCH$_3$	OH	H	301	Red
Delphinidin (Dp)	OH	OH	OH	303	Bluish red
Petunidin (Pt)	OCH$_3$	OH	OH	317	Bluish red
Malvidin (Mv)	OCH$_3$	OH	OCH$_3$	331	Bluish red

FIGURE 6.1 Structure of common anthocyanins.

extraction (SFE) and pressurised liquid extraction (PLE) have also been assayed to extract anthocyanins, because solvent extraction may cause partial hydrolysis of acylated anthocyanin. However, these techniques are still of limited use because PLE involves high temperature and high pressure that may cause anthocyanin degradation, and SFE is found to suit mostly non-polar compounds.

6.4.3 RECOVERY AND PRESERVATION OF ANTHOCYANINS

The recovery of anthocyanin after extraction depends primarily on the types and concentration of solvents, time, temperature and solvent to solid ratio. In general, acidified methanol gives the highest recovery solvent extraction. Yet, because of its toxicity, other solvents or techniques are being developed as a substitute. For example, Hua et al. (2013) could recover up to 96.09% of anthocyanin extracted from fruit pulp retrieved after juice production by using aqueous two-phase extraction containing 30% (w/w) ethanol and 19% ammonium sulphate. After extraction, anthocyanins can be purified and recovered through solid phase extraction using SPE cartridge, solid phase micro-extraction (SPME) by C18 cartridge or HPLC. Nevertheless, SPME application is limited by the capability to hold only small amounts of anthocyanin due to the small volume of coated polymer. HPLC is also not popular due to its high cost. Various types of resin on column chromatography have been alternatively selected for collecting large amount of extracted anthocyanins. After loading anthocyanins to the cartridge or column, they will usually be eluted using acidified alcohol. It is recommended to preserve the purified anthocyanin extracts in a cold, dark and oxygen-free environment. Freeze drying of purified anthocyanin followed by storage in a dark and cold place is a common practice to prevent the loss of anthocyanins.

6.4.4 APPLICATIONS/USES OF ANTHOCYANINS IN FOOD PRODUCTS AND FACTORS AFFECTING THEIR STABILITY

Food and dietary supplements are the most common application of anthocyanins. The use of anthocyanin in food is as food colourant in various products such as soft drinks, jelly and soup. The use of anthocyanin-derived colorants is approved as a natural dye by the Codex Alimentarius Commission (Codex), European Union (EU) and US Food and Drug Administration (FDA). They are given INS and E-number: INS or E 163. In EU, sources of anthocyanins can be from grape skin, blackcurrant, purple corn, red cabbage, black carrot and purple sweet potatoes while the United States has more strict use of anthocyanin colourants, which must be sourced from grape colour extract and grape skin extract. Dietary supplements of anthocyanin from various fruit source are widely found in marketplace (Lee 2016). Numerous scientific reviews of the potential health benefits of anthocyanins owing to their anticancer, anti-inflammatory, protective effect on cardiometabolic and neuronal health has raised interest among health-conscious consumers for decades (Faria et al. 2010; Huang et al. 2014; Burton-Freeman et al. 2016). However, the anthocyanins in a product may present in much lower concentrations than expected because the anthocyanin itself is sensitive to various processing conditions.

The anthocyanin structure determines its stability: the increase in number and position of hydroxyl will improve its stability, while more methoxyl groups weaken its stability. Acylation clearly increases anthocyanin stability. The classic examples of plants that contain a high amount of acylated anthocyanin are *Ipomoea tricolor*, *Zebrina pendula* and *Clitoria ternatea* and the anthocyanins extracted from them are highly stable (Teh and Francis 1988). Sweet potatoes and red radish contain a higher number of acylated anthocyanins than those from grapes, strawberries and raspberries, so these are more stable to heat and UV light (Hayashi et al. 1996). Changes of pH from acidic to basic will transform anthocyanins that exist in stable flavylium cation (at pH less than 3) form to unstable ionic chalcone (beyond pH 6). High temperature causes hydrolysis of sugar residues and formation of furfural and hydroxymethylfurfural, which has been shown to accelerate anthocyanin degradation (Oancea et al. 2012). Storage of product at low temperatures is an appropriate approach to protect anthocyanins. Blueberries can be stored at $-18°C$ for up to 3 months without significant change in anthocyanin level, while drying could cause more than 40% loss (Lohachoompol et al. 2004). Oxygen increases the rate of degradation by a direct and indirect oxidation mechanism, and oxygen and ascorbic acid also act synergistically to cause high rates of anthocyanin degradation (Jackman and Smith 1996). Radiation causes instability of anthocyanin pigment. Anthocyanins from *Tibouchina semidecandra* stored in the dark at 25°C kept their colour for up to 26 days versus only 10 days if exposed to light during storage (Janna et al. 2007).

6.5 BENEFICIAL EFFECTS OF BIOACTIVE PHYTOCHEMICALS FOR HUMAN HEALTH

Plants have long been used as health foods and sources of medicinal properties. An impressive number of modern drugs have been isolated or derived from natural sources, based on their use in traditional medicine or their ethnopharmacological use, which is also channelled into the discovery of new biologically active molecules (Houghton 1995). In Thai traditional medicine, the theory recommended using the taste technique for indicating pharmacological properties, that is, plants with a bitter taste were used as antipyretic, antidiabetic or hepatotonic drugs (Subcharoen 1998). This theory was proved by many studies to be true. Bitter gourd or bitter melon (*Momordica charantia* L) is used as a vegetable in Thai cuisine and has a bitter taste. It is also used in Thai traditional medicine to treat diabetic patients and was found to have hepatotonic and antidiabetic activities (Cortez-Navarrete et al. 2018). Cucurbitane-type triterpenoid isolated from *M. charantia* has potential for the prevention and management of diabetes by improving insulin sensitivity and glucose homeostasis (Han et al. 2018). Neem (*Azadirachta indica* var. *siamensis* Valeton) is used as a food and has a bitter taste. It is used to reduce fever in Thai traditional medicine. Many studies have shown its antipyretic (Okpanyi and Ezeukwu 1981; Ashorobi 1998) and antidiabetic activity (Satyanarayana et al. 2015). Astringent tasting foods in Thai traditional medicine were used for antidiarrheal treatment and wound healing. Guava leaves (*Psidium guajava* Linn), which have an astringent taste, are used as an antidiarrheal remedy (Katpunyapong et al. 1998; Ojewole et al. 2008). The leaves are rich in tannins and phenolic compounds (Simão et al. 2017). Knowledge of the principles of folk medicine is important for investigators studying bioactive compounds (Nakanishi 1999).

6.5.1 TESTING OF BENEFICIAL EFFECTS OF BIOACTIVE PHYTOCHEMICALS FOR HUMAN HEALTH

Nowadays, the study of bioactive compounds from plants requires the development of bioassay techniques, especially *in vitro* methods that allow large numbers of plant extracts to be screened for activity – especially cytotoxic compounds against many types of cancer cell lines. *In vitro* assays are particularly useful for bioassay-guided fractionation of plant extracts. It is not always possible to test against cancer in animal models. *In vitro* assays are more sensitive to most antitumor agents than *in vivo* assays and also cost less and require less test material and time. Development of methods for initial screening by the US National Cancer Institute (NCI) started in 1955. The initial screening programme or primary screening used the *in vivo* L-1210 and P388 mouse leukaemia models for selection of anticancer compounds. NCI developed *in vitro* assay using Sulphorhodamine B assay (SRB) for screening cytotoxic activity against cancer cell lines in 1990. This program could screen 20,000 compounds per year (Skehan et al. 1990).

Inflammation is a complex pathophysiological process mediated by a variety of signalling molecules produced by macrophages, leukocytes and mast cells, and so forth. Macrophages play a central role in host defence against foreign agents by releasing various pro-inflammatory cytokines and inflammatory mediators such as nitric oxide (NO), tumour necrosis factor-alpha (TNF-α) and cyclooxygenase (COX-2; Saha et al. 2004). NO, an inorganic free radical, is synthesised from the amino acid L-arginine by a family of nitric oxide synthases (NOS). In the NOS family, inducible nitric oxide synthase (iNOS) is a main source of NO produced by macrophages during inflammation. Overproduction of NO has been involved in many diseases such as cancer, asthma, rheumatoid arthritis and atherosclerosis (Lee et al. 2013; Sowndharajan et al. 2016). Griess assay has been used to determine the inhibition of nitric oxide formation in RAW 264.7 cells induced by lipopolysaccharide (LPS) and interferon-gamma (INF-γ; Zhu et al. 2002). This assay was used to test for chronic inflammation and it showed high benefits for screening in natural products.

6.5.2 THE EFFICACY OF KEY BIOACTIVE COMPOUNDS FROM FOODS IN TERMS OF ANTICANCER AND ANTI-INFLAMMATORY EFFECTS

Benjakul (BJK), a Thai traditional medicine preparation, has long been used for balanced health, control of abnormalities in the body, carminative effects and the relief of flatulence. This preparation is a food preparation. It is composed of five plants: *Piper interruptum* Opiz., *Piper longum* L., *Piper sarmentosum* Roxb., *Plumbago indica* L. and *Zingiber officinale* Roscoe. The ethanol extracts of BJK, its five individual plants and pure constituents of BJK were investigated for their anti-inflammatory activity using LPS-induced nitric oxide (NO) and tumour necrosis factor-alpha (TNF-α) in RAW 264.7 cells. The ethanol extracts of BJK exhibited potent NO inhibitory effect (IC_{50} = 16.60 μg/mL), but were inactive on TNF-α release. Determination of the anti-inflammatory activity by measuring the inhibition of NO production showed that plumbagin and 6-shogaol exhibited higher values than crude BJK with IC_{50} values of 0.002 and 0.92 μg/mL, respectively. In particular, plumbagin also showed higher anti-inflammatory activity than prednisolone, positive control, with IC_{50} value of 0.59 μg/mL. Also 6-shogaol showed an inhibitory effect on TNF-α release (IC_{50} = 9.16 μg/mL). These preliminary results may provide some scientific support for the use of BJK for inflammatory disorders through the inhibition of NO production. (Makchuchit et al. 2017). BJK also showed high cytotoxicity against breast cancer cell (MCF-7) and its components extracts when using the SRB assay. The extraction method imitated folk doctors' use of maceration in ethanol and boiling in water. The results showed that the ethanol extract of *Piper chaba*, *Zingiber officinale* and BJK displayed high cytotoxic activity against breast cancer cell (IC_{50} = 35.17, 31.15 and 33.20 μg/mL, respectively), but the water extract showed no cytotoxic activity against breast cancer cells. Two compounds (piperine and 6-shogaol as 7.48% and 0.54% w/w of crude extract) were isolated from the ethanol extract of BJK by bioassay guide fractionation and they were also tested for cytotoxic activity. It was found that piperine and 6-shogaol had cytotoxicity against MCF7 with IC_{50} value of 9.8 and 10.18 μg/mL (Sakpakdeejaroen and Itharat 2009). These five plants and BJK were also investigated for cytotoxic activity against four human cancer cell lines: large lung carcinoma (CORL23), cervical cancer cell lines (Hela), liver cancer cell line (HepG2) and also tested against one normal lung fibroblast cell (MRC-5) using the SRB assay. The extraction method imitated folk doctors who use maceration in ethanol and boiling in water. The ethanol extract of BJK showed specific cytotoxic against lung cancer cell (IC_{50} = 19.8 μg/mL). Three compounds [gingerol, plumbagin and piperine as 0.54%, 4.18% and 7.48% w/w of crude extract] were isolated from the ethanol extract of BJK by bioassay guided fractionation and they were also tested for cytotoxic activity (Ruangnoo et al. 2012). It was found that plumbagin showed the highest cytotoxic activity against CORL-23, HepG2, Hela and MRC-5 (IC_{50} = 2.55, 2.61, 4.16 and 11.54 μM). These results could support using BJK to treat cancer patients and its three compounds could be markers for standardisation of this preparation. Piperine has been identified as the main compound and plumbagin as the most cytotoxic compound. The study also developed a reversed-phase high-performance liquid chromatography (HPLC) method for quality control such as chemical fingerprint, quantification and stability of the ethanol extract of BJK preparation. Reversed-phase HPLC was performed with a gradient mobile phase composed of water and acetonitrile, and peaks were detected at 256 nm. Based on the validation results, this analytical method is a precise, accurate and stable method to quantify determination of piperine and plumbagin, which are the cytotoxic compounds isolated from the ethanol extract of BJK preparation. The stability of the ethanol extract of the BJK preparation was evaluated under accelerated conditions (45 $\pm$ 2°C with 75 $\pm$ 5% RH for 4 months). The results indicated that piperine appears to be a stable compound (Itharat and Sakpakdeejaroen 2010). BJK ethanol extract also inhibited an increase in tumour size in mice induced by a tumour promoter.

6.5.3 CLINICAL STUDIES RELATED TO EFFECTS OF BIOACTIVE EXTRACT ON CANCER AND INFLAMMATION

BJK extract was also investigated in a clinical study. The safety study of BJK extract tablets included 20 normal volunteers. The volunteers were divided into 2 groups, 10 samples for each, which contained 100 and 200 mg orally, respectively. The tablet was taken 3 times a day after meal for 14 days. The safety of the BJK extract tablets was determined by physical examination and laboratory tests, including liver function test (LFT), renal function test (RFT), lipid profile, blood sugar, haematology and malondialdehyde assay, before and after administering BJK extract tablets on day 0, day 1, day 7, day 14 and 2 weeks after stopping tablet intake (D_{1m}). Twenty-three subjects took BJK extract tablets with conventional medicine. The results showed neither of the two groups of volunteers had any severe adverse event (SAE). The results of this study indicated that the tablets of BJK extract 100 and 200 mg taken 3 times a day continually for 14 days did not yield clinical signs revealed by abnormalities or laboratory tests (Amorndoljai et al. 2011). The clinical efficacy and safety of BJK in stage 4 non-small cell lung cancer patients was also studied. This trial was approved by the Medical Ethics Committee of the Faculty of Medicine, Thammasat University. Four volunteer patients who met the inclusion criteria, received a BJK capsule of 100 mg/capsule. They took 2 capsules 3 times a day for 24 weeks. This was followed up with assessment of the history of capsule intake, physical examination, laboratory tests and assessment of quality of life before and during treatment every 4 weeks. The results show that the intake of BJK capsules did not produce any side effect on the ECOG (Eastern Cooperative Oncology Group) performance scale and O_2 saturation, which is a test that measures the amount of oxygen being carried by red blood cells. The response of volunteers to the test showed that the disease stabilised up to 4 months, in later stages. The quality of life of the volunteers improved after the test, however. As for the safety aspect, the volunteers had symptoms of sweating and some stomach discomfort, but no renal toxicity was detected after taking BJK for 5 months. BJK can increase quality of life, and stabilise the disease for up to 4 months (Pagarang et al. 2017). BJK ethanol extract also showed good anti-inflammatory and analgesic activities in *in vivo* studies. Thus, the investigation of the clinical efficacy and safety of the BJK extract for treating primary osteoarthritis of the knee (OA knee) was compared with the standard NSAIDs, diclofenac. A clinical phase 2 trial, double blind, randomised controlled study was conducted. Eighty-four patients diagnosed with primary OA knee were randomly treated with either BJK remedy extract or diclofenac for 28 days. The BJK group received 100 mg of BJK extract/capsule 3 times per day, orally after meals, while the other group received 25 mg of diclofenac sodium capsules 3 times per day, orally after meals. All patients were followed up at 14 and 28 days. The changing of the visual analogue scale (VAS) for pain, 100-metre walk times, the Modified Thai WOMAC Index (Western Ontario and McMaster Universities) Arthritis Index scores and the global assessment were used for evaluation of efficacy. For safety issues, clinical signs and symptoms, complete physical examination and renal and liver function were evaluated. The results revealed that 77 patients completed the intervention, 39 patients for the BJK extract group and 38 patients for diclofenac group. For efficacy, all patients from both groups reported a decrease in VAS pain score and 100-metre walking times, but only the diclofenac group showed significant reduction of both measurements when compared to baseline (day 0). The modified Thai WOMAC score in both groups showed a significantly reduction from baseline. However, all efficacy outcomes were not significantly different between the two groups. For safety outcomes, the patients from both groups had no severe adverse events reported. The blood chemistry showed no toxicity in renal and liver functions after taking BJK extract for 28 days, while the patients who took diclofenac showed significant increase in both their renal and liver function chemistry levels. Moreover, Blood Urine Nitrogen (BUN) was significantly different between the two groups. The BJK remedy extract showed equal clinical efficacy in relieving symptoms of OA knee when compared with diclofenac and improved the quality of life in OA patients with less systemic side effects when compared with diclofenac. Using BJK is a good alternative for treating osteoarthritis of the knee (Rachawat et al. 2017). The clinical studies of BJK, a combination of herbs with various bioactive compounds, demonstrated their benefits for human health.

6.6   CONCLUDING REMARKS

This chapter describes three examples of bioactive compounds that are of importance in functional foods. The first group of compounds is found in honey and bee products. It includes substances found in plants and also those produced by bees such as propolis and royal jelly. They show antimicrobial properties, are anti-inflammatory agents and can inhibit enzymatic browning. The second group is lutein, a plant pigment that is a naturally occurring carotenoid and is found mostly in dark, leafy vegetables and selected fruits. Lutein is the major carotenoid pigment accumulated in the human macula lutea, the area responsible for high-resolution vision. The third group comprises antioxidants such as phenolic compounds and fruit colourants (anthocyanins and carotenoids). Their sources are mainly edible berries.

The three groups of bioactive compounds are characterised by their main source, followed by the extraction method and then by description of their applications and factors affecting their stability in food products.

The last section dealt with the techniques used to study the potential beneficial effects of bioactive phytochemicals for human health. Special consideration is given to bioassays that are used to screen the plant extracts for their activity. A second aspect that is considered is the testing for the anticancer and anti-inflammatory effects of plants that are used as food but are also known as medicinal plants. Finally, the chapter includes the description of clinical tests that compare the food extracts with pharmaceuticals following a series of standard tests used in the development of new drugs.

REFERENCES

Abdel-Aal, E. S. M., Young, J. C., Akhtar, H. and Rabalski, I. (2010). Stability of lutein in wholegrain bakery products naturally high in lutein or fortified with free lutein. *Journal of Agricultural and Food Chemistry*, **58**(18), 10109–10117.

Adebolu, T. (2005). Effect of natural honey on local isolates of diarrhea-causing bacteria in southwestern Nigeria. *African Journal of Biotechnology*, **4**(10), 1172–1174.

Aga, H., Shibuya, T., Sugimoto, T., Kurimoto, M. and Nakajima, S. H. (1994). Isolation and identification of antimicrobial compounds in Brazilian propolis. *Bioscience, Biotechnology, and Biochemistry*, **58**, 945–946.

Ahn, M. R., Kumazawa, S., Hamasaka, T., Bang, K. S. and Nakayama, T. (2004). Antioxidant activity and constituents of propolis collected in various areas of Korea. *Journal of Agricultural and Food Chemistry*, **52**(24), 7286–7292.

Alreshoodi, F. M. and Sultanbawa, T. (2015). Antimicrobial activity of royal jelly. *Anti-infective Agents*, **13**, 50–59.

Alves-Rodrigues, A. and Shao, A. (2004). The science behind lutein. *Toxicology Letters*, **150**(1), 57–83.

Amorndoljai, P., Kiatinun, S. and Sompan, N. (2011). Study on safety of Benjakul extract tablet in normal volunteers. *Thammasat Medical Journal*, **11**(2), 195–202.

Amoros, M., Sauvager, F., Girre, L. and Cormier, M. (1992). In vitro antiviral activity of propolis. *Apidologie*, **23**(3), 231–240.

Arunkumar, R., Prashanth, K. V. H. and Baskaran, V. (2013). Promising interaction between nanoencapsulated lutein with low molecular weight chitosan: Characterization and bioavailability of lutein *in vitro* and *in vivo*. *Food Chemistry*, **141**(1), 327–337.

Aryana, K. J., Barnes, H. T., Emmick, T. K., McGrew, P. and Moser, B. (2006). Lutein is stable in strawberry yogurt and does not affect its characteristics. *Journal of Food Science*, **71**(6), S467–S472.

Ashorobi, R. B. (1998). Antipyretic effects of *Azadirachta indica* in bacteria endotoxin induced fever in the rat. *Phytotherapy Research*, **12**(1), 41–43.

Bankova, V. (2005). Chemical diversity of propolis and the problem of standardization. *Journal of Ethnopharmacology*, **100**(1–2), 114–117.

Biesalski, H.-K., Dragsted, L. O., Elmadfa, I. et al. (2009). Bioactive compounds: Definition and assessment of activity. *Nutrition*, **25**(11–12), 1202–1205.

Boon, C. S., McClements, D. J., Weiss, J. and Decker, E. A. (2010). Factors influencing the chemical stability of carotenoids in foods. *Critical Reviews in Food Science and Nutrition*, **50**(6), 515–532.

Britton, G., Liaaen-Jensen, S. and Pfander, H. (2004). *Carotenoids Handbook*. Basel, Switzerland: Birkhauser Verlag.

Burton-Freeman, B. M., Sandhu, A. K. and Edirisinghe, I. (2016). Red raspberries and their bioactive polyphenols: Cardiometabolic and neuronal health links. *Advances in Nutrition*, **7**, 44–65.

Cantrill, R., Meyland, I. and Dessipri, E. (2016). Lutein esters from *Tagetes erecta*: Chemical and Technical Assessment (CTA). Rome, Italy: Food and Agriculture Organization of the United Nations.

Caparica-Santos, C. and Marcucci, M. C. (2007). Quantitative determination of trans-10-hydroxy-2-decenoic acid (10-HDA) in Brazilian royal jelly and commercial products containing royal jelly. *Journal of Apicultural Research*, **46**(3), 149–153.

Chen, L., Mehta, A., Berenvaum, M., Zangerl, A. R. and Engeseth, J. (2000). Honeys from different floral sources as inhibitors of enzymatic browning in fruit and vegetable homogenates. *Journal of Agricultural and Food Chemistry*, **48**, 4997–5000.

Chen, L., Sanguandeekul, R., Zhang, F., Deaowanish, S., Thapa, R. and Wongsiri, S. (2009). Advance in propolis research in China. *Journal of Royal Institute of Thailand*, **12**, 136–151.

Cortez-Navarrete, M., Martínez-Abundis, E., Pérez-Rubio, K. G., González-Ortiz, M. and Villar, M. M. (2018). *Momordica charantia* administration improves insulin secretion in type 2 diabetes mellitus. *Journal of Medicinal Food*. doi:10.1089/jmf.2017.0114.

Crombie, L. B. (2004). Method for extracting lutein from green plant materials. US Patent 6,737,552.

Cushnie, T. P. T. and Lamb, A. J. (2005). Detection of galangin-induced cytoplasmic membrane damage in *Staphylococcus aureus* by measuring potassium loss. *Journal of Ethnopharmacology*, **101**, 243–248.

de Sá, M. D. and Rodriguez-Amaya, D. B. (2003). Carotenoid composition of cooked green vegetables from restaurants. *Food Chemistry*, **83**(4), 595–600.

Dwyer, J. H., Navab, M., Dwyer, K. M., Hassan, K., Sun, P., Shircore, A., Hama-Levy, S. et al. (2001). Oxygenated carotenoid lutein and progression of early atherosclerosis: The Los Angeles atherosclerosis study. *Circulation*, **103**(24), 2922–2927.

Faria, A., Pestana, D., Teixeira, D., de Freitas, V., Mateus, N. and Calhau, C. (2010). Blueberry anthocyanins and pyruvic acid adducts: Anticancer properties in breast cancer cell lines. *Phytotherapy Research*, **24**(12), 1862–1869.

Fernandez-Lopez, J., Viuda-Martos, M., Sendra, E., Sayas-Barbera, E., Navarro, C. and Perez-Alvarez, J. A. (2007). Orange fibre as potential functional ingredient for dry-cured sausages. *European Food Research and Technology*, **226**(1–2), 1–6.

Fernández-Sevilla, J. M., Acién Fernández, F. G. and Molina Grima, E. (2010). Biotechnological production of lutein and its applications. *Applied Microbiology and Biotechnology*, **86**(1), 27–40.

Fiorani, M., Accorsi, A., Blasa, M., Diamantini, G. and Piatti, E. (2006). Flavonoids from Italian multifloral honeys reduce the extracellular ferricyanide in human red blood cells. *Journal of Agricultural and Food Chemistry*, **54**, 8328–8334.

Fujiwara, S., Imai, J., Fujiwara, M., Yaeshima, T., Kawashima, T., Kawashima, T. and Kobayashi, K. (1990). A potent antibacterial protein in royal jelly. Purification and determination of the primary structure of royalisin. *The Journal of Biological Chemistry*, **265**, 11333–11337.

Gheldof, N., Wang, X. H. and Engeseth, N. J. (2002). Identification and quantification of antioxidant components of honeys from various floral sources. *Journal of Agricultural and Food Chemistry*, **50**(21), 5870–5877.

Granado-Lorencio, F., López-López, I., Herrero-Barbudo, C., Blanco-Navarro, I., Cofrades, S., Pérez-Sacristán, B., Delgado-Pando, G. et al. (2010). Lutein-enriched Frankfurter-type products: Physicochemical characteristics. *Food Chemistry*, **120**(3), 741–748.

Guaadaoui, A., Benaicha, S., Elmajdoub, N., Bellaoui, M. and Hamal, A. (2014). What is a bioactive compound? A combined definition for a preliminary consensus. *International Journal of Nutrition and Food Sciences*, **3**(3), 174–179.

Guedes de Pinho, P., Silva Ferreira, A. C., Mendes Pinto, M., Gomez Benitez, J. and Hogg, T. A. (2001). Determination of carotenoid profiles in grapes, musts, and fortified wines from Douro varieties of *Vitis vinifera*. *Journal of Agricultural and Food Chemistry*, **49**(11), 5484–5488.

Guo, H., Kouzuma, Y. and Yonekura, M. (2009). Structures and properties of antioxidative peptides derived from royal jelly protein. *Food Chemistry*, **113**, 238–245.

Han J. H., Tuan N. Q., Park, M. H., Quan, K. T., Oh, J., Heo, K. S., Na, M. et al. (2018). Cucurbitane triterpenoids from the fruits of *Momordica charantia* improve insulin sensitivity and glucose homeostasis in streptozotocin-induced diabetic mice. *Molecular Nutrition and Food Research*. doi:10.1002/mnfr.201700769.

Houghton, P. (1995). The role of plants in traditional medicine and current therapy. *The Journal of Alternative and Complementary Medicine*, **1**(3), 131–143.

Hua, Z., Yuesheng, D., Ge, X., Menglu, L., Liya, D., LiJia, A. and Zhilong, Z. (2013). Extraction and purification of anthocyanins from the fruit residues of *Vaccinium uliginosum* Linn. *Journal of Chromatography & Separation Techniques*, **4**(2), 167. doi:10.4172/2157-7064.1000167.

Huang, W. Y., Liu, Y. M., Wang, J., Wang, X. N. and Li, C. Y. (2014). Anti-inflammatory effect of the blueberry anthocyanins malvidin-3-glucoside and malvidin-3-galactoside in endothelial cells. *Molecules*, **19**(8), 12827–12841.

Huang, Y. M., Dou, H. L., Huang, F. F., Xu, X. R., Zou, Z. Y. and Lin, X. M. (2015). Effect of supplemental lutein and zeaxanthin on serum, macular pigmentation, and visual performance in patients with early age-related macular degeneration. *BioMed Research International*, **2015**(564738), 1–8.

Hayashi, K., Ohara, N. and Tsukui, A. (1996). Stability of anthocyanins in various vegetables and fruits. *Food Science and Technology*, **2**(1), 30–33.

Itharat, A. and Sakpakdeejaroen, I. (2010). Determination of cytotoxic compounds of Thai traditional medicine called Benjakul using HPLC. *Journal of the Medical Association of Thailand*, **93**(Suppl. 7), 198–203.

Jackman, R. L. and Smith, J. L. (1996). *Anthocyanins and betalains*. In: G. A. F. Hendry and J. D. Houghton, Eds., *Natural Food Colorants*, 2nd edition. New York: Blackie Academic and Professional, pp. 244–296.

Janna, O., Khairul, A. and Maziah, M. (2007). Anthocyanin stability studies in *Tibouchina semidecandra* L. *Food Chemistry*, **101**(4), 1640–1646.

Kaczor, A. and Pacia, M. Z. (2016). Impact of stress factors on carotenoid composition, structures, and bioavailability in microbial sources. In: A. Kaczor, and M. Barańska, Eds., *Carotenoids: Nutrition, Analysis and Technology*. Oxford, UK: John Wiley & Sons, pp. 241–260.

Katpunyapong, W., Siriwatanakul, Y., Itharat, A. and Ngampongsai, W. (1998). Effect of *Andrographis paniculata* and *Psidium guajava* for growth and performance of using feed additive in Piglets. *Journal of Thai Traditional Medicine*, **5**, 33–42.

Khachik, F., Goli, M. B., Beecher, G. R., Holden, J., Lusby, W. R., Tenorio, M. D. and Barrera, M. R. (1992). Effect of food preparation on qualitative distribution of major carotenoids constituents of tomatoes and several green vegetables. *Journal of Agricultural and Food Chemistry*, **40**(3), 390–398.

Khalil, M., Raila, J., Ali, M., Islam, K. M. S., Schenk, R., Krause, J. P., Schweigert, F. J. and Rawel, H. (2012). Stability and bioavailability of lutein ester supplements from Tagetes flower prepared under food processing conditions. *Journal of Functional Foods*, **4**(3), 602–610.

Kimura, M. and Rodriguez-Amaya, D. B. (2003). Carotenoid composition of hydroponic leafy vegetables. *Journal of Agricultural and Food Chemistry*, **51**(9), 2603–2607.

Landrum, J. T. and Bone, R. A., (2001). Lutein, zeaxanthin, and the macular pigment. *Archives of Biochemistry and Biophysics*, **385**(1), 28–40.

Larsen, E. and Christensen, L. P. (2005). Simple saponification method for the quantitative determination of carotenoids in green vegetables. *Journal of Agricultural and Food Chemistry*, **53**(17), 6598–6602.

Lee, J. (2016). Anthocyanin analyses of *Vaccinium* fruit dietary supplements. *Food Science and Nutrition*, **4**(5), 742–752.

Lee, J., Yang, G., Lee, K., Lee, M. H., Eom, J. W., Ham, I. and Choi, H.-Y. (2013). Anti-inflammatory effect of *Prunus yedoensis* through inhibition of nuclear factor-κB in macrophages, *BMC Complementary and Alternative Medicine*, **13**(92), 1–9.

Li, B., Ahmed, F. and Bernstein, P. S. (2010). Studies on the singlet oxygen scavenging mechanism of human macular pigment. *Archives of Biochemistry and Biophysics*, **504**(1), 56–60.

Lohachoompol, V., Srzednicki, G. and Craske, J. (2004). The change of total anthocyanins in blueberries and their antioxidant effect after drying and freezing. *Journal of Biomedicine and Biotechnology*, **2004**(5), 248–252.

Ma, Q., Xu, X., Gao, Y., Wang, Q. and Zhao, J. (2008). Optimisation of supercritical carbon dioxide extraction of lutein esters from marigold (*Tagetes erect* L.) with soybean oil as a co-solvent. *International Journal of Food Science and Technology*, **43**(10), 1763–1769.

Makchuchit, S., Rattarom, R. and Itharat, A. (2017). The anti-allergic and anti-inflammatory effects of Benjakul extract (a Thai traditional medicine), its constituent plants and its some pure constituents using in vitro experiments. *Biomedicine & Pharmacotherapy*, **89**, 1018–1026.

Marcucci, M. C., Ferreres, F., Garc-Viguera, C., Bankova, V. S., De Castro, S. L., Dantas, A. P., Valente, P. H. M. and Paulino, N. (2001). Phenolic compounds from Brazilian propolis with pharmacological activities. *Journal of Ethnopharmacology*, **74**, 105–112.

Mares-Perlman, J. A., Fisher, A. I., Palta, M., Block, G., Millen, A. E. and Wright, J. D. (2001). Lutein and zeaxanthin in the diet and serum and their relation to age-related maculopathy in the third national health and nutrition examination survey. *American Journal of Epidemiology*, **153**(5), 424–432.

Mirzoeva, O. K. and Calder, P. C. (1996). The effect of propolis and its components on eicosanoid production during the inflammatory response. *Prostaglandins, Leukotrienes & Essential Fatty Acids*, **55**, 441–449.

Müller, H. (1997). Determination of the carotenoid content in selected vegetables and fruit by HPLC and photodiode array detection. *Zeitschrift für Lebensmitteluntersuchung und Forschung*, **204**(2), 88–94.

Nagai, T. and Inoue, R. (2004). Preparation and functional properties of water extract and alkaline extract of royal jelly. *Food Chemistry*, **84**, 181–186.

Nagai, T., Inoue, R., Kanamori, N., Suzuki, N. and Nagashima, T. (2006). Characterization of honey from different floral sources. Its functional properties and effects of honey species on storage of meat. *Food Chemistry*, **97**, 256–262.

Nakanishi, K. (1999). An historical perspective of natural products chemistry. In: U. Sankawa, ed., *Comprehensive Natural Products Chemistry. Vol. I. Polyketides and Other Secondary Metabolites Including Fatty Acids and Their Derivatives*. Amsterdam, the Netherlands: Elsevier. pp. 23–30.

Oancea, S., Stoia, M. and Coman, D. (2012). Effects of extraction conditions on bioactive anthocyanin content of *Vaccinium corymbosum* in the perspective of food applications. *Procedia Engineering*, **42**, 489–495.

Ojewole, J. A., Awe, E. O. and Chiwororo, W. D. (2008). Antidiarrhoeal activity of *Psidium guajava* Linn. (Myrtaceae) leaf aqueous extract in rodents. *Journal of Smooth Muscle Research*, **44**(6), 195–207.

Okpanyi, S. N. and Ezeukwu, G. C. (1981). Anti-inflammatory and antipyretic activities of *Azadirachta indica*. *Planta Medica*, **41**, 34–39.

Osztmianski, J. and Lee, C. Y. (1990). Inhibition of polyphenols oxidase activity and browning by honey. *Journal of Agricultural and Food Chemistry*, **38**, 1892–1895.

Pagarang, C., Rattanabanjerdkul, H. and Itharat, A. (2017). Case studies of Benjakul recipes in treating stage 4 non – small cell lung cancer. *Thammasat Medical Journal*, **17**(2), 172–181.

Palumpitag, W., Prasitchoke, P., Goto, M. and Shotipruk, A. (2011). Supercritical carbon dioxide extraction of marigold lutein fatty acid esters: Effects of co-solvents and saponification conditions. *Separation Science and Technology*, **46**(4), 605–610.

Parada, J. and Aguilera, J. M. (2007). Food microstructure affects the bioavailability of several nutrients. *Journal of Food Science*, **72**(2), R21–R32.

Pasupuleti, V. R., Sammugam, L., Ramesh, N. and Gan, S. H. (2017). Honey, propolis, and royal jelly: A comprehensive review of their biological actions and health benefits. *Oxidative Medicine and Cellular Longevity*, **2017**, Article ID 1259510. doi:10.1155/2017/1259510.

Paulino, N., Coutinho, L. A., Coutinho, J. R., Vilela, G. C., da Silva Leandro, V. P. and Paulino, A. S. (2015). Antiulcerogenic effect of Brazilian propolis formulation in mice. *Pharmacology & Pharmacy*, **6**(12), 580–588.

Pereira, E. M. R., da Silva, J. L. D. C., Silva, F. F., De Luca, M. P., Lorentz, T. C. M. and Santos, V. R. (2011). Clinical evidence of the efficacy of a mouthwash containing propolis for the control of plaque and gingivitis: A phase II study. *Evidence-Based Complementary and Alternative Medicine*, **2011**, Article ID: 750249.

Perry, A., Rasmussen, H. and Johnson, E. (2009). Xanthophyll (lutein, zeaxanthin) content in fruits, vegetables and corn and egg products. *Journal of Food Composition and Analysis*, **22**(1), 9–15.

Pietta, P. G. (2000). Flavonoids as antioxidants. *Journal of Natural Products*, **63**(7), 1035–1042.

Pietta, P. G., Gardana, C. and Pietta, A. M. (2002). Analytical methods for quality control of propolis. *Fitoterapia*, **73**(1), 7–20.

Rachawat, P., Pinsornsak, P., Kanokkangsadal, P. and Itharat, A. (2017). Clinical efficacy and safety of Benjakul remedy extract for treating primary osteoarthritis of knee compared with diclofenac: Double blind, randomized controlled trial. *Evidence-Based Complementary and Alternative Medicine*, **2017**, 9593580. doi:10.1155/2017/9593580.

Roberts, R. L., Green, J., Lewis, B. and Metrics, P. X. (2009). Lutein and zeaxanthin in eye and skin health. *Clinics in Dermatology*, **27**(2), 195–201.

Ruangnoo, S., Itharat, A., Sakpakdeejaroen, I., Rattarom, R., Tappayutpijam, P. and Pawa, K. K. (2012). In vitro cytotoxic activity of Benjakul herbal preparation and its active compounds against human lung, cervical and liver cancer cells. *Journal of the Medical Association of Thailand*, **95**(Suppl 1), S127–S134.

Saha, K, Lajis, N. H., Israf, D. A., Hamzah, A. S., Khozirah, S., Khamis, S. and Syahida, A. (2004). Evaluation of antioxidant and nitric oxide inhibitory activities of selected Malaysian medicinal plants. *Journal of Ethnopharmacology*, **92**(2–3), 263–267.

Sakpakdeejaroen, I. and Itharat, A. (2009). Cytotoxic compounds against breast adenocarcinoma cells (MCF-7) from Pikutbenjakul. *Thai Journal of Health Research*, **23**(2), 71–76.

Satyanarayana, K., Sravanthi, K., Shaker, I. A. and Ponnulakshmi, R. (2015). Molecular approach to identify antidiabetic potential of *Azadirachta indica*. *Journal of Ayurveda and Integrative Medicine*, **6**(3), 165–174. doi:10.4103/0975-9476.157950.

Seddon, J. M., Ajani, U. A., Sperduto, F. L. D., Hiller, R., Blair, N., Burton, T. C., Farber, M. D. et al. (1994). Dietary carotenoids, vitamins A, C, and E, and advanced age-related macular degeneration. *The Journal of the American Medical Association*, **272**(18), 1413–1420.

Selway, J. W. T. (1986). Antiviral activity of flavones and flavans. In: V. Cody, E. Middleton, and J. B. Harborne, Eds., *Plant Flavonoids in Biology and Medicine: Biochemical, Pharmacological and Structure Activity Relationships*. New York: Alan R. Liss, Inc., pp. 75–125.

Simão, A. A., Marques, T. R., Marcussi, S. and Corrêa, A. D. (2017). Aqueous extract of *Psidium guajava* leaves: Phenolic compounds and inhibitory potential on digestive enzymes. *Anais da Academia Brasileira de Ciências*, **89**(3 Suppl), 2155–2165. doi:10.1590/0001-3765201720160067.

Šivel, M., Kráčmar, S. Fišera, M., Klejdus, B. and Kubáň, V. (2014). Lutein content in marigold flower (*Tagetes erecta* L.) concentrates used for production of food supplements. *Czech Journal of Food Sciences*, **32**(6), 521–525.

Skehan, P., Storeng, R., Scudiero, D., Monks, A., McMahon, J., Vistica, D., Warren, J. T. et al. (1990). New colorimetric cytotoxicity assay for anticancer-drug screening. *Journal of the National Cancer Institute*, **82**, 1107–1112.

Skrovankova, S., Sumczynski, D., Mlcek, J., Jurikova, T. and Sochor, J. (2015). Bioactive compounds and antioxidant activity in different types of berries. *International Journal of Molecular Science*, **16**, 24673–24706.

Sowndharajan, K., Santhanam, R., Hong, S., Jhoo, J.-W. and Kim S. (2016). Suppressive effects of acetone extract from the stem bark of three *Acacia* species on nitric oxide production in lipopolysaccharide-stimulated RAW 264.7 macrophage cells. *Asian Pacific Journal of Tropical Biomedicine*, **6**(8), 658–664.

Subcharoen, P. (1998). *Anticancer: Thai Traditional Medicine as Alternative Self-Care for Treated Cancer Patients*, 18. Bangkok, Thailand: Thai traditional Medicine Institute, Ministry of Public Health.

Teh, L. S., Francis and F. J. (1988). A research note stability of anthocyanins from *Zebrina pendula and Ipomoea tricolor* in a model beverage. *Journal of Food Science*, **53**(5), 1580–1581.

Teo, A., Lee, S. J., Goh, K. K. T. and Wolber, F. M. (2017). Kinetic stability and cellular uptake of lutein in WPI-stabilised nanoemulsions and emulsions prepared by emulsification and solvent evaporation method. *Food Chemistry*, **221**, 1269–1276.

Vishwanathan, R., Wilson, T. A. and Nicolosi, R. J. (2009). Bioavailability of a nanoemulsion of lutein is greater than a lutein supplement. *Nano Biomedicine and Engineering*, **1**(1), 57–73.

Viuda-Martos, M., Ruiz-Navajas, Y., Fernández-López, J. and Pérez-Alvarez, J. A. (2008). Functional properties of honey, propolis, and royal jelly. *Journal of Food Science*, **73**(9), 117–124.

Yue, X., Xu, Z., Prinyawiwatkul, W. and King, J. M. (2006). Improving extraction of lutein from egg yolk using an ultrasound-assisted solvent method. *Journal of Food Science*, **71**(4), C239–C241.

Zaripheh, S., Erdman, J. W. (2002). Factors that influence the bioavailability of xanthophylls. *Journal of Nutrition*, **132**(3), 531S–534S.

Zhu, F. G., Reich, C. F. and Pisetsky, D. S. (2002). Inhibition of murine macrophage nitric oxide production by synthetic oligonucleotides. *Journal of Leukocyte Biology*, **71**(4), 686–694.

7 Biomarkers for Quality Control of Chinese Tonifying Herbs and Herbal Health Products

Pou Kuan Leong and Kam Ming Ko

CONTENTS

7.1 THEORETICAL BASIS OF CHINESE MEDICINE

7.1.1 THE YIN-YANG THEORY AND HEALTH STATUS

Traditional Chinese medicine (TCM) views the human body as an organic entity made of various organs that function in a mutually interdependent manner (O'Brien and Xue 2003). The Yin-Yang theory, which originated from ancient Chinese philosophy, is central to the conceptual framework of TCM. According to the Yin-Yang theory, the functioning of the human body is governed by the interplay of two complementary, but opposing, forces, namely, Yin and Yang. The dynamic equilibrium between Yin and Yang determines the physiological status of the human body (Liu and Liu 2009). Any disturbance in the balance of Yin and Yang can lead to various pathological conditions. For example, an absolute excess of Yin can lead to an over-consumption of Yang, and vice versa;

a relative excess of Yin or Yang is referred to as Yang deficiency or Yin deficiency, respectively. Within this philosophical framework, TCM classifies bodily structures, explains clinical symptoms and guides the treatment of diseases on the basis of the Yin-Yang theory (Zhang and Wu 1991).

According to TCM theory, the interaction between Yin (postnatal essence or Yin Qi) and Yang (pre-natal essence or Yang Qi) generates *Zheng* Qi, which is regarded as 'the Qi of the body', maintains life activities and defends against pathogens, as well as adapting to changes in the body due to inter-nal and external factors. *Zheng* Qi can flow through meridians and thereby energise physiological activities. TCM theory also states that ageing and ageing-associated disorders can be caused by the gradual depletion of *Zheng* Qi, and the complete deprivation of *Zheng* Qi, which is mainly due to the exhaustion of prenatal essence, will ultimately result in death (Leong et al. 2015). As the prenatal essence is inherited from parents and cannot be replenished after birth, a sufficient supply of postnatal essence is essential to minimise the utilisation of prenatal essence for the generation of *Zheng* Qi. In addition, while exhaustive sexual activity and the Yin-Yang imbalance of body functioning cause an over-consumption of prenatal essence, the maintenance of an optimal Yin-Yang balance in body function (in particular that of the 'Spleen' for digestion and absorption) and a healthy lifestyle (diet and physical exercise) is crucial in acquiring sufficient postnatal essence and hence preserving the prenatal essence in humans. In this regard, the use of Chinese tonifying herbs or herbal health products aim to re-establish the Yin-Yang balance in the body and thereby prevent the over-consumption of prenatal essence.

According to TCM theory, Blood, a thick red liquid circulating in circulatory vessels, is viewed as one of the basic substances essential for supporting life activities in humans. Blood circulation in the body is dependent on the driving action of Qi and it exerts a strong nourishing effect on various organs. The interrelationship between Qi and Blood exemplifies the importance of harmony between Yin (Blood) and Yang (Qi) in determining optimal physiological function. In addition, any internal or external causes of diseases (i.e. pathogenic factors) can be classified as Yin or Yang on the basis of their pathological characteristics. Various modalities of interventions (therapeutic and toni-fying) in TCM, including the use of herbal formulations and acupuncture, can also exert Yin/Yang-modulatory actions, thereby producing beneficial effects in Yin/Yang-deficiency disorders (Zhang and Wu 1991).

7.1.2 Various Functional Categories of Chinese Tonifying Herbs for Safeguarding Health

Within the framework of TCM theory, disease is primarily caused by a Yin-Yang imbalance in the body, and therefore any factor that can disrupt this balance can lead to a sub-healthy or even pathological condition. In the aetiology of diseases caused by external pathogens, the antagonistic interaction between *Zheng* Qi and pathogens can result in an 'excessive' syndrome (characterised by acute and short-lived symptoms) or a 'deficiency' syndrome (characterised by chronic and long-lived symptoms; Geng et al. 1991). Therapeutic and/or tonifying interventions using TCM aim to get rid of the pathogens and re-establish the Yin-Yang balance in the body, thereby restoring *Zheng* Qi to a normal level. In doing so, the prescription of Chinese herbal formulations and acupuncture are common approaches for the treatment of diseases in TCM. Fundamentally, the practice of TCM in the treatment of diseases favours prevention over treatment. As such, a sub-healthy status (a malfunctioning body condition prior to the development of a disease state) of an individual should be remedied in a timely manner by using Chinese tonifying herbs or formulations. While Chinese herbs are broadly divided into therapeutic and tonifying groups in terms of their pharmacological actions, tonifying herbs can be classified into four functional categories: Yang-invigorating, Yin-nourishing, Qi-invigorating and Blood-enriching, with respect to their mode of action in enhancing the physiological functions under sub-optimal body conditions (Ko et al. 2006; see Figure 7.1). With regard to the Yin-Yang theory, Qi-invigorating and Blood-enriching actions are classified under the Yang and Yin categories, respectively.

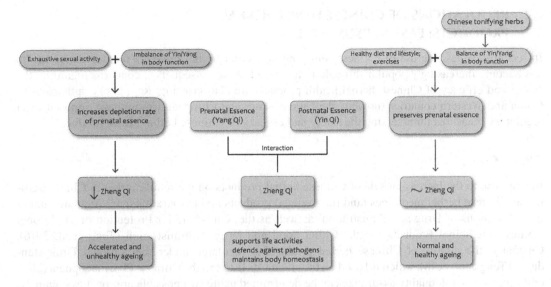

FIGURE 7.1   Factors affecting the strength of Zheng Qi.

In recent years, pharmacological investigations of Chinese tonifying herbs have demonstrated that Yang/Qi-invigorating herbs can increase mitochondrial ATP generation capacity, whereas Yin/Blood-tonifying herbs can produce immunomodulatory effects and/or enhance the production of red blood cells (Ko and Leung 2007; Lee et al. 2014). Interestingly, while Yang-invigorating herbs are able to stimulate mitochondrial electron transport and hence ATP generation by fluidising the mitochondrial inner membrane, the increase in mitochondrial ATP generation induced by Qi herbs appears to be an event secondary to the enhancement of cellular glutathione redox status, which counteracts the inhibition of mitochondrial electron transport by reactive oxygen species. In this regard, the pharmacological profile of Chinese tonifying herbs fits in well with the current approach in preventive health in modern (Western) medicine, which emphasises antioxidation and immunomodulation as well as homeostasis (via neuroendocrinological regulation) in the prevention of disease (Figure 7.2).

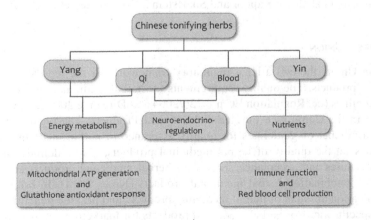

FIGURE 7.2   Modes of action by Chinese tonifying herbs.

7.2 REGULATIONS OF CHINESE HERBS/HERBAL PRODUCTS: EAST *VERSUS* WEST

In recent decades, the use of Chinese tonifying herbs and herbal products for preventive health has become increasingly popular throughout the world. As a consequence, concerns regarding the safety and efficacy of Chinese herbal health products are also growing. Regulatory authorities in China and Western countries (notably, the United States and European Union) have imposed strict regulatory measures for assessing the safety and efficacy of Chinese herbal health products.

7.2.1 CHINA

In response to the increasing sale of Chinese herbal products on the retail market in China, traditional Chinese herbal medicines (and their related products and preparations) are regulated under the 'Provisions of Drug and Registration' as well as the 'Guideline for Protection of Traditional Chinese Medicinal Products' by the China Food and Drug Administration (Teng et al. 2016). Currently, the quality of Chinese herbal products is regulated under the National Drug standards (Teng et al. 2016), which is based on the standards listed in the Chinese Pharmacopoeia (2015 edition). In general, quality assurance can be determined using two possible approaches – namely, the use of chemical markers and fingerprinting. While the chemical marker approach relies on the identification and quantification of individual compound(s) in an herbal preparation, the fingerprinting approach makes use of unique chromatographic profile/patterns determined by liquid and/or gas chromatography analysis of an herbal preparation (Zhang et al. 2011). A manufacturer is required to submit evidence for assuring the quality and safety of an herbal product before its approval for marketing.

7.2.2 UNITED STATES

Currently, herbal products have been increasingly accepted and utilised in the United States for disease prevention and auxiliary treatment. In the United States, herbal medicines/products are classified as dietary supplements and are regulated by the Food and Drug Administration and Federal Trade Commission under the United States federal government. As far as the quality and consistency of herbal supplements are concerned, manufacturers are required to follow current good manufacturing practices (cGMPs) under the 'Dietary Supplement and Nonprescription Drug Consumer Protection Act' in the United States (Kapoor and Sharfstein 2016; Pawar and Grundel 2017). Chemical fingerprinting and DNA barcoding (which will be discussed in the following section) are commonly used methods to ensure the quality and reduce the incidence of adulteration in herbal products (Newmaster et al. 2013; Kapoor and Sharfstein 2016; Parveen et al. 2016).

7.2.3 EUROPEAN UNION

In the European Union, there is a legal regulatory framework for the regulation of (traditional) herbal medicinal products. The quality requirements for herbal medicinal products are laid down in scientific guidelines (i.e. Regulation EC no. 726/2004 and Directive 2004/24/EC) by the Quality Drafting Group in the Committee on Herbal Medicinal Products. The Quality Drafting Group has developed a number of guidelines for quality assurance of herbal medicinal products, such as: (1) guidelines on the quality of herbal medicinal products, (2) guidelines on specifications such as test procedures and acceptance criteria for herbal medicinal products and (3) guidelines on the quality of combination herbal medicinal products (Kroes 2014). In brief, the guidelines outline the application dossiers of herbal medicinal products and provide general rules for setting and justifying specifications of herbal medicinal products for marketing authorisation. The guidelines also emphasise the validation and documentation of the manufacturing process of these products (Kroes 2014). The ultimate goal of such guidelines is to assure the quality of herbal medicinal products, which are manufactured by authorised manufacturers under good manufacturing practices (GMPs), in the European market.

7.3   CURRENT APPROACHES IN QUALITY CONTROL FOR CHINESE HERBS AND HERBAL FORMULATIONS

7.3.1   Approaches to Quality Control of Chinese Herbs

7.3.1.1   Botanical, Macroscopic and Microscopic Authentication Methods

Botanical authentication refers to the comparison between the herbal sample under consideration and an authenticated reference specimen. Macroscopic authentication is the assessment of the macroscopic and sensory characteristics of the processed whole plant or plant part (i.e. herb). In case the macroscopic characteristics are indistinguishable, microscopic authentication can be performed by examination of the whole, fragmented or powdered herb under the microscope. These methods have the advantage of being very cost-effective and time-efficient (Zhao et al. 2011). However, authenticated reference specimens should be readily available and stored under ideal conditions to avoid any degradation or contamination (Techen et al. 2004). A limitation is that these methods are only applicable to herbs that possess morphologically distinct properties (Smillie and Khan 2010), meaning that they may not be applicable in the case of closely related herbal species.

7.3.1.2   DNA-Based Methods (DNA Fingerprinting; Next-Generation Sequencing)

To complement the limitations of authentication methods based on morphological and histological properties, DNA-based analysis is an ideal method to detect adulteration of Chinese herbs of closely related species (Heubl 2010). With the technique of polymer chain reaction (PCR), only a small quantity of DNA-containing sample is required for authentication (Nybom et al. 2014). For the herb with an unknown DNA sequence, the random amplified polymorphic DNA technique using the amplified fragmented length polymorphism technique or the inter-simple sequence repeat method can be used to generate PCR fragments from the genomic DNA of the herbal sample (Nybom et al. 2014). Following electrophoretic separation and visualisation, a multi-locus banding pattern (i.e. a DNA fingerprint) can be obtained for authentication purposes. For herbs with a well-defined genome, the PCR-restriction fragment length polymorphism method, in which the amplified specific DNA sequences are digested by restriction enzymes, can be used to generate a DNA fingerprint (Heubl 2010). With the advances in DNA technology, DNA fingerprinting techniques have been replaced by DNA sequencing (Nybom et al. 2014). The combination of a PCR-based method and Sanger's method of DNA sequencing results in a new technique called 'DNA barcoding' (Sucher et al. 2012), which makes use of short and standardised genomic regions as taxon barcodes for the distinguishing of different, but closely related, species. In the past decade, the revolutionary next-generation sequencing, which offers a number of advantages over the Sanger sequencing (such as higher sensitivity, faster running time, massive and parallel sequencing reactions and clonal expansion of DNA templates), has been shown to be a cost-effective and time-efficient method for the authentication of Chinese herbs and herbal products (Ronaghi et al. 1998; Nyrén 2007). However, the major limitation of DNA authentication is that it is impossible to distinguish between plant parts of the same Chinese tonifying herb. In addition, a low-quality DNA preparation can arise from poor DNA extraction of the dried or processed herb or interference by secondary herbal metabolites (Smillie and Khan 2010).

7.3.1.3   Spectroscopic Methods (IMR and NMR)

Infrared (IR; vibrational) spectrometry measures changes in the molecular dipole moment associated with a chemical bond vibration within the molecules in an herbal sample (Rohman et al. 2014). The characteristic peaks and bands in the IR spectrum correspond to specific functional groups of molecules in the herbal sample and hence the IR spectrum of an herbal sample, which may contain a number of individual phytochemicals, can serve as a unique fingerprint for authentication (Rohman et al. 2014). Regarding the unique IR spectroscopic fingerprint of an herbal sample, IR spectrometry can be used to differentiate closely related herbal species, to identify adulterants and for quality control of herbal raw materials, intermediate herbal preparations and final herbal products (Guo et al. 2011; Gad et al. 2013). The advantages of IR spectrometry are rapidity, robustness, time-efficiency and that it is non-invasive and non-destructive to the herbal samples (Guo et al. 2011).

Nuclear magnetic resonance (NMR) spectroscopy, which examines the nuclei of a given molecule under a magnetic field, can be used for the structural analysis of chemical compounds in an herbal sample. NMR spectroscopy can differentiate chemical components in different crude herbal extracts (van der Kooy et al. 2009). Similar to IR spectrometry, NMR spectroscopy, with the use of authentic reference standards, can differentiate closely related herbal species, herbal species from different geographic origins and adulterated herbal preparations (van der Kooy et al. 2009; Chen et al. 2014). NMR spectroscopy also allows the quantitative analysis of the active components of herbal samples (Liu et al. 2014). Although results obtained from NMR spectroscopy are reproducible and the analytical process is of high throughput, a major drawback of NMR spectroscopy is its relatively low sensitivity and resolution (Pferschy-Wenzig and Bauer 2015).

7.3.1.4 Chromatographic Methods (HPLC-MS/GC-MS)

Chromatographic methods (such as thin-layer chromatography, high-performance chromatography, capillary electrophoresis and gas chromatography) are commonly used methods in the authentication, determination of adulterant and quality control of herbal samples (Pferschy-Wenzig and Bauer 2015). Among the aforementioned chromatographic methods, high-performance chromatography is the most popular technique by virtue of its ease of operation, high resolution, high selectivity and high sensitivity (Tistaert et al. 2011). In addition, a number of analytical approaches are available for tracing the chromatographic records, including UV absorbance, fluorescence and light scattering methods (Pferschy-Wenzig and Bauer 2015). UV absorbance detection can be used to analyse phytochemicals possessing particular chromophoric groups. While fluorescent phytochemicals can be analysed by fluorescence detection, phytochemicals without any chromophore and/or fluorescent groups can be examined by light scattering detection, which measures the amount of light scattered by the molecules in the mobile phase. In principle, mass spectrometric detection can be applied to any kind of phytochemical that can be ionised by electron bombardment. Liquid chromatography, coupled with mass spectrometry (LC-MS), can provide high sensitivity and selectivity for the phytochemical analysis of herbal samples. Therefore, LC-MS is frequently used for marker- and fingerprint-based qualitative and quantitative analyses of herbal samples/products (Steinmann and Ganzera 2011; Wu et al. 2013).

7.3.2 Methods for Identification of Chemical Markers in Chinese Herbs

As a reliable chemical marker of Chinese herbs, its content should be relatively high in the herb and its pharmacological properties should be relevant to its therapeutic or tonifying action(s) Wu et al. (2018). The evaluation of the quality of Chinese herbs presents a number of difficulties and challenges because of their unique modes of action and complex chemical composition. Given that the pharmacological action of a Chinese herb is likely produced by more than one component, it is not a scientifically sound approach to focus on a single compound for the quality assurance of efficacy. In addition, herbs from closely related plant species (e.g. *Schisandra chinensis* Fructus and *Schisandra sphenanthera* Fructus), herbs derived from different plant parts (e.g. cylindrical and upper part [head], axial root [body] and branch roots [tails] of *Angelicae sinensis* Radix) or herbs processed by different methods (e.g. Chinese Ginseng Radix and Korean red) can be regarded as different categories of Chinese herbs with different pharmacological properties. This further hinders the identification of a specific chemical marker for Chinese herbs. To cope with the aforementioned challenges, Xin et al. (2018) have recently proposed the use of biomarkers for implementing quality control of Chinese herbs. In brief, the chemical constituents of an herb or herbal formulation are analysed in relation to their clinical indication(s) using network pharmacology, which entails the identification of biological response-relevant signalling pathways and target proteins using techniques in bioinformatics. Upstream pharmacological targets are arranged into relevant signalling pathways in order to identify the downstream targets, with the latter serving as candidate biomarkers. Finally, the biological effect of an herb or herbal formulation, which determines its particular clinical indication, is validated by *in vitro* cell-based bioassay, which is performed in parallel with the measurement of the above mentioned biomarkers.

7.4 BIOMARKERS OF CHINESE TONIFYING HERBS AND HERBAL HEALTH PRODUCTS

As mentioned earlier, Chinese tonifying herbs and herbal health products can be classified into four functional categories: Yang-invigorating, Qi-invigorating, Yin-nourishing and Blood-enriching. They can be used alone or in combination with other tonifying herbs (belonging to the same or to different functional categories) in order to replenish the 'deficiency' of body function (Yang, Yin, Qi, Blood) in various clinical situations. With regard to pharmacological actions in relation to Western medicine, while Yang-invigorating herbs act primarily by stimulating mitochondrial ATP generation, Qi-invigorating herbs enhance cellular glutathione redox status, with a resultant increase in mitochondrial ATP generation capacity (unpublished data). As such, Yang and Qi herbs differ in the time-course of stimulating mitochondrial ATP generation (as assessed by *in vitro* cell-based assay), in that a 4-h pre-incubation (but not 16-h for Qi herb extracts) with Yang herb extracts can cause an increase in mitochondrial ATP generation in cultured cardiomyocytes. However, the stimulation of mitochondrial ATP generation by Qi herbal extracts (but not Yang herbal extracts) is associated with an enhancement of cellular glutathione redox status. Experimental findings therefore support the use of mitochondrial ATP generation and cellular glutathione redox status as biomarkers for Yang-invigorating and Qi-invigorating herbs/herbal health products, respectively (Figure 7.3). While the characteristic pharmacological activity of Yin-nourishing herbs can be measured by the stimulation of mouse splenocyte proliferation (Ko and Leung 2007), blood-enriching herbs can increase the production of erythropoietin (EPO) in cultured liver and kidney cells (Zheng et al. 2012). Therefore, splenocyte proliferation and EPO production can be used as biomarkers for Yin-nourishing and Blood-enriching herbs, respectively (Figure 7.3).

7.4.1 Biomarker Measurement for Yang-Invigorating Herbs and/or Herbal Health Products – Mitochondrial ATP-Generation Capacity Assay

For the measurement of mitochondrial ATP generation capacity (ATP-GC), H9c2 cells, which are embryonic myoblasts derived from rat myocardium, were seeded at a density of 2.5×10^4 cells/well onto 24-well microtiter plates. Forty-eight hours post-seeding, cells were pre-incubated

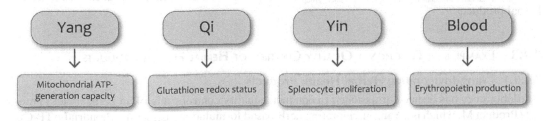

FIGURE 7.3 Biomarkers for quality control of Chinese tonifying herbs/herbal products.

with the extract of an herbal health product-containing medium (at concentrations of 30, 100 and 300 μg/mL) at 37°C for 4 h. The herbal product extract–containing medium was prepared by adding the sample solution in dimethylsulphoxide (DMSO) to the culture medium, with the final concentration of DMSO being less than 0.2% (v/v). The control group was given vehicle [DMSO (0.2%, v/v, final concentration)] only. After a 4-h incubation with the extract-containing medium, the removal of the medium was followed by cell membrane permeabilisation with digitonin (50 μg/mL) in an incubation buffer (120 mM KCl, 5 mM KH_2PO_4, 2 mM EGTA, 10 mM HEPES, 0.1 mM $MgCl_2$, 0.5% BSA, pH 7.4). Pyruvate (15 mM), malate (5 mM) and ADP (10 μM) were added to initiate mitochondrial ATP generation at 37°C, which was monitored at increasing time intervals ranging from 0 to 15 min. The reaction was terminated by the addition of 60 μL of perchloric acid (30%, w/v), and the reaction mixtures were centrifuged at 540 ×g for 10 min at 4°C, and the supernatants were analysed for ATP content by the luciferase assay (ATPlite, PerkinElmer Inc., MA, USA). The ATP-GC of non-extract pre-incubated cells was estimated by determining the area under the curve of a graph (AUC_1) plotting ATP generated (nmol/mg protein) *versus* time (0–15 min) and expressed in arbitrary units. For the herbal extract–pre-incubated cells, AUC_1 values at increasing incubation times (7.5 and 15 min) were normalised to a respective mean control value from non-herbal extract–incubated cells and expressed as a per cent of control. The area under the curve (AUC_2) of the graph plotting per cent control values against incubation time (7.5–15 min) was computed and expressed in arbitrary units. The ATP-GC value of the experimental sample is expressed as AUC_2. The area under the curve (AUC_3) of a graph plotting AUC_2 values against herbal extract concentration was calculated and expressed in arbitrary units. The ratio of $AUC_{3\text{herbal extract-incubated group}}$ to $AUC_{3\text{vehicle group}}$ was expressed as the stimulation index for each batch of herbal product.

7.4.2 Biomarker Measurement for Yin-Nourishing Herbs and/or Herbal Health Products – Mouse Splenocyte Proliferation Assay

Primary splenocytes, which consist of T-and B-lymphocytes, were isolated from female ICR mice under aseptic conditions, as described in Ko and Leung (2007). Isolated splenocytes were incubated with herbal product extract-containing medium [at 30, 100 and 300 μg/mL, 0.2% DMSO in the culture medium (v/v)] for 48 h prior to the cell proliferation assay. The control group contained vehicle [DMSO (0.2%, v/v, final concentration)] only. At 28 h post-incubation with the herbal product extract–containing medium, bromodeoxyuridine (BrdU, 10 μM) was co-incubated with the splenocytes for 20 h prior to the measurement of cell proliferation. The proliferation of splenocytes was assessed using a BrdU cell proliferation assay kit (Cell Signaling Technology Inc., MA, USA) according to the manufacturer's instructions. The procedure is based on the principle of enzyme-linked immunosorbent assay. The extent of splenocyte proliferation was determined by measuring the absorbance at 450 nm using a Victor V3 Multi-Label Counter (Perkin Elmer, Turku, Finland).

The absorbance of the herbal extract–incubated group was normalised relative to the vehicle control and expressed as per cent stimulation. The area under the curve (AUC) of a graph plotting per cent stimulation against log (concentrations of herbal extract) was determined. The ratio of $AUC_{\text{herbal extract-incubated group}}$ to $AUC_{\text{vehicle group}}$ was expressed as the stimulation index for the tested herbal product.

7.4.3 Examples of Functional Quality Control of Herbal Health Products

7.4.3.1 Yang-Invigorating Herbal Health Products

Our laboratory has been commissioned to conduct a quality control study of an herbal health product (Product M, which is a Yang-invigorating herb-based formulation) using mitochondrial ATP-GC as biomarker. The results obtained from various batches of product M are listed in Table 7.1.

TABLE 7.1

Quality Biomarkers of Various Batches of Product M

Batch No.	Stimulation Indices
1	1.20
2	1.23
3	1.19
4	0.97
5	1.19
6	1.18
7	1.10
8	1.19
9	1.12

TABLE 7.2

Quality Biomarkers of Various Batches of Product C on ATP-GC and Splenocyte Proliferation

Batch No.	Stimulation Indices	
	ATP-GC	Splenocyte Proliferation
1	1.16	1.39
2	1.16	1.51
3	1.19	1.13
4	1.21	1.18

7.4.3.2   Yang-Invigorating and Yin-Nourishing Herbal Health Products

The measurement of biomarkers of a health product containing an extract of cultured mycelium of *Cordyceps sinensis* (Product Cs) was also performed. Based on Chinese medicine theory, *Cordyceps sinensis* can produce both Yang-invigorating and Yin-nourishing actions. A previous study in our laboratory has demonstrated Yang-invigorating and Yin-nourishing actions produced by *Cordyceps sinensis* (both wild type and cultured mycelium) using the ATP-GC assay (Yang-invigorating) and splenocyte proliferation assay (Yin-nourishing), respectively (Ko and Leung 2007). Results obtained from various batches of Product C are shown in Table 7.2.

7.5   CONCLUSIONS

The use of chemical markers, including the application of fingerprinting techniques, is not optimal for the quality control of Chinese herbs or herbal products, all of which possess complex chemical compositions. A major drawback of the chemical marker analytical procedure is its inability to ascertain the functional characteristics of the herb or herbal product in its entirety due to the presence of multiple active chemical components. Here, we propose the adoption of biomarkers for the quality control of Chinese tonifying herbs or herbal health products, which are purported to produce health-promoting actions (namely, Yang-invigorating, Qi-invigorating, Yin-nourishing and Blood-enriching) in the context of Chinese medicine. Using pharmacological assays for measuring various tonifying actions of Chinese herbs (Yang, Qi, Yin and Blood), biomarkers can be used to monitor the functionally relevant biological activity of Chinese tonifying herbs or herbal health products. Results obtained from a proof-of-concept study on two Chinese tonifying herbal products indicate that the use of functional biomarkers is practical to monitor batch-to-batch variations in biomarker(s).

REFERENCES

Chen, Y., Song, Y., Wang, Y. et al. (2014). Metabolic differentiations of *Pueraria lobata* and *Pueraria thomsonii* using 1H NMR spectroscopy and multivariate statistical analysis. *Journal of Pharmaceutical and Biomedical Analysis*, **93**, 51–58.

Gad, H. A., El-Ahmady, S. H., Abou-Shoer, M. I. and Al-Azizi, M. M. (2013). Application of chemometrics in authentication of herbal medicines: A review. *Phytochemical Analysis*, **24**, 1–24.

Geng, J., Huang, W., Ren, T. and Ma, X. (1991). *Practical Traditional Chinese Medicine & Pharmacology*. Beijing, China: New World Press.

Guo, L.P., Huang, L. Q., Zhang, X. P. et al. (2011). Application of near-infrared spectroscopy (NIRS) as a tool for quality control in Traditional Chinese Medicine (TCM). *Current Bioactive Compounds*, **7**, 75–84.

Heubl, G. (2010). New aspects of DNA-based authentication of Chinese medicinal plants by molecular biological techniques. *Planta Medica*, **76**, 1963–1974.

Kapoor, A. and Sharfstein, J. M. (2016). Breaking the gridlock: Regulation of dietary supplements in the United States. *Drug Testing and Analysis*, **8**, 424–430.

Ko, K. M., Leon, T. Y., Mak, D. H., Chiu, P. Y., Du, Y. and Poon, M. K. (2006). A characteristic pharmacological action of 'Yang-invigorating' Chinese tonifying herbs: Enhancement of myocardial ATP-generation capacity. *Phytomedicine*, **13**, 636–642.

Ko, K. M. and Leung, H. Y. (2007). Enhancement of ATP generation capacity, antioxidant activity and immunomodulatory activities by Chinese Yang and Yin tonifying herbs. *Chinese Medicine*, **2**, 3.

Kroes, B. H. (2014). The legal framework governing the quality of (traditional) herbal medicinal products in the European Union. *Journal of Ethnopharmacology*, **158 Pt B**, 449–453.

Lee, H. W., Kim, H., Ryuk, J. A., Kil, K. J. and Ko, B. S. (2014). Hemopoietic effect of extracts from constituent herbal medicines of Samul-tang on phenylhydrazine-induced hemolytic anemia in rats. *International Journal of Clinical and Experimental Pathology*, **7**, 6179–6185.

Leong, P. K., Wong, H. S., Chen, J. and Ko, K. M. (2015). Yang/Qi invigoration: An herbal therapy for chronic fatigue syndrome with yang deficiency? *Evidence-Based Complementary and Alternative Medicine*, **2015**, 945901.

Liu, Y., Chen, S., McAlpine, J. B. et al. (2014). Quantification of a botanical negative marker without an identical standard: Ginkgotoxin in Ginkgo biloba. *Journal of Natural Products*, **77**, 611–617.

Liu, Z. and Liu, L. (2009). *Essentials of Chinese Medicine*. London, UK: Springer.

Newmaster S. G., Grguric, M., Shanmughanandhan, D., Ramalingam, S. and S. Ragupathy. (2013). DNA barcoding detects contamination and substitution in North American herbal products. *BMC Medicine*, **11**, 222.

Nybom, H., Weisig, K. and Rotter, B. (2014). DNA fingerprinting in botany: Past, present, future. *Investigative Genetics*, **5**, 1.

Nyrén, P. (2007). The history of pyrosequencing. *Methods in Molecular Biology*, **373**, 1–14.

O'Brien, K. A. and Xue, C. C. (2003). The theoretical framework of Chinese medicine. In P. C. Leung, C. C. Xue and Y. C. Chen, eds., *A Comprehensive Guide to Chinese Medicine*, Singapore: World Scientific Publishing Co. Pte. Ltd., pp. 47–84.

Parveen, I., Gafner, S., Techen, N., Murch, S. J. and Khan, I. A. (2016). DNA barcoding for the identification of botanicals in herbal medicine and dietary supplements: Strengths and limitations. *Planta Medica*, **82**, 1225–1235.

Pawar, R. S., and Grundel, E. (2017). Overview of regulation of dietary supplements in the USA and issues of adulteration with phenethylamines (PEAs). *Drug Testing and Analysis*, **9**, 500–517.

Pferschy-Wenzig, E. M. and Bauer, R. (2015). The relevance of pharmacognosy in pharmacological research on herbal medicinal products. *Epilepsy and Behavior*, **52**, 344–362.

Rohman, A., Nugroho, A., Lukitaningsih, E. and Sudjadi. (2014). Application of vibrational spectroscopy in combination with chemometrics techniques for authentication of herbal medicine. *Applied Spectroscopy Reviews*, **49**, 603–613.

Ronaghi, M., Uhlén, M. and Nyrén, P. (1998). DNA sequencing: A sequencing method based on real-time pyrophosphate. *Science*, **281**, 363–365.

Smillie, T. J. and Khan, I. A. (2010). A comprehensive approach to identifying and authenticating botanical products. *Clinical Pharmacology & Therapeutics*, **87**, 175–186.

Steinmann, D. and Ganzera, M. (2011). Recent advances on HPLC/MS in medicinal plant analysis. *Journal of Pharmaceutical and Biomedical Analysis*, **55**, 744–757.

Sucher, N. J., Hennell, J. R. and Carles, M. C. (2012). *Plant DNA Fingerprinting and Barcoding: Methods and Protocols. Methods in Molecular Biology*, vol. 862. New York: Humana Press.

Techen, N., Crockett, S. L., Khan, I. A. and Scheffler, B. E. (2004). Authentication of medicinal plants using molecular biology techniques to complement conventional methods. *Current Medicinal Chemistry*, **11**, 1391–1401.

Teng, L., Zu, Q., Li, G., Yu, T., Job, K. M., Yang, X., Di, L., Sherwin, C. M. and Enioutina, E. Y. (2016). Herbal medicines: Challenges in the modern world. Part 3. China and Japan. *Expert Review of Clinical Pharmacology*, **9**, 1225–1233.

Tistaert, C., Dejaegher, B. and Vander Heyden, Y. (2011). Chromatographic separation techniques and data handling methods for herbal fingerprints: A review. *Analytica Chimica Acta*, **690**, 148–161.

van der Kooy, F., Maltese, F., Choi, Y. H., Kim, H.K. and Verpoorte, R. (2009). Quality control of herbal material and phytopharmaceuticals with MS and NMR based metabolic fingerprinting. *Planta Medica*, **75**, 763–775.

Wu, H., Guo, J., Chen, S. et al. (2013). Recent developments in qualitative and quantitative analysis of phytochemical constituents and their metabolites using liquid chromatography–mass spectrometry. *Journal of Pharmaceutical and Biomedical Analysis*, **72**, 267–291.

Wu, X., Zhang, H., Fan, S. et al. (2018). Quality markers based on biological activity: A new strategy for the quality control of traditional Chinese medicine. *Phytomedicine*, **44**, 103–108.

Zhang, D. and Wu, X. (1991). Chapter 5 Qi, Blood, body fluid, essence of life and spirit. In Y. Liu, ed., *The Basic Knowledge of Traditional Chinese Medicine*. Hong Kong: Hai Feng Publishing Co., pp. 49–53.

Zhang, Y., Sun, S., Dai, J. et al. (2011). Quality control method for herbal medicine – Chemical fingerprint analysis. In Y. Shoyama, ed., *Quality Control of Herbal Medicines and Related Areas*. IntechOpen. doi:10.5772/23962.

Zhao, Z., Liang, Z. and Ping, G. (2011). Macroscopic identification of Chinese medicinal materials: Traditional experiences and modern understanding. *Journal of Ethnopharmacology*, **134**, 556–564.

Zheng, K. Y., Zhang, Z. X., Guo, A. J. et al. (2012). Salidroside stimulates the accumulation of HIF-1α protein resulted in the induction of EPO expression: A signaling via blocking the degradation pathway in kidney and liver cells. *European Journal of Pharmacology*, **679**, 34–39.

8 Nelumbo nucifera
Pharmacological Profile, Metabolite Profiling and Therapeutic Uses

Pulok K. Mukherjee, Debayan Goswami,
Bhaskar Das and Subhadip Banerjee

CONTENTS

8.1   NELUMBO NUCIFERA – AN OVERVIEW

Nelumbo nucifera, also called the Indian lotus, is a giant aquatic herb with stout crawling chromatic white-coloured rhizomes that has primarily been used as food throughout the Asian continent, and its medicinal values are represented in Ayurvedic and traditional Chinese medicine.

Nelumbo nucifera comes under the family Nymphaceace, which has various local tribal names (Indian lotus, bean of India, Chinese water lily and sacred lotus) and several botanical names (*Nelumbium nelumbo, N. speciosa, N. speciosum* and *Nymphaea nelumbo*) (Harer 1985; Karki et al. 2012, 2013).

Ancient medical literature assigned the Sanskrit name 'Kamala' and there are two forms – one with white flowers commonly called 'Pundarika' or 'sveta kamala' and the other with pink or reddish pink flowers called 'Rakta Kamala' (Chopra et al. 1958). Every part of the plant has a distinct name and almost all parts are used medicinally – the whole plant with flowers is known as 'Padmini'; the rhizome is known as 'Kamalakand'; the tender leaves as 'Sambartika'; the peduncle as 'mrinal' or 'Visa'; the stamens as 'Kirijalaka'; the torus as 'Padmakosa'; the seeds as 'Karnika' or 'Padmaksya' and the honey formed in the flowers by the bees feeding upon padma is known as 'Makaranda' or 'Padma- Madhu' (CCRAS 1982).

N. nucifera is a native of China, Japan and India. It is commonly found growing in ponds and lakes and is often cultivated for its elegant, sweet-scented flower. It is the 'National Flower of India' and is also cultivated in China and Japan (CSIR 1966). Leaves, flowers, rhizomes, roots, fruits and seeds of *N. nurcifera* have been claimed to possess various medicinal values.

N. nucifera has been widely used by indigenous communities as a diuretic, cardiac tonic, vasodilator, antitumour, antibacterial, antihelminthic and in the treatment of strangury, vomiting, skin diseases and nervous exhaustion (Mukherjee et al. 2009). The tremendous potential of *N. nucifera* and its different parts, from root to shoot, has been well documented in traditional systems of medicine including Ayurveda and Chinese traditional medicine (Duke 2002). Following the traditional claims, considerable efforts have been made by researchers to verify its utility through scientific pharmacological screenings. Pharmacological studies have shown that *N. nucifera* possesses various notable pharmacological activities like anti-ischemic, antioxidant, anticancer, antiviral, anti-obesity, lipolytic, hypocholesterolaemic, antipyretic, hepatoprotective, hypoglycaemic, antidiarrhoeal, antifungal, antibacterial, anti-inflammatory and diuretic (Mukherjee et al. 2009). A wide variety of phytoprinciples have also been isolated from the plant.

With the advancement of scientific exploration of traditional medicines, several classes of plant species have been studied in order to evaluate their therapeutic potential and to isolate the lead compounds. *Nelumbo nucifera* has witnessed a pharmacological and toxicological evaluation of these claims pointing to some important therapeutic benefits of this traditional drug, which are highlighted in this chapter.

This chapter deals with a critical assessment of the currently available information on ethnobotanical and ethnomedical uses, pharmacognosy and medicinal uses as recorded in traditional systems of medicine. It also reviews secondary metabolites, pharmacological and toxicological studies of this useful plant.

8.2   PHYSICAL CHARACTERISTICS AND DESCRIPTION

Nelumbo nucifera is a large aquatic rhizomatous herb consisting of a slender, elongated, creeping stem with nodal roots. The lotus is a perennial plant with both aerial and floating orbicular leaves. Aerial leaves are cup shaped and floating leaves have a flat shape. Its petioles are considerably long and rough with distinct prickles. Flowers vary in colour from white to rosy and are pleasantly sweet-scented, solitary and hermaphrodite. Flower average diameter is 10–25 cm, and it is ovoid and glabrous. The fruit contains black seeds that are hard and ovoid and arranged in whorls; seeds ripen and are released as a result of the bending down of the pod to the water. Tuberous roots are 8 inches long and 2 inches in diameter. The smooth outer skin of the lotus root is green in colour; however, the inner part possesses numerous large air pockets running throughout the length of the tuber that assist in flotation (Mukherjee et al. 1996a, 2009).

8.3   ETHNOPHARMACOLOGICAL USES

Traditional knowledge of the medicinal uses of lotus plant is demonstrated by many scientific investigations. Rhizomes are prescribed for piles as demulcents – beneficial in dysentery, chronic dyspepsia – nutritive, diuretic and cholagogue (Kirtikar and Basu 1975; Chatterjee and Pakrashi 1991). The stem is used in indigenous Ayurvedic medicine as a diuretic, antihelminthic and to treat strangury, vomiting, leprosy, skin disease and nervous exhaustion. The leaves are used for the treatment of haematemesis, epistaxis, hemoptysis, haematuria, metrorrhagia and hyperlipidaemia (Onishi et al. 1984). Young leaves are mixed with sugar for rectal prolapse therapy. Leaves boiled with goat's milk and *Mimosa pudica* are used as an antidiarrhoeal. Natural remedies obtained from leaf paste are effective in fever and inflammed skin. Leaves can be used for treatment of metrorrhagia, haematemesis, haemoptysis, haematuria and epistaxis (Ou 1989). Astringent properties are attributed to leaves used to treat strangury, fever and sweating and as styptic (Anonymous 1997). The flowers are useful to treat diarrhoea, cholera, fever and gastric ulcers. Flower consumption can promote conception and are also important to treat fever, diarrhoea, hyperdipsia, cholera and hepatopathy (Chopra et al. 1956). The flowers and leaves are of importance in treating bleeding disorders. The seeds and fruits are used as a health food in Asia and to treat many ailments including poor digestion, enteritis, chronic diarrhoea, insomnia, palpitations, spermatorrhoea, leucorrhoea, dermatopathy, halitosis, menorrhagia, leprosy, antiemetic, antidote, tissue inflammation, cancer, diuretic, refrigerant, fever and heart complaints (Chopra et al. 1956; Varshney and Rzóska 1976). In traditional folk medicine, the seeds are used for the treatment of poison and diseases of the skin and usually prescribed as a refrigerant and diuretic to children (Chopra et al. 1956). The seeds and fruits are also astringent in nature and can be used for the treatment of various skin diseases, hyperdipsia, halitosis and menorrhagia (Nadkarni 1982). Mixed honey and lotus seed powder is useful in treating cough. Ghee and lotus roots, milk and gold potentiate strength and virility. Lotus seeds have been used as antimicrobials due to their antimicrobial properties (Mukherjee et al. 1995b; Mukherjee 2002). Lian Zi Xin, a Chinese drug, is prepared using embryos of lotus seeds, which are useful in insomnia, various cardiovascular diseases (e.g. hypertension and arrhythmia), nervous disorders and high fevers with restlessness (Chen et al. 2007c).

8.4   PHYTOCHEMICAL AND METABOLITE PROFILING

A large number of phytochemical constituents have been isolated from various parts of *Nelumbo nucifera*.

Normally lotus seeds are rich in protein, amino acids, unsaturated fatty acids and minerals (Wu et al. 2007). Lotus seeds were also found to contain a variety of minerals like Cr (0.0042%), Na (1.00%), K (28.5%), Ca (22.10%), Mg (9.20%), Cu (0.0463%), Zn (0.0840%), Mn (0.356%) and Fe (0.1990%). Other relevant nutritional values include total ash (4.50%), moisture (10.50%), crude carbohydrate (1.93%), crude fibre (10.60%), fat (72.17%), protein (2.70%) and energy value (348.45 cal/100 g) (Indrayan et al. 2005). The major secondary metabolites present in the seeds are liensinine (**1**), isoliensinine (**2**), neferine (**3**), nuciferine (**4**), lotusine (**5**), demethylcoclaurine (**6**), pronuciferine (**7**), armepavine (**8**), dauricine (**9**), nelumboferine (**10**), methylcorypalline (**11**), rhamnetin (**12**), oleanolic acid (**13**) and gallic acid (**14**) (Chopra et al. 1956; Furukawa et al. 1965; Koshiyama et al. 1970; Liu et al. 2006; Rai et al. 2006; Chen et al. 2007c; Sridhar and Bhat 2007; Mukherjee et al. 2009; Kredy et al. 2010; Zhang et al. 2012; Nishimura et al. 2013; Yang and Chen 2013; Addelhamid et al. 2015).

Liensinine (1)   Isoliensinine (2)

Neferine (3)

Nuciferine (4)

Lotusine (5)

Demethylcoclaurine (6)

Pronuciferine (7)

Armepavine (8)

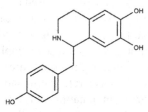

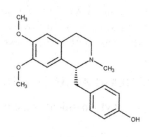

Nelumboferine (10)

Dauricine (9)

Methylcorypalline (11)

Rhamnetin (12)

Oleanolic acid (13)

Gallic acid (14)

The major components found in the leaf extract were nuciferine (**4**), dehydronuciferine (**15**), rutin (**16**), anonaine (**17**), dehydroanonaine (**18**), β-sitosterol (**19**), asimilobine (**20**), and roemarin (**21**) (Kunitomo et al. 1973; Luo et al. 2005; Ohkoshi et al. 2007; Zhao et al. 2013; Grienke et al. 2015). Non-phenolic bases including roemerine (**21**), nuciferine (**4**), nornuciferine (**22**), anonaine (**17**) and liriodenine (**23**), while phenolic bases like norarmepavine (**24**) are also found in *N. nucifera* leaf extract (Kunitomo et al. 1973; Do et al. 2013; Li et al. 2014). From leaves and petioles, lirinidine (**25**), astragalin (**26**), caaverin (**27**), lysicamine (**28**), cepharadione (**29**), oleracein E (**30**), epicatechin (**31**), taxifolin (**32**) and alphitolic acid (**33**) were isolated (Shoji et al. 1987; Ohkoshi et al. 2007; Kim et al. 2009; Li et al. 2014; Lin et al. 2014; Liu et al. 2014; Sharma et al. 2016; Tang et al. 2017).

The leaves also contain flavonoinds like isoquercitrin (**34**) and leucocyanidin (**35**) (Nakaoki 1962; Ohkoshi et al. 2007).

Nuciferine (4)

Dehydronuciferine (15)

Rutin (16)

Anonaine (17)

Dehydroanonaine (18)

β-sitosterol (19)

Asimilobine (20)

Roemerin (21)

Nornuciferine (22)

Liriodenine (23)

Norarmepavine (24)

Lirinidine (25)

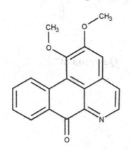

Astragalin (26)

Caaverine (27)

Lysicamine (28)

Cepharadione (29)

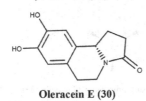

Oleracein E (30)

Epicatechin (31)

Taxifolin (32)

Alphitolic acid (33)

Isoquercitrin (34)

Leucocyanidin (35)

Several flavonoids have been identified in the flowers and stamens of *N. nucifera*. Some of them are kaempferol, quercetin, luteolin 7-glucoside, isorhamnetin 3-glucoside and delphinidin 3-*O* glucoside (Lim et al. 2006; Xingfeng et al. 2010; Chen et al. 2013; Zhou et al. 2013; Lee et al. 2015a). Some non-flavonoid compounds including *N*-methylasimilobine, *N*-methylcoclaurine, norjuziphine, arbutin and *N*-methylisococlaurine has also been identified in flower and stamen extract (Mukherjee et al. 2009; Nakamura et al. 2013; Velusami et al. 2013; Morikawa et al. 2016).

Kaempferol (36)

Quercetin (37)

Luteolin 7-glucoside (38)

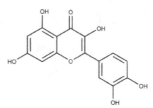

Isorhamnetin 3-glucoside (39)

Delphinidin 3-Oglucoside (40)

_N_-methylasimilobine (41)

_N_-methylcoclaurine (42)

Norjuziphine (43)

Arbutin (44)

N-methylisococlaurine (45)

The rhizome of the lotus contains abundant amounts of starch grains throughout the tissue. Fresh rhizome contains 31.2% of starch, which shows no characteristic taste or odour (Mukherjee et al. 1995a). Isolated lotus starch has been evaluated for its binding and disintegration property compared to maize and potato starch, which has been proved to be superior as an adjuvant in preparation of tablet (Mukherjee et al. 1996a). It has been reported that 50% (v/v) alcohol is responsible for the maximum extraction of the constituents (Mukherjee et al. 1993). The methanolic extract of the rhizome has been found to possess betulinic acid, a steroidal triterpenoid – betulinic acid (**45**) (Mukherjee et al. 1997b). It also contains betulin (**46**), maslinic acid (**47**) and hyptatic acid (**48**) (Kim et al. 2009; Chaudhuri and Singh 2012). Rhizome extract has also been reported to contain a small amount of catechin.

The fresh rhizome contains water (83.80%), fat (0.11%), reducing sugar (1.56%), sucrose (0.41%), crude protein (2.70%), starch (9.25%), fibre (0.80%), ash (1.10%) and calcium (0.06%), along with vitamins including thiamine (0.22 mg/100 g), riboflavin (0.6 mg/100 g), niacin (2.10 mg/100 g), ascorbic acid (1.5 mg/100 g) and amino acids like asparagine (2%). The oxalate content of the rhizome was found to be 84.3 mg/100 g (Kaul and Verma, 1967; Mukherjee et al. 1996b). The percentage concentration of various elements was found to be Ca (1.15%), Cu (0.0015%), Fe (0.053%), Mg (0.398%), Zn (0.032%), Ba (0.00064%), K (0.756%) and Na (0.10%); Shi-Ying and Charles 1986).

Betulinic acid (45)

Betulin (46)

Maslinic acid (47)

Hyptatic acid A (48)

The other parts of *N. nucifera*, such as the stem, contain norarmepavine (Duan et al. 2013), the roots consisted of rutin and hyperin (**49**) (Guon and Chung 2016), the plumule contains higenamine (**50**) (Zhou et al. 2013) and the pollen contains β-amyrin (**51**) (Xu et al. 2011).

Hyperin (49)

Higenamine (50)

β-Amyrin (51)

8.5 PHARMACOLOGICAL ACTIVITIES

8.5.1 ANTIOXIDANT ACTIVITY

Several studies have demonstrated the antioxidant activity of *Nelumbo nucifera*. Lotus seed extracts were found to exhibit free radical scavenging properties and protective effects against reactive nitrogen, sodium nitroprusside (SNP), peroxynitriteinduced cytotoxicity and DNA damage in macrophage RAW 264.7 cell lines (Yen et al. 2006). Hydroalcoholic extract of *Nelumbo nucifera* (HANN) seeds showed significant DPPH (1,1-diphenyl-2-picrylhydrazyl) free radical scavenging activity with IC_{50} values of 6.12 ± 0.41 µg/mL and nitric oxide (NO) scavenging activity with IC_{50} value of 84.86 ± 3.56 µg/mL *in vitro*, which was better than rutin used as standard. Administration of HANN to Wistar strain rats at doses of 100 and 200 mg/kg body weight showed a substantial dose-dependent increase of superoxide dismutase (SOD) and catalase enzyme level and fall in the level of thiobarbituric acid reactive substances (TBARS) compared to CCl4 and tocopherol (50 mg/kg) treatment in both the liver and kidney (Rai et al. 2006).

Several compounds isolated from lotus leaves exhibited antioxidant activity as measured by antiradical scavenging (2,2- azinobis [3-ethyl-benzothiazoline-6-sulphonic acid] and 2,2-diphenyl-1 picrylhydrazyl [DPPH]) assay and ferric reducing power antioxidant assay (Liu et al. 2014). Similarly the Korean traditional lotus liquor (Yunyupju) prepared from lotus blossom and leaves possessed strong DPPH and superoxide radical scavenging activities with IC_{50} values of 17.9 µg and 1 mg, respectively (Lee et al. 2005). The ethyl acetate fraction and essential oil showed IC_{50} values of 191 and 450 µg/mL in DPPH assay, 123 and 221 µg/mL in ABTS assay, and 69 and 370 µg/mL in superoxide assay (Khan et al. 2015). Lee et al. (2015b) revealed the antioxidant activity using cell free and cell assays. The IC_{50} values for DPPH scavenging activity of water and methanolic extracts were found to be 1699.47 and 514.36 µg/mL, respectively. In addition, the extracts inhibited vascular endothelial growth factor (VEGF)-induced reactive oxygen species (ROS) production in human umbilical vein endothelial cells (HUVECs).

The IC_{50} values for hydroxyl radical scavenging activity and superoxide radical scavenging activities of procyanidins, isolated from the non-edible parts of lotus seed pod were determined to be 10.5 and 17.6 mg/L, respectively (Ling et al. 2005). Butanol extract of leaves inhibited free radicals and suppressed intracellular ROS generation in hydrogen peroxide-treated cells and increased cell viability (Je and Lee 2015). Isorhamnetin glycosides from the stamens showed antioxidant activities (Hyun et al. 2006). *N. nucifera* showed significant hypocholesterolaemic and antioxidant properties by modulating erythrocyte function and structural abnormalities (Sasikumar et al. 2012). Also four different chemical analyses resulted in high antioxidant activity from the rhizome knot (Hu and Skibsted 2002).

8.5.2 SKIN PROTECTIVE EFFECT

Studies have revealed the extract of leaves reduced ultraviolet-B (UVB)-mediated wrinkle formation and subcutaneous fat *in vivo* when applied topically. The extract also inhibited UVB-induced expression of IL-6, IL-8 and MCP3 in mouse skin fibroblasts, against photoageing-related disorders (Park et al. 2016). Consumption of lotus seed tea resulted in higher moisture content, thinner epidermis and lowered protein oxidation of skin tissue in the UVB-irradiated skin of rats, which could be due to its potential antioxidative activity (Kim and Moon 2015). Similarly, extracts from leaves, seeds and flowers exhibited 56%, 49% and 54% inhibition of elastase resulting in anti-wrinkle effects, respectively (Kim et al. 2011). In addition, hyperoside (a bioactive constituent of *N. nucifera*) inhibited tyrosinase activity and melanin synthesis in alpha-melanocyte-stimulating hormone stimulated B16F10 melanoma cells (Jung et al. 2014).

8.5.3 NEUROLOGICAL DISORDERS

The literature suggests that dichloromethane, ethyl acetate and *n*-butanol fractions and alkaloids derived from seeds showed promising butylcholinesterase (BChe) and β-site amyloid precursor protein-cleaving enzyme 1 (BACE1) activities, suggesting prevention and treatment of Alzheimer's disease (AD; Jung et al. 2015). Neferine isolated from lotus showed antioxidant, anti-inflammatory and inhibitory effects against cholinesterases and BACE1 to prevent amnesia (Jung et al. 2010). Furthermore hydroethanolic extract of rhizome restored the brain-derived neurotrophic factor in the hippocampus to promote proliferation and neuroblast differentiation as evidenced by increased Ki67-positive cells, doublecortin-immunoreactive cells and brain-derived neurotrophic factor level in the hippocampus of the extract-treated groups (Yoo et al. 2011).

The active constituents such as liensinine, vitexin, quercetin 3-*O*-glucoside and northalifoline were explored for their ChEs- and BACE1-inhibitory activities (Jung et al. 2015). Nuciferine showed a similar receptor profile to aripiprazole-like antipsychotic drugs, where it was found to block head-switch responses and enhanced amphetamine-induced locomotor activity (Farrell et al. 2016). Hydroalcoholic extract of flowers inhibited acetylcholinesterase and monoamine oxidases (MAO-A and MAO-B) in the hippocampus of stress-induced rats (Prabsattroo et al. 2016). Moreover, it was demonstrated that lotus leaf alkaloid extract binds to Gama-Amino Butyric Acid (GABA) receptor and activates the monoaminergic system, resulting in sedative-hypnotic and anxiolytic effects. It was also observed that total alkaloids from lotus leaf increases GABA in the brain, resulting in a sedative-hypnotic effect (Yan et al. 2015). Compounds such as liensinine, isoliensinine and neferine isolated from lotus seed embryo have shown antidepressant effects in mice as evident from forced swimming tests (Sugimoto et al. 2015). In another study, allantoin treatment in scopolamine-treated mice increased the expression levels of phospho PI3K, AKT and GSK to improve the cognitive function observed in AD (Ahn et al. 2014).

8.5.4 Hepatoprotective Effect

Ethanolic extract of lotus seeds showed significant hepatoprotective activity against CCl_4-induced cytotoxicity in rat hepatocytes by inhibiting cellular leakage of AST and the cell death (Sohn et al. 2003; Jung et al. 2015). Adding to that, hydroalcoholic extract administration of seeds alleviated the levels of Super-oxide Dismutase (SOD) and catalase, thus protecting CCl_4-induced liver and kidney damage in Wistar rats (Rai et al. 2006). Neferine was also found to inhibit CCl_4-induced hepatic fibrosis in mice, partly due to lowered expression of TGF-β1 in the liver (Chen et al. 2015). Another study revealed haemoglobin-induced linoleic acid peroxidation was inhibited by Korean traditional lotus liquor made from lotus blossom and leaves (Lee et al. 2005). It was found that lotus germ oil inhibited hydrogen peroxide–induced apoptosis in PC-12 cells and also protected mice from CCl_4-induced injury (Lv et al. 2012). It has also been reported that butanol extract of leaves protected H_2O_2-induced hepatic damage in cultured hepatocytes by increasing the expression of SOD-1, CAT and HO-1 (Je and Lee 2015). Nuciferine isolated from leaves also inhibited cytochrome P450 *in vitro* (Hu et al. 2010). The authors further discovered that nuciferine, when co-administered with phenacetin, changed the pharmacokinetic profile of phenacetin, suggesting that the compounds isolated from lotus may interfere with the bioavailability of prescribed drugs. Moreover, Ye et al. (2014) observed that lotus leaves contain alkaloid compounds that have a potent inhibitory effect on CYP2D6 enzymes. Consistent with this, neferine has been reported to inhibit CYP2D6 (Zhao et al. 2012, 2015). In another study, armepavine has been found to be effective against hepatic fibrosis induced by thioacetamide in rats. The treatment of armepavine inhibited protein expression of α-smooth muscle actin, collagen type I and angiopoietin-1, H_2O_2 production and nuclear translocation of NF-κB, JunD and C/EBPβ in TNF-α stimulated hepatic stellate cells (HSC-T6; Weng et al. 2012).

8.5.5 Pulmonary Fibrosis

The effect of isoliensinine, a bisbenzylisoquinoline alkaloid extracted from the seed embryo of *N. nucifera*, on bleomycin-induced pulmonary fibrosis was first investigated by Xiao et al. (2006). Administration of isoliensinine remarkably suppressed the increase in hydroxyproline content and abated the lung histological injury induced by bleomycin by enhancing SOD activity and suppressing the overexpression of TNF-α and TGF-β1. It was further explored that the anti-inflammation, antioxidation and NF-κB inhibitory mechanisms of neferine might have protected bleomycine-induced pulmonary fibrosis in mice (Zhao et al. 2010). Given the apparent contribution of oxidative stress in pulmonary fibrosis, this antioxidant property could be beneficial in the prevention of pulmonary fibrosis.

8.5.6 Antidiabetic Effect

Hydroalcoholic and alkaloidal extracts of lotus revealed potent aldose reductase inhibitory activity (Gupta et al. 2014). Lotus stamens were examined for their possible inhibitory activity on aldose reductase and isolated alkaloids from the ethyl acetate soluble fraction of the methanolic extract demonstrated potent aldose reductase inhibitory activity (Lim et al. 2006; Veeresham et al. 2014). Natural products are reported to have blood glucose lowering effects in streptozotocin-induced hyperglycaemic rats (Sharma and Rhyu 2015). In one study, Mukherjee et al. reported that the rhizome suppressed blood glucose levels in normal, glucose-fed hyperglycaemic and streptozotocin-induced hyperglycaemic rats. Further, they found improved glucose tolerance and potentiated action of exogenously injected insulin by ethanolic extract of rhizomes (Mukherjee et al. 1997b). The presence of high fibre might have decreased intestinal glucose absorption in diabetic rats. Lotus plumule polysaccharide slightly enhanced the basal insulin secretion and regulated different lipid profiles in non-obese diabetes (NOD) mice by increasing the number of pancreatic islet cells (Liao and Lin 2013b). Consistently, Huang et al. discovered that among various constituents of *N. nucifera*, catechin decreased hyperglycaemia as insulin secretagogues. They further discovered that nuciferine acted on K-ATP channels and amplified the protein kinase A and protein kinase C signaling pathways to elicit greater insulin response as demonstrated in isolated islets (Huang et al. 2011). In addition, Sharma et al. recently reported that aqueous extract from *N. nucifera* leaves enhanced insulin secretion and protected pancreatic beta cells from cytokine-induced toxicity (Sharma et al. 2016).

8.5.7 Anti-obesity Effect

In a study, ethanolic extract of *N. nucifera* seeds decreased body weight and serum lipid levels in high-fat diet-induced obese rats by inhibiting adipogenic factors, such as PPAR-γ, GLUT4, and leptin (You et al. 2014a). In line with this study, kaempferol, isolated from aqueous extract of *N. nucifera* leaves, reduced the expression of different adipogenic transcription factors and their target genes. Kaempferol was shown to interact with VAL324, THR279 and LEU321 residues of PPAR-γ to activate it. More interestingly, the PPAR-γ binding activity of kaempferol was stronger than a well-known PPAR-γ agonist fenofibrate (Lee et al. 2015a). Ohkoshi et al. found that a hydroalcoholic extract of *N. nucifera* leaves stimulated lipolysis in the white adipose tissue of mice through the beta-adrenergic receptor pathway (Ohkoshi et al. 2007). Flavonoids from *N. nucifera* leaves including quercetin, catechin, hyperoside, isoquercitrin and astragalin exhibited lipolytic activity in visceral adipose tissue. The anti-obesity effect of hydroalcoholic extract *N. nucifera* leaves was further elucidated using both mouse and rat models. The mice treated with *N. nucifera* showed decreased body weight, adipose tissue weight and triacylglycerol. The mechanism involved in reducing body weight was impaired digestion, impaired absorption of lipids and carbohydrates, and upregulation of energy expenditure in skeletal muscle cells (Ono et al. 2006). Pronuciferine and nuciferine isolated from *N. nucifera* leaves have been reported to decrease lipid accumulation, total TG content and glucose uptake by increasing AMPK activation in insulin resistant 3 T3-L1 adipocytes (Ma et al. 2015). Moreover, quercetin, a major flavonoid present in *N. nucifera* extract, was reported to have an anti-obesity effect in high-fat diet induced mice by regulating the transcription level of lipogenesis-related genes in the liver (Jung et al. 2013). The treatment of lotus plume polysaccharides in NOD mice decreased blood glucose in both fasting and glucose tolerance tests. Similarly, serum glucose, insulin, total lipid, TG, TC and low-density lipoprotein were found to be decreased in *N. nucifera*-treated NOD mice. The underlying mechanism behind those effects was found to be increased number of islet cells and basal insulin (Liao and Lin 2013a). Oligomeric procyanidins from *N. nucifera* seed pod have been reported to inhibit AGE formation through activation of RAGE-MAPK and NF-κB signaling in high-fat diet rats (Wu et al. 2015b). Tsuruta et al. reported that *N. nucifera* root powder suppressed the progression of non-alcoholic fatty liver disease in db/db mice as evidenced by decreased body and liver weight, liver TG and the markers of liver injury, such as GPT and ALP. The study further noted that *N. nucifera* increased the level of adiponectin and suppressed the expression of lipogenic (ACC1 and FAS) and the inflammatory genes (CRP, MCP-1, and TNF-α; Tsuruta et al. 2012). Wu et al. (2010) further supported these finding by demonstrating that flavonoid-rich fraction of *N. nucifera* regulated body weight by adjusting lipid composition, FAS, HMGCoA and AMPK activities in the liver. In addition, one of the studies revealed that *N. nucifera* not only regulates the different process of adipocyte life cycle but also decreases lipid accumulation without attenuating the total number of fat cells. The study showed that *N. nucifera* leaf extract decreased adipocyte differentiation capacity by attenuating ADD1/SREBP-C signal (Siegner et al. 2010). Tsuruta et al. (2011) reported that polyphenols from dietary lotus root powder could ameliorate hepatic steatosis in db/db mice via the suppression of hepatic lipogenesis. Several papers reported that the mixture of *N. nucifera* leaf extract with other natural remedies synergistically decreased the lipid profiles and body weight in high-fat diet induced obese animals, suggesting that *N. nucifera* can also be consumed as a mixed natural remedy (Du et al. 2010; Sharma et al. 2015). Similarly, You et al. (2014b) reported that ethanolic extract of *N. nucifera* seed inhibited adipogenesis in human pre-adipocytes and decreased body weight and lipid biomarkers in high-fat diet-induced obese rats. In addition, *N. nucifera* leaves have been reported to have anti-obesity effects. Aqueous extract of petals of *N. nucifera* inhibited lipase enzyme activity, adipogenesis, and adipolysis via regulating 5-HT2C and CNR2, which are the central players in obesity (Velusami et al. 2013).

8.5.8 CARDIOPROTECTIVE EFFECT

Vascular smooth muscle cell (VSMC) migration from the media to the intima and subsequent proliferation are the primary events in the development of neointima formation in atherosclerosis and restenosis after angioplasty (Reidy 1992; Ross 1993). Targeting VSMC proliferation and migration represents one of the therapeutic strategies in the prevention and treatment of atherosclerosis and associated diseases, including restenosis. Although several drugs have been identified to inhibit VSMC proliferation and migration *in vitro*, their therapeutic significance *in vivo* has not yet been established (Miller and Megson 2007; Karki et al. 2013). One of our previous studies revealed that administration of aqueous extract of *N. nucifera* leaves significantly suppressed neointima formation in rat carotid artery balloon injury model. *N. nucifera* inhibited TNF-α-induced ERK and JNK activation to inhibit VSMC proliferation. In addition, aqueous extract of *N. nucifera* leaves inhibited TNF-α-induced secretion of MMP-9 to inhibit VSMC migration (Karki et al. 2012). In a similar study, *N. nucifera* leaves showed potent anti-atherosclerotic activity in a rabbit model of atherosclerosis (Ho et al. 2010). However, the extract contained thousands of different chemical entities present in a wide range of concentrations, for most of which the therapeutic activity has not been well studied. To have a greater insight into the mechanisms of the antirestenotic effect of *N. nucifera* extract, various fractions from *N. nucifera* were tested for their inhibitory activity on VSMC proliferation and migration. Alkaloid rich fraction and neferine isolated from alkaloid rich fraction possessed the strongest effect on inhibition of VSMC proliferation and migration. Neferine inhibited cell cycle regulators including cyclin E, cyclin D, CDK2 and CDK4 to induce cell cycle arrest to regulate VSMC proliferation (Jun et al. 2016). Neferine can prevent foam cell formation by inhibition of low-density lipoprotein oxidation and platelet aggregation (Feng et al. 1998). In addition, neferine and liensinine are effective in preventing the onset of re-entrant ventricular tachyarrhythmias (Qian 2002). Neferine has been reported to inhibit angiotensin II–stimulated VSMC proliferation through induction of heme oxygenase-1 (Li et al. 2010) and downregulation of fractalkine gene expression (Zheng et al. 2014). Nuciferine from lotus leaf increased the phosphorylation of eNOS at Ser (1177), thereby increasing the cytosolic NO level to promote vasorelaxation in HUVEC cells. Under endothelium-free conditions, nuciferine attenuated calcium-induced contraction, suggesting that nuciferine may have a therapeutic effect on vascular diseases associated with aberrant vasoconstriction (Wang et al. 2015b). Similarly, anti-angiogenic activity of *N. nucifera* leaf aqueous and methanolic extracts was evaluated in a chick chorioallantoic membrane model using fertilised chicken eggs. The treatment of the *N. nucifera* extracts significantly suppressed VEGF-induced angiogenesis (Lee et al. 2015c). Chen et al. found that neferine isolated from green seed embryo of *N. nucifera* increased the concentration of cAMP in rabbit corpus cavernosum tissue by inhibiting phosphodiesterase activity in a dose-dependent manner (Chen et al. 2008). Neferine relaxes corpus cavernosum smooth muscle cells by inhibiting calcium elevation in the cells by blocking the voltage-dependent calcium channel, alpha 1 adrenoceptor operated calcium channel and calcium release from intracellular calcium pool (Chen et al. 2007a). Furthermore, Mutreja et al. (2008) found that a hydroalcoholic extract of *N. nucifera* seeds has an anti-estrogenic effect without altering the general physiology of reproductive system.

8.5.9 TREATMENT FOR ERECTILE DYSFUNCTION

Neferine showed the effects on basal concentration of cyclic adenosine monophosphate and cyclic guanosine monophosphate (Chen et al. 2008). Neferine potentiated cAMP concentration dose dependently; however, this effect was not suppressed by inhibiting adenylyl cyclase in rabbit corpus cavernosum *in vitro*. Neferine dose dependently increased cAMP accumulation catalyzed by a stimulator of cAMP production, namely, prostaglandin E1 (PGE1). The level of cGMP was not affected by guanylyl cyclase inhibitor and sodium nitroprusside. Neferine enhances the concentration of cAMP in tissue of rabbit corpus cavernosum notably by suppressing activity of phosphodiesterase (Chen et al. 2008). In another study, Chen et al. (2007) further highlighted treatment of erectile dysfunction of the *in vitro* relaxation mechanisms of neferine on the rabbit corpus cavernosum tissue and *in vitro* effects of neferine on cytosolic-free calcium concentration in corpus cavernosum smooth muscle cells of rabbits.

8.5.10 ANTI-FERTILITY ACTIVITY

The petroleum ether extract of the seed has been reported to possess anti-fertility activity in female albino mice at a dose of 3 mg/kg. It blocked the oestrus cycle at the metoestrus stage compared with ethyl oleate (0.1 mL/20 g). The extract significantly reduced uterine weight and affected the oestrus cycle by blocking biogenesis of ovarian steroids at an intermediate stage (Mazumder et al. 1992).

8.5.11 ANTIDIARRHOEAL ACTIVITY

The antidiarrhoeal potential of *N. nucifera* rhizome extract has been reported. The extract produced significant inhibitory effects against castor oil–induced diarrhoea and PGE2-induced enteropooling; the propulsive movements of charcoal meal were also reduced significantly (Mukherjee et al. 1995a). The observed antidiarrhoeal effect was reconfirmed by Talukder and Nessa (1998) in a rat model.

8.5.12 DIURETIC ACTIVITY

The methanolic extract of the rhizome induced significant diuresis in rats at doses of 300, 400 and 500 mg/kg. There was a dose-dependent increase in the volume of urine, with Na+ and Cl⁻ excretion, accompanied by a significant excretion of K+. The increase in volume of urine was less than with the standard diuretic Furosemide (20 mg/kg; Mukherjee et al. 1996b).

8.5.13 ANTIVIRAL EFFECT

Jiang et al. (2011) found that antioxidant components isolated from lotus rhizomes strongly inhibited HIV-1 enzyme. The authors in their *in vivo* studies discovered that antioxidants from *N. nucifera* rhizome exhibited positive regulation on IL-2, IL-4 and IL-10 and inhibited HIV-1 directly by inhibiting TNF-α. Liu et al. (2007) reported that ethanolic extract of *N. nucifera* leaves inhibited phytohaemagglutinin-induced primary human peripheral blood mononuclear cells (PBMCs) proliferation and cytokine expression by regulating Itk and PLC gamma activation in a PI3K-dependent manner, demonstrating the immunomodulatory effects of *N. nucifera*. The potential benefit of (S)-armepavine on systemic lupus erythematosus was studied on MRL/MpJlpr/lpr mice, a model to study human systemic lupus erythematosus.

The administration of (S)-armepavine prevented lymphadenopathy and extended the lifespan of MRL/MpJ-lpr/lpr mice. Consequently, (S)-armepavine impaired the production of IL-2 and IFN-γ in human PBMCs (Liu et al. 2006). Earlier, Liu et al. (2004) found that impaired production of cytokines after (S)-armepavine treatment was due to blunting of membrane-proximal effectors such as Itk and PLC-γ in a PI3K-dependent manner. In a different study by Kashiwada et al. (2005), the authors reported that (+)-1(R)-coclaurine and (−)-1(S)-norcoclaurine, quercetin 3-O-b-ᴅ-glucuronide, aporphine, liensinine, neferine and isoliensinine from *N. nucifera* leaves possessed potent anti-HIV activity. Similarly, ethanolic extract of *N. nucifera* seeds has been reported to inhibit herpes simplex type 1 (HSV-1) replication through the inhibition of immediate early transcripts, such as ICP0 and ICP4 mRNA and the blocking of all downstream viral product accumulation and progeny HSV-1 production (Kuo et al. 2005). In a different study, aqueous extract of *N. nucifera* and luteolin has been shown inhibitory effect against rotavirus (Knipping et al. 2012).

8.5.14 ANTIBACTERIAL AND ANTIFUNGAL EFFECTS

Lin et al. (2014) isolated ten aporphine derivatives from *N. nucifera* and discovered their anthelmintic activities against *A. simplex* and *H. nana*. Moreover, Brindha et al. tested the efficacy of hydroethanolic extract of *N. nucifera* flower against five important bacterial strains and two fungal strains. The minimum inhibitory concentration for *N. nucifera* flower extract against *Escherichia coli* and *Staphylococcus aureus* was found to be 430 and 450 μg, respectively. The moderate zone of inhibition was found against *Klebsiella pneumonia* and *Pseudomonas aeruginosa*. Similarly, the extract possessed antifungal activity against *Aspergillus niger* and *Monascus purpureus* (Brindha and Arthi 2010). *N. nucifera* inhibited quorum-sensing, an intercellular signalling and gene regulated mechanism, which is used by a number of opportunistic bacteria in determining virulence of gene expression, in *Chromobacterium violaceum* and *Pseudomonas aeruginosa* suggesting *N. nucifera* may be a source to combat pathogenic bacteria and reduce development of antibiotic resistance (Koh and Tham 2011).

8.5.15 ANTI-INFLAMMATORY AND ANTI-PYRETIC EFFECTS

Tissue inflammation is a harmful response that produces tissue injury and may cause serious diseases such as asthma, atopic dermatitis and rheumatoid arthritis (Hanada and Yoshimura 2002). Cytokines secreted by T cells such as IL-4, IL-10 and INF-γ in response to antigen stimulation play a key role in atopic dermatitis, diabetes, lung inflammation and asthma (Goodman et al. 1996). Ethanolic extract from *N. nucifera* leaves significantly suppressed phytohaemaglutinin-stimulated PBMC proliferation by inducing cell cycle arrest and the gene expression of IL-4, IL-10 and INF-γ (Liu et al. 2004). Methanolic extract of *N. nucifera* rhizome and the isolated betulinic acid have been reported to possess anti-inflammatory activity similar to that of the prototype anti-inflammatory drugs phenylbutazone and dexamethasone in a carrageenin and serotonin-induced rat paw edema model (Mukherjee et al. 1997a). Furthermore, purified active lotus plumule polysaccharides showed strong ant-inflammatory activities in mouse primary splenocytes stimulated with LPS via inhibiting TLR-2 and/or TLR-4 expressions (Liao and Lin 2013b). Consistently, purified fractions of lotus plumule polysaccharide showed strong anti-inflammatory activities in LPS stimulated macrophages. Nuciferine decreased hyperuricaemia in potassium oxonate-induced rats by regulating urate transport related proteins, such as URAT1, GLUT9, ABCG2 and OAT1 (Wang et al. 2015a). Inflammasomes are a multimeric protein complex that are assembled after recognition of various pathogen-associated molecular patterns or danger-associated molecular patterns to activate caspase-1 activation thereby leading to the production of matured pro-inflammatory cytokines IL-1β and IL-18 that play an important role in the regulation of different inflammation-associated chronic diseases (Strowig et al. 2012; Karki et al. 2015). Interestingly, Wang et al. discovered that nuciferine regulates TLR-4/Myd88/NF-κB-mediated signaling and NLRP3 activation in hyperuricaemic mice. Their *in vivo* study was further supported by impaired production of IL-1β in renal tubular epithelial cells stimulated by uric acid. Therefore, this study for the first time claimed that nuciferine regulates NLRP3 inflammasome to control inflammatory diseases (Wang et al. 2015a). Similarly, hyperoside, an active constituent found in the leaves of *N. nucifera*, inhibited caspase-1 cleavage to inhibit inflammasome dependent cytokines IL-1β in human mast cell line-1 (HMC-1; Han et al. 2014). Atopic dermatitis, a chronic inflammatory skin disease, is caused by distorted immunological response (DaVeiga 2012). We reported that aqueous extract from *N. nucifera* leaves attenuated the development of atopic dermatitis–like skin lesions in NC/Nga mice (Karki et al. 2012). Neferine has been shown to have a protective effect on NO production in HUVEC stimulated by lysophosphatidylcholine via modulating DDAH-ADMA pathway (Peng et al. 2011). *N. nucifera* rhizome inhibited histamine release, reduced NO production, and stabilised erythrocyte membrane (Mukherjee et al. 2010). The anti-pyretic potential of ethanolic extract from *N. nucifera* stalks was evaluated on normal body temperature and yeast induced pyrexia in rats. It was found that the extract caused significant lowering of body temperature in both models, and the results were similar to that of standard antipyretic drug, paracetamol (Sinha et al. 2000). The immune-modulatory activity of *N. nucifera* rhizome was evaluated, and the study found that a treatment of rhizome inhibited mast cell degranulation and LPS-induced activation of macrophages (Mukherjee et al. 2010). Kaempferol isolated from methanolic extract of flavonoid rich *N. nucifera* stamens inhibited Fc epsilon RI expression in human basophilic KU812F cells suggesting that it may exert anti-allergic effect (Shim et al. 2009). The finding was further supported by negative regulatory activity of kaempferol isolated from *N. nucifera* stamens on basophil activation via the suppression of Fc epsilon RI expression. Moreover, kaempferol inhibited degranulation by reducing the level of β-hexosamindase through inhibition of Lyn, Syk and ERK1/2 activation (Shim et al. 2015).

8.5.16 ANTICANCER ACTIVITY

Progression of cancer depends on the interplay between proliferative and apoptotic signalling. Liu et al. discovered that nuciferine inhibited nicotine-induced non-small cell lung cancer by inhibiting proliferative Wnt/B-catenin signalling pathway and its downstream targets including c-myc, cyclin D and VEGFA. Furthermore, the pro-apoptotic effect of nuciferine was based on decreased ratio of Bcl-2/Bax expression. Tumour weight and size were also decreased in xenograft model nude mice (Liu et al. 2015). Similarly, Zhang et al. (2015a) revealed the anticancer effects of three major bisbenzylisoquinoline alkaloids – isoliensinine, liensinine, and neferine – in triple-negative breast cancer cells. Cell apoptosis in hepatocellular carcinoma was triggered by isoliensinine by inducing p65 dephosphorylation at Ser536 and inhibition of NF-kB activation (Shu et al. 2015). In depth investigation suggests that isoliensinine stimulates PP2A-dependent p65 dephosphorylation at Ser536 by promoting p65/PP2A interaction and impairing PP2A/I2PP2A interaction resulting in suppression of pro-survival pathway NFkB activation in HCC cells (Shu et al. 2016). Neferine-treated HepG2 cells showed increased levels of LDH and NO in their culture medium, indicating more cell death upon neferine treatment. Furthermore, neferine caused mitochondrial membrane damage to induce cell death by initiating apoptotic caspase cascades (Poornima et al. 2013a). The mitochondrial characteristics in cancerous cells like membrane potential, ATP production were preserved by *N. nucifera* seeds. It also reduced cellular apoptosis; inhibited p53, Bax, and caspase 3 activities; and induced Bcl-2 production in antimycin A induced mitochondria-mediated cell death (Im et al. 2013). Neferine from lotus seed embryos inhibited the proliferation of human osteosarcoma cells by attributing cell cycle arrest at G1 phase (Zhang et al. 2012). Wu et al. recently found the anticancer effect of 7- hydroxydehydronuciferine (7-HDNF) on melanoma using an *in vivo* xenograft mice model. Flow cytometric analysis revealed that 7-HDNF increased cell cycle arrest at G2/M phase. The authors found that 7-HDNF induced the formation of autophagic intracellular vacuoles and the augmentation of acidic vesicular organelles (AVO). The treatment of 7-HDNF increased the expression of autophagy-related proteins, such as ATG-6, ATG-3, ATG-7, ATG-16 and ATG-5, in A375. S2 cells (Wu et al. 2015a). Je and Lee (2015) reported that *N. nucifera* leaf extract inhibited VEGF-induced angiogenesis *in vitro* and *in vivo*. In addition, aqueous extract of *N. nucifera* leaves has been reported to inhibit the proliferation and migration of epidermal carcinoma cell line A431 and human breast cancer cell line MDA-MB-231 (Karki et al. 2008b).

Duan et al. reported the autophagic effect of procyanidins from *N. nucifera* seed pod (LSPCs) on HepG2 cells. LSPCs-induced autophagy and autophagic cell death were driven by the ROS generation in HepG2 cells (Duan et al. 2016). In addition, Poornima et al. reported that neferine treatment inhibited A549 cell proliferation by inducing acidic vesicular accumulation, an indication of autophagy. The study found that neferine-mediated autophagy was dependent on inhibition of PI3K/AKT/mTOR signaling pathways (Poornima et al. 2013b). Neferine induces autophagy via p38 MAPK/JNK activation and inhibits the mTOR signaling to suppress the growth of ovarian cancer cells (Xu et al. 2016). Guon et al. reported that treatment of hyperoside and rutin isolated from the roots of *N. nucifera* activated mitochondria-dependent apoptotic pathway via modulation of Bcl2-associated X protein and B-cell lymphoma 2 expression to induce cell death in HT-29 human colon cancer cells, suggesting that hyperoside and rutin may be useful in the prevention of colon cancer (Guon and Chung 2016). It has been shown that the aqueous extract of *N. nucifera* leaves has been shown to inhibit angiogenesis in a chicken chorioallantoic membrane model and growth of tumour in a xenograft model. The inhibitory mechanism of *N. nucifera* is associated with its ability to downregulate connective tissue growth factor-induced PI3K/AKT/ERK signalling (Chang et al. 2016). In line with this, inhibition of CT26 (colorectal cancer cells) tumour growth in nude mice by nuciferine is mediated through inhibiting the PI3K/AKT signalling pathway (Qi et al. 2016).

8.6 CLINICAL TRIALS AND THERAPEUTIC IMPLICATIONS

Although much has been explored about *Nelumbo nucifera*, still there are few studies on its application on clinical trials because of limited information on ADME (absorption, distribution, metabolism and excretion) and toxicity. Taking the cue from the above, some of the clinical aspects of *N. nucifera* are provided in this section.

A clinical trial was conducted to study the efficacy of *Nelumbo nucifera* gaertn. (rhizome powder) in the management of type 2 diabetes mellitus on 120 patients diagnosed with the disease, by the Department of Kayachikitsa, Government Ayurvedic College Hospital, Guwahati. It was observed that the trail of *Nelumbo nucifera* was very effective in controlling blood sugar level. The level of fasting blood sugar and postprandial blood sugar was significantly reduced upon treatment with *Nelumbo nucifera* rhizome powder (Ahmed and Sarma 2017). The level of glycosylated haemoglobin was significantly reduced, showing good glycaemic control. Thus the folkloric use and preclinical studies of *N. nucifera* for the management of diabetes were found to be effective in clinical trial as well.

In another study it was found that emulsions prepared from extracts of *N. nucifera* and green tea displayed synergistic/additive effects in reducing the facial sebum levels in patients. Apart from that, it has also been found that this formulation reduced melanin contents while improving hydration of skin without causing erythema (Mahmood and Akhtar 2013; Mahmood et al. 2013).

Extensive basic and clinical studies on higenamine (**50**) (a compound isolated from *N. nucifera*) showed valuable therapeutic effects on different disorders. Higenamine appears to be a useful pharmacological stress agent in myocardial perfusion imaging (MPI). A phase 2 trial was conducted to compare higenamine stress MPI with an adenosine stress test (Yanrong et al. 2014). Their study suggested that higenamine SPECT was comparable with adenosine SPECT at detecting areas of the heart with reduced blood flow. They also found a similar effect on the detection of left anterior descending coronary artery, left circumflex coronary artery and right coronary artery.

Higenamine is of great value for treating bradyarrhythmia. Several clinical studies exploring the effect of higenamine on bradyarrhythmia have been documented. A multicenter study in China showed that intravenous infusion of 2.5 mg higenamine could increase heart rate, promoting conduction of sinus and AV node and enhancing the contraction of the myocardium and thus improve sinoatrial block and AV block in patients with bradyarrhythmia induced by different diseases such as CADs, myocarditis and cardiomyopathy. One small clinical study assessed the effects of intravenous higenamine infusion on bradyarrhythmia in 14 patients. The total effect rate was 77.0% with transient side effects. Specifically, higenamine had a marked therapeutic effect on sick sinus syndrome (SSS) for which Western medicine has a poor curative effect. The compound markedly improved the function of atrionector and atrioventricular node by shortening the sinus cycle length and reducing sinus node recovery time and total sinoatrial conduction time in patients with SSS (Zhang et al. 2017).

Apart from its clinical implications *Nelumbo nucifera* is widely accepted for its role as a functional food or supplement. Dietary fibre incorporation in meat products appeals to many health-conscious consumers looking for low- and reduced-fat food. Dietary fibre can act as a valuable extender, with innumerable functions including binder and fat replacer in the development of various novel meat products. Dietary fibre–enriched chicken patties were developed by incorporation of fresh lotus stem paste (Bharti et al. 2017). The incorporation of dietary fibre into meat products resulted in a supplementary nutritional surge for the consumers.

In another study, lotus root samples were fermented with brown sugar to develop a new functional syrup and/or beverage from *Nelumbo nucifera*, which showed that fermented lotus root sugar syrup samples containing phenolic and flavonoid compounds exhibited remarkable antioxidant and tyrosinase inhibitory activities compared to control (brown sugar broth). Moreover, total phenolic and flavonoid contents of lotus root sugar syrup samples increased with the fermentation period. Sugar-fermented lotus root could be a readily accessible fermented herbal syrup supplement with potential as a natural bioactive product with potent antioxidant and melanin-reducing effects (Shukla et al. 2015).

The comprehensive scrutiny of the literature on *N. nucifera* in terms of phytochemical, pharmacological, clinical and therapeutic evidence revealed sporadic information on phytoconstituents, ethnopharmacological activity, preclinical and clinical research. All parts of *N. nucifera*, from root to fruit, have been experimentally validated for a multitude of structural features of their phytochemical secondary metabolites, which impart innumerable versatile, potent and unprecedented biological properties, medicinal uses and sensory evaluations (Karki et al. 2008; Mukherjee et al. 2009). Emerging evidence from different disciplines suggests a great potential for *N. nucifera* in the prevention and treatment of life-threatening diseases like cancer (Zhang et al. 2015b), obesity (You et al. 2014a), inflammation (Liu et al. 2014) and infection (Knipping et al. 2012). Lotus can also serve as a potential candidate for functional food supplements like nutraceuticals. Further exploration of its potential features – including clinical trials and human applications – are necessary.

REFERENCES

Addelhamid, M. S., Kondratenko, E. I. and Lomteva, N. A. (2015). GC-MS analysis of phytocomponents in the ethanolic extract of *Nelumbo nucifera* seeds from Russia. *Journal of Applied Pharmaceutical Science*, **5**, 115–118.

Ahmed, N. and Sarma, B. P. (2017). A study on the efficacy of *Nelumbo nucifera* gaertn in the management of type-2 diabetes mellitus. *Journal of Science*, **2**, 10–13.

Ahn, Y. J., Park, S. J., Woo, H. et al. (2014). Effects of allantoin on cognitive function and hippocampal neurogenesis. *Food and Chemical Toxicology*, **64**, 210–216.

Anonymous. (1966). *The Wealth of India*. Vol. III, P.ID, CSIR, New Delhi, 7. Chaudhuri, P. and Singh, D. (2012). A new triterpenoid from the rhizomes of Nelumbo nucifera. *Natural Product Research*. 27. doi: 10.1080/14786419.2012.676549.

Anonymous. (1982). *Pharmacognosy of Indigenous Drugs*. Vol. 11, New Delhi: CCRAS, 806.

Bharti, S. K., Pathak, V., Goswami, M., Sharma, S., Ojha, S. and Anita. (2017). Quality assessment of *Nelumbo nucifera* supplemented functional muscle food. *Journal of Entomology and Zoology Studies*, **5**(4), 445–451.

Brindha, D. and Arthi, D. (2010). Antimicrobial activity of white and pink nelumbo nucifera gaertn flowers. *JPRHC*, **2**(2), 147–155.

Chang, C. H., Ou, T. T., Yang, M. Y., Huang, C. C. and Wang, C. J. (2016). Nelumbo nucifera Gaertn leaves extract inhibits the angiogenesis and metastasis of breast cancer cells by downregulation connective tissue growth factor (CTGF) mediated PI3K/AKT/ERK signaling. *Journal of Ethnopharmacology*, **188**, 111–122.

Chatterjee, A. and Pakrashi, S. C. (1991). *The Treatise on Indian Medicinal Plants*, vol. 1. New Delhi, India: Publication and Information Directorate, 94–96.

Chaudhuri, P. K. and Singh, D. (2012). A new triterpenoid from the rhizomes of *Nelumbo nucifera*. *Natural Product Research*, **27**, 532–536.

Chen, J., Liu, J. H., Jiang, Z. J. et al. (2007a.) Effects of neferine on cytosolic free calcium concentration in corpus cavernosum smooth muscle cells of rabbits. *Andrologia*, **39**(4), 141–145.

Chen, J., Liu, J. H., Wang, T., Xiao, H. J., Yin, C. P. and Yang, J. (2008). Effects of plant extract neferine on cyclic adenosine monophosphate and cyclic guanosine monophosphate levels in rabbit corpus cavernosum in vitro. *Asian Journal of Andrology*, **10**(2), 307–312.

Chen, J., Qi, J., Chen, F. et al. (2007b). Relaxation mechanisms of neferine on the rabbit corpus cavernosum tissue in vitro. *Asian Journal of Andrology*, **9**(6), 795–800.

Chen, M. S., Zhang, J. H., Wang, J. L., Gao, L., Chen, X. X. and Xiao, J. H. (2015). Anti-fibrotic effects of neferine on carbon tetrachlorideinduced hepatic fibrosis in mice. *American Journal of Chinese Medicine*, **43**, 231–240.

Chen, S., Fang, G., Xi, H. et al. (2012). Simultaneous qualitative assessment and quantitative analysis of flavonoids in various tissues of lotus (*Nelumbo nucifera*) using high-performance liquid chromatography coupled with triple quad mass spectrometry. *Analytica Chimica Acta*, **724**, 127–135.

Chen, S., Xiang, Y., Deng, J., Liu, Y. and Li, S. (2013). Simultaneous analysis of anthocyanin and non-anthocyanin flavonoid in various tissues of different lotus (*Nelumbo*) cultivars by HPLC-DAD-ESI-MSn. *PLoS ONE*, **8**(4), e62291.

Chen, Y., Fan, G., Wu, H., Wu, Y. and Mitchell, A. (2007c). Separation, identification and rapid determination of liensine, isoliensinine and neferine from embryo of the seed of *Nelumbo nucifera* Gaertn. by liquid chromatography coupled to diode array detector and tandem mass spectrometry. *Journal of Pharmaceutical and Biomedical Analysis*, **43**, 99–104.

Chopra, R. N., Nayar, S. L. and Chopra, I. C. (1956). *Glossary of Indian Medicinal Plants*. New Delhi, India: Council of Scientific and Industrial Research, p. 174.

Chopra, R. N. et al. (1958). *Indigenous Drugs of India,* 2nd ed. Calcutta, India: U N Dhur and Sons Pvt., 679.

DaVeiga, S. P. (2012). Epidemiology of atopic dermatitis: A review. *Allergy and Asthma Proceedings: The Official Journal of Regional and State Allergy Societies*, **33**, 227–234.

Do, T. C., Nguyen, T. D., Tran, H., Stuppner, H. and Ganzera, M. (2013). Analysis of alkaloids in Lotus (*Nelumbo nucifera* Gaertn.) leaves by non-aqueous capillary electrophoresis using ultraviolet and mass spectrometric detection. *Journal of Chromatography A*, **1302**, 174–180.

Du, H., You. J. S., Zhao, X., Park, J. Y., Kim, S. H. and Chang, K. J. (2010). Antiobesity and hypolipidemic effects of lotus leaf hot water extract with taurine supplementation in rats fed a high fat diet. *Journal of Biomedical Science*, **17**(Suppl 1), S42.

Duan, X. H., Pei, L. and Jiang, J. Q. (2013). Cytotoxic alkaloids from stems of *Nelumbo nucifera*. *Zhongguo Zhong Yao Za Zhi*, **38**(23), 4104–4108.

Duan, Y., Xu, H., Luo, X., Zhang, H., He, Y., Sun, G. and Sun, X. (2016). Procyanidins from Nelumbo nucifera Gaertn: Seedpod induce autophagy mediated by reactive oxygen species generation in human hepatoma G2 cells. *Biomedicine Pharmacotherapy*, **79**, 135–152. doi:10.1016/j.biopha.2016.01.039.

Duke, J. A. et al. (2002). *Handbook of Medicinal Herbs*, 2nd ed. Boca Raton, FL: CRC Press, 473.

Farrell, M. S., McCorvy, J. D., Huang, X. P. et al. (2016). In vitro and in vivo characterization of the alkaloid nuciferine. *PLoS One*, **11**, e0150602.

Feng, Y., Wu, J., Cong, R., Wang, C., Zong, Y. and Feng, Z. (1998). The effect of neferine on foam cell formation by anti-low density lipoprotein oxidation. *Journal of Tongji Medical University*, **18**, 134–136.

Furukawa, H., Yang, T. H. and Lin, T. J. (1965). On the alkaloids of *Nelumbo nucifera* Gaertn. XI. Alkaloids of loti embryo. 4. Structure of lotusine, a new water soluble quaternary base. *Journal of the Pharmaceutical Society of Japan*, **85**, 472–475.

Goodman, R. B., Strieter, R. M., Martin. D. P., Steinberg. K. P., Milberg, J. A., Maunder, R. J., Kunkel, S. L., Walz, A., Hudson, L. D. and Martin, T. R. (1996). Inflammatory cytokines in patients with persistence of the acute respiratory distress syndrome. *American Journal of Respiratory and Critical Care Medicine*, **154**, 602–611.

Grienke, U., Mair, C. E., Saxena, P. et al. (2015). Human ether-a-go-go related gene (hERG) channel blocking aporphine alkaloids from lotus leaves and their quantitative analysis in dietary weight loss supplements. *Journal of Agricultural and Food Chemistry*, **63**, 5634–5639.

Guon, T. E. and Chung, H. S. (2016). Hyperoside and rutin of Nelumbo nucifera induce mitochondrial apoptosis through a caspase-dependent mechanism in HT-29 human colon cancer cells. *Oncology Letters*, **11**(4), 2463–2470.

Gupta, S., Singh, N. and Jaggi, A. S. (2014). Evaluation of in vitro aldose reductase inhibitory potential of alkaloidal fractions of Piper nigrum, Murraya koenigii, Argemone mexicana, and Nelumbo nucifera. *Journal of Basic and Clinical Physiology and Pharmacology*, **25**, 255–265.

Han, N.-R., Go, J.-H., Kim, H.-M. and Jeong, H.-J. (2014). Hyperoside regulates the level of thymic stromal lymphopoietin through intracellular calcium signalling. *Phytotherapy Research: PTR*. **28**. 10.1002/ptr.5099.

Harer, W. B. (1985). Pharmacological and biological properties of the Egyptian lotus. *Journal of the American Research Center in Egypt*, **22**, 49–54.

Ho, H. H., Hsu, L. S., Chan, K. C., Chen, H. M., Wu, C. H. and Wang, C. J. (2010). Extract from the leaf of nucifera reduced the development of atherosclerosis via inhibition of vascular smooth muscle cell proliferation and migration. *Food and Chemical Toxicology: An International Journal Published for the British Industrial Biological Research Association*, **48**, 159–168.

Hu, M. and Skibsted, L. (2002). Antioxidative capacity of rhizome extract and rhizome knot extract of edible lotus (*Nelumbo nuficera*). *Food Chemistry*, **76**(3)L, 327–333.

Huang, C. F., Chen, Y. W., Yang, C. Y., Lin, H. Y., Way, T. D., Chiang, W. and Liu, S. H. (2011). Extract of lotus leaf (Nelumbo nucifera) and its active constituent catechin with insulin secretagogue activity. *Journal of Agricultural and Food Chemistry*, **59**, 1087–1094.

Hyun, S. K., Jung, Y. J., Chung, H. Y., Jung, H. A. and Choi, J. S. (2006). Isorhamnetin glycosides with free radical and ONOO- scavenging activities from the stamens of Nelumbo nucifera. *Archives of Pharmacal Research*, **29**, 6.

Indrayan, A. K., Sharma, S., Durgapal, D., Kumar, N. and Kumar, M. (2005). Determination of nutritive value and analysis of mineral elements for some medicinally valued plants from Uttaranchal. *Current Science*, **89**(7), 1252–1255.

Im, A. R., Kim, Y. H., Uddin, M. R., Chae, S. W., Lee, H. W., Jung, W. S., Kim, Y. H., Kang, B. J., Kim, Y. S. and Lee, M. Y. (2013). Protection from antimycin A-induced mitochondrialdysfunction by Nelumbonucifera seed extracts. *Environmental Toxicology and Pharmacology*, **36**, 19–29.

Je, J. Y. and Lee, D. B. (2015). *Nelumbo nucifera* leaves protect hydrogen peroxide-induced hepatic damage via antioxidant enzymes and HO-1/Nrf2 activation. *Food & Function*, **6**, 1911–1918.

Jiang, Y., Ng, T. B., Liu, Z., Wang, C., Li, N., Qiao, W. and Liua, F. (2011). Immunoregulatory and anti-HIV-1 enzyme activities of antioxidant components from lotus (Nelumbo nucifera Gaertn.) rhizome. *Bioscience Reports*, **31**, 381–390.

Jiangsu New Medical College. (1997). *Dictionary of Chinese Materia Medica*. Shanghai, China: Peoples Publishing House.

Jun, M. Y., Karki, R., Paudel, K. R., Sharma, B. R., Adhikari, D. and Kim, D. W. (2016). Alkaloid rich fraction from Nelumbo nucifera targets VSMC proliferation and migration to suppress restenosis in balloon-injured rat carotid artery. *Atherosclerosis*, **248**, 179–189.

Jung, C. H., Cho, I., Ahn, J., Jeon, T. I. and Ha, T. Y. (2013). Quercetin reduces high-fat diet-induced fat accumulation in the liver by regulating lipid metabolism genes. *Phytotheraphy Research* **27**, 139–143.

Jung, H. A., Jin, S. E., Choi, R. J. et al. (2010). Anti-amnesic activity of neferine with antioxidant and anti-inflammatory capacities, as well as inhibition of ChEs and BACE1. *Life Sciences*, **87**, 420–430.

Jung, H. A., Karki, S., Kim, J. H. and Choi, J. S. (2015). BACE1 and cholinesterase inhibitory activities of *Nelumbo nucifera* embryos. *Archives of Pharmacal Research*, **38**, 1178–1187.

Jung, S. Y., Jung, W. S., Jung, H. K. et al. (2014). The mixture of different parts of *Nelumbo nucifera* and two bioactive components inhibited tyrosinase activity and melanogenesis. *Journal of Cosmetic Science*, **65**, 377–388.

Karki, R, Jeon, E. R. and Kim, D. W. (2013). Nelumbo nucifera leaf extract inhibits neointimal hyperplasia through modulation of smooth muscle cell proliferation and migration. *Nutrition*. **29**, 268–275.

Karki, R., Jung, M. A., Kim, K. J. and Kim, D. W. (2012). Inhibitory effect of nelumbo nucifera (Gaertn.) on the development of atopic dermatitis-like skin lesions in NC/Nga, ice. *Evidence based Complementary and Alternative Medicine*, eCAM, 153568.

Karki, R., Man, S. M., Malireddi, R. K., Gurung, P., Vogel, P., Lamkanfi, M., Kanneganti, T. D. (2015). Concerted activation of the AIM2 and NLRP3 inflammasomes orchestrates host protection against Aspergillus infection. *Cell Host & Microbe*, **17**, 357–368.

Kashiwada, Y., Aoshima, A., Ikeshiro, Y., Chen, Y. P., Furukawa, H., Itoigawa, M., Fujioka, T., Mihashi, K., Cosentino, L. M., Morris-Natschke, S. L. and Lee, K. H. (2005). Anti-HIV benzylisoquinoline alkaloids and flavonoids from the leaves of Nelumbo nucifera, and structure-activity correlations with related alkaloids. *Bioorganic & Medicinal Chemistry*, **13**, 443–448.

Kaul, S. and Verma, S. L. (1967). Oxalate contents of foods commonly used in Kashmir. *Indian Journal of Medical Research*, **55**, 5.

Khan, S., Khan, H., Ali, F., Ali, N., Khan, F. U. and Khan, S. U. (2015). Antioxidant, cholinesterase inhibition activities and essential oil analysis of *Nelumbo nucifera* seeds. *Natural Product Research*, **30**, 1335–1338.

Kim, K. H., Chang, S. W., Ryu, S. Y., Choi, S. U. and Lee, K. R. (2009). Phytochemical constituents of *Nelumbo nucifera*. *Natural Product Sciences*, **15**, 90–95.

Kim, S. Y. and Moon, G. S. (2015). Photoprotective Effect of lotus (*Nelumbo nucifera* Gaertn.) seed tea against UVB irradiation. *Preventive Nutrition and Food Science*, **20**, 162–168.

Kim, T., Kim, H. J. and Cho, S. K. (2011). *Nelumbo nucifera* extracts as whitening and anti-wrinkle cosmetic agent. *Korean Journal of Chemical Engineering*, **28**, 424–427.

Kirtikar, K. R. and Basu, B. D. (1975). *Indian Medicinal Plants*, 2nd ed. New Delhi, India: International Book Distributors, 116–120.

Knipping, K., Garssen, J. and Land, B. (2012). An evaluation of the inhibitory effects against rotavirus infection of edible plant extracts. *Virology Journal*, **9**, 137.

Koh, K. H. and Tham, F. Y. (2011). Screening of traditional Chinese medicinal plants for quorum-sensing inhibitors activity. *Journal of Microbiology, Immunology and Infection*, **44**, 144e148.

Koshiyama, H., Ohkuma, H., Kawaguchi, H., Hsu, H. and Chen, Y. (1970). Isolation of 1-(p-Hydroxybenzyl)-6,7-dihydroxy-1,2,3,4-tetrahydroisoquinoline (demethylcoclaurine), an active alkaloid from *Nelumbo nucifera*. *Chemical and Pharmaceutical Bulletin*, **18**(12), 2564–2568.

Kredy, H. M., Huang, D., Xie, B. et al. (2010). Flavonols of lotus (*Nelumbo nucifera*, Gaertn.) seed epicarp and their antioxidant potential. *European Food Research and Technology*, **231**, 387–394.

Kunitomo, J., Yoshikawa, Y., Tanka, S. et al. (1973). Alkaloids of *Nelumbo nucifera*. *Physical Chemistry A*, **12**, 699–701.

Kuo, Y. C., Lin, Y. L., Liu, C. P. and Tsai, W. J. (2005). Herpes simplex virus type 1 propagation in HeLa cells interrupted by Nelumbo nucifera. *Journal of Biomedical Science*, **12**, 1021–1034.

Lee, B., Kwon, M., Choi, J. S., Jeong, H. O., Chung, H. Y. and Kim, H. R. (2015a). Kaempferol isolated from *Nelumbo nucifera* inhibits lipid accumulation and increases fatty acid oxidation signaling in adipocytes. *Journal of Medicinal Food*, **18**, 1363–1370.

Lee, D. B., Kim, D. H. and Je, J. Y. (2015b). Antioxidant and cytoprotective effects of lotus (*Nelumbo nucifera*) leaves phenolic fraction. *Preventive Nutrition and Food Science*, **20**: 22–28.

Lee, H. K., Choi, Y. M., Noh, D. O. and Suh, H. J. (2005). Antioxidant effect of Korean traditional lotus liquor (Yunyupju). *International Journal of Food Science & Technology*, **40**, 7.

Lee, J. S., Shukla, S., Kim, J. A. and Kim, M. (2015c). Anti-angiogenic effect of Nelumbo nucifera leaf extracts in human umbilical vein endothelial cells with antioxidant potential. *PLoS One*, **10**(2), e0118552. doi:10.1371/journal.pone.0118552.

Li, X. C., Tong, G. X., Zhang, Y., Liu, S. X., Jin, Q. H., Chen, H. H. and Chen, P. (2010). Neferine inhibits angiotensin II-stimulated proliferation in vascular smooth muscle cells through heme oxygenase-1. *Acta Pharmacologica Sinica*. **31**, 679–686.

Li, S. S., Wu, J., Chen, L. G. et al. (2014). Biogenesis of C-glycosyl flavones and profiling of flavonoid glycosides in lotus (*Nelumbo nucifera*). *PLoS One*, **9**, e108860.

Liu, C. P. et al. (2004). The extracts from Nelumbo nucifera suppress cell cycle progression, cytokine genes expression, and cell proliferation in human peripheral blood mononuclear cells. *Life Sciences*, **75**, 699–716.

Liu, C. P. et al. (2007). (S)-armepavine inhibits human peripheral blood mononuclear cell activation by regulating Itk and PLCg activation in a PI-3K-dependent manner. *Journal of Leukocyte Biology*, **81**, 1276–1286.

Liu, W., Yi, D. D., Guo, J. L., Xiang, Z. X., Deng, L. F. and He, L. (2015). Nuciferine, extracted from Nelumbo nucifera Gaertn, inhibits tumor-promoting effect of nicotine involving Wnt/β-catenin signaling in non-small cell lung cancer. *Journal of Ethnopharmacology*, **165**, 83–93.

Lim, S. S., Jung, Y. J., Hyun, S. K., Lee, Y. S. and Choi, J. S. (2006). Rat lens aldose reductase inhibitory constituents of *Nelumbo nucifera* stamens. *Phytotherapy Research*, **20**, 825–830.

Lin, R. J., Wu, M. H., Ma, Y. H., Chung, L. Y., Chen, C. Y. and Yen, C. M. (2014). Anthelmintic activities of aporphine from *Nelumbo nucifera* Gaertn. cv. Rosa-plena against Hymenolepis nana. *International Journal of Molecular Sciences*, **15**, 3624–3639.

Ling, Z. Q., Xie, B. J. and Yang, E. L. (2005). Isolation, characterization, and determination of antioxidative activity of oligomeric procyanidins from the seedpod of *Nelumbo nucifera* Gaertn. *Journal of Agricultural and Food Chemistry*, **53**, 2441–2445.

Liu, C. M., Kao, C. L., Wu, H. M. et al. (2014). Antioxidant and anticancer aporphine alkaloids from the leaves of *Nelumbo nucifera* Gaertn. cv. Rosa-plena. *Molecules*, **19**, 17829–17838.

Liu, C. P., Tsai, W. J., Shen, C. C. et al. (2006). Inhibition of (S)-armepavine from *Nelumbo nucifera* on autoimmune disease of MRL/MpJlpr/lpr mice. *European Journal of Pharmacology*, **531**, 270–279.

Luo, X., Chen, B., Liu, J. and Yao, S. (2005). Simultaneous analysis of Nl-nornuciferine, O-nornuciferine, nuciferine, and roemerine in leaves of *Nelumbo nucifera* Gaertn by high-performance liquid chromatography-photodiode array detection- electrospray mass spectrometry. *Analytica Chimica Acta*, **538**, 129–133.

Lv, L., Jiang, C., Li, J. and Zheng, T. (2012). Protective effects of lotus (*Nelumbo nucifera* Gaertn) germ oil against carbon tetrachloride induced injury in mice and cultured PC-12 cells. *Food and Chemical Toxicology*, **50**, 1447–1453.

Ma, C., Li, G., He, Y., Xu, B., Mi, X., Wang, H. and Wang, Z. (2015). Pronuciferine and nuciferine inhibit lipogenesis in 3T3-L1 adipocytes by activating the AMPK signaling pathway. *Life Sciences*, **136**, 120–125.

Mahmood, T. and Akhtar, N. (2013). Combined topical application of lotus and green tea improves facial skin surface parameters. *Rejuvenation Research*, **16**, 91–97.

Mahmood, T., Akhtar, N. and Moldovan, C. (2013). A comparison of the effects of topical green tea and lotus on facial sebum control in healthy humans. *Hippokratia*, **17**, 64–67.

Mazumder, U. K., Gupta, M. A., Pramanik, G. et al. (1992). Antifertility activity of seed of *Nelumbo nucifera* in mice. *Indian Journal of Experimental Biology*, **30**, 533–534.

Miller, M. R. and Megson, I. L. (2007). Recent developments in nitric oxide donor drugs. *British Journal of Pharmacology*, **151**, 305–321.

Morikawa, T., Kitagawa, N., Tanabe, G. et al. (2016). Quantitative determination of alkaloids in lotus flower (flower buds of *Nelumbo nucifera*) and their melanogenesis inhibitory activity. *Molecules*, **21**, 930.

Mukherjee, P. K. (2002). *Quality Control of Herbal Drugs: An Approach to Evaluation of Botanicals*, 1st ed. New Delhi, India: Business Horizons.

Mukherjee, P. K. et al. (1993). Studies on some co-chemicals properties tinctures of Nelumbo nucifera Gaertn (Family: Nymphaeaceae). *Res Ind*, 1993; **38**, 264–265.

Mukherjee, P. K., Balasubramanian, R., Saha, K., Saha, B. P. and Pal, M. (1996a). A review on *Nelumbo nucifera* gaertn. *Ancient Science of Life*, **15**(4), 268–276.

Mukherjee, D., Biswas, A., Bhadra, S., Pichairajan, V., Biswas, T., Saha, B. P. and Mukherjee, P. K. (2010). Exploring the potential of Nelumbo nucifera rhizome on membrane stabilization, mast cell protection, nitric oxide synthesis, and expression of costimulatory molecules. *Immunopharmacology and Immunotoxicology*, **32**, 466–472.

Mukherjee, P. K., Das, J., Saha, K. et al. (1996b). Diuretic activity of the rhizomes of *Nelumbo nucifera* Gaertn (Fam. Nymphaeaceae). *Phytotherapy Research*, **10**, 424–425.

Mukherjee, P. K., Das, J. B., Balasubramanian, R. et al. (1995a). Antidiarrhoeal evaluation of *Nelumbo nucifera* rhizome extract. *Indian Journal of Experimental Biology*, **27**, 262–264.

Mukherjee, P. K., Mukherjee, D., Maji, A. K., Rai, S. and Heinrich, M. (2009). The sacred lotus (*Nelumbo nucifera*)-phytochemical and therapeutic profile. *Journal of Pharmacy and Pharmacology*, **61**, 407–422.

Mukherjee, P. K., Saha, K., Das, J., Pal, M. and Saha, B. P. (1997a). Studies on the anti-inflammatory activity of rhizomes of Nelumbo nucifera. *Planta Medica*, **63**, 367–369.

Mukherjee, P. K., Saha, K., Giri, S. N., Pal, M. and Saha, B. P. (1995b). Antifungal screening of *Nelumbo nucifera* (Nymphaeaceae) rhizome extract. *Indian Journal of Microbiology*, **35**, 327–330.

Mukherjee, P. K., Saha, K., Pal, M. and Saha, B. P. (1997b). Effect of Nelumbo nucifera rhizome extract on blood sugar level in rats. *Journal of Ethnopharmacology*, **58**, 207–213.

Mutreja, A., Agrawal, M., Kushwaha, S. and Chuhan, A. (2008). Effect of Nelumbo nucifera seeds on the reproductive organs of female rats. *Iranian Journal of Reproductive Medicine*, **6**, 7–12.

Nadkarni, A. K. (1982). *The Indian Materia Medica*, vol. 1. Bombay, India: Popular Prakashan Pvt.

Nakamura, S., Nakashima, S., Tanabe, G. et al. (2013). Alkaloid constituents from flower buds and leaves of sacred lotus (*Nelumbo nucifera*, Nymphaeaceae) with melanogenesis inhibitory activity in B16 melanoma cells. *Bioorganic & Medicinal Chemistry*, **21**, 779–787.

Nakaoki, T. (1962). Medicinal resources XIX. Flavonoid of the leaves of *Nelumbo nucifera*. *Chemical Abstracts*, **56**, 1527d.

Nishimura, K., Horii, S., Tanahashi, T., Sugimoto, Y. and Yamada, J. (2013). Synthesis and pharmacological activity of alkaloids from embryo of lotus, *Nelumbo nucifera*. *Chemical and Pharmaceutical Bulletin*, **61**, 59–68.

Ohkoshi, E., Miyazaki, H., Shindo, K., Watanabe, H., Yoshida, A. and Yajima, H. (2007). Constituents from the leaves of *Nelumbo nucifera* stimulate lipolysis in the white adipose tissue of mice. *Planta Medica*, **73**, 1255–1259.

Onishi, E. et al. (1984). Comparative effects of crude drugs on serum lipids. *Chemical and Pharmaceutical Bulletin*, **32**, 646–650.

Ono, Y., Hattori, E., Fukaya, Y., Imai, S. and Ohizumi, Y. (2006). Anti-obesity effect of Nelumbo nucifera leaves extract in mice and rats. *Journal of Ethnopharmacology*, **106**, 238–244.

Ou, M. (1989). *Chinese-English Manual of Common-Used in Traditional Chinese Medicine*. Hong Kong: Joint Publishing Company.

Park, K. M., Yoo, Y. J., Ryu, S. and Lee, S. H. (2016). *Nelumbo nucifera* leaf protects against UVB-induced wrinkle formation and loss of subcutaneous fat through suppression of MCP3, IL-6 and IL-8 expression. *Journal of Photochemistry and Photobiology B*, **161**, 211–216.

Peng, Z. Y., Zhang, S. D., Liu, S. and He, B. M. (2011). Protective effect of neferine on endothelial cell nitric oxide production induced by lysophosphatidylcholine: The role of the DDAH-ADMA pathway. *Canadian Journal of Physiology and Pharmacology*, **89**, 289–294.

Prabsattroo, T., Wattanathorn, J., Somsapt, P. and Sritragool, O. (2016). Positive modulation of pink *Nelumbo nucifera* flowers on memory impairment, brain damage, and biochemical profiles in restraint rats. *Oxidative Medicine and Cellular Longevity*, **2016**, 1–11.

Qi, Q., Li, R., Li, H., Cao, Y., Bai, M., Fan, X., Wang, S., Zhang, B. and Li, S. (2016). Identification of the anti-tumor activity andmechanisms of nuciferine through a networkpharmacology approach. *Acta Pharmacologica Sinica*, **37**(7), 963–972.

Rai, S., Wahile, A., Mukherjee, K., Saha, B. P. and Mukherjee, P. K. (2006). Antioxidant activity of *Nelumbo nucifera* (sacred lotus) seeds. *Journal of Ethnopharmacology*, **104**(3), 322–327.

Reidy, M. A. (1992). Factors controlling smooth-muscle cell proliferation. *Archives of Pathology & Laboratory Medicine*, **116**, 1276–1280.

Ross, R. (1993). The pathogenesis of atherosclerosis: A perspective for the 1990s. *Nature*, 362, 801–809.

Sasikumar, D., Mathi, S., Awdah Masoud, A. H. and Ramesh, T. (2012). Physiological and beneficial role of *Nelumbo nucifera* on hypercholesterolemia in rats exposed to cigarette smoke. *Journal of Pharmacy Research*, **5**(1), 425–427.

Sharma, B. R., Kim, M. S. and Rhyu, D. Y. (2016). *Nelumbo nucifera* leaf extract attenuated pancreatic β-cells toxicity induced by interleukin-1β and interferon-γ, and increased insulin secretion of pancreatic β-cells in streptozotocin-induced diabetic rats. *Journal of Traditional Chinese Medicine*, **36**, 71–77.

Sharma, B. R., Oh, J., Kim, H. A., Kim, Y. J., Jeong, K. S., and Rhyu, D. Y. (2015). Anti-obesity effects of the mixture of eriobotrya japonica and nelumbo nucifera in adipocytes and high-fat diet-induced obese mice. *The American Journal of Chinese Medicine*, **43**, 681–694.

Shim, S. Y., Choi, J. S. and Byun, D. S. (2009). Kaempferol isolated from Nelumbo nucifera stamens negatively regulates Fcepsilon RI expression in human basophilic KU812F cells. *Journal of Microbiology and Biotechnology*, **19**, 155–160.

Shi-Ying, X. and Charles, F. S. (1986). Gelatinization properties of Chinese water chestnut, starch and lotus root starch. *Journal of Food Science*, **51**, 445–449.

Shoji, N., Umeyama, A., Saito, N. et al. (1987). Asimilobine and lirinidine, serotonergic receptor antagonists, from *Nelumbo nucifera*. *Journal of Natural Products*, **50**, 773–774.

Shu, G., Yue, L., Zhao, W., Xu, C., Yang, J., Wang, S. and Yang, X. (2015). Isoliensinine, a Bioactive Alkaloid Derived from Embryos of Nelumbo nucifera, Induces Hepatocellular Carcinoma Cell Apoptosis through Suppression of NF-kappaB Signaling. *Journal of Agricultural and Food Chemistry*, **63**, 8793–8803.

Shu, G., Zhang, L., Jiang, S., Cheng, Z., Wang, G., Huang, X. and Yang, X. (2016). Isoliensinine induces dephosphorylation of NF-kB p65 subunit at Ser536 via a PP2A-dependent mechanism in hepatocellular carcinoma cells: Roles of impairing PP2A/I2PP2A interaction. *Oncotarget*, **7**(26), 40285–40296. doi:10.18632/oncotarget.9603.

Shukla, S., Lee, J. S., Park, J., Hwang, D., Park, J. H. and Kim, M. (2015). Quantitative analysis of functional components from *Nelumbo nucifera* root fermented broth with antioxidant and tyrosinase inhibitory effects. *Journal of Food Biochemistry*, **40**, 248–259.

Siegner, R., Heuser, S., Holtzmann, U., Sohle. J., Schepky, A., Raschke, T., Stab, F., Wenck, H. and Winnefeld, M. (2010). Lotus leaf extract and L-carnitine influence different processes during the adipocyte life cycle. *Nutrition & Metabolism*, **7**, 66. doi:10.1186/1743-7075-7-66.

Sinha, S., Mukherjee, P. K., Mukherjee, K., Pal, M., Mandal, S. C. and Saha, B. P. (2000). Evaluation of anti-pyretic potential of Nelumbo nucifera stalk extract. *Phytotherapy Research*, **14**, 272–274.

Sohn, D. H., Kim, Y. C., Oh, S. H., Park, E. J., Li, X. and Lee, B. H. (2003). Hepatoprotective and free radical scavenging effects of *Nelumbo nucifera*. *Phytomedicine*, **10**, 165–169.

Sridhar, K. R. and Bhat, R. (2007). Lotus: A potential nutraceutical source. *Journal of Agricultural Science and Technology*, **3**, 143–155.

Strowig, T., Henao-Mejia, J., Elinav, E. and Flavell, R. (2012). Inflammasomes in health and disease. *Nature*, **481**, 278–286.

Sugimoto, Y., Nishimura, K., Itoh, A. et al. (2015). Serotonergic mechanisms are involved in antidepressant-like effects of bisbenzylisoquinolines liensinine and its analogs isolated from the embryo of *Nelumbo nucifera* Gaertner seeds in mice. *Journal of Pharmacy and Pharmacology*, **67**, 1716–1722.

Talukder, M. J. and Nessa, J. (1998). Effect of *Nelumbo nucifera* rhizome extract on the gastrointestinal tract of rat. *Bangladesh Medical Research Council Bulletin*, **24**, 6–9.

Tang, X., Tang, P. and Liu, L. (2017). Molecular structure–Affinity relationship of flavonoids in lotus leaf (*Nelumbo nucifera* Gaertn.) on binding to human serum albumin and bovine serum albumin by spectroscopic method. *Molecules*, **22**, 1036.

Tsuruta, Y., Nagao, K., Kai, S., Tsuge, K., Yoshimura, T., Koganemaru, K. and Yanagita, T. (2011). Polyphenolic extract of lotus root (edible rhizome of Nelumbo nucifera) alleviates hepatic steatosis in obese diabetic db/db mice. *Lipids in Health and Disease*, **10**, 202.

Tsuruta, Y., Nagao, K., Shirouchi, B., Nomura, S., Tsuge, K., Koganemaru, K. and Yanagita, T. (2012). Effects of lotus root (the edible rhizome of Nelumbo nucifera) on the deveolopment of non-alcoholic fatty liver disease in obese diabetic db/db mice. *Bioscience, Biotechnology, and Biochemistry*, **76**, 462–466.

Varshney, C. K. and Rzóska, J. (1976). *Aquatic Weeds in South East Asia*, 1st ed. New Delhi, India: Springer, 39.

Veeresham, C., Rama Rao, A. and Asres, K. (2014). Aldose reductase inhibitors of plant origin. *Phytotherapy Research*, **28**(3), 317–333.

Velusami, C. C., Agarwal, A. and Mookambeswaran, V. (2013). Effect of *Nelumbo nucifera* petal extracts on lipase, adipogenesis, adipolysis, and central receptors of obesity. *Evidence-Based Complementary and Alternative Medicine*. doi:10.1155/2013/145925.

Weng, T. C., Shen, C. C., Chiu, Y. T., Lin, Y. L. and Huang, Y. T. (2012). Effects of armepavine against hepatic fibrosis induced by thioacetamide in rats. *Phytotherapy Research*, **26**, 344–353.

Wu, J. Z. et al. (2007). Evaluation of the quality of lotus seed of Nelumbo nucifera Gaertn: From outer pace mutation. *Food Chemistry*, **105**, 540–547.

Wu, P. F., Chiu, C. C., Chen, C. Y., and Wang, H. M. (2015a). 7-Hydroxydehydronuciferine induces human melanoma death via triggering autophagy and apoptosis. *Experimental Dermatology*, **24**, 6.

Wu, Q., Li, S., Li, X., Sui, Y., Yang, Y., Dong, L., Xie, B. and Sun, Z. (2015b). Inhibition of advanced glycation endproduct formation by lotus seedpod oligomeric procyanidins through RAGE-MAPK signaling and NF-κB activation in gigh-fat-diet rats. *Journal of Agricultural and Food Chemistry*, **63**, doi:10.1021/acs.jafc.5b01082.

Wu, C. H., Yang, M. Y., Chan, K. C., Chung, P. J., Ou, T. T. and Wang, C. J. (2010). Improvement in high-fat diet-induced obesity and body fat accumulation by a Nelumbo nucifera leaf flavonoid-rich extract in mice. Journal of Agricultural and Food Chemistry, **58**, 7075–7081.

Xingfeng, G., Daijie, W., Wenjuan, D., Jinhua, D. and Xiao, W. (2010). Preparative isolation and purification of four flavonoids from the petals of *Nelumbo nucifera* by high-speed counter-current chromatography. *Phytochemical Analysis*, **21**, 268–272.

Xiao, J. H., Zhang, Y. L., Feng, X. L., Wang, J. L. and Qian, J. Q. (2006). Effects of isoliensinine on angiotensin II-induced proliferation of porcine coronary arterial smooth muscle cells. *Journal of Asian Natural Products Research*, **8**, 209–216.

Xu, S., Sun, Y., Jing, F., Duan, W., Du, J. and Wang, X. (2011). Separation and purification of flavones from *Nelumbo nucifera* Gaertn. By silica gel chromatography and high-speed counter-current chromatography. *Se Pu*, **29**, 1244–1248.

Xu, L., Zhang, X., Li, Y., Lu, S., Lu, S., Li, J., Wang, Y., Tian, X., Wei, J. J., Shao, C. and Liu, Z. (2016). Neferine induces autophagy of human ovarian cancer cells via p38 MAPK/ JNKactivation. *Tumour Biology*.doi:10.1007/s13277-015-4737-8.

Yan, M. Z., Chang, Q., Zhong, Y. et al. (2015). Lotus leaf alkaloid extract displays sedative-hypnotic and anxiolytic effects through GABAA receptor. *Journal of Agricultural and Food Chemistry*, **63**, 9277–9285.

Yang, T. H. and Chen, C. M. (2013). On the alkaloids of *Nelumbo nucifera* Gaertn. studies on the alkaloids of loti embryo. *Journal of the Chinese Chemical Society*, **17**, 235–242.

Yanrong, D., Fang, L., Qian, W., Dianfu, L., Mingqing, L., Yimin, L. and Bilu, L. (2014). Efficacy and safety of a novel pharmacological stress test agent-higenamine in radionuclide myocardial perfusion imaging: Phase II clinical trial. *Chinese Journal of Nuclear Medicine and Molecular Imaging*, **34**(1), 34–38.

Ye, L. H., He, X. X., Kong, L. T., Liao, Y. H., Pan, R. L., Xiao, B. X., Liu, X. M. and Chang, Q. (2014). Identification and characterization of potent CYP2D6 inhibitors in lotus leaves. *Journal of Ethnopharmacology*, **153**, 190–196.

Yen, G. C., Duh, P. D., Su, H. J., Yeha, C. T. and Wu, C. H. (2006). Scavenging effects of lotus seed extracts on reactive nitrogen species. *Food Chemistry*, **94**, 596–602.

Yoo, D. Y., Kim, W., Yoo, K. Y. et al. (2011). Effects of *Nelumbo nucifera* rhizome extract on cell proliferation and neuroblast differentiation in the hippocampal dentate gyrus in a scopolamine-induced amnesia animal model. *Phytotherapy Research*, **25**, 809–815.

You, J. S., Lee, Y. J., Kim, K. S., Kim, S. H. and Chang, K. J. (2014a). Anti-obesity and hypolipidaemic effects of Nelumbo nucifera seed ethanol extract in human pre-adipocytes and rats fed a high-fat diet. *Journal of the Science of Food and Agriculture*, **94**, 568–575.

You, J. S., Lee, Y. J., Kim, K. S., Kim, S. H. and Chang, K. J. (2014b). Ethanol extract of lotus (Nelumbo nucifera) root exhibits an anti-adipogenic effect in human pre-adipocytes and antiobesity and anti-oxidant effects in rats fed a high-fat diet. *Nutrition Research*, **34**, 258–267.

Zhang, N., Lian, Z., Peng, X., Li, Z. and Zhu, H. (2017). Applications of Higenamine in pharmacology and medicine. *Journal of Ethnopharmacology*, **196**, 242–252.

Zhang, X., Liu, Z., Xu, B., Sun, Z., Gong, Y., and Shao, C. (2012). Neferine, an alkaloid ingredient in lotus seed embryo, inhibits proliferation of human osteosarcoma cells by promoting MAPK-mediated p21 stabilization. *European Journal of Pharmacology*, **677**, 47–54.

Zhang, Y. I., Lu, X. U., Zeng, S., Huang, X., Guo, Z., Zheng, Y., Tian, Y. and Zheng, B. (2015b). Nutritional composition, physiological functions and processing of lotus (Nelumbo nucifera Gaert.) seeds: A review. *Phytochemistry Reviews*, **14**, 14.

Zhang, X., Wang, X., Wu, T., Li, B., Liu, T., Wang, R., Liu, Q., Liu, Z., Gong, Y. and Shao, C. (2015a). Isoliensinine induces apoptosis in triple-negative human breast cancer cells through ROS generation and p38 MAPK/JNK activation. *Scientific Reports*, **5**, 12579.

Zhao, Y., Hellum, B. H., Liang, A. and Nilsen, O. G. (2015). Inhibitory mechanisms of human CYPs by three alkaloids isolated from traditional Chinese herbs. *Phytotherapy Research*, **29**, 825–834.

Zhao, Y., Hellum, B. H., Liang, A. H. and Nilsen, O. G. (2012). The in vitro inhibition of human CYP1A2, CYP2D6 and CYP3A4 by tetrahydropalmatine neferine and berberine. *Phytotherapy Research*, **26**(2), 277–283.

Zhao, L., Wang, X., Chang, Q., Xu, J., Huang, Y., Guo, Q., Zhang, S., Wang, W., Chen, X. and Wang, J. (2010). Neferine, a bisbenzylisoquinline alkaloid attenuates bleomycin-induced pulmonary fibrosis. *European Journal of Pharmacology*, **627**, 304–312.

Zhao, X. L., Wang, Z. M., Ma, X. J., Jing, W. G. and Liu A. (2013). Chemical constituents from leaves of *Nelumbo nucifera. Zhongguo Zhong Yao Za Zhi*, **38**, 703–708.

Zheng, L., Cao, Y., Liu, S., Peng, Z. and Zhang, S. (2014). Neferine inhibits angiotensin II-induced rat aortic smooth muscle cell proliferation predominantly by downregulating fractalkine gene expression. *Experimental and Therapeutic Medicine*, **8**, 1545–1550.

Zhou, M., Jiang, M., Ying, X. et al. (2013). Identification and comparison of anti-inflammatory ingredients from different organs of Lotus nelumbo by UPLC/Q-TOF and PCA coupled with a NFkappa B reporter gene assay. *PLoS One*, **8**, e81971.

Section II

Safety

9 Safety and Toxicity of Medicinal Plants
Concerns and Overview

Neeraj Tandon and Satyapal Singh Yadav

CONTENTS

9.1 INTRODUCTION

Medicinal plants have been used in the treatment of human ailments since time immemorial. The earliest recorded medicinal use of plants is in the *Veda-Rigveda*, which goes back to 4500–1500 BCE, listing 67 Indian plants for their therapeutic value as medicine. Other ancient literary works, including the *Yajurveda, Atherveda, Caraka Saṃhitā* (~1000 BC) and *Suśruta Saṃhitā* have recorded medicinal values for several hundred plants. The *Caraka Saṃhitā* mentions 341 medicinal plants and the *Suśruta Saṃhitā* describes 395 medicinal plants. The traditional systems of medicine in many other countries (Persian, Egyptian, Chinese, Arabian, etc.) also document the use of medicinal plants for a variety of human ailments.

With the renewed interest in the usage of plants as medicines, nutraceuticals, food supplements, cosmetics and household remedies globally, there is a growing concern to know about the safety of medicinal plants and other traditional medicines, which include plants as the main components. Increased usage of medicinal plants necessitates us knowing about their safety, whether it is proven in humans or backed by prevailing scientific methods.

9.2 WHAT MAKES PLANTS ACT AS A MEDICINE?

Plant produces secondary metabolites as a by-product of its metabolic pathway that either help in their growth and development or are produced to help in defence from herbivores, pests and pathogens. These synthesised metabolites belong to several chemical classes of compounds like alkaloids, glycosides, terpenes, flavonoids and steroids, and most of these classes of phytochemicals are bioactive in humans and act as a medicine in a manner similar to modern drugs. Many modern drugs like atropine, metformin, morphine, aspirin, cocaine, codeine, digoxin, quinine, pilocarpine, paclitaxel, artemisinin and silymarin were originally plant derived secondary metabolites.

9.3 SAFETY/TOXICITY OF MEDICINAL PLANTS/HERBAL MEDICINES: WHAT IS THE EVIDENCE?

The general perception and belief considering herbal medicines as safe in the modern scientific era would be illogical in absence of scientific proof of safety. Herbal medicine and medicinal plants are comprised of many kinds of phytochemicals that make them act as medicines, but similar to modern medicine these may also produce unwanted effects in humans, thus making them unsafe or even sometimes toxic (Niggemann and Grüber 2003).

Most of the plants which are toxic to humans, basically contain inherent toxic principle(s) like pyrrolizidine alkaloids, colchicine, alpha gliadin, cyanogenic glycosides, thiocyanates and lectins. There are handful of plants that contain toxic concentrations of poisonous constituent(s) and some of these have been well known for causing health hazards, like anticholinergic poisoning with *Atropa belladonna* due to the presence of atropine and other alkaloids (Ulbricht et al. 2004); severe gastro-enteritis and internal bleeding with *Arnica montana* due to helenalin; cardiotoxicity and neurotoxic-ity with *Aconitum* species due to aconitine (Tak et al. 2016); cardiotoxicity with *Digitalis* species due to digoxin-like glycosides; hepatotoxicity with pyrrolizidine alkaloid–containing plants such as *Senecio, Crotalaria, Cynoglossum, Amsinckia, Heliotropium* and *Echium* species (Stegelmeier 2011); and teratogenicity and other toxicity of Solanaceous plants due to presence of toxic alkaloid chaconine, solasodine and solanine (Crawford and Kocan 1993). However, with the discovery of new phytochemicals may further enhance this list of toxic plants.

Commonly used medicinal plants even may also cause various adverse effects in humans. One such important example is the commonly used household spice, garlic which was reported to induce many adverse effects like gastrointestinal discomfort, mild nausea, gastric reflux, heartburn, constipation, bloating/flatulence, mouth ulcers, breathing difficulty, burping, change of taste, head-ache, itching and skin rash in clinical trials (Bordia 1981; Gardner et al. 2007; Ried et al. 2013). Similarly numerous other commonly used medicinal plants have been reported to produce varying adverse effects in clinical trials. Interestingly, the intensity of most of these adverse events ranged from mild to moderate. However, serious adverse effects were also reported with medicinal plants, including hypotension and syncope reported with *Wrightia antidysenterica* (Linn.) R. Br. bark treatment in patients with amoebiasis and giardiasis (Chaturvedi and Singh 1983). Table 9.1 tabu-lates adverse events for 36 such commonly used Indian medicinal plants that have been reported in clinical studies.

9.4 FACTORS INVOLVED IN DETERMINING THE SAFETY OF MEDICINAL PLANTS

Intrinsic and extrinsic factors of both plants and humans play a key role in determining the toxicity and safety of any medicinal plant. The mere presence of toxic compound(s) in a plant does not ascer-tain its toxic effect in humans. The resultant safety and toxicity of any medicinal plant besides the presence of intrinsic toxic constituent(s) also depend upon several extrinsic factors related to any plant. The important aspect that determines safety/toxicity beside the quantity of toxic constituent(s) present in any medicinal preparation is their final bioavailable concentration that reaches in sys-temic circulation and to target organ(s) after interaction with various coexisting chemicals and with the biological barriers and metabolic system. Various external factors that alter the composition of constituents and resultant toxicity, include the part of the plant used, locality of the plant, season and time of collection, storage and processing of collected plant material, nature of the extract or plant preparation used in formulation, dosage and manner in which it is prescribed and used, pre-scriber's understanding of the disease and finally health status of the end users. It is necessary to understand and evaluate all these contributory factors connected with the plant before labelling any plant or its preparation as safe or unsafe, even in the scenario when it has been found toxic in experi-ments or has shown significant adverse effects in humans. Hence to understand the complexity of

TABLE 9.1

Adverse Events of Commonly Used Medicinal Plants Reported in Clinical Studies

Botanical Name of the Medicinal Plant	Popular Name of the Plant (Part Used)	Adverse Events	References
Allium sativum Linn.	Garlic (clove/bulb)	Gastrointestinal discomforts, mild nausea, gastric reflux, heartburn, constipation, bloating/flatulence, mouth ulcer, breathing difficulty, burping, garlic like breath and body odour, garlic like taste, headache, rash and itching	Bordia (1981); Gardner et al. (2007); Ried et al. (2013)
Andrographis paniculata (Burm. f.) Wall. ex Nees	Kalmegh (whole plant)	Nausea, gastric irritation/discomforts, diarrhoea, cramps, fatigue, headache, skin rash	Calabrese et al. (2000); Agarwal et al. (2005); Saxena et al. (2010); Sandborn et al. (2013)
Azadirachta indica A. Juss.	Neem (seed, leaf, stem bark)	Reye's syndrome and death in children, ventricular fibrillation, cardiac arrest, toxic optic neuropathy, poisoning with seed oil in children and adults	Sinniah and Baskaran (1981); Sinniah et al. (1982); Sundaravalli et al. (1982); Sivashanmugham et al. (1984); Balakrishnan et al. (1986); Lai et al. (1990); Dhongade et al. (2008); Bhaskar et al. (2010); Mishra and Dave (2013); Suresha et al. (2014)
Bacopa monnieri (Linn.) Wettst.	Brahmi (whole plant)	Epigastric pain, nausea, vomiting, fullness, bloating of abdomen, diarrhoea, GIT cramps, skin rash	Raghav et al. (2006); Calabrese et al. (2008); Dave et al. (2008); Stough et al. (2008); Morgan and Stevens (2010)
Berberis aristata DC.	Indian barberry (stem)	Abdominal discomfort	Di Pierro et al. (2013)
Boerhavia diffusa Linn.	Punarnava (whole plant)	Reduction in RBC, haemoglobin, vital capacity	Appa Rao et al. (1967)

(Continued)

TABLE 9.1 (*Continued*)

Adverse Events of Commonly Used Medicinal Plants Reported in Clinical Studies

Botanical Name of the Medicinal Plant	Popular Name of the Plant (Part Used)	Adverse Events	References
Boswellia serrata Roxb. ex Colebr.	Shallaki/Salai guggul (oleo-gum resin)	Nausea, vomiting, abdominal/epigastric pain, lack of appetite hyperacidity, diarrhoea, itching, general weakness, headache, mild fever	Gupta et al. (1998); Gerhardt et al. (2001); Madisch et al. (2007); Sander et al. (1998); Kimmatkar et al. (2003); Sontakke et al. (2007); Sengupta et al. (2008); Vishal et al. (2011)
Cassia fistula Linn.	Golden shower tree, Amaltas (fruit pod)	Diarrhoea, mucus like stool, abdominal pain	Barkatullah et al. (1997); Kaur and Chandola (2010)
Centella asiatica (Linn.) Urb.	Indian pennywort, Gotu kola (whole plant)	Nausea, gastric pain	Bosse et al. (1979); Marastoni et al. (1982); Shin et al. (1982); Pointel et al. (1987)
Cinnamomum verum J. Presl syn. *C. zeylanicum* Blume	Dalchini, Cinnamon (stem bark)	Skin rash, urticaria	Altschuler et al. (2007); Crawford (2009)
Commiphora wightii (Arn.) Bhandari	Guggul, Indian bdellium (oleo-gum resin)	Nausea, vomiting, hypersensitivity skin rash, headache, hiccups, loose stools, eructation, thyroid disorders, anorexia, irregular menstruation, restlessness	Malhotra and Ahuja (1971); Sharma et al. (1973); Malhotra et al. (1977); Pandit and Shukla (1981); Arora et al. (1982); Chandrasekaran et al. (1994); Beg et al. (1998); Szapary et al. (2003); Nohr et al. (2009); Yousefi et al. (2013)
Crocus sativus Linn.	Saffron, Kesar (Style and Stigma)	Anxiety, nausea, decreased as well as increased appetite, sedation, headache and hypomania	Noorbala et al. (2005); Akhondzadeh et al. (2005, 2010)
Curcuma longa Linn.	Turmeric, Haldi (rhizome)	Diarrhoea, nausea, epigastric burning, gastritis, bloating, skin itchiness, dryness of mouth and throat, headache, mild giddiness and tranquilising effect	Victor et al. (1972); Jain et al. (1979); Joshi et al. (2003); Kuptniratsaikul et al. (2009); Appelboom and Mélot (2013); Kim et al. (2013); Henrotin et al. (2013); Appelboom et al. (2014)
Cyperus rotundus Linn.	Nut grass, Nagarmotha (tuberous root/rhizome)	Nausea and suppression of appetite	Bambhole and Jiddewar (1984)

(Continued)

TABLE 9.1 (*Continued*)
Adverse Events of Commonly Used Medicinal Plants Reported in Clinical Studies

Botanical Name of the Medicinal Plant	Popular Name of the Plant (Part Used)	Adverse Events	References
Eclipta prostrata (Linn.) Linn.	False daisy, Bhrangaraja (whole plant)	Headache	Dube et al. (1982)
Embelia ribes Burm. f.	Vidanga (fruit)	Diarrhoea	Srivastava and Datey (1962)
Eucalyptus globulus Labill.	Eucalyptus (mature leaf)	Heartburn, nausea, diarrhoea, stomach ache and exanthema	Kehrl et al. (2004); Fischer and Dethlefsen (2013)
Euphorbia neriifolia Linn.	Milkhedge (stem, latex)	Corrosive effect of latex of the plant upon contact with skin and mucous membrane	Naik (2009)
Ficus religiosa Linn.	Pipal tree (bark)	Itching	Virani et al. (2010)
Gloriosa superba Linn.	Langli, Kalihari (tuberous root)	Nausea, vomiting, diarrhoea and abdominal pain	Ide et al. (2010); Senthilkumaran et al. (2011); Peranantham et al. (2014)
Glycyrrhiza glabra Linn.	Licorice, Mulethi	Diarrhoea, heaviness of head, giddiness, headache, increase in body weight and myalgia, acute renal failure, hypokalaemia, hypertension, water retention (oedema), hypokalaemic rhabdomyolysis, hypokalaemic paralysis/acute myopathy, torsades de pointes, acute adrenal crisis, hypercalcaemia and pseudoaldosteronism	Tewari and Trembalowicz (1968); Conn et al. (1968); Engqvist et al. (1973); Habibullah et al. (1979); Caradonna et al. (1992); Shintani et al. (1992); Heikens et al. (1995); Arase et al. (1997); Isaia et al. (2008); Manns et al. (2012); Daniş et al. (2015)
Momordica charantia Linn.	Bitter gourd, Karela (fruit and seed)	Headache, nausea, vomiting, abdominal discomfort, increased frequency of stools, occasional feeling of bilious and bitter taste in mouth	Vad (1960); Waheed et al. (2008)
Mucuna pruriens (Linn.) DC.	Cowhage, Kaunch (seed)	Nausea, vomiting, gastric pain, dizziness, giddiness, sweating, flatulence, diarrhoea, dry mouth, skin rash/pruritus and blue-black urine	Vaidya et al. (1978); Anonymous (1995); Katzenschlager et al. (2004)

(*Continued*)

TABLE 9.1 (Continued)

Adverse Events of Commonly Used Medicinal Plants Reported in Clinical Studies

Botanical Name of the Medicinal Plant	Popular Name of the Plant (Part Used)	Adverse Events	References
Myristica fragrans Houtt.	Nutmeg, Jaiphal (fruit and seed kernels)	Weak pulse, hypothermia, delirium, vertigo nausea and abusive	Kalbhen (1971); Forrest and Heacock (1972); Hallström and Thuvander (1997)
Nardostachys jatamansi (D. Don) DC.	Nardus root, Jatamansi (rhizome/root)	Nausea, anorexia, vertigo and mild sedation	Vakil and Dalal (1955a, 1955b); Arora (1965)
Narthex asafoetida Falc. ex Lindl	Hing, Devil's dung (Oleo-gum resin)	Methemoglobinaemia	Kelly et al. (1984)
Picrorhiza kurroa Royle ex Benth.	Hellebore, Kutki (whole plant)	Gastric irritation, vomiting, diarrhoea, griping pain, anorexia, severe giddiness, itching, and cutaneous rash	Chaturvedi and Singh (1966); Rajaram (1975); Vegnanarayan et al. (1982); Doshi et al. (1983)
Plectranthus amboinicus (Lour.) Spreng.	Country borage, Indian borage, Pattaajvaayana (leaf)	Allergic contact dermatitis	Chang et al. (2005)
Plumbago zeylanica Linn.	Lead wort, Chitra (root)	Abortifacient effect	Tiwari et al. (1982)
Rauvolfia serpentina Linn. Benth. ex Kurz	Sarpagandha, Chota chand (root)	Lethargy, muscular relaxation, drowsiness, nasal congestion or stuffiness, rhinorrhoea, increased frequency of bowel movements, diarrhoea, dizziness, decreased libido and potential tendency to gain weight, nightmares or disturbing dreams, agitated depression and dyspnoea at rest	Bhatia (1942); Vakil (1949); Livesay et al. (1954); Locket (1955); Forster and Holzmman (1966); Smith et al. (1969); PVAMC (1982)
Terminalia arjuna (Roxb.) Wight & Arn.	Arjuna (stem bark)	Constipation and fullness of abdomen	Dixit et al. (2009)
Tinospora cordifolia (Willd.) Miers	Guduchi, Giloe (stem)	Anorexia, nausea, vomiting, headache, giddiness and insomnia	Gulati et al. (1982); Kalikar et al. (2008)
Trigonella foenum-graecum Linn.	Fenugreek, Methi (seed)	Mild diarrhoea, flatulence, gastrointestinal discomfort, stomach ache, fullness of stomach and increased satiety state	Sharma et al. (1990, 1991); Sharma et al. (1996); Prasanna (2000); Mathern et al. (2009); Poole et al. (2010)
Withania somnifera (Linn.) Dunal	Indian ginseng, Ashwagandha (root)	Nasal congestion (rhinitis), constipation, cough, cold, drowsiness and decreased appetite	Chandrasekhar et al. (2012); Raut et al. (2012)

(Continued)

TABLE 9.1 (*Continued*)

Adverse Events of Commonly Used Medicinal Plants Reported in Clinical Studies

Botanical Name of the Medicinal Plant	Popular Name of the Plant (Part Used)	Adverse Events	References
Wrightia antidysenterica (Linn.) R. Br.	Ester tree, Conessi bark tree, Kurchi, Inderjav (stem bark and seed)	Nausea, vomiting, burning sensation in head, abdomen and feet, dryness of mouth, flatulence, constipation, agitation, nervousness, fatigue and insomnia, vertigo, hypotension, syncope	Lavier et al. (1948); Chaturvedi and Singh (1983); Pal et al. (2009)
Zingiber officinale Roscoe	Ginger, Adrak (rhizome)	Heartburn, nausea, bloating/gas, somnolence, headache, gastric irritation	Nanda et al. (1993); Phillips et al. (1993); Riebenfeld and Borzone (1999); Eberhart et al. (2003); Wigler et al. (2003); Zick et al. (2009); Fahimi et al. (2011); Zakeri et al. (2011); Ryan et al. (2012); Yekta et al. (2012); Kalava et al. (2013); van Tilburg et al. (2014)

this phenomenon, one has to follow a multidisciplinary approach and require expertise and understanding of the botanical, phytochemical, pharmaceutical and pharmacological aspects, besides the clinical expertise with a careful judgement while labelling any medicinal plant as safe or toxic. Historical evidence of safe use of medicinal plants has many differences in their method of preparation and manner of use for traditional medicines. In preparation of traditional medicines, various strategies and procedures are followed like use of particular part (fruit, seed, leaf, root, bark, etc.) of the plant; following specific procedures of handling and processing like *sodhana* (detoxification), *kshirpaka* (boiling with milk); rendering plants nontoxic by removing the undesired chemicals or reducing the quantity that induces toxicity; use of polyherbal preparations to synergise the therapeutic effects without inducing toxicity; following a specific procedure such as *koshtashuddi* (enema, bowel cleansing/evacuation) before taking these medicines, and so forth. However, many currently used plant preparations may not be following the proper documented traditional method(s) while preparing or using them as medicine.

Often the toxic constituents of a plant also vary in different parts of the plant, for example toxic amount of atropine and hyoscyamine in *Datura stramonium* Linn. or *Atropa belladonna* Linn. are present in higher amounts in fruits and seeds compared to the leaves and thus selection of plant parts for preparing medicine also determines its safety or toxicity. Altogether different to above scenario, using the whole plant or its part(s) as a whole often retains a pool of chemicals that interfere with each other in both a favourable and unfavourable manner. Interesting cases were reported in this context. One such interesting example is of the Saffron where reduction in the toxic effects of safranal was seen, when an equivalent amount of safranal was administered through whole extract of saffron, another important case reported was the reduction of toxic effects of reserpine due to the presence of ajmaline and rescinnamine in the Rauvolfia root extract. Another important example reported in this context is of Momordica, where administration of whole fruit extract of *Momordica charantia* Linn. was found devoid of anti-implantation and abortifacient effects in mice and had no effect on isolated rat uterus (Dhawan et al. 1980); whereas administration of its purified constituents, α- and β-momorcharins led to fetal death and abortion of fetuses in mice (Chan et al. 1984).

Long-term intake of substandard or spurious preparations of plants is also responsible to produce toxicity due to use of different species, the presence of heavy metals, solvent residue, aflatoxins or pesticide residue over and above the prescribed limits. Other human-related factors that alter the safety of any medicinal plant preparation are its route of administration or exposure, the amount ingested out of prescribed limit, the bioavailable fraction of toxic constituent(s) that reaches systemic circulation after interactions with biological processes of absorption, distribution, metabolism and excretion, and with other interfering constituents of the same or other plant ingredients of a preparation and finally the herb–drug, herb–herb and herb–food interactions. Thus, the resultant toxicity/safety depends upon various parameters leading from the net effect of the cocktail of phytochemicals, including concentration of inherited toxicant and other intrusive parameters.

9.5 COMPLEXITY AND LIMITATION IN THE ASSESSMENT OF SAFETY OF MEDICINAL PLANTS

Unlike the synthetic drugs that represent a single pure chemical entity, a plant drug is a complex mixture of wide variety of primary and secondary plant metabolites. These secondary metabolites, categorised under several phytochemical classes such as alkaloids, flavonoids, glycosides, terpenoids, tannins, steroids, saponins, alkamides, lignans, lectins, polypeptides and non-protein amino acids are often associated with biological activities and sometimes may also be associated with toxicities in living beings, including humans. However, this inherent property of some of the chemicals (e.g. pyrrolizidine group of alkaloids, cyanogenetic and mustard glycosides, phytoestrogens like coumestrol, etc.) that produce toxicity often varies from plant to plant and also in different parts of the same plant depending upon the concentration present.

Different animal species have different susceptibilities to toxic phytoconstituents. The phyto-constituents that exhibit toxicity in one animal species may not necessarily replicate the same effects in other animal species or human being; due to changes in ADME parameters of different species. For example, *Atropa belladonna*, which causes severe poisoning in humans, is often consumed by cattle and rabbits without causing any symptoms of poisoning in them (Lee 2007). The toxic doses of some plants are estimated to be 20 times higher for sheep than those that kill cattle (Stegelmeier 2011).

General toxicity studies undertaken on a plant often represents contradictory or equivocal results, thereby making it difficult to draw any conclusion based on the diverse results reported. This may occur because of involvement of a multitude of confounding factors such as use of different species of animals, different parts of the plant, geographical location, time and season of collection of plant material, soil characteristics, pathogenicity or growth status of plant (young or old), processing and storage of the collected plant material, contaminants such as pathogenic microbes, aflatoxins, heavy metal and pesticide residues, methods and solvents used for preparation of the extract etc. There may also be a scenario where results of such studies are either under- or overexpressed.

Furthermore, in some plant species the poisonous constituent(s) occur throughout the plant, whereas in others, these may be present in one part of the plant and also may vary in another part of the plant. The varying concentrations present in the different plant materials also result in varying biological effects when administered in living beings. However, it is finally the bioavailable concentration of the phytochemical(s) in living beings that determines the overall effects. Standardised extracts offer the added advantage of definite levels of certain key constituents and most of the toxicity reported for herbal preparations is either because it is not a standardised preparation or because it has a different type of phytochemicals, thus making it difficult to correlate the data of therapeutic studies with the toxicological dose of a plant. This results in variation of dose for toxicity, which is often the case. Additionally, a toxic signal generated in conventional toxicity studies in animal species does not necessarily result in toxicity in humans, since the dose used in the toxicity studies is at least 5–10 times higher than the therapeutic dose.

Another difficulty arises due to numerous types of phytoconstituents present in a plant, which usually interfere and influence each other pharmacodynamically and/or pharmacokinetically in a positive or negative manner. Thus the mere presence of a toxic compound, even in toxicologically significant amounts, may not always have similar profiles of efficacy and safety as it has in the whole plant material/crude extract. For example the toxic effects of safranal are reduced when an equivalent amount of safranal is administered through whole extract of saffron (Ziaee et al. 2014) and the reduction of toxic effects of reserpine due to the presence of ajmaline and rescinnamine in the *Rauvolfia* root extract has been noted (Chopra et al. 1948). The situation becomes more complex when two or more plants are mixed together (polyherbal preparations) and the cocktail often results in a pool of chemicals, so the resultant effect cannot be attributed to any particular ingredient.

Herbal medicines are sometimes adulterated with modern drugs like corticosteroids, NSAID and others. Patients taking these illicit medicines are at risk of severe adverse effects, including potentially fatal complications (Niggemann and Grüber 2003; Chong et al. 2015). Thus to determine safety and whether to label any medicinal plants to be toxic or safe is a complex scenario.

9.6 MEDICINAL PLANTS AND PREGNANCY

The use of medicinal plants preparations/herbal medicines during pregnancy should be given utter importance and this significant issue should not be forbidden at all. The traditional practice of using herbal medicines in pregnancy has certain historical limitations. Most of classical preparations utilise medicinal plants in limited amount and in combination with many other herbs. In these preparations, individual plants may have little or negligible adverse impact; however the scenario would be different if these are used individually or in higher quantity. Evidence exists on the abortifacient effects of herbs/medicinal plants in animals. Some commonly used medicinal plants like *Acacia catechu* (Linn. f.) Willd. (Giri et al. 1987); *Azadirachta indica* A. Juss. (Talwar et al. 1997; Mukherjee et al. 1999); *Cuminum cyminum* Linn. (Al-Khamis et al. 1988); *Cyperus rotundus* Linn. (Muzaffer et al. 1982); *Gloriosa superba* Linn. (Tewari et al. 1972; Malpani et al. 2011); *Justicia adhatoda* Linn. (Sethi et al. 1987); *Plumbago zeylanica* Linn. (Devarshi et al.1991; Gupta et al. 2011); *Salacia reticulata* Wight (Ratnasooriya et al. 2003); *Terminalia arjuna* (Roxb.) Wight & Arn. (Yadav et al. 1980; Gupta et al. 1989) have shown abortifacient effects in experimental animals. Therefore, the prescriber of medicinal plants needs to be cautious while prescribing such herbs in pregnancy.

9.7 HERB–DRUG INTERACTIONS

With the increasing concurrent usage of herbal medicines with modern drugs over the last few decades, many cases of potential herb-drugs interactions have been reported among their users. The true prevalence of herb–drug interactions is although unknown; however the reported figures are far below to realistic one. This could be a result of many reasons, including under-reporting, unidentified cases, or not understood by treating physicians, or patients often do not report the use of the other system of medicine to their treating physicians. The situation gets further complicated among users of traditional formulations, which often contain more than one ingredient, resulting in difficulty in establishing a direct correlation to the interacting ingredient. These interactions occur at two different levels, one being the pharmacodynamic type, which interferes with the bioactivity of the drug in synergistic or antagonistic ways, and the other being the pharmacokinetic type, which alters the blood levels of the interacting drugs by interfering at the levels of ADME (absorption, distribution, metabolism and excretion). Examples of potential pharmacodynamic type herb–drug interactions that have been reported with some commonly used medicinal plants in humans are listed in Table 9.2.

9.8 SUMMARY

The increasing usage of herbal and traditional medicines in the recent past, also increases the risks of their impending adverse effects. The general perception or advocates of traditional medicines to consider these safe is not realistic and would be irrational in light of available information. No medicine is thought to be spared of adverse effects, and a drug devoid of any adverse effect is also usually devoid of desired main effect. Growing scientific evidence indicates that herbal medicines/medicinal plants are also not spared of adverse effects and these may also have potential to induce adverse effects ranging from negligible discomfort to severe and life-threatening events. In recent years, numerous case reports and some controlled studies have been published on the adverse effects of herbal medicines. Certainly, some adverse events seen with the use of herbal medicines may not have a definite relation to the herbal medicines, but these cannot be ignored in absence of any other possible cause. Cases of organ toxicities to liver, kidneys and heart have also been reported associated with the use of various herbal preparations. Cases of toxic hepatitis reported with the intake of rhizome of *Dioscorea bulbifera* Linn. (Liu 2002), whole herb of *Centella asiatica* (Linn.) Urb. (Jorge and Jorge 2005), leaf of *Gymnema sylvestre* (Retz.) R. Br. ex Sm. (Shiyovich et al. 2010) are a few such examples. Herbs may also cause potential mutagenicity in humans. For example *Gmelina arborea* Roxb. leaf showed genotoxicity in mice (Sahu et al. 2010). Further general consideration of medicinal plants as safe may also impact outcomes in pregnancy. Special precaution needs to be taken while prescribing medicinal plants during pregnancy, because many herbs possess abortifacient qualities or fetal toxicity and may even be contraindicated in pregnancy. Herbs like *Azadirachta indica* Linn., *Gloriosa superba* Linn., *Justicia adhatoda* Linn, and the bark of *Alstonia scholaris* (Linn.) R. Br. showed retardation of growth and congenital malformations in litters of pregnant mice (Jagetia and Baliga 2003).

TABLE 9.2

Pharmacodynamic Herb–Drug Interactions of Commonly Used Medicinal Plants Reported in Humans

Plant Name (Part)	Interacting Modern Drug	Effect of Interaction	References
Allium sativum Linn. (clove)	Warfarin	Decreased platelet aggregation and increased risk of bleeding	Peng et al. (2004)
Azadirachta indica A. Juss. (leaf)	Insulin and other antidiabetic drugs	Reduction in dose of insulin and other oral antidiabetic drugs	Bhargava (1986, (1987); Shukla et al. (1973)
Glycyrrhiza glabra Linn. (rhizome)	Nitrofurantion	Reduction in the nitrofurantoin induced gastrointestinal adverse effects	Lahri et al. (1980); Datla et al. (1981)
Momordica charantia Linn. (fruit)	Metformin and glibenclamide	Synergistic blood glucose lowering effect of metformin and glibenclamide in type 2 diabetic patients	Tongia et al. (2004)
	Chlorpropamide	Reduction in dose of chlorpropamide and glycosuria in a diabetic female after eating curry made up of fruit for several days	Aslam and Stockley (1979)
Sesamum indicum Linn. (seed and seed oil)	Nifedipine	Significant enhancement of antihypertensive effect of nifedipine and reduction in its dosage requirement after dietary substitution of edible oil by sesame oil in hypertensive patients	Sankar et al. (2004a, 2004b)
Tinospora cordifolia (Willd.) Miers (stem/aerial parts)	Choloroquine	Additive antimalarial effect of chloroquine through accelerated subsidence of haemolytic state, marked reduction in spleen size and serum IgM levels with increase in haemoglobin levels of malaria patients	Singh (2005)
Trigonella foenum-graecum Linn. (seed)	Sulphonylureas	Additional reduction of blood glucose of type 2 diabetic patients	Lu et al. (2008)
	Insulin	Significant reduction in the requirement of insulin by type 1 diabetic patients	Sharma (1986)
Zingiber officinale Roscoe (rhizome)	Nifedipine	Synergistic platelet antiaggregation effect with nifedipine in both normal volunteers and hypertensive patients	Young et al. (2006)

Contact allergy, dermatitis type reactions and respiratory allergy/fibrotic lung diseases may also reported to occur among handlers of medicinal plants, and their sensitising capacity may even lead to IgE-mediated clinical symptoms (Gomes et al. 2010).

Herb–drug interactions, the prevalence of which although is exactly not known, however this may also be increasing with the increasing concurrent use of herbal products with modern drugs over the last few decades. Many herbs have been reported to significantly influence the pharmacodynamics or pharmacokinetics of modern drugs when used together.

Adulteration of herbal medicines with steroids and other modern drugs is also an important issue and must also be look at seriously, as it may potentially cause adverse effects that are not known and related the plant, and may lead to unknown herb–drug interactions among their users.

Thus, the pattern of adverse effects with medicinal plants is no different to what has been observed with modern drugs. Finally, one has to be judicious while labelling any medicinal plant safe or toxic, because it has many complexities and various scenarios that need to be looked into from all angles – including the source of the material used, processing and preparation methods and the clinical indications and general health of the user in order to minimize the adverse health effects.

REFERENCES

Agarwal, R., Sulaiman, S. A. and Mohamed, M. (2005). Open label clinical trial to study adverse effects and tolerance to dry powder of the aerial part of *Andrographis paniculata* in patients with type 2 diabetes mellitus. *Malaysian Journal of Medical Sciences,* **12**, 13–19.

Akhondzadeh, S., Sabet, M. S., Harirchian, M. H. et al. (2010). A 22-week, multicenter, randomized, double-blind controlled trial of *Crocus sativus* in the treatment of mild-to-moderate Alzheimer's disease. *Psychopharmacology,* **207**, 637–643.

Akhondzadeh, S., Tahmacebi-Pour, N., Noorbala, A. A. et al. (2005). *Crocus sativus* L. in the treatment of mild to moderate depression: A double-blind, randomized and placebo-controlled trial. *Phytotherapy Research,* **19**, 148–151.

Al-Khamis, K. I., Al-Said, M. A., Islam, M. W., Tariq, M., Parmar, N. S. and Ageel, A. M. (1988). Antifertility, anti-implantation and abortifacient activity of the aqueous extract of *Cuminum Cyminum*: *Fitoterapia,* **59**, 5–9.

Altschuler, J. A., Casella, S. J., Mackenzie, T. A. and Kurtis, K. M. (2007). The effect of cinnamon on A1c among adolescents with type 1 diabetes. *Diabetes Care,* **30**, 813–816.

Anonymous. (1995). An alternative medicine treatment for Parkinson's disease: Results of a multicenter clinical trial. HP-200 in Parkinson's Disease Study Group. *Journal of Alternative and Complementary Medicine,* **1**, 249–255.

Appa Rao, M. V. R., Usha, S. P., Rajagopalan, S. S. and Sarangan, R. (1967). Six month's result of double blind clinical trial to study effect of Mandookparni and Punarnava on normal adults. *Journal of Research in Indian Medicine,* **2**, 79.

Appelboom, T. and Mélot, C. (2013). Flexofytol, a purified curcumin extract, in fibromyalgia and gout: A retrospective study. *Open Journal of Rheumatology and Autoimmune Disease,* **3**, 104–107.

Appelboom, T., Maes, N. and Albert, A. (2014). A new curcuma extract (Flexofytol®) in osteoarthritis: Results from a Belgian real-life experience. *Open Rheumatology Journal,* **8**, 77–81.

Arase, Y., Ikeda, K., Murashima, N. et al. (1997). Long-term efficacy of glycyrrhizin in chronic hepatitis C patients. *Cancer,* **79**, 1494–1500.

Arora, R. B. 1965. *Nardostachys jatamansi,* a chemical, pharmacological and clinical appraisal, Special Report Series. *Indian Council of Medical Research,* **51**, 1–77.

Arora, R. B., Sharma, J. N. and Shastri, H. (1982). Beneficial effect of fraction A of gum-guggul in arthritic syndrome and liver function in clinical and experimental arthritis. *Rheumatism,* **18**, 9–16.

Aslam, M. and Stockley, I. H. (1979). Interaction between curry ingredient (Karela) and drug (chlorpropamide). *Lancet,* **1**(8116), 607.

Balakrishnan, V., Pillai, N. R. and Santhakumari, G. (1986). Ventricular fibrillation and cardiac arrest due to neem leaf poisoning. *Journal of the Association of Physicians of India,* **34**, 536.

Bambhole, V. D. and Jiddewar, G. G. (1984). Evaluation of *Cyperus rotundus* in the management of obesity and high blood pressure of human subjects. *Nagarjun,* **27**(5), 110–113.

Barkatullah, M., Siddiqui, M. H. and Hakim, M. H. (1997). Clinical evaluation of *Laooq-e-khiyar* shamber in *Zeequn-nafas shobi* (bronchial asthma). *Hamdard Medicus,* **40**(1), 98–101.

Beg, M., Afzaal, S. and Akhter, N. (1998). Hypolipidaemic and cardioprotective effectiveness of Gugulip in nephrotic syndrome. *Indian Medical Gazette,* **132**(2), 35–38.

Bhargava, A. K. (1986). A note on the use of neem oil (*Azadirachta indica*) as antihyperglycaemic agent in human volunteers of secondary diabetes. *Journal of Veterinary Medicine and Allied Science,* **5**, 45–48.

Bhargava, A. K. (1987). Neem oil as a synergist to antidiabetic drugs for management of secondary hyperglycemia. *Neem Newsletter,* **4**(3), 31–32.

Bhaskar, M. V., Pramod, S. J., Jeevika, M. V., Chandan, P. K. and Shetteppa, G. (2010). MR imaging findings of neem oil poisioning. *American Journal of Neuroradiology,* **31**, E60–E61.

Bhatia, B. B. (1942). On the use of *Rauwolfia serpentina* in high blood pressure. *Journal of the Indian Medical Association,* **11**, 262–268.

Bordia, A. (1981). Effect of garlic on blood lipid in patients with coronary heart disease. *The American Journal of Clinical Nutrition,* **34**, 2100–2103.

Bosse, J. P., Papillon, J., Frenette, G., Dansereau, J., Cardotte, M. and Le Lorier, J. (1979). Clinical study of a new antikeloid agent. *Annals of Plastic Surgery,* **3**, 13–21.

Calabrese, C., Berman, S. H., Babish, J. G. et al. (2000). A phase I trial of andrographolide in HIV positive patients and normal volunteers. *Phytotherapy Research,* **14**, 333–338.

Calabrese, C., Gregory, W. L., Leo, M., Kramer, D., Bone, K. and Oken, B. (2008). Effects of a standardized *Bacopa monnieri* extract on cognitive performance anxiety and depression in the elderly a random- ized, double-blind, placebo-controlled trial. *Journal of Alternative and Complementary Medicine*, **14**, 707–713.

Caradonna, P., Gentiloni, N., Servidei, S., Perrone, G. A., Greco, A. V. and Russo, M. A. (1992). Acute myop- athy associated with chronic licorice ingestion reversible loss of myoadenylate deaminase activity. *Ultrastructural Pathology*, **169**, 529–535.

Chan, W. Y., Tam, P. P. and Yeung, H. W. (1984). The termination of early pregnancy in the mouse by beta- momorcharin. *Contraception*, **29**, 91–100.

Chandrasekaran, A. N., Porkodi, R., Radhamadhavan, Parthiban, M. and Bhatt, N. S. (1994). Study of Ayurvedic drugs in rheumatoid arthritis: Comparison with auranofin. *Indian Practitioner*, **57**, 489–502.

Chandrasekhar, K., Kapoor, J. and Anishetty, S. (2012). A prospective, randomized double-blind, placebo- controlled study of safety and efficacy of a high concentration full-spectrum extract of Ashwagandha root in reducing stress and anxiety in adults. *Indian Journal of Psychological Medicine*, **34**, 255–262.

Chang, S. L., Chang, Y. C., Yang, C. H. and Hong, H. S. (2005). Allergic contact dermatitis to *Plectranthus amboinicus* masquerading as chronic leg ulcer. *Contact Dermatitis*, **53**, 356–357.

Chaturvedi, G. N. and Singh, K. P. (1983). Side effects of a traditional indigenous drug-kutaja (*Holarrhena antidysenterica*). *Indian Journal of Physiology and Pharmacology*, **27**, 255–256.

Chaturvedi, G. N. and Singh, R. H. (1966). Jaundice of infectious hepatitis and its treatment with an indig- enous drug, *Picrorhiza kurroa*. *Indian Journal of Medical Research*, **1**, 1–13.

Chong, Y. K., Ching, C. K., Ng, S. W. and Mak, T. W. (2015). Corticosteroid adulteration in proprietary Chinese medicines: A recurring problem. *Hong Kong Medical Journal*, **21**, 411–416.

Chopra, R. N., Bose, B. C., Gupta, J. C. and Chopra, I. C. (1948). Alkaloids of *Rauwolfia serpentina*: A com- parative study of their pharmacological action and their role in experimental hypertension. *Indian Journal of Medical Research*, **30**, 319–324.

Conn, J. W., Rovner, D. R. and Cohen, E. L. (1968). Licorice-induced pseudoaldosteronism. *JAMA*, **205**, 492–496.

Crawford, L. and Kocan, R. M. (1993). Steroidal alkaloid toxicity to fish embryos. *Toxicology Letters*, **66**(2), 175–181.

Crawford, P. (2009). Effectiveness of cinnamon for lowering hemoglobin A1C in patients with type 2 diabetes: A randomized, controlled trial. *Journal of the American Board of Family Medicine*, **22**, 507–512.

Daniş, R., Ruhi, Ç., Berketoğlu, N., Kaya, A. V., Yilmazer, B. and Kaya, S. (2015). Licorice ingestion: An unusual cause of rhabdomyolysis and acute renal failure. *Turkish Nephrology, Dialysis and Transplantation Journal*, **24**, 106–109.

Datla, R., Rao, S. R. and Murthy, K. J. R. (1981). Excretion studies of nitrofurantoin and nitrofurantoin with declycyrrhizinated liquorice. *Indian Journal of Physiology and Pharmacology*, **25**, 59–63.

Dave, U. P., Wasim, P., Joshua, J. A., et al. (2008). BacoMind®: A cognitive enhancer in children requiring individual's education programme. *Journal of Pharmacology and Toxicology*, **3**, 302–310.

Devarshi, P., Patil, S. and Kanase, A. (1991). Effect of *Plumbago zeylanica* root powder induced preimplan- tationary loss and abortion on uterine luminal proteins in albino rats. *Indian Journal of Experimental Bioliogy*, **29**, 521–522.

Dhawan, B. N., Dubey, M. P., Mehrotra, B. N., Rastogi, R. P. and Tandon, J. S. (1980). Screening of Indian plants for biological activity: Part IX. *Indian Journal of Experimental Bioliogy*, **18**, 594–606.

Dhongade, R. K., Kavade, S. G. and Damle, R. S. (2008). Neem oil poisioning. *Indian Paediatrics*, **45**, 56–57.

Di Pierro, F., Putignano, P., Villanova, N., Montesi, L., Moscatiello, S. and Marchesini, G. (2013). Preliminary study about the possible glycemic clinical advantage in using a fixed combination of *Berberis aristata* and *Silybum marianum* standardized extracts versus only *Berberis aristata* in patients with type 2 dia- betes. *Clinical Pharmacology: Advances and Applications*, **5**, 167–174.

Dixit, R., Joshi, V. K. and Reddy, K. V. V. B. (2009). Arjuna kshirapaka in hridroga (heart disease). *Journal of Research in Ayurveda and Siddha*, **30**(2), 1–10.

Doshi, V. B., Shetye, V. M., Mahashur, A. A. and Kamat, S. R. (1983). *Picrorrhiza kurroa* in bronchial asthma. *Journal of Postgraduate Medicine*, **29**, 89–95.

Dube, C. B., Kumar, D. and Srivastav, P. S. (1982). A trial of Bhringaraja Ghanasatwavati on the patients of Kostha-Shakhasrita kamala. *Journal of the National Integrated Medical Association*, **24**, 265–269.

Eberhart, L. H., Mayer, R., Betz, O. et al. (2003). Ginger does not prevent postoperative nausea and vomiting after laparoscopic surgery. *Anesthesia & Analgesia*, **96**, 995–998.

Engqvist, A., von Feilitzen, F., Pyk, E. and Reichard, H. (1973). Double-blind trial of deglycyrrhizinated liquorice in gastric ulcer. *Gut*, **14**, 711–715.

Fahimi, F., Khodadad, K., Amini, S., Naghibi, F., Salamzadeh, J. and Baniasadi, S. (2011). Evaluating the effect of *Zingiber officinalis* on nausea and vomiting in patients receiving cisplatin based regimens. *Iranian Journal of Pharmaceutical Research*, **10**, 379–384.

Fischer, J. and Dethlefsen, U. (2013). Efficacy of cineole in patients suffering from acute bronchitis: A placebo-controlled double-blind trial. *Cough*, **9**(1), Article No. 25.

Forrest, J. F. and Heacock, R. A. (1972). Nutmeg and Mace, the psychotropic spices from *Myristica fragrans*. *Lloydia*, **35**, 440–449.

Forster, G. and Holzmman, M. (1966). Zur ajmaline terapic von herzhythmusstorugen. *J Suisse Med*, **97**, 185.

Gardner, C. D., Lawson, L. D., Block, E., et al. (2007). Effect of raw garlic versus commercial garlic supplements on plasma lipid concentrations in adults with moderate hypercholesterolemia. *Archives of Internal Medicine*, **167**, 346–353.

Gerhardt, H., Seifert, F., Buvari, P., Vogelsang, H. and Repges, R. Z. (2001). Therapy of active Crohn disease with *Boswellia serrata* extract H 15. *Zeitschrift für Gastroenterologie*, **39**, 11–17.

Giri, A. K., Banerjee, J. S., Talukdar, G. and Sharma, A. (1987). Induction of sister chromatid exchange and dominant lethal mutation by 'Katha' (catechu) in male mice. *Cancer Letters*, **36**, 189–196.

Gomes, J., Pereira, T., Vilarinho, C., Duarte Mda, L. and Brito, C. (2010). Contact dermatitis due to *Centella asiatica*. *Contact Dermatitis*, **62**, 54–55.

Gulati, O. D., Shah, C. P., Kanani, R. C., Pandya, D. C. and Shah, D. S. (1982). Clinical trial of *Tinospora cordifolia* in rheumatoid arthritis. *Rheumatism*, **17**, 143–148.

Gupta, D. N., Keshri, G., Lakshmi, V. and Kapil, R. S. (1989). Post coital contraceptive efficacy of *Terminalia arjuna* in albino rats. *Fitoterapia*, **60**, 275–276.

Gupta, I., Gupta, V., Parihar, A., et al. (1998). Effects of *Boswellia serrata* gum resin in patients with bronchial asthma: Result of a double-blind, placebo-controlled, 6 week clinical study. *European Journal of Medical Research*, **3**, 511–514.

Gupta, S., Ahirwar, D., Sharma, N. K., Jhade, D. and Ahirwar, B. (2011). Effect of plumbagin free alcohol extract of *Plumbago zeylanica* Linn. root on reproductive system of female Wistar rat. *Asian Pacific Journal of Tropical Medicine*, **4**, 978–984.

Habibullah, C. M., Chandra, V., Padmanabham, C. and Datla, R. (1979). A double blind trial of deglycyrrhizinated liquorice in peptic ulcer. *Indian Practioner*, **32**, 119–122.

Hallström, H. and Thuvander, A. (1997). Toxicological evaluation of myristicin. *Natural Toxins*, **5**, 186–192.

Heikens, J., Fliers, E., Endert, E., Ackermans, M. and Van-Montfrans, G. (1995). Liquorice-induced hypertension- a new understanding of an old disease: Case report and brief review. *The Netherlands Journal of Medicine*, **47**, 230–234.

Henrotin, Y., Priom, F. and Mobasheri, A. (2013). Curcumin: A new paradigm and therapeutic opportunity for the treatment of osteoarthritis – Curcumin for osteoarthritis management. *Springerplus*, **2**, Article No. 56.

Ide, N., Suzuki, A., Suzuki, E. and Gotou, S. (2010). Case of colchicine intoxication caused by tubers of *Gloriosa superba*. *Chudoku Kenkyu*, **23**, 243–245.

Isaia, G. C., Pellissetto, C., Ravazzoli, M. and Tamone, C. (2008). Acute adrenal crisis and hypercalcemia in a patient assuming high liquorice doses. *Minerva Medica*, **99**, 91–94.

Jagetia, G. C. and Baliga, M. S. (2003). Induction of developmental toxicity in mice treated with *Alstonia scholaris* (Sapthaparni) *in utero*. *Birth defects research. Part B, Developmental and Reproductive Toxicology*, **68**, 472–478.

Jain, J. P., Bhatnagar, L. S and Parsai, M. R. (1979). Clinical trials of Haridra (*Curcuma longa*) in cases of Tamak *Sawasa* and *kasa*. *Journal of Research in Indian Medicine, Yoga and Homoeopathy*, **14**(2), 110–120.

Jorge, O. A. and Jorge, A. D. (2005). Hepatotoxicity associated with the ingestion of *Centella asiatica*. *Revista Española de Enfermedades Digestivas*, **97**, 115–124.

Joshi, J., Ghaisas, S., Vaidya, A. et al. (2003). Early human safety study of turmeric oil (*Curcuma longa* oil) administered orally in healthy volunteers. *Journal of the Association of Physicians of India*, **5**, 1055–1060.

Kalava, A., Darji, S. J., Kalstein, A., Yarmush, J. M., Schianodicala, J. and Weinberg, J. (2013). Efficacy of ginger on intraoperative and postoperative nausea and vomiting in elective cesarean section patients. *European Journal of Obstetrics, Gynecology and Reproductive Biology*, **169**, 184–188.

Kalbhen, D. A. (1971). Nutmeg as a narcotic. A contribution to the chemistry and pharmacology of nutmeg (*Myristica fragrans*). *Angewandte Chemie International Edition in English*, **10**, 370–374.

Kalikar, M. V., Thawani, V. R., Varadpande, U. K., Sontakke, S. D., Singh, R. P. and Khiyani, R. K. (2008). Immunomodulatory effect of *Tinospora cordifolia* extract in human immune deficiency virus positive patients. *Indian Journal of Pharmacology*, **40**, 107–110.

Katzenschlager, R., Evans, A., Manson, A. et al. (2004). *Mucuna pruriens* in Parkinson's disease: A double blind clinical and pharmacological study. *Journal of Neurology, Neurosurgery, and Psychiatry*, **75**, 1672–1677.

Kaur, M. and Chandola, H. M. (2010). Role of Rasayana in cure and prevention of recurrence of Vicharchika (Eczema). *Ayu*, **31**, 33–39.

Kehrl, W., Sonnemann, U. and Dethlefsen, U. (2004). Therapy for acute nonpurulant rhinosinusitis with cineole: Results of a double-blind, randomized, placebo-controlled trial. *Laryngoscope*, **114**, 738–742.

Kelly, K. J., Neu, J., Camitta, B. M. and Honig, G. R.(1984)). Methemoglobinemia in an infant treated with the folk remedy glycerited asafoetida. *Pediatrics*, **73**, 717–719.

Kim, S. W., Ha, K. C., Choi, E. K. et al. (2013). The effectiveness of fermented turmeric powder in subjects with elevated alanine transaminase levels: A randomized controlled study. *BMC Complementary and Alternative Medicine*, **13**, Article No. 58.

Kimmatkar, N., Thawani, V., Hingorani, L. and Khiyani, R. (2003). Efficacy and tolerability of *Boswellia serrata* extract in treatment of osteoarthritis of knee- A randomized double blind placebo controlled trial. *Phytomedicine*, **10**, 3–7.

Kuptniratsaikul, V., Thanakhumtorn, S., Chinswangwatanakul, P., Wattanamong Konsil, L. and Thamlikitkul, V. (2009). Efficacy and safety of *Curcuma domestica* extracts in patients with knee osteoarthritis. *Journal of Alternative and Complementary Medicine*, **15**, 891–897.

Lahri, K., Raju, D. S. N. and Rao, P. R. (1980). Influence of deglycyrrhizinated liquorice on the bioavalability of nitrofurantoin. *Eastern Pharmacist*, **23**, 191–193.

Lai, S. M., Lim, K. W. and Cheng, H. K. (1990). Margosa oil poisioning as a cause of toxic encephalopathy. *Singapore Medical Journal*, **31**, 463–465.

Lavier, G., Crosnier, R. and Merle, F. (1948). Traitment de l'amibiase par La conessine. *Bulletin de la Société de Pathologie Exotique*, **41**, 548–553.

Lee, M. R. (2007). Solanaceae IV: Atropa belladonna, deadly nightshade. *Journal of the Royal College of Physicians of Edinburgh*, **37**(1), 77–84.

Liu, J. R. (2002). Two cases of toxic hepatitis caused by *Dioscorea bulbifera* L. *Adverse Drug Reactions*, **2**, 129–130.

Livesay, W. R., Moyer, J. H. and Miller, S. I. (1954). Treatment of hypertension with *Rauwolfia serpentina* alone and combined with other drugs: Results in eighty-four cases. *JAMA*, **155**, 1027–1035.

Locket, S. (1955). Oral preparations of *Rauwolfia serpentina* in treatment of essential hypertension. *BMJ*, **1**(4917), 809–813.

Lu, F. R., Shen, L., Qin, Y., Gao, L, Li, H. and Dai, Y. (2008). Clinical observation on *Trigonella foenumgraecum* L. total saponins in combination with sulfonylureas in the treatment of type 2 diabetes mellitus. *Chinese Journal of Integrated Medicine*, **14**, 56–60.

Madisch, A., Miehlke, S., Eichele, O. et al. (2007). *Boswellia serrata* extract for the treatment of collagenous colitis: A double-blind, randomized, placebo-controlled, multicenter trial. *International Journal of Colorectal Disease*, **22**, 1445–1451.

Malhotra, S. C. and Ahuja, M. M. S. (1971). Comparative hypolipidaemic effectiveness of gum guggulu (*Commiphora mukul*) fraction 'A', ethyl-p-chlorophenoxyisobutyrate and Ciba-13437-Su. *Indian Journal of Medical Research*, **59**, 1621–1632.

Malhotra, S. C., Ahuja, M. M. S. and Sundaram, K. R. (1977). Long-term clinical studies on the hypolipidemic effects of *Commiphora mukul* (guggulu) and clofibrate *Indian Journal of Medical Research*, **65**, 390–395.

Malpani, A. A., Aswar, U. M., Kushwaha, S. K., Zambare, G. N. and Bodhankar, S. L. (2011). Effect of the aqueous extract of *Gloriosa superba* Linn. (Langli) roots on reproductive system and cardiovascular parameters in female rats. *Tropical Journal of Pharmaceutical Research*, **10**, 169–176.

Manns, M. P., Wedemeyer, H., Singer, A. et al. (2012). Glycyrrhizin in patients who failed previous interferon alpha-based therapies: Biochemical and histological effects after 52 weeks. *Journal of Viral Hepatitis*, **19**, 537–546.

Marastoni, F., Baldo, A., Redaelli, G. and Ghiringhelli, L. (1982). *Centella asiatica* extract in venous pathology of the lower limbs and its evaluation as compared with tribenoside. *Minerva Cardioangiologica*, **30**, 201–207.

Mathern, J. R., Raatz, S. K., Thomas, W. and Slavin, J. L. (2009). Effect of fenugreek fiber on satiety, blood glucose, insulin response and energy intake in obese subjects. *Phytotherapy Research*, **23**, 1543–1548.

Mishra, A. and Dave, N. (2013). Neem oil poisoning: Case report of an adult with toxic encephalopathy. *Indian Journal of Critical Care Medicine*, **17**, 321–322.

Morgan, A. and Stevens, J. (2010). Does *Bacopa monnieri* improve memory performance in older persons? Results of a randomized, placebo-controlled, double-blind trial. *Journal of Alternative and Complementary Medicine*, **16**, 753–759.

Mukherjee, S., Garg, S. and Talwar, G. P. (1999). Early post implantation contraceptive effects of purified fraction of neem (*Azadirachta indica*) seeds, given orally in rats: Possible mechanism involved. *Journal of Ethnopharmacology*, **67**, 287–296.

Muzaffer, A., Pillai, N. R. and Purushothaman, K. K. (1982). Examination of biochemical parameter after administration of gangetin in female albino rats. *Journal of Reasearch in Ayurveda and Siddha*, **2**, 172–175.

Naik, B. S. (2009). Common milk hedge (*Euphorbia neriifolia*) juice ingestion: A clinical case report. *Journal of Indian Society of Toxicology*, **5**(2), 61–62.

Nanda, G. C., Tekari, N. S. and Kishore, P. (1993). Clinical evaluation of shunthi (*Zingiber officinale*) in the treatment of Grhaniroga. *J Res Indian Med Yoga Homoeop*, **14**(1–2), 34–44.

Niggemann, B. and Grüber, C. (2003). Side-effects of complementary and alternative medicine. *Allergy*, **58**, 707–716.

Nohr, L. A., Rasmussen, L. B. and Strand, J. (2009). Resin from the mukul myrrh tree, guggul, can it be used for treating hypercholesterolemia? A randomized, controlled study. *Complementary Therapies in Medicine*, **17**, 16–22.

Noorbala, A. A., Akhondzadeh, S., Tahmacebi-Pour, N. and Jamshidi, A. H. (2005). Hydro-alcoholic extract of *Crocus sativus* L. versus fluoxetine in the treatment of mild to moderate depression: A double-blind, randomized pilot trial. *Journal of Ethnopharmacology*, **97**, 281–284.

Pal, A., Sharma, P. P. and Mukherjee, P. K. (2009). A clinical study of kutaja (*Holarrhena antidysenterica* Wall.) on Shoni tarsha. *AYU*, **30**, 369–372.

Pandit, M. M. and Shukla, C. P. (1981). A study of shuddha guggulu on rheumatoid arthritis. *Rheumatism*, **16**, 54–67.

Peng, C. C., Glassman, P. A., Trilli, L. E., Hayes-Hunter, J. and Good, C. B. (2004). Incidence and severity of potential drug-dietary-supplement interactions in primary care patients: An exploratory study of 2 outpatient practices. *Archives of Internal Medicine*, **164**, 630–36.

Peranantham, S., Manigandan, G. and Shanmugam, K. (2014). Fatal *Gloriosa superba* poisoning: A case report. *International Journal of Medicine and Pharmaceutical Science*, **4**(10), 21–24.

Phillips, S., Ruggier, R. and Hutchinson, S. E. (1993). *Zingiber officinale* (ginger): An antiemetic for day case surgery. *Anaesthesia*, **48**, 715–717.

Pointel, J. P., Boccalon, H., Clorec, M., Ledevehat, C. and Joubert, M. (1987). Titrated extract of *Centella asiatica* (TECA) in the treatment of venous in sufficiency of the lower limbs. *Angiology*, **38**, 46–50.

Poole, C., Bushey, B., Foster, C., et al. (2010). The effect of a commercially available botanical supplement on strength, body composition, power output, and hormonal profiles in resistance trained males. *Journal of the International Society of Sports Nutrition*, **7**, Article No. 34.

Prasanna, M. (2000). Hypolipidemic effect of fenugreek: A clinical study. *Indian Journal of Pharmacology*, **32**, 34–36.

PVAMC (Participating Veterans Administration Medical Centers). (1982). Low doses v standard dose of reserpine. A randomized, double-blind, multiclinic trial in patients taking chlorthalidone. *JAMA*, **248**, 2471–2477.

Raghav, S., Singh, H., Dalal, P. K., Srivastava, J. S. and Asthana, O. P. (2006). Randomized controlled trial of standardized *Bacopa monnieri* extract in age-associated memory impairment. *Indian Journal of Psychiatry*, **4**, 238–242.

Rajaram, D. (1975). A preliminary clinical trial of *Picrorhiza kurroa* in bronchial asthma. *Indian Journal of Pharmacology*, **7**, 95–96.

Ratnasooriya, W. D., Jayakody, J. R. A. C. and Premakumara, G. A. S. (2003). Adverse pregnancy outcome in rats following exposure to a *Salacia reticulata* (Celastraceae) root extract. *Brazilian Journal of Medical and Biological Research*, **36**, 931–935.

Raut, A. A., Rege, N. N., Tadvi, F. M., Solanki, P. V., Kene, K. R., Shirolkar, S. G., Pandey, S. N., Vaidya, R. A. and Vaidya, A. B. (2012). Evaluation of safety, tolerability and activity of Ashwagandha (*Withania somnifera*) in healthy volunteers. *Journal of Ayurveda and Integrative Medicine*, **3**, 111–114.

Riebenfeld, D. and Borzone, L. (1999). Randomized double blind study comparing ginger (Zintona®) and dimehydrinate. *HealthNotes Review of Complementary and Integrative Medicine*, **6**, 98–101.

Ried, K., C. Toben and P. Fakler. (2013). Effect of garlic on serum lipids: An updated meta-analysis. *Nutrition Reviews*, **71**, 282–299.

Ryan, J. L., Heckler, C. E., Roscoe, J. A. et al. (2012). Ginger (*Zingiber officinale*) reduces acute chemotherapy-induced nausea: A URCC CCOP study of 576 patients. *Supportive Care in Cancer*, **20**, 1479–1489.

Sahu, R., Divakar, G. and Divakar, K. (2010). *In vivo* rodent micronucleus assay of *Gmelina arborea* Roxb. (gambhari) extract. *Journal of Advanced Pharmaceutical Technology & Research*, **1**(1), 22–29.

Sandborn, W. J., Targan, S. R., Byers, V. S. et al. (2013. *Andrographis paniculata* extract (HMPL-004) for active ulcerative colitis. *American Journal of Gastroenterology*, **108**, 90–98.

Sander, O., Herborn, G. and Rau, R. (1998). Is H15 (resin extract of *Boswellia serrata*, 'incence') a useful supplement to establish drug therapy of chronic polyarthritis? Result of a double-blind pilot study. *Zeitschrift für Rheumatologie*, **57**, 11–16.

Sankar, D., Sambandam, G., Rao, M. R. and Pugalendi, K. V. (2004a). P1176 sesame oil exhibits additive effect on nifedipine and modulates oxidative stress and electrolytes in hypertensive patients. *Journal of Pediatric Gastroenterology and Nutrition*, **39**, S504.

Sankar, D., Sambandam, G., Rao, M. R. and Pugalendi, K. V. (2004b). Impact of sesame oil on nifedipine in modulating oxidative stress and electrolytes in hypertensive patients. *Asia Pacific Journal of Clinical Nutrition*, **13**, S107.

Saxena, R. C., Singh, R., Kumar, P., et al. (2010). A randomized double-blind placebo-controlled clinical evaluation of extract of *Andrographis paniculata* (Kamcold) in patients with uncomplicated upper respiratory tract infection. *Phytomedicine*, **17**, 178–185.

Sengupta, K., Alluri, K. V., Satish, A. R. et al. (2008). A double blind, randomized, placebo controlled study of the efficacy and safety of 5-loxin® for treatment of osteoarthritis of knee. *Arthritis Research & Therapy*, **10**(4), R85.

Senthilkumaran, S., Balamurugan, N., Rajesh, N. and Thirumalaikolundu-Subramanian, P. (2011). Hard facts about loose stools: Massive alopecia in *Gloriosa superba* poisoning. *International Journal of Trichology*, **3**, 126–127.

Sethi, N., Nath, D., Shukla, S. C., Dayal, R. and Sinha, N. (1987). Abortifacient activity of a medicinal plant *Adhatoda vasica* in rats. *Arogya Journal of Health Sciences*, **13**, 99–101.

Sharma, J. N., Sharma, J. N., Shastri, H. D. and Arora, R. B. (1973). Beneficial effect of fraction A of gum guggulu in arthritis and liver functions-a clinical appraisal. *Rheumatism*, **8**, 21–53.

Sharma, R. D. (1986). Effect of fenugreek seeds and leaves on blood glucose and serum insulin responses in human subjects. *Nutrition Research*, **6**, 1353–1364.

Sharma, R. D., Sarkar, A., Hazara, D. K., et al. (1996). Hypolipidaemic effect of fenugreek seeds: A chronic study in non-insulin dependent diabetic patients. *Phytotherapy Research*, **10**, 332–334.

Sharma, R. D., Raghuram, T. C. and Rao, V. D. (1991). Hypolipidaemic effect of fenugreek seeds. A clinical study. *Phytotherapy Research*, **5**, 145–147.

Sharma, R. D., Raghuram, T. C. and Rao, N. S. (1990). Effect of fenugreek seeds on blood glucose and serum lipids in type 1 diabetes. *European Journal of Clinical Nutrition*, **44**, 301–306.

Shin, H. S., Choi, G., Lee, M. and Park, K. N. (1982). Clinical trials of madecassol (*Centella asiatica*) on gastrointestinal ulcer patients. *Korean Journal of Gastroenterology*, **14**, 49–56.

Shintani, S., Murase, H., Trukagoshi, H. and Shiigai, T. (1992). Glycyrrhizin (licorice)-induced hypokalemic myopathy. *European Neurology*, **32**, 44–51.

Shiyovich, A., Sztarkies, I. and Nesher, L. (2010). Toxic hepatitis induced by *Gymnema sylvestre*, a natural remedy for type 2 diabetes mellitus. *American Journal of Medical Sciences*, **340**, 514–517.

Shukla, R., Singh, S. and Bhandar, G. R. (1973). Preliminary clinical trial on antidiabetic action of *Azadirachta indica*. *Med Surg*, **13**, 11–12.

Singh, R. K. (2005). *Tinospora cordifolia* as an adjuvant drug in the treatment of hyper-reactive malarious splenomegaly—Case reports. *Journal of Vector Borne Diseases*, **42**, 36–38.

Sinniah, D. and Baskaran, G. (1981). Margosa oil poisoning as a cause of Reye's syndrome. *Lancet*, **317**(8218), 487–489.

Sinniah, D., Baskaran, G., Looi, L. M. and Leong, K. L.(1982). Reye like syndrome due to Margosa oil poisoning: Report of a case with postmortem findings. *American Journal of Gastroenterology*, **77**, 158.

Sivashanmugham, R., Bhaskar, N. and N. Banumathi, N. (1984). Ventricular fibrillation and cardiac arrest due to neem leaf poisioning. *Journal of the Association of Physicians of India*, **32**, 610–611.

Smith, W. M., Thurm, R. H. and Bromer, L. (1969). Comparative evaluation of *Rauwolfia* whole root and reserpine. *Clinical Pharmacology & Therapeutics*, **10**, 338–343.

Sontakke, S., Thawani, V., Pimpalkhute, S., Kabra, P., Babuhulkar, S. and Hingorani, L. (2007). Open, randomized, controlled clinical trial of *Boswellia serrata* extract as compared to valdecoxib in osteoarthritis of knee. *Indian Journal of Pharmacology*, **39**, 27–29.

Srivastava, B. N. and Datey, M. D. (1962). *Embelia ribes* as an anthelmintic for ascariasis. *Current Medical Practice*, **6**(2), 73–75.

Stegelmeier, B. L. (2011). Pyrrolizidine alkaloid: Containing toxic plants (*Senecio, Crotalaria, Cynoglossum, Amsinckia, Heliotropium*, and *Echium* spp.). *Veterinary Clinics of North America: Food Animal Practice*, **27**(2), 419–442.

Stough, C., Downey, L. A. and Lloyd, J. (2008). Examining the nootropic effects of a special extract of *Bacopa monniera* [sic] on human cognitive functioning: 90 day double-blind placebo- controlled randomized trial. *Phytotherapy Research*, **22**, 1629–1634.

Sundaravalli, N., Bhaskar, R. B. and Krishnamoorthy, K. A. (1982). Neem oil poisioning. *Indian Journal of Pediatrics*, **49**, 357–359.

Suresha, A. R., Rajesh, P., Anil Raj, K. S. and Torgal, R. (2014). A rare case of toxic optic neuropathy secondary to consumption of neem oil. *Indian Journal of Ophthalmology*, **62**, 337–339.

Szapary, P. O., Walfe, M. L., Bloedon, L. T., et al. (2003). Guggulipid for the treatment of hypercholesterolemia: A randomized controlled trial. *JAMA*, **290**, 765–772.

Tak, S., Lakhotia, M., Gupta, A., Sagar, A., Bohra, G. and Bajari, R. (2016). Aconite poisoning with arrhythmia and shock. *Indian Heart Journal*, **68**(Suppl 2), S207–S209.

Talwar, G. P., Shah, S., Mukherjee, S. and Chabra, R. (1997). Induced termination of pregnancy by purified extracts of *Azadirachta indica* (Neem): Mechanisms involved. *American Journal of Reproductive Immunology*, **37**, 485–491.

Tewari, P. V., Sharma, P. V., Prasad, D. N. and Chaturvedi, C. (1972). Experimental studies on the ecobolic properties of *Goriosa superba* Linn. *Indian Journal of Medical Research*, **7**(2), 27–38.

Tewari, S. N. and Trembalowicz, F. C. (1968). Some experience with deglycyrrhizinated liquorice in the treatment of gastric and duodenal ulcers with special reference to its spasmolytic effect. *Gut*, **9**, 48–51.

Tiwari, K. C., Majumder, R. and Bhattacharjee, S. (1982). Folklore information from Assam for family planning and birth control. *International Journal of Crude Drug Research*, **20**, 133–137.

Tongia, A., Tongia, S. K. and Dave, M. (2004). Phytochemical determination and extraction of *Momordica charantia* fruit and its hypoglycemic potentiation of oral hypoglycemic drug in diabetes mellitus (NIDDM). *Indian Journal of Physiology and Pharmacology*, **48**, 241–244.

Ulbricht, C., Basch, E., Hammerness, P., Vora, M., Wylie J. Jr., and Woods, J. (2004). An evidence-based systematic review of belladonna by the natural standard research collaboration. *Journal of Herbal Pharmacotherapy*, **4**(4), 61–90.

Vad, B. G. (1960). Place of *Momordica charantia* in the treatment of diabetes mellitus. *Maharashtra Medical Journal*, **6**, 733–745.

Vaidya, A. B., Rajagopalan, T. G., Mankodi, N. A. et al. (1978). Treatment of Parkinson's disease with the cowhage plant *Mucuna pruriens* Bak. *Neurology India*, **26**, 171–176.

Vakil, R. J. (1949). A clinical trial of *Rauwolfia serpentina* in essential hypertension. *British Heart Journal*, **11**, 350–355.

Vakil, R. J. and Dalal, S. R. (1955a). A clinical trial of *Nardostachys jatamansi* in neurocirculatory asthenia: (A preliminary report). *Indian Practitioner*, **8**, 227–230.

Vakil, R. J. and Dalal, S. R. (1955b). Further clinical trials of the *Nardostachys jatamansi* plant. *Indian Practitioner*, **8**, 715–718.

van Tilburg, M. A., Palsson, O. S., Ringel, Y. and Whitehead, W. E. (2014). Is ginger effective for the treatment of irritable bowel syndrome? A double blind randomized controlled pilot trial. *Complementary Therapies in Medicine*, **22**, 17–20.

Vegnanarayan, R., Dange, S. V., Vaidya, S. D. and Balwani, J. J. (1982). Study of *Picrorhiza kurroa* (PK 300) in cases of bronchial asthma. *Bombay Hospital Journal*, **24**(2), 15/81–18/84.

Victor, G., Manickavasagam, V. C., Murugesan, V. and Rex, P. M. (1972). Effect of *Curcuma longa* (edible turmeric) on serum cholesterol level in the human being. *Antiseptic*, **69**, 163–169.

Virani, N. V., Chandola, H. M., Vyas, S. N. and Jadeja, D. B. (2010). Clinical study on erectile dysfunction in diabetic and non-diabetic subjects and its management with *Ficus religiosa* Linn. *Ayu*, **31**, 272–279.

Vishal, A. A., Mishra, A. and Raychaudhuri, S. P. (2011). A double blind, randomized, placebo controlled clinical study evaluates the early efficacy of Alfapin® in subjects with osteoarthritis of knee. *International Journal of Medical Sciences*, **8**, 615–622.

Waheed, A., Miana, G. A., Sharafatullah, T. and Ahmad, S. I. (2008). Clinical investigation of hypoglycemic effect of unripe fruit on *Momordica charantia* in type-2 (NIDDM) diabetes mellitus. *Pakistan Journal of Pharmacology*, **25**(1), 7–12.

Wigler, I., Grotto, I., Caspi, D. and Yaron, M. (2003). The effects of Zintona EC (a ginger extract) on symptomatic gonarthritis. *Osteoarthritis and Cartilage*, **11**, 783–789.

Yadav, B. L., Mathur, R. and Gupta, R. B. (1980). Antifertility activity of *Terminalia arjuna* W. & A. in female albino rats. *Probe*, **19**, 196–198.

Yekta, Z. P., Ebrahimi, S. M., Hosseini, M. et al. (2012). Ginger as a miracle against chemotherapy-induced vomiting. *Iranian Journal of Nursing and Midwifery Research*, **17**, 325–329.

Young, H. Y., Liao, J. C., Chang, Y. S., Luo, Y. L., Lu, M. C. and Peng, W. H. (2006). Synergistic effect of ginger and nifedipine on human platelet aggregation a study in hypertensive patients and normal volunteers. *American Journal of Chinese Medicine*, **34**, 545–551.

Yousefi, M., Mahdavi, M. R., Hosseini, S. M. et al. (2013). Clinical evaluation of *Commiphora mukul*, a botanical resin, in the management of hemorrhoids: A randomized controlled trial. *Pharmacognosy Magazine*, **9**(36), 350–356.

Zakeri, Z., Izadi, S., Bari, Z., Soltani, F., Narouie, B. and Ghasemi-Rad, M. (2011). Evaluating the effects of ginger extract on knee pain, stiffness and difficulty in patients with knee osteoarthritis. *Journal of Medicinal Plants Research*, **5**, 3375–3379.

Ziaee, T., Razavi, B. M. and Hosseinzadeh, H. (2014). Saffron reduced toxic effects of its constituent, safranal, in acute and subacute toxicities in rats. *Jundishapur Journal of Natural Pharmaceutical Products*, **9**(1), 3–8.

Zick, S. M., Ruffin, M. T.,Lee, J., et al. (2009). Phase II trial of encapsulated ginger as a treatment for chemotherapy induced nausea and vomiting. *Supportive Care in Cancer*, **17**, 563–572.

10 Approaches to Safety Evaluation of Botanicals and Processed Botanicals Known in Traditional Knowledge

D.B. Anantha Narayana and Sharanbasappa Durg

CONTENTS

10.1 BACKGROUND

Use of botanicals in traditional medicines is quite well known, has a long history of safe usage and is acknowledged for its efficacy. Such usage in a well-documented nature, prescribed by traditional qualified physicians, has a history of usage both in Indian traditional medicine (Ayurveda, Unani and Siddha [AUS]) healthcare systems as well as traditional Chinese medicine (TCM). The Ayurvedic system is considered to have originated with the first treatise of Ayurveda, the *Charaka Samhita* (the Sanskrit word *Saṃhitā* meaning treatise, pharmacopoeia or medical compendium, written by the sage Charaka), which dates to around 1000 BCE (Tripathi, 2010). Subsequent to this, a large number of other treatises have been documented in Ayurveda that describe holistic healthcare science, descriptions of health and diseases, diagnostic methods, surgery procedures, treatment with diet, behavioural aspects and medicines. The last such treatment included medicines prepared using botanicals in an elaborate

TABLE 10.1

A Few Authoritative Books of Traditional Healthcare and Medicines

Authoritative Books	System of Healthcare	Author	Year
Charak Samhita	Ayurveda	Compiled by Maharshi Atreya	Around 1000 BC
Sushrut Samhita	Ayurveda	Compiled by legendary surgeon Sushruta	Around 1500–1000 BC (completed by 2nd AD)
Madhava Nidana	Ayurveda	Madhavakara	Around Seventh Century AD
Bhavaprakasha	Ayurveda	Bhavamisra	Around Sixteenth Century AD
Astanga Hridayam	Ayurveda	Compiled by Vagbhatta	Around Sixth Century AD
Sharanghadhara Samhita	Ayurveda	Sharangadhara	Around Thirteenth Century AD
Bhava Prakasa Nighantu (Addendum)	Ayurveda	Bhavamisra	Around Sixteenth Century AD
Shen Nong Ben Cao Jing	Traditional Chinese medicine	Shen Nong	25 –220 AD
Ben Cao	Traditional Chinese medicine	Wu Jin	220–280 AD
Ben Cao Jing Ji Zhu	Traditional Chinese medicine	Tao Hongjing	c. 452–536
Xin Xiu Ben Cao	Traditional Chinese medicine	Over 20 scholars led by Su Jing	659 AD
Ben Cao Tu Jing	Traditional Chinese medicine	Su Song	1061
Chong Guang Bu Zhu Shen Nong Ben Cao Bing Tu Jing	Traditional Chinese medicine	Chen Cheng	1092

pharmaceutical approach called 'Bheshaj Kalpana' (Reddy 2015). Similarly, TCM *Materia Medica* has been documented since c. 425–536 (Gurib-Fakim 2006; Liao 2006). The drugs listed in such traditional medicine books demonstrate the long history of safe use, as any drug to enter one such *Materia Medica* is known to have undergone usage and observation for at least 50–60 years. Only those that have been found to have a good safety profile either as such or after specified processing methods deserved an entry in to such books. Other traditional systems of healthcare that are not so well documented continue to be used, including the Bhutanese system of medicine, Kampo medicine in Japan, African traditional medicine, Australian and Southeast Asian traditional medicine, to name a few. Table 10.1 lists a few authoritative books on traditional healthcare and medicine.

While botanical medicines from such systems continue to be used, advances in biological and chemical sciences have led to the development of drugs of synthetic origin that have undergone extensive scientific evaluation for safety and efficacy. Such drugs and pharmaceuticals have overtaken the use of botanical medicines due to a variety of reasons (Butler 2008; Rishton 2008).

The literature reports that 50% or even higher leads for an effective drug had their origin in botanicals, either known in traditional knowledge or in ethno-medicines (Gurib-Fakim 2006; Butler 2008). The leads from such origins were later developed through synthetic chemistry to obtain related compounds that provide better safety and efficacy through the drug development processes (Paterson and Anderson 2005). However, during the 1990s, the consumer push in the United States to 'go back to nature', consumers wanted to take preventive and protective care through natural remedies on their own, without the need for approval from the US Food and Drug Administration (FDA) for such ingredients and products, culminating in the enactment of the Dietary Supplement Health and Education Act (DSHEA) in 1994 (US FDA 1994). The DSHEA heralded a new category of healthcare products called supplements or nutraceuticals. The authors believe more than 65%

of supplements and nutraceuticals use botanicals or their extracts or purified fractions and single compounds from botanicals to maintain health and to provide various types of health benefits, including disease risk reduction. The remaining 35% of this category includes vitamins, minerals, amino acids, enzymes, pro- and pre-biotics and such other non-botanically based ingredients.

The DSHEA triggered a movement from an illness-centric drug-based approach to a wellness centred approach through diet, exercise, mediation and use of botanically based supplements/ nutraceuticals. Most nations followed, enacting similar regulatory provisions to promote supplements and nutraceuticals in their countries. The latest of these regulations was the notification of functional foods, supplements, nutraceuticals, foods for specified dietary use, foods for specific medical purposes and novel foods (referred to as nutraceutical regulation in the rest of the chapter) by India in November 2016 (India. Food Safety Standards Authority 2016), which was updated in December 2017 (India. Food Safety Standards Authority 2017).

Even a cursory view of these developments – especially the wellness centric products – reveals the use of a large number of botanicals or processed botanicals. The botanicals could fall into many categories, and in particular those listed below:

1. Botanicals known and documented in the traditional knowledge literature of that country.
2. Botanicals known and documented in the traditional knowledge literature of that country and prepared following the processes as described in the traditional knowledge literature.
3. Botanicals known in ethno-medicine and prepared following the ethno-medical practices.
4. Botanicals known in oral traditions and grandmother remedies and prepared following processes as described in them.
5. Botanicals not falling in any of the categories listed above, but originating from a country other than the country where it is used (vis-à-vis a botanical known in Nigeria, not listed in 1–4 above, but intended for use in India or China).
6. Botanicals falling in categories 1–5 above, but:
   6.1. A different species is used.
   6.2. A different part of the plant is used.
   6.3. An entirely different process is used to prepare the ingredient for use as a healthcare product.
   6.4. It is used in a different route of administration not known in 1–5 above.
   6.5. It is processed using current pharmaceutical processing involving organic solvents leading to fractionation. It is common knowledge that the processing of botanicals in traditional knowledge documents never would have used organic solvents like methanol, ethyl acetate, acetone, hexane, isopropyl alcohol, petroleum ether, propylene glycol, DMSO (dimethyl sulfoxide), supercritical fluid extraction using liquid CO_2 and other such solvents, as these entered into science only in the eighteenth century at the earliest. The sole exception could be use of self-generated alcohol (ethanol) for extraction of botanicals, like in wine, which was known and documented in the 'Bheshaj Kalpana' books of Ayurveda (Reddy 2015).
   6.6. Processed using fractional distillation or fractionation of fatty acids employed in processing distilled oils or vegetable oils from botanicals.
   6.7. Processed with multi-step fractionation leading to obtaining single chemical compound in its pure form possessing health benefit properties.

These descriptions, although they are understood scientifically, in a regulatory context each of these botanicals and outputs may fall into different categories. They may be classified as either a traditional ASU drug, a TCM, a botanical drug, a phytopharmaceutical, a health supplement, a nutraceutical or a new chemical entity (NCE), depending on the nature and extent of processing. A broad understanding applies that modified processed material or a fractionated material or a NCE would fall into a drug category under regulations whenever the intentions of use are to treat or mitigate or diagnose or cure a disease or a disorder. If processed as per traditional documented processes and intended for use as per traditional knowledge, they would be classified as an ASU drug (in India as per Indian Drug Regulations) or TCM (in the Republic of China as per State FDA Regulations applicable to TCM). Figures 10.1 through 10.3 illustrate this in a representative way.

Often debates and discussions revolve around the need, nature, extent and types of evaluation required for obtaining knowledge of safety profile of botanicals. Most regulators and scientists

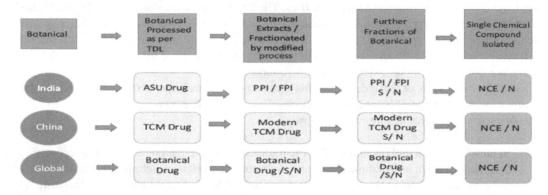

FIGURE 10.1   A schematic diagram of botanicals, processes, categories. (*Abbreviations*: TDL, Traditional documented literature; ASU, Ayurveda, Siddha Unani; PPI/FPI, Phytopharmaceutical ingredient/Formulation of PPI; TCM, Traditional Chinese medicine; S, Supplements; N, Nutaraceuticals; NCE, New chemical entity.)

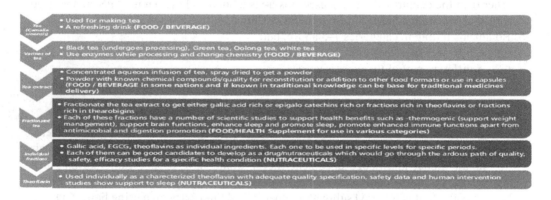

FIGURE 10.2   A schematic diagram of tea (*Camellia sinensis*), processing steps and categories.

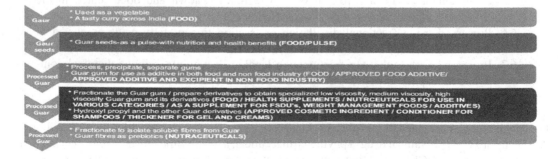

FIGURE 10.3   A schematic diagram of gaur beans (*Cyamopsis tetragonoloba*), processing steps and categories.

would look for traditional and conventional toxicology data for all botanicals, adopting the same or similar acute/chronic toxicity studies, protocols commonly adopted for synthetic drugs. From such toxicology data, many would demand data on carcinogenicity, effect on chromosomes and three-generation teratology information. This chapter provides different insights to deal with the safety assessment of botanicals and the need for innovative strategies. It is neither logical nor scientific to demand a conventional toxicology and safety profile data by putting all botanicals on the same platform as a synthetic drug. There is a need to recognise, where available, the long history of safe use (HoSU) data. While recognising the HoSU application would be a logical approach, identifying gaps in the safety profile, finding specific concern areas and demanding appropriate limited safety data would also be required.

10.2 TRADITIONAL USAGE

As stated above, Ayurveda traces its usage as far as 1000 BCE (Tripathi 2010). Similarly TCM has its *Materia Medica* documentation going back to c. 425–536 (Liao 2006). This literature documents that each ingredient or recipe of botanicals underwent a long duration of usage in patients before they satisfied the requirement of entry into one of the *Materia Medica* treatises. Traditional physicians are known to have used botanical processed in one or more methods for use in their patients and carefully observed both the safety and efficacy aspects. Efficacy was observed with interpretations of the diagnostic methodological philosophy of Ayurveda (vis-à-vis Tridosha theory of effect on three humours namely Vata, Pitta and Kapha) or TCM (vis-à-vis the theory of *yin* and *yang*). A number of publications and historical documents corroborate that discussions and conferences were common amongst these physicians and the exchange of safety and efficacy information flowed freely amongst them, leading to cross-utilisation and multi-centric experience generation. A research-minded Ayurvedic physician notes that, on average, it took 4 or 5 decades of usage and observation before a botanical or a processed botanical or a recipe was accepted with a known safety profile and found entry into the documentation. The very fact that most of the botanicals documented either in Ayurvedic or TCM books are safely used even today provides confidence as to their safety. It is important that such safety profiles would apply to the correct botanical, the correct part to be used, in the right dose, duration and route of usage prepared, adopting the processes given in the textual references. Table 10.2 provides a few examples to describe the HoSU.

TABLE 10.2
A Few Examples of Botanicals: Processing and Differentiation

Botanical Documented in Traditional Text	Part of Plant, Processed Material and Dose (HoSU)	Part of Plant, Processed Material and Not Documented (Has No History of Usage)	Reference
Tomato (*Solanum lycopersicum*)	Fruits, juice, cooked fruits as puree, and dried powder: fried with oil or clarified butter	Leaves, stalk, root	Standard food processing methods for tomato, including grandmother recipes and commercial production
Brinjal (*Solanum melongena*)	Fruits, cooked fruit: fried with oil or clarified butter	Leaves, stalk, root	Standard food processing methods for brinjal, including grandmother recipes and commercial production

(Continued)

TABLE 10.2 (*Continued*)
A Few Examples of Botanicals: Processing and Differentiation

Botanical Documented in Traditional Text	Part of Plant, Processed Material and Dose (HoSU)	Part of Plant, Processed Material and Not Documented (Has No History of Usage)	Reference
Ashwagandha (*Withania somnifera*)	Roots, root bark, stem: as dried powder (Churna): aqueous extract concentrate (Quatha): pasty mass obtained by frying with clarified butter (Avaleha or Ghritha): medicated wine-like preparation processed by allowing fermentation and self-generation of alcohol during extraction of an aqueous decoration of the botanical	Leaves, fruit, seed: fractionated extract using organic solvents	Ayurvedic Pharmacopoeia of India (Volume 1), Ministry for Health and Family Welfare (2010a); Chunekar and Pandeya (2010)
Brahmi (*Bacopa monnieri*)	Leaves as dried powder (Churna): aqueous extract concentrate (Quatha): pasty mass obtained by frying with clarified butter (Avaleha or Ghritha): medicated wine-like preparation processed by allowing fermentation and self-generation of alcohol during extraction of an aqueous decoration of the botanical	Root, stem, flowers and seed: fractionated extract using organic solvents	Ayurvedic Pharmacopoeia of India (Volume 2), Ministry for Health and Family Welfare (2010b); Chunekar and Pandeya (2010)

10.3 DEFINITION OF TRADITIONAL PROCESSING AND MODIFIED PROCESSING

BOX 10.1 LIST OF TERMINOLOGIES AND THEIR DEFINITION/DESCRIPTION

Terminology	Definition/Description
Active ingredients	Refer to the ingredients of herbal medicines with therapeutic activity. In herbal medicines where the active ingredients have been identified, the preparation of these medicines should be standardised to contain a defined amount of the active ingredients, if adequate analytical methods are available. In cases where it is not possible to identify the active ingredients, the whole herbal medicine may be considered one active ingredient.
Characterising a compound or marker	A natural constituent of a plant part that may be used to assure the identity or quality of a plant material or preparation, but is not necessarily responsible for the plant's biological or therapeutic activity.
Complementary medicine	The terms 'complementary medicine' or 'alternative medicine' refer to a broad set of healthcare practices that are not part of that country's own tradition or conventional medicine and are not fully integrated into the dominant healthcare system. They are used interchangeably with traditional medicine in some countries.

(Continued)

BOX 10.1 (Continued) LIST OF TERMINOLOGIES AND THEIR DEFINITION/DESCRIPTION

Terminology	Definition/Description
Herbs	Include crude plant material such as leaves, flowers, fruit, seed, stems, wood, bark, roots, rhizomes or other plant parts, which may be entire, fragmented or powdered.
Herbal materials	Include, in addition to herbs, fresh juices, gums, fixed oils, essential oils, resins and dry powders of herbs. In some countries, these materials may be processed by various local procedures, such as steaming, roasting, or stir baking with honey, alcoholic beverages or other materials.
Herbal medicines	Plant-derived materials or products with therapeutic or other human health benefits that contain either raw or processed ingredients from one or more plants. In some traditions, materials of inorganic or animal origin may also be present, although for the purpose of this document, the focus will be on plant materials only.
Herbal preparations	The basis for finished herbal products that may include comminuted or powdered herbal materials, or extracts, tinctures and fatty oils of herbal materials. They are produced by extraction, fractionation, purification, concentration or other physical or biological processes. They also include preparations made by steeping or heating herbal materials in alcoholic beverages and/or honey or in other materials.
Finished herbal products	Herbal preparations made from one or more herbs. If more than one herb is used, the term mixture herbal product can also be used. Finished herbal products and mixture herbal products may contain excipients in addition to the active ingredients. However, finished products or mixture products to which chemically defined active substances have been added, including synthetic compounds and/or isolated constituents from herbal materials, are not considered to be herbal.
Ingredient	The substance in the herbal formulation that may not be a purified chemical component.
Medicinal herbal products	Finished, labelled pharmaceutical products in dosage forms that contain one or more of the following: powdered plant materials, extracts, purified extracts, or partially purified active substances isolated from plant materials. Medicines containing plant material combined with chemically defined active substances, including chemically defined, isolated constituents of plants, are not considered to be herbal medicines.
Medicinal plant	A plant that has been used for medical purposes at one time or another, and that, although not necessarily a product or available for marketing, is the original material of herbal medicines.
Processed plant materials	Plant materials treated according to traditional procedures to improve their safety and efficacy, to facilitate their clinical use, or to make medicinal preparations.
Raw plant materials	Fresh or dry plant materials that are marketed whole or simply cut into small pieces.
Traditional and complementary medicine practices	Include medication therapy and procedure-based healthcare therapies such as herbal medicines, naturopathy, acupuncture and manual therapies such as chiropractic, osteopathy as well as other related techniques including qigong, tai chi, yoga, thermal medicine and other physical, mental, spiritual and mind-body therapies.
Traditional and complementary medicine practitioners	Can be traditional medicine practitioners, complementary medicine practitioners, conventional medicine professionals and healthcare workers such as doctors, dentists, nurses, midwives, pharmacists and physical therapists who provide traditional medicine/complementary and alternative medicine services to their patients.

(Continued)

**BOX 10.1 (Continued)   LIST OF TERMINOLOGIES
AND THEIR DEFINITION/DESCRIPTION**

Terminology	Definition/Description
Traditional and complementary medicine products	Include herbs, herbal materials, herbal preparations and finished herbal products that contain parts of plants, other plant materials or combinations thereof as active ingredients. In some countries herbal medicines may contain, by tradition, natural organic or inorganic active ingredients that are not of plant origin (e.g. animal and mineral materials).
Traditional and complementary medicine	Merges the terms traditional medicine and complementary medicine, encompassing products, practices and practitioners.
Traditional medicine	Traditional medicine has a long history. It is the sum total of the knowledge, skill and practices based on the theories, beliefs and experiences indigenous to different cultures, whether explicable or not, used in the maintenance of health as well as in the prevention, diagnosis, improvement or treatment of physical and mental illness.
Traditional use	The use of herbal medicines by practitioners of a traditional system of medicine, where: a. The use is well-established and widely acknowledged, i.e. the use represents the accumulated experience of many practitioners over an extended period of time; b. The use of the herbal medicine, including dosage, indication and administration route is well-established and documented; and c. The use is generally and currently regarded as safe.

Source: World Health Organization, *Guidelines for the Appropriate Use of Herbal Medicines*, World Health Organization, Geneva, Switzerland, 1998; World Health Organization, *WHO-Geneva*, 1, 1–74, 2000; World Health Organization, *WHO Traditional Medicine Strategy 2014–2023*, World Health Organization, Geneva, Switzerland, 2013.

10.4   GENERATING SIMILARITY AND DISSIMILARITY DATA

Traditional texts describe a number of ways in which botanicals are processed for consumption either as food items or during preparation of foods or specifically described processes for preparing a supplement or a traditional medicine preparation. Most modern pharmaceutical processing and unit operations can be traced to one or more processes either described in traditional texts or followed in cultural/grandmother cooking and processing methods. Having greater exposure to Indian traditional medicine processes, namely the 'Bheshaj Kalpana' of Ayurveda, attempts to give a number of terminologies and their definitions/descriptions of traditional processing have been tabulated in Table 10.3 and modified processes adopted even at industrial scale corresponding to each of the traditional processing methods are described. Many modified processes may not really offer significant changes in the processed material or output, while many of them result in significant changes in the chemistry/physico-chemical properties of the processed material. It must be determined whether materials obtained from these three different broad types of outputs comply with HoSU description or are very similar to HoSU material or are entirely different and dissimilar to HoSU material. This understanding is very important for safety assessment of botanical and processed material. Keeping in mind the constraints of space for the chapter, a non-exhaustive and typical tabulation has been made and interested readers would need to refer to authoritative texts, formularies or books on 'Bheshaj Kalpana'. A similar approach would be fully applicable to other traditional knowledge–based processing, including TCM and these are not described here. Processing in homeopathic practice is also not covered here.

TABLE 10.3
A Few Examples of Botanicals: Traditional and Modified Processing

Botanicals and Its Parts	Traditional Processing (Definition/Description)	Modified Processing	Author Insights
Fresh leaves	Juices (*Swaras*[a]) – by crushing the fresh leaves with limited quantity of water or with prescribed quantity of water at cold or room temperature. Occasionally crushing is improved with grinding including mechanical grinders. The resultant juice is strained or filtered	Normally no modified processing is used	*Swaras* is the term used in traditional texts that literally means 'its own nutrients or its own juice'. The texts give descriptions of the amount of water to be used. It also describes a process where dried leaves are soaked in water, stirred and strained which also meets the need of *swaras* in those cases where fresh leaves are not available or cannot be processed in fresh condition
Dried plant parts	Cold infusion (*Swaras* or *Him*) Warm infusion (*Phant*) Hot infusion (*Phant*) Decoction (Kwath /*Quath*/*Kashaya*) Cold or hot maceration The above are self-explanatory and basis the part of the plant the ratio of solvent most commonly water may vary (for softer botanicals part lesser quantity of water and for harder parts like bark and roots larger quantity of water) The resultant solution is strained or filtered. Traditional processes describe consuming the liquid extract as such (*Him*/*Phant*/*Quath*) or after concentrating it to the specified reduced quantities (*Quath* or *kashya*). Traditional processes also describe – concentration to liquid extracts (*quath*), further concentration to yield soft extracts / semi solid mass (*Sattava* or *Ghana sattava*), or adsorption to inert material to obtain powders (*Sattava* or *Ghana sattava*)	Modified processes include – liquid extracts adsorbed on inert substance to be sun dried or tray dried either in forced air or vacuum; liquid extracts processed in a spray drier to obtain powders; liquid extracts processed in falling film evaporator and drum driers; liquid extracts dried to obtain powders using freeze-drying or lyophilisation technologies where the botanical components in the water do not get heated at all Use of solvents other than water – the list of solvents available are exhaustive and most common ones are – ethanol, ethanol-water mixture, hexane, methanol, acetone, isopropyl alcohol, ethyl acetate, propylene glycol and others. Additionally counter current extraction with mixture of solvents also adopted	Except lyophilisation process most of the botanicals processed by the methods in the first paragraph under modified processes column would show close similarity of the produced to that of a traditional processed material. In those cases extrapolation of the history of long and safe use and the safety profile is justified and only on a case to case basis generation of safety data to fill concern areas or gaps in safety profile would be needed In case of botanicals processed using the solvents and processes described in the second paragraph under modified process theoretically extrapolation of the history of long and safe use and the safety profile is not justified unless establishment of similarities and dissimilarities between a HoSU process and the modified process is generated. In those solvent extracts involving multiple steps of fractionation extrapolation of HoSU safety profile would be unscientific. (See section under approaches to safety assessment for further guidance)

(Continued)

TABLE 10.3 (*Continued*)

A Few Examples of Botanicals: Traditional and Modified Processing

Botanicals and Its Parts	Traditional Processing (Definition/Description)	Modified Processing	Author Insights
Fresh or dried plant parts	Distilled in presence of water and the condensate is collected which is normally a mixture of the distillate oil either floating on water or partially dissolved in water (*Ark* or *Ark taila*). Allowing settlement would provide the distilled oil to separate as a layer yielding distilled oils Depending on the solubility the water would yield an aromatic water with a yield of clearly separated essential oil Oils obtained by this process are generally not vegetable or fixed oils consisting of chemistry primarily made of fatty acids. Such oils are composed of organic compounds like terpenes, cineoles, etc.	The distilled oil is further processed to fractionate one or more group of individual chemical compounds. In specific cases the fractionated compounds may further be processed with one or more synthetic steps to obtain new derivatives It could also be a single step fractionation to only remove an identified component of the distilled oils and obtain an oil with modified composition from that occurring in nature	Most traditional fixed oils listed in traditional texts describe only crude vegetable oils or fats at the most undergoing straining or clarification. Even steps of de-waxing are not common in such processes. The crude oils hence had their own dark colours, odour and waxy nature. Even the list of such oils in traditional texts in India is limited to sesame oil, coconut oil, castor oil, cottonseed oil, mustard oil, neem oil, karanj oil and almond oil. The first three oils were most commonly used either alone or in combination both as healthy diet and for processing of botanicals for preparing medicated oils. These oils and the medicated oils listed in traditional texts have HoSU status
Seeds and fruits of botanicals	Expressed mechanically to yield fixed oils that are then strained (*Taila*). These fixed oils are crude in nature and traditionally one or more step of simple clarification and straining are described. Historically the mechanical expression could either be done in cold condition or in slightly warmed condition (cold pressed)	Improved extraction of oil or fat using hydraulic press and such other high-pressure equipment. Improving yields of extraction by treating the marc (the cold pressed fruit or seed in which there is still some oil or fat) and extracting with hexane and evaporating away the hexane (solvent extracted oil)	

(*Continued*)

TABLE 10.3 *(Continued)*
A Few Examples of Botanicals: Traditional and Modified Processing

Botanicals and Its Parts	Traditional Processing (Definition/Description)	Modified Processing	Author Insights
	In some cases the seed or fruit are boiled with copious amount of water and allowed to cool. After cooling the fat separated is collected removing by suitable decantation or straining the water In specific cases the seed or fruit is crushed and mixed with sand/mud/other adsorbents for specified periods and then the fat or oil is extracted. The fruit is then used for producing an extract or an herbal preparation	The obtained oil or fat is processed through steps like – de-waxing, bleaching, deodorisation, refining, and ultra-filtration Still further processing by fractionating, inter esterification	It is only in the later century that other vegetable oils and their RBD (refined, bleached and deodorised) varieties entered the list namely – ground nut oil (pea nut oil), rice bran oil, corn oil, palm oil, palm fat, sun flower oil, safflower oil and others. These oils by virtue of their extensive studies by food scientists and technologists as well as long term usage in large population also have HoSU status However, use of mineral oils produced out of petroleum refining do not fall in the list of these oils

Note: The above-tabulated matter typically provides insights as to what can be considered traditionally processed material having HoSU status not needing detailed safety or toxicology data generation. It also provides insights to when and in what conditions a modified processed materials can still be very similar to a traditionally processed material and the HoSU status can be extrapolated. Certain type and nature of modifications in the process can make the material largely dissimilar to HoSU material in which case generation of detailed pharmacology and toxicology data would be required.

[a] Terms given in italics and in parenthesis are the original terms in the oriental language of Sanskrit described in traditional Ayurvedic texts.

The descriptions in the above sections would give innovative approaches to the safety evaluation of botanicals. Since large proportions of botanicals in any part of the globe have some usage history, blind adoption of modern toxicology evaluation processes for botanicals would not be logical or scientifically necessary. It is to be recognised that a history of long usage provides adequate insights to the safety profile of the botanical materials and a logical and stepwise approach to decide the nature and extent of safety assessment and data requirement should be the order of the day. More so in those botanicals that have documented history of usage and processes like those seen in Ayurveda, Unani, Siddha, homeopathy, TCM to name a few. Perhaps as the basis for such an understanding, the Traditional Medicine Directive of the EU states that limited or nil data would be required for approval of botanicals and traditional medicines in the EU if 'the material has 30 years of documented usage in any part of the globe with at least 15 years of documented usage in one or the other nation within EU' (European Commission 1997; The European Parliament and The Council of the European Union 1997, 2015; Qu et al. 2018). Due to the growth of the botanicals industry in the last 3 decades and the development of technology to produce standardised botanical extracts that are commercially produced and used, their safety assessment also requires a different approach. Many nations accept the safety profile of such botanicals if they are standardised, chemistry information and technical specifications are available, produced under hygienic conditions and have been in commerce for 10–15 years and detailed toxicology data are not demanded. The presence of a pharmacopoeial monograph also supports such acceptance without detailed toxicology data. All these approaches are logical and adequately scientific. The key in such cases is the botanical or the processes adopted have a long history.

Even in those cases where processes are modified that appear to be different from the traditional processes, a number of innovative approaches are being developed by scientists in the assessment of safety of botanicals. The primary objective is to give weightage to long history of use and to avoid unnecessary conventional toxicology data generation that is time consuming, expensive and complicated. The pressure of environmentalists and animal enthusiasts is also forcing the reduction in testing involving animals and leading to the development of alternatives to animal testing. In fact, testing of any ingredient – including botanicals – on animals for safety data for use in any cosmetic preparation has already been prohibited (European Commission 2016). A few innovative approaches are described in this context.

10.4.1 Approach 1: Preparing a Document to Describe the HoSU Data

There are no standard methods or processes that detail preparation of a document on HoSU data. Often applicants wishing to get regulatory approval quote traditional documented literature and give the name of the authoritative documented traditional books of either ASU or TCM or other books recognised in the nation. For example, the Indian Drugs and Cosmetics Act, 1940 and Rules, 1945 amended till current date, has in its First Schedule a list of books recognised as official books under the law for Ayurveda, Siddha and Unani (India. Director General of Health Services 2016; Deshpade and Nilesh 2018). This Schedule provides these books and the botanicals and recipes documented in them HoSU status and any firm or physician manufacturing them as per processes in these books do not need to generate any fresh safety or efficacy data. Such a provision was also applicable as long as the dose, duration of treatment/use and the indications of use were the same as in these books. The provisions further permitted new combinations of these botanicals under similar conditions. Similar provisions are applicable to TCMs codified and documented in the official *Materia Medica* of China. These provisions not only recognise but also provide regulatory approval from the wisdom of the Parliaments of these two countries. Applicants must provide the textual references and photocopies along with English certified translations in support of HoSU status. Different nations and national regulatory authorities treated such data differently and most often termed them inadequate. However, in the last decade, recognition of HoSU is slowly increasing in many parts of the globe. The authors tried to provide an approach that can be more descriptive and informative than just citing a book reference. In this approach, not only the information from the traditional documented literature (TDL) is described in greater detail, but current usage of the botanicals in products that are licensed under regulations and being marketed either as a traditional drug or under other categories are also documented. It also suggests more information by way of data generation on the use of the botanical in current treatment by experienced physicians, obtained through structured interviews. A criterion of basic qualification to practice as a physician followed by a minimum number of years of practice experience can be laid down for deciding which physicians would be interviewed. The below description/information provides a brief document covering this approach and all the three sections of the HoSU document for the botanical Haritaki (*Terminalia chebula*; one of the myrobalans).

10.4.1.1   Description of the Botanical and Its Use in TDL

Description: Haritaki, commonly known as 'Chebulic myrobalan' in English and Harad in Hindu, is a brown or brownish black dried fruit that is oval in shape and irregular. The surface is mostly smooth and has ridges in some places. It has a characteristic odour. It is astringent in taste. It has a seed inside and most often the outer rind is used and the seeds are not. Each dried fruit is slightly larger than or of the same size as a fresh grapefruit.

Use in TDL

1. In most parts of India, a pinch of Haritaki powder is given to children to improve their immunity, digestion, expel gas and to treat common cold and cough. In South India, the fruit is ground with a little water on a stone plate commonly used for making sandalwood paste to make a wet paste. This paste is applied to the forehead or stomach of infants and children to reduce fever or gripping pain and gas in the stomach. This is a common grandmother remedy. It is also common to prepare a dilute infusion of the fruit and give a spoonful for such conditions orally.

2. *Bhavaprakasha*, an authoritative Ayurvedic text (Srikantha Murthy 2008), has an entire chapter titled 'Haritakyadi Varga' (dealing with Haritaki-like botanicals), which provides detailed descriptions of Haritaki and its medicinal properties, preparations, indications and contraindications.

3. In the same chapter referenced above, there is also a description of Triphala (a recipe), which made of three fruits, that is equal quantities of Amla (*Emblica officinalis*), Haritaki (*Terminalia chebula*) and Bibhitaki (*Terminalia belerica*). This is a common powder used for gastrointestinal (GI) tract health, as a mild laxative, bowel regulator, a *rasayana* (immunomodulator) and good for eyes and vision. The dose is normally 3–6 g of Triphala powder taken 2–3 times a day with water.

4. Another authoritative book, the *Ayurvedic Formulary of India* (AFI), describes Triphaladi taila (a medicated oil) prepared as per traditional processing (India. Department of Indian Systems of Medicine and Homeopathy 2003). In traditional processing of such medicated oil, normally one part of herb is cooked with 4 parts of sesame oil and 8 or 16 parts of an infusion or decoction of herbs. A paste of the herb with water is also added to this recipe during cooking. Cooking is continued until all the water in the infusion or decoction is completely removed. The resultant oil is then cooled and strained or filtered and the marc is pressed to get the adhered oil out and mixed with the filtrate. This recipe uses 38 hers for preparing the oil, of which Haritaki is an important one. This oil is stored in bottles and used externally in the *Abhyangam* process (commonly referred to as whole body massage). This is indicated in treatment of *siroroga* (problems of head), *khalitya* (loss of hair and low hair growth), *palitya* (greying of hair) and other indications.

5. The texts also describe plain Triphala taila, prepared using the same process as described in the above text AFI, but using only the three herbs of Triphala stated above. This taila has indications for headaches, scalp health, hair growth and hair loss and to delay greying of hair.

6. As per *Bhavaprakash Nighantu* (BPN), it has a number of multiple usages (Chunekar and Pandeya 2010). Most importantly a statement of this text clearly states 'it does not cause any type of troubles or side effects'. So much so that in one other text describing the property of this botanical, a Sanskrit verse is quoted by most which read as below:

Yasyagruhematanaasti ITasyagruheharitaki II
Maatakinchitakupita INa Haritaki II

This translates as 'in absence of a mother in the house, keep Haritaki. Even mothers may be annoyed or angry sometimes, but Haritaki will never be'. This speaks volumes about the safety profile of Haritaki. This book also describes a number of all-round health benefits and uses for Haritaki.

7. BPN also provides a Haritaki recipe in the texts called *pathya kwath* (patya is another name for Haritaki). This *kwath* is prepared by grinding Haritaki to coarse and large sized pieces, boiling with 16 parts water, continuing to heat and concentrate to a quarter of the original volume. Cool and strain or filter the result and the filtrate is the *kwath*, which is administered orally as per texts. In this reference of this recipe, the ratio of herb to water for extraction can be obtained.

Note: Many of the references on the lines above can be quoted in the document and provide the doses, process for preparation, usage, indications and other information including any contraindications or special advisories provided in the authoritative books. In absence of access to TCM *Materia Medica* and inability to read texts written in Mandarin language, similar information on myrobalan and its usage in China has not been given, but including those references would add value to the document. Likewise, information in texts of healthcare or medicine from other parts of the globe where myrobalans are available and used would add value to the HoSU document.

10.4.1.2 Description of the Current Usage of the Botanical Either Individually or in Combination in Products Marketed under Regulatory Licenses

In this section, information/data on marketed preparations should be provided. Where possible, exposure computation may be provided, which adds value for the safety assessment. A few examples are given to demonstrate the same.

Example 10.1

1. Haritaki being a component of Triphala churna (powder) would contain a third of the quantity of the churna. Such churna preparations are marketed across India packed in wide-mouthed bottles with lid (50, 100 and 500 g packs). These are licensed under the Indian Drugs Regulations as an ASU medicine. The dose of the churna, as per text, is 3–6 g, two or three times a day. This means that if the churna is taken even at a dose of 3 g thrice a day, this would be 9 g/day for the churna, which would be 3 g of Haritaki/day. If the dose of the churna rises to 6 g per dose, then the total consumption would be 6 g/day of Haritaki.

2. Triphala is also sold compressed as tablets after binding suitably with permitted binders and other tableting excipients. Due to technological reasons, such tablets available in market are normally about 600 mg average weight, providing about 350–400 mg of Triphala, which means that the dose would be about 8–10 tablets a day to get 3 g of Triphala/day – this would still provide only 1 g Haritaki/day. Such tablets are available both with the traditional name and some of them being sold under brand names. A reference to Ayurvedline (Nayak 2014) shows that more than 50 firms market either Triphala churna or Triphala tablets. In the absence of authentic market data on volumes and value, exact figures on consumption of these preparations are difficult to provide (where such data are available, these must be provided).

3. The Triphala tablets described above limit the consumption of the full recommended dose as the number of tablets to be consumed is large per day and becomes consumer unfriendly. Several firms have prepared Triphala *kwath* with water, concentrated and then granulated for compression. Based on extractive value, the Triphala becomes more concentrated by this method and in such cases the labels of these products suggest 3 tablets twice a day as dosage (with the knowledge of the actual extractive values, calculations can be done to find the equivalent of raw herb provided in each tablet).

Note: Along similar lines, detailed tabulated information can be prepared giving the brand name of the product, presentation as dosage form, composition, recommended daily dose, proportion of the botanical under consideration for which HoSU data is being made and, where required, computation of the equivalent to the raw botanical quantity.

Example 10.2

A hypothetical example given below for Triphala tablet consumption as described under 10.1(2) above.

- Tablets sold in a strip pack of 10, packed in box of 10 strips. Equal to 100 tablets per box.
- Cost of 1 box above is 110.00 INR.
- Sales turnover of such packs per annum = 25,00,000 INR.
- Consumption per day of tablets is 10 tablets
- Consumption for 6 months = 1800 tablets
- Number of packs sold = 22,730 per annum × 100 tablets each (sales turnover/cost per pack)

This means about 1260 persons consume Triphala tablets for a 6-month period, which is the estimated population exposure.

Note: Along the lines of the above, computations can be made for 10.1(1) and 10.1(3) and additional marketed products data that are provided in the document could give a cumulative approximate population exposure.

10.4.1.3 Current Usage and Experience by Practicing Physicians

In order to get current usage in medical practice, interviews – either face to face or written questionnaire or over the telephone – can be conducted to obtain information from practicing physicians. There must be predetermined, agreed-upon criteria concerning the qualifications and experience of the physicians to be interviewed and whose input and data are considered. For example, minimum degree holders of Ayurvedic science with at least 5 years of clinical practicing experience may be a good minimum criteria. It is important to draw a short list of focused questions in order to elicit information. Given below is an approach to such data collection for Haritaki.

Questions for interview:

1. Do you prescribe Haritaki individually?
2. What is the dose that you prescribe?
3. For what indications have you used it?
4. How long do you ask for it to be consumed?
5. Do you see good response?
6. Can you tell us for how long and approximately how many patients you have prescribed Haritaki?
7. Please give us any common safety concerns experienced in the users.
8. Do you prescribe it for pregnant women and/or lactating mothers?
9. Do you prescribe this for children also? If so, for what age group?
10. Without giving your identity, would you permit the data to be added to a collation document being prepared?

The responses obtained can be tabulated as below and a typical example of 10 physicians is given in Box 10.2.

BOX 10.2   QUESTIONS FOR INTERVIEW –
A TYPICAL EXAMPLE OF 10 PHYSICIANS

S. No.	Physician (Qualification and Years of Experience)	Q 1	Q 2	Q 3	Q 4	Q 5	Q 6	Q 7[a]	Q 8[b]	Q 9[c]	Q 10
1	BAMS, 6 years	Y	1–2 g	A, BR, HL, R	3–6 months	Y	3 years, >100	N	Y	N	Y
2	MD, 10 years	Y, occasionally	1 g	BR, HL	Continuous with gap of a week every 2 months	Y	7 years, >500	N	Y	N	Y
3	BAMS, 5 years	Y	3 g	BR, HL	3–6 months	Y	2 years, >50	N	Y	N	Y
4	MD, PhD, 6 years	Y	2–5 g	BR, HL, R	1 year	Y	2 years, >50	N	Y	N	Y
5	BAMS, 7 years	Y	2–5 g	BR, HL	3 months	Y	5 years, >150	N	Y	N	Y
6	MD, 3 years	Y	3 g	BR, HL, R	4 months	Y	1 year, >50	N	Y	N	Y
7	BAMS, 2 years	Y	3 g	BR, HL	3 months	Y	1 year, >50	N	Y	N	Y
8	BAMS, 20 years	Y	3 g	BR, HL, R	3–6 months	Y	5 years, >500	N	Y	N	Y
9	MD, 2 years	Y	5 g	BR, HL	3 months	Y	6 months, >20	N	Y	N	Y
10	BAMS, 11 years	Y	5 g	BR, HL	1 year	Y	5 years, >200	N	Y	N	Y

Abbreviations: A, Acidity; BR, Bowel regulation; HL, Hair loss; N, No; R, *Rasayana* (Immunomodulation); Y, Yes.

[a] Most physicians stated not having seen any side effects. In rare cases, where users did not comply with the dose prescribed and took higher doses, the experience of loose stools were seen probably due to laxative effect of Haritaki at higher doses.

[b] Physicians stated that they use Haritaki in pregnant women complaining of constipation due to iron preparations being prescribed during second trimester. Some of the physicians noted that use of Haritaki during lactating period also promotes lactation to some extent.

[c] Most physicians stated using Haritaki only in children above 10 years of age.

Narayana and colleagues have given an example of a similar nature and especially related to the dose of any botanical; Tulsi (*Ocimum sanctum*) can be seen in the published study (Narayana et al. 2014). Further, Narayana pointed out the most common research/scientific imprecisions occurring while working on botanicals for safety, quality and efficacy data (Narayana 2016a, 2016b).

10.4.2   APPROACH 2: ESTABLISHING SIMILARITY/DISSIMILARITY DATA OF THE BOTANICAL PREPARED USING MODIFIED PROCESS IN COMPARISON TO A HOSU MATERIAL

Currently botanicals are analysed by a battery of tests with a view to obtain and use standard botanicals that can provide batch-to-batch uniformity. This intention of obtaining uniformity is primarily to guarantee safety and efficacy through the quality control analysis. Available scientific approaches adopted for such testing involves the confirmation of identity, tests for physico-chemical quality, confirmation of absence or below acceptable limits of contaminants and an assay for presence and quantitative levels of marker compounds (India; Indian Pharmacopeia Commission 2018). The marker compounds may be either bioactive markers or simply analytical markers. Ability to analyse for one marker compound has now grown into the specification and quantification of a number of marker compounds (as many as eight in some herbs). In specific cases, testing for negative markers have also been adopted, as in the monograph on Kalmegh (*Andrographis paniculata*, Nees), in Indian Pharmacopoeia 2018, a test and limit have been prescribed for 14-deoxy-11,12-didehydroandrographalide content.

The above concept and approach is widely accepted globally and is reflected in quality specifications/monographs in various pharmacopoeias.

10.4.2.1 Need for New Thinking

The approach discussed above is based on an assumption that the safety and efficacy of a botanical can be linked to one or more marker compounds and their levels, apart from other parameters listed above. Most scientists believe and adopt tests for quantitative levels of marker compounds. This approach suffers from a lack of appreciation that in a botanical or processed botanical the safety and efficacy can be linked to only analysable organic compounds. It does not consider components of the botanicals that are not analysed in these specifications such as carbohydrates, starches, proteins, amino acids, fibres, vitamin like or metabolites of vitamins, minerals and metals that exist in the botanical and their role towards safety and efficacy. Most of these components do not form any part of the specifications either for qualitative or for quantitative estimations.

However advancement of scientific knowledge as well as the availability of a large number of solvents and vehicles other than those known during the time of traditional knowledge development has changed the scenario. Contemporary biological and chemical sciences have now given new processes and fractionation ability, which have been adopted by pharmaceutical technologies with a belief that fractionated botanicals provide higher potency. In such a scenario, analysis for the marker compounds discussed above may have limitations in that these marker compounds may be present in the current day solvent extraction or fractionation processes, while the traditionally processed botanical may not even show those marker compounds.

Another scenario often faced in an industrial setup is of supply chain management. The buying department only looks at marker compound–based specification as a requirement and in times of constraints or when the current supplier is not able to supply the material or for cost reduction purposes, opts to buy from other suppliers. The new supply may not fully comply with marker compound–based specification, which creates a serious situation in the firm. If this new supplier provides adequate safety profile data, firms often consider switching to the new supplier without much ado. Most often the finished supply specification is only looked into and no review of the process by which the material is produced takes place. A simple example could be – aqueous-extracted material, ethanolic extracted material, hydroethanolic extracted material, methanolic extracted material with or without steps of defatting, fractionation – each of these processes would yield differences in the presence and quantity of the markers. The ability to extrapolate the safety profile compared to a material processed as per traditional methods (e.g. HoSU) is the important aspect to be kept in mind. Readers of cutting edge research are aware of the time, energy and cost of generating complete safety data for any processed botanical.

10.4.2.2 A New Approach

This approach involves an attempt to generate multiple data points that can capture not just marker compounds but attempt to cover many components of the botanical or processed botanical. These data points can be plotted using appropriate statistical tools, one of which is becoming popular as Principle Components Analysis (PCA; Roussal 2010).

For data generation in this approach limitation to a chromatographic technique of marker compound analysis (HPLC [high-performance liquid chromatography] or GC [gas chromatography] or MPLC [medium pressure liquid chromatography]) is not adopted. The botanical or processed botanical is analysed by all analytical techniques to detect and get data of the range of components in the botanicals. These can include UV (ultraviolet–visible) spectra, IR (infrared) spectra, NMR (nuclear magnetic resonance), mass spectra, XRD (X-ray powder diffraction), XRF (X-ray fluorescence) spectra, ICP (inductively coupled plasma; either OES [optical emission spectrometry] or MS [mass spectroscopy]) or fluorescence spectra, powdered microscopy for various features to name a few.

Such data generation may be done with a sample that adopted a traditional processing method (with HoSU), a sample from an approved supplier, a sample from a new supplier, a sample produced by a modified or a new process and such other variations. The output of multiple point data generated is then plotted using the PCA technique that provides a comparative similarity or dissimilarity plots. If the new supplier or modified process material shows closely similar PCA output, it would be logical either to extrapolate the history of safe profile or to consider the new supplier's material to be closely similar to the current used material and switch to use the same. Of course this approach would require analysing the botanical by multiple analytical tools/equipment, but the savings of the need to generate exhaustive safety data outweighs the multiple testing otherwise needed.

As an example, the UV spectra, IR spectra, HPLC, NMR and mass data for 3 samples of *Terminalia chebula* (Haritaki, commonly called as Chebulic myrobalan) processed by different methods are provided here (Table 10.4; Figure 10.4). Also given are data from the physico-chemical analysis and quantitative testing for few marker compounds in the samples, performed using standard testing methods (Table 10.5). A typical PCA chart (Figure 10.5) is also provided as an example of how the similarity plots on a statistical tool adopted by this analysis (detailed references for exact analysis of the samples whose data is given here has not been provided).

The results of the PCA data will give information about the similarity or dissimilarity of the samples in comparison to the HoSU processed material. One can decide the acceptable similarity score as a part of decision-making – say any data that shows a similarity scope of above 90% as compared to the HoSU sample could be approvable for either switching to the new processed material or the new supplier material, without the need for any new safety assessment. As with other methodologies, generation of more data of this approach is necessary. A comparative study of pharmacological or biological activity of botanicals that are analysed by the current

TABLE 10.4
Sample Information

S. No.	Sample Name	Description
1	Sample 01	Traditionally prepared *Terminalia chebula* extract (HoSU extract).
		100 g of *Terminalia chebula* dry fruits were taken and boiled with 1.6 L of water till the extract was concentrated to 0.4 L. Filtered the extract and further completely dried under vacuum at 70°C. The yield of prepared extract was 45%.
2	Sample 02	HoSU extract prepared commercially using water as solvent, verified from manufacturer.
		Process method: RM is extracted with water, concentrated, spray dried and blended.
3	Sample 03	Methanolic extract prepared commercially, verified from manufacturer.
		Process method: RM is extracted with methanol, concentrated, vacuum dried and blended. The residual solvent levels comply with the pharmacopoeial limits.

marker compound approach or by the similarity analysis approach briefly described in this chapter would provide adequate basis for switching over to the new technique.

10.4.3 Approach 3: Preparing a Review Document on Published Scientific Literature to Support Data on Safety and Other Aspects of the Botanical

Before embarking on actual safety/toxicology studies on the botanical, the next part of the approach is to prepare a document that captures and reviews current published scientific literature on the botanical. This document can be along similar lines to the way one prepares a document for

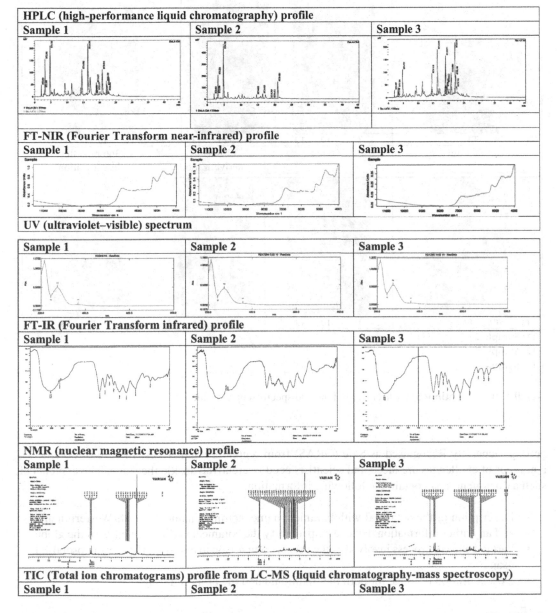

FIGURE 10.4 Chromatographic and spectroscopic profiles. *(Continued)*

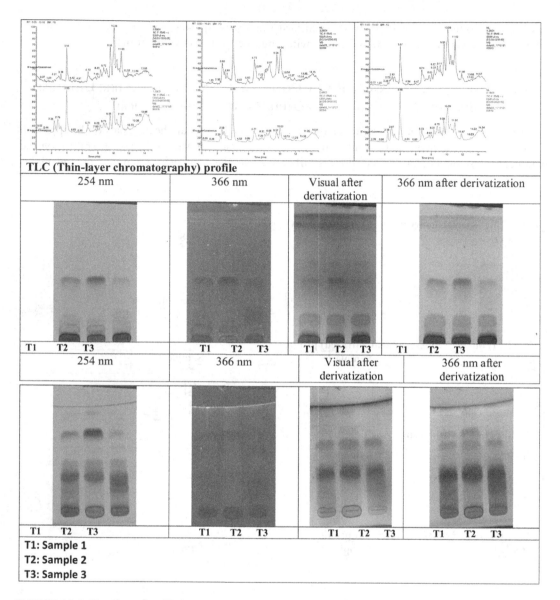

FIGURE 10.4 (Continued) Chromatographic and spectroscopic profiles.

getting Generally Recognised as Safe (GRAS) from regulatory authorities. In case of botanicals, a number of challenges are faced and scientists need to creatively tackle the same. The contents of such a document may contain the following information:

- Description of the botanical with botanical name, common name, English/Western name and any other information that can help identify the botanical in different parts of the globe
- Part to be used, process involved in the usage, comparison to traditional usage and proposed usage
- Dose, duration of usage for both the traditional and the proposed usage

TABLE 10.5

Quantification Results

Test Parameters	Sample 1	Sample 2	Sample 3
Ash value (%w/w)	3.0	8.0	2.1
Acid insoluble ash (%w/w)	0.15	0.50	0.50
Assay by UV (%w/w)			
Total polyphenol content	67.41	67.28	84.16
Assay by HPLC (%w/w)			
Chebulic acid	20.95	34.9	5.49
Gallic acid	4.65	12.13	2.58
Corilagin	5.28	1.59	4.76
TGG	10.67	2.37	9.47
Chebulagic acid	3.23	0.46	11.1
Ellagic acid	2.34	0.07	1.93
Chebulinic acid	3.78	15.42	13.44

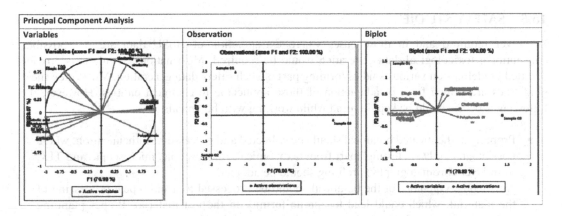

FIGURE 10.5   Principal component analysis plot (typical).

- Indications known and intended for use
- Published scientific literature giving adequate and crisp information on reported safety studies. These studies may be classified and given under headings such as *in vitro*, *in vivo* and any human data. Where available, any computational docking or predictive studies on safety may also be included. These information need to be properly referenced and important publications and full-length papers should be provided. Abstracts of published studies may also be included. In this section, it is important to clearly describe the botanical, part used, process adopted, dose tested, design of experiment, positive or negative control studied, interpretation and conclusions of the author, along with the data. If the study material has been tested for chemistry, details of the same should be given as well.

- Published scientific literature giving adequate information on pharmacology or pharmacodynamic or pharmacokinetic studies that would add value to the review of the safety
- Information on any regulatory aspects of the botanical, including listing or approval of the botanical under any category
- Information on pharmacopoeial monographs, if available
- Information on marketed products that have regulatory approvals giving the strength, nature, dose, duration of use and health benefits or indications of use
- Information on side effects, adverse events, advisories or cautions for usage, including those that apply to vulnerable populations
- All information in the document should be adequately referenced and the document must be reviewed by a competent scientist with his/her signature along with a brief CV of the reviewer

Challenges faced in preparing such a document include limited information available that can be accessed online or digitally, more information available in published books, some of which could be in languages other than English and some of the information may be in traditional texts that can only be read and interpreted by an expert on traditional knowledge.

Providing a well-written review document could assist in reducing the need for detailed toxicological studies, thus saving time and cost.

10.5   SAFETY STUDIES

Wherever required and in those cases where extrapolation of HoSU data are not possible, conventional toxicological data generation would be required. Most nations' regulations provide detailed guidelines on various studies forming part of such safety data generation. Most often these guidelines are drawn from or adaptation of those applicable to chemical entities. However, the following aspects should be kept in mind while working with botanicals:

- Properly authenticated botanical should be collected and processed. Authentication, where possible, using DNA testing apart from taxonomical, macroscopic, microscopic and TLC (thin-layer chromatography) profiling should be adopted.
- An adequate quantity of the botanical should be processed to avoid repeat processing of the material, which could lead to non-uniformity in the test material. Proper planning and computation of the total test material requirement for all studies, control sample requirements, requirements for quality assurance testing is recommended. A proper scaled up batch to obtain this total quantity should be taken under hygienic and good manufacturing practice procedures and properly documented.
- Adequate testing for quality, freedom from contaminants and compliance to microbial quality should be performed on the scaled up production and records of such testing and report properly documented.
- The produced material should be properly packed and stored in predefined conditions to protect the material.
- Documentation on issue for different testing to be prepared and preserved.
- Where a number of processing steps are involved, the document should record the yield at each stage and back calculate the quantity of the raw herb that should be prepared and kept. This will become the guide for computing the processed material quantity to be used for testing in animal toxicology or carcinogenicity and other studies where dose of the botanical would normally be available for the raw herb. Extractive value could be the other alternative for such computation.
- Most botanicals and processed botanicals provide challenges for administration to animals due to their insoluble nature in water, taste and quick settling nature. Wherever

suspending agents or solubilisers are used, the design of such studies should be carefully selected. Similar challenges occur when testing botanicals *in vitro*, due not only to poor solubility, but also due to the colour of the material, which may interfere with the parameters measured.

It is not possible to give details of conventional toxicology studies. However, common oversights occur in the design of such studies, especially related to dose computations. Standard guidelines are available for computing human equivalent dose (HED) for safety studies of traditional botanicals and/or their products (US Department of Health and Human Services 2005). Reproduced below is one such guideline (Table 10.6; Figure 10.6). Further, standard guidelines are available that help in computing the number of days that the botanical needs to be fed to specific laboratory animal in relation to complete human dosage regimen for the botanical. Improper computations in both the above designs are common missteps that generate unusable data.

TABLE 10.6
Calculating Human Equivalent Dose for Safety Studies of Traditional Botanicals and/or Their Products Based on Body Surface Area

Species	Weight (Kg)	Working Weight Range (Kg)	Body Surface Area (m²)	To Convert Animal Dose in mg/kg to Dose in mg/m², Multiply by k_m	To Convert Animal Dose in mg/kg to HED[a] in mg/kg, Either:	
					Divide animal dose by	Multiply animal dose by
Human						
Adult	60		1.62	37	–	–
Child[b]	20		0.80	25	–	–
Mouse	0.02	0.011–0.034	0.007	3	12.3	0.081
Hamster	0.08	0.047–0.157	0.016	5	7.4	0.135
Rat	0.15	0.08–0.27	0.025	6	6.2	0.162
Ferret	0.30	0.16–0.54	0.043	7	5.3	0.189
Guinea pig	0.40	0.208–0.700	0.05	8	4.6	0.216
Rabbit	1.8	0.90–3.0	0.15	12	3.1	0.324
Dog	10	5–17	0.50	20	1.8	0.541
Primates:						
Monkeys[c]	3	1.4–4.9	0.25	12	3.1	0.324
Marmoset	0.35	0.14–0.72	0.06	6	6.2	0.162
Squirrel monkey	0.60	0.29–0.97	0.09	7	5.3	0.189
Baboon	12	7–23	0.60	20	1.8	0.541
Micro-pig	20	10–33	0.74	27	1.4	0.730
Mini-pig	40	25–64	1.14	35	1.1	0.946

[a] Assumes 60 Kg human. For species not listed or for weights outside the standard ranges, HED can be calculated from the following formula:

HED = animal dose in mg/kg × (animal weight in kg/human weight in kg)$^{0.33}$.

[b] This km value is provided for reference only since healthy children will rarely be volunteers for phase 1 trials.

[c] For example, cynomolgus, rhesus, and stumptail.

$$\text{HED} \left(\frac{mg}{kg} \right) = \text{Animal dose} \left(\frac{mg}{kg} \right) \text{multipled by } \frac{\text{Animal km}}{\text{Human km}}$$

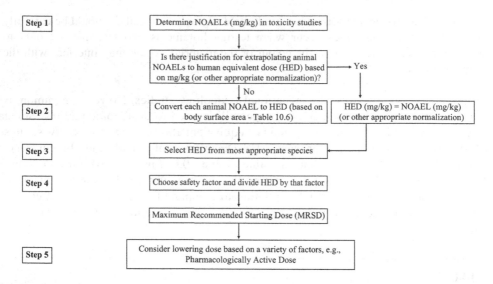

FIGURE 10.6 Steps to estimate starting dose in human studies. (*Abbreviation*: NOAEL, No observed adverse effect level.)

10.6 GUIDELINES FOR TOXICOLOGY EVALUATION

Schedule Y of the Drugs and Cosmetics Act, 1940 and Rules, 1945 of India gives conditions and durations of toxicology study (India; Director General of Health Services 2016; Deshpade and Nilesh 2018) to be conducted based on intended duration of treatment, including systemic/local/special toxicity (Table10.7a–c and repeated-dose toxicity studies) (Table 10.8). Reference to this Schedule is recommended to get complete details of the safety studies required by regulatory authorities while reviewing their application.

TABLE 10.7

(a) Systemic Toxicity Studies; (b) Local Toxicity Studies; (c) Special Toxicity Studies

Route of Administration	Duration of Proposed Human Administration	Human Phase(s) for Which Study Is Proposed to Be Conducted	Long-Term Toxicity Requirements
		a: Systemic Toxicity Studies	
Oral or Parenteral or Transdermal	Single dose or several doses in 1 day, up to 1 week	I, II, III	2 species, 2 weeks
	>1 week but up to 2 weeks	I, II, III	2 species, 4 weeks
	Up to 2 weeks	Marketing permission	2 species, 4 weeks
	>2 weeks but up to 4 weeks	I, II, III	2 species, equal to duration of human exposure
		Marketing permission	2 species, 12 weeks
	>4 weeks but up to 12 weeks	I, II, III	2 species, equal to duration of human exposure
		Marketing permission	2 species, 24 weeks

(Continued)

TABLE 10.7 (*Continued*)
(a) Systemic Toxicity Studies; (b) Local Toxicity Studies; (c) Special Toxicity Studies

Route of Administration	Duration of Proposed Human Administration	Human Phase(s) for Which Study Is Proposed to Be Conducted	Long-Term Toxicity Requirements
		a: Systemic Toxicity Studies	
	>12 weeks but up to 24 weeks	I, II, III	2 species, equal to duration of human exposure
		Marketing permission	2 species, rodent 24 weeks, non-rodent 36 weeks
	>24 weeks	I, II, III	2 species, rodent 24 weeks, non-rodent
		Marketing permission	36 weeks
Inhalation (general anaesthetics, aerosols)	Up to 2 weeks	I, II, III	2 species, 1 month (exposure time 3 h/day, 5 day/week)
	Up to 4 weeks	I, II, III	2 species, 12 weeks (exposure time 6 h/day, 5 day/week)
	>14 weeks	I,II,III	2 species, 24 weeks (exposure time 6 h/day, 5 day/week)
		b: Local Toxicity Studies	
Dermal	Up to 2 weeks	I, II	1 species, 4 weeks
		III	2 species, 4 weeks
	>2 weeks	I, II, III	2 species, 12 weeks
Ocular or Otic or Nasal	Up to 2 weeks	I, II	1 species, 4 weeks
		III	2 species, 4 weeks
	>2 weeks	I, II, III	2 species, 12 weeks
Vaginal or Rectal	Up to 2 weeks	I, II	1 species, 4 weeks
		III	2 species, 4 weeks
	>2 weeks	I, II, III	2 species, 12 weeks

c: Special Toxicity Studies

Male Fertility Study:
  Phase III in male volunteers/patients
Female Reproduction and Developmental Toxicity Studies:
  Segment II studies in 2 species; Phase II, III involving female patients of childbearing age
  Segment I study; Phase III involving female patients of childbearing age
  Segment III study; Phase III for drugs to be given to pregnant or nursing mothers for long periods or where there are indications of possible adverse effects on fetal development
Allergenicity/Hypersensitivity:
  Phase I, II, III – when there is a cause of concern or for parenteral drugs (including dermal application)
Photo-allergy or dermal photo-toxicity:
  Phase I, II, III – if the drug or a metabolite is related to an agent causing photosensitivity or the nature of action suggests such a potential
Genotoxicity:
  In vitro studies – Phase I
  Both *in vitro* and *in vivo* – Phase II, III
Carcinogenicity:
  Phase III – when there is a cause for concern, or when the drug is to be used for more than 6 months

TABLE 10.8
Repeated-Dose Toxicity Studies

	14–28 Days				84–182 Days			
	Rodent (Rat)		Non-Rodent (Dog or Monkey)		Rodent (Rat)		Non-Rodent (Dog or Monkey)	
Group	Male	Female	Male	Female	Male	Female	Male	Female
Control	6–10	6–10	2–3	2–3	15–30	15–30	4–6	4–6
Low dose	6–10	6–10	2–3	2–3	15–30	15–30	4–6	4–6
Intermediate dose	6–10	6–10	2–3	2–3	15–30	15–30	4–6	4–6
High dose	6–10	6–10	2–3	2–3	15–30	15–30	4–6	4–6

10.7 SCOPE FOR FURTHER FUTURE DEVELOPMENT

Currently, most studies on the generation of safety profile information and data on botanicals and their processed materials, in the absence of regulatory guidelines, adopt and stick to conventional toxicology studies that are meant for new chemical entities. There is also discussion in scientific circles on the need for generating carcinogenicity, teratogenicity and chromosomal aberration data on these botanicals, especially for those where there is known history of use. In conventional toxicology studies (reference Schedule Y) the dose, duration, routes of administration, animal species to be used (more than one) and number of animals in each group and of either sex are prescribed. Many scientists who have knowledge and expertise on botanicals with a history of use question whether all these requirements are necessary and whether testing on one species of animal in limited numbers for acute, sub-chronic, chronic and repeat dose administration studies might not be adequate. The science and regulatory understanding will emerge in the coming years, especially with botanical drugs being approved by the USFDA, as well as the growing momentum in the area of nutraceutical development. This subject itself justifies a complete chapter and is not covered here. The authors of this chapter strongly recommend the development of future regulatory provisions with cross-functional and cross-system scientists, physicians and regulators. Such cross-functional teams would need to recognise the strengths and weaknesses of each other's systems of healthcare practice, recipes, botanicals and competency in current biomedical and analytical science testing. Such interactions would lead to justifiable data generation saving time, energy and cost.

ACKNOWLEDGEMENTS

Approach 2 in principle is based on the concept and methods worked out by a team of scientists, including the first author along with a full team of Unilever R&D, Colworth/Shanbrook, UK, and Unilever R&D Bangalore, led by Paul Roussal. Thanks to the editorial group of Cutting Edge, Spinco Biotech, Chennai, India, and Mr Murali B, et al. for granting permission to use material from the paper published in Volume 7, Issue 9, January 2018, pp. 9–14. The data on Haritaki used in Approach 1, except the NMR spectra, were generated by M/S Natural Remedies, Bangalore, India. Acknowledgements are due to Ayurvidye Trust, Bangalore, India, for sponsoring the cost of NMR testing of the samples.

REFERENCES

Butler, M. S. (2008). Natural products to drugs: Natural product-derived compounds in clinical trials. *Natural Product Reports,* **25**(3), 475. doi:10.1039/b514294f.

Chunekar, K. C., and Pandeya, G. S. (2010). *Bhavaprakash Nighantu.* Varanasi, India: Chaukhamba Bharathi Academy.

Deshpade, S. W., and Nilesh, G. (2018). *Drugs & Cosmetics Act, 1940 and Rules, 1945.* Mumbai, India: Susmit Publishers.

European Commission. (1997). 'Human Consumption to a Significant Degree' Information and Guidance Document. Available from: https://ec.europa.eu/food/sites/food/files/safety/docs/novel-food_guidance_human-consumption_en.pdf.

European Commission. (2016). Report from the Commission to the European Parliament and the Council on the Development, Validation and Legal Acceptance of Methods Alternative to Animal Testing in the Field of Cosmetics (2013–2015). http://eur-lex.europa.eu/legal-content/EN/TXT/PDF/?uri=CELEX:52016DC0599&from=EN.

European Parliament and The Council of the European Union. (1997). Regulation (EC) No 258/97 of the European Parliament and of the Council of 27 January 1997 Concerning Novel Foods and Novel Food Ingredients. *Official Journal of the European Communities,* **40**, 1–6. https://eur-lex.europa.eu/legal-content/EN/TXT/PDF/?uri=CELEX:31997R0258&from=EN.

European Parliament and The Council of the European Union. (2015). Regulation (EU) 2015/2283 of the European Parliament and of the Council of 25 November 2015. *Euratom,* **327**, 1–22.

Gurib-Fakim, A. (2006). Medicinal plants: Traditions of yesterday and drugs of tomorrow. *Molecular Aspects of Medicine,* **27**(1), 1–93. doi:10.1016/j.mam.2005.07.008.

India. Department of AYUSH. (2010a). *The Ayurvedic Pharmacopoeia of India.* Vol. 1. Ministry of Health and Family Welfare, Government of India.

India. Department of AYUSH. (2010b). *The Ayurvedic Pharmacopoeia of India.* Vol. 2. Ministry of Health and Family Welfare, Government of India.

India. Department of Indian Systems of Medicine and Homeopathy, Ministry of Health and Family Welfare. (2003). *The Ayurvedic Formulary of India.* 2nd edition. New Delhi, India: The Controller of Publications.

India. Director General of Health Services, Ministry of Health and Family Welfare. (2016). *Drugs and Cosmetics Act, 1940 and Rules, 1945.* Central Drugs Standard Control Organisation, New Delhi, India. Available from: http://cdsco.nic.in/writereaddata/2016Drugs and Cosmetics Act 1940 & Rules 1945.pdf.

India. Food Safety Standards Authority. (2016). *Food Safety and Standards (Health Supplements, Nutraceuticals, Food for Special Dietary Use, Food for Special Medical Purpose, Functional Food and Novel Food) Regulations 2016.* Ministry of Health and Family Welfare, Government of India.

India. Food Safety Standards Authority. (2017). *Food Safety and Standards (Health Supplements, Nutraceuticals, Food for Special Dietary Use, Food for Special Medical Purpose, Functional Food and Novel Food) Regulations 2016.* Ministry of Health and Family Welfare, Government of India.

India. Indian Pharmacopeia Commission, Ministry of Health and Family Welfare. (2018). Herbs, Processed Herbs and Herbal Products. In *Indian Pharmacopoeia,* pp. 3165–3283. Ghaziabad, India.

Liao, Y. (2006). *Traditional Chinese Medicine.* Cultural China Series. China International Press. https://books.google.co.in/books?id=DgT6xWMgu4QC.

Murthy, S. (2008). *Bhavaprakasa of Bhavamisra.* Volume 1. Varanasi, India: Chowkhamba Krishnadas Academy.

Narayana, D. B. A. (2016a). Evidence for ayurvedic products' efficacy: The devil is in details. *Ancient Science of Life,* **35**(4), 193–194. doi:10.4103/0257-7941.188176.

Narayana, D. B. A. (2016b). Improving quality of research on herbals and its reporting. *Ancient Science of Life,* **36**(1), 1–2. doi:10.4103/0257-7941.195413.

Narayana, D. B. A., Manohar, R., Mahapatra, A., Sujithra, R. M. and Aramya, A. R. (2014). Posological considerations of Ocimum sanctum (Tulasi) as per ayurvedic science and pharmaceutical sciences. *Indian Journal of Pharmaceutical Sciences,* **76**(3), 240–245.

Nayak, B. (2014). *Ayurvedline: Ayurvedic Drug Index.* XV. Bangalore, India: Seetharam Prasad.

Paterson, I. and Anderson, E. A. (2005). Chemistry. The renaissance of natural products as drug candidates. *Science,* **310**(5747), 451–453. doi:10.1126/science.1116364.

Qu, L., Zou, W., Wang, Y. and Wang, M. (2018). European regulation model for herbal medicine: The assessment of the EU monograph and the safety and efficacy evaluation in marketing authorisation or registration in member states. *Phytomedicine,* **42**(March), 219–25. doi:10.1016/j.phymed.2018.03.048.

Reddy, K. R. C. (2015). *Bhaisajya Kalpana Vijnanam.* Varanasi, India: Chaukhambha Sanskrit Bhawan.

Rishton, G. M. (2008). Natural products as a robust source of new drugs and drug leads: Past successes and present day issues. *American Journal of Cardiology,* **101**(10A), 43D–49D. doi:10.1016/j.amjcard.2008.02.007.

Roussal, P. (2010). "Poster Presented in the One Day Symposium on Assessment of Safety of Naturals, Unilever Research."

Tripathi, B. (2010). *Chaukhamba Ayurvijnan Granthamala.* Vol. I & II. Varanasi, India: Chaukhamba Surabharati Prakashan.

USA. Food and Drug Administration (USFDA). (1994). *Dietary Supplement Health and Education Act of 1994.* US Department of Health and Human Services, no. 1. Available from: https://ods.od.nih.gov/About/DSHEA_Wording.aspx.

USA. Food and Drug Administration (USFDA). (2005). *Guidance for Industry: Estimating the Maximum Safe Starting Dose in Initial Clinical Trials for Therapeutics in Adult Healthy Volunteers.* Center for Drug Evaluation and Research (CDER). Available from: https://www.fda.gov/downloads/drugs/guidances/ucm078932.pdf.

World Health Organization. (1998). *Guidelines for the appropriate use of herbal medicines.* Geneva, Switzerland: World Health Organization.

World Health Organization. (2000). *General guidelines for methodologies on research and evaluation of traditional medicine.* Geneva, Switzterland: World Health Organization.

World Health Organization. (2013). *WHO Traditional Medicine Strategy 2014–2023.* Geneva, Switzerland: World Health Organization.

Section III

Regulation

Section II

Regulation

11 Korea's Health Functional Food Classification

Shin Seung Chul

CONTENTS

11.1 KOREA CLASSIFIES HEALTH FUNCTIONAL FOODS AS FOOD

According to this, the expression of having the effect of treatment or the prevention of diseases cannot be used on health functional food (HFF).

Although it is categorised as food, unlike general food management, an HFF is a food produced by using materials or ingredients that have helpful functionality for the human body. Thus, HFFs should be passed as having a certain level of functionality after evaluating their functionality and safety, and HFFs are managed by stricter standards, specifications and manufacturing standards than normal food.

11.2 THE POLICY ENVIRONMENT FOR HEALTH FUNCTIONAL FOODS IN KOREA

As in other developed countries, Korea has become increasingly concerned for self-care management due to increased chronic diseases caused by dietary habit such as diabetes, geriatric diseases and ageing society. In line with this, Korea's economic scale and level of medical care have developed rapidly over the past several decades, and as a result of this, people have become more interested in maintaining health, improving physical functioning and healthy ageing beyond merely supplementing food for survival or epicureanism.

Due to these economic and technological changes in the environment, the demand for *health functional foods* has increased, and the market for HFF in Korea is also growing rapidly. The Korean HFF market grew at a compound annual growth rate (CAGR) of 11.3% from 2010 to 2015, and its performance rate for production and imports in 2015 grew 16.7% year-on-year to about $2 billion. Domestic production was about $1.6 billion and imports were about $400 million.

As the market for HFF expands, the need for policy management, such as securing safety and protecting consumers' interests, is increasing.

11.3 THE ORGANISATION AND LAW FOR HEALTH FUNCTIONAL FOODS

11.3.1 HEALTH FUNCTIONAL FOODS ACT

As the distribution of HFFs has expanded, *Health Functional Foods Act* 2002 was enacted to manage HFFs separately that had been managed in the same way as normal foods. Previously, an HFF was classified as 'Special purpose food' or 'Dietary supplements' in the Food Sanitation Act. However, safety management of foreign dietary supplements was difficult, and there was a problem that the function of health food was exaggerated to mislead consumers. To solve these problems, the government enacted laws and ordinances and strengthened the safety management of HFFs by strengthening inspection of foreign dietary supplements, prohibiting customs clearance and establishing grounds for punishment for false/exaggerative advertisement.

11.3.2 THE HEALTH FUNCTIONAL FOODS MANAGEMENT ORGANISATION

The Health Functional Foods Act is under the responsibility of the Ministry of Food and Drug Safety (MFDS), and each of its laws is managed functionally by the various departments in MFDS.

The Health Functional Food Policy Division is in charge of establishing management plans for HFFs and revising laws and ordinances, as well as overseeing safety management for adverse events, hazardous functional foods collection, good manufacturing practice certification and the monitoring of false/exaggerative advertising. The Food Standard Planning office is in charge of standards and specifications of HFFs, including presence of heavy metals, rate of rancidity and re-evaluation of *functional ingredients*. The Nutritional and Functional Food Research Team in the National Institute of Food and Drug Safety Evaluation is responsible for evaluating the safety and functionality of the *functional ingredients* when applying for other ingredients not notified as *functional ingredients*.

The MFDS has six local authorities. Each provincial office carries out tasks such as accepting a report of business and monitoring HFFs in the administrative area. The *Health Functional Foods Act* requires the Health Functional Food Deliberation Committee to conduct investigations and deliberation at the request of the Minister of Drug Administration. The Health Functional Food Deliberation Committee is divided into six sub-committees: (1) Policy, (2) Approval of Functional Ingredients and Standards, (3) Functionality Claim Labelling and Advertisement Review, (4) Human Body Study Evaluation, (5) Abnormal Case Evaluation and (6) Re-evaluation of Functional Ingredients.

11.3.3 HEALTH FUNCTIONAL FOODS MANAGEMENT POLICY

If we look at changes in HFF policy so far, the policy has shifted toward strengthening overall safety management. Since the law was enacted in 2002 and enforced in 2004, the monitoring of false/exaggerative advertising has been conducted since 2006, and media such as the Internet, newspapers and broadcasting have been monitored as well.

In addition, the MFDS introduced the *good manufacturing practice (GMP)*, which is the management to produce high-quality HFFs. The approved formulation types for HFFs were expanded further to capsules, tablets, syrups, gels and jellies in 2008. To protect consumers, as the regulations on false/exaggerative advertising became stronger, the MFDS introduced the pre-advertising review system in 2010. In 2013, the MFDS reorganised its internal organisation by launching the *illegal food monitoring team* to strengthen the crackdown on false/exaggerative advertising. Recently, the MFDS introduced the *re-evaluation* system for HFFs in 2017.

11.4 FUNCTIONAL INGREDIENT AND NUTRIENT MANAGEMENT

11.4.1 APPROVAL OF FUNCTIONAL INGREDIENTS

Functional ingredients are classified into announced and individually approved. Functional ingredients include food materials widely recognised to be functional such as red ginseng and green tea. Essential nutrients such as vitamins and minerals are also classified into announced ingredients.

If a seller wants to manufacture and process other food materials and sell them as health functional foods, he or she must obtain individual approval. A manufacturer or importer submits data on functional, safety, and standard and applies for approval.

The approval requires the following ten items: (1) the summary of the entire submission, (2) origin, development status, domestic and overseas approval and use status, (3) data on manufacturing methods, (4) data on the characteristics of the functional ingredient, (5) data on standards, test methods and report for functional ingredients, (6) data on standards and test methods for toxic substances, (7) data related to safety, (8) data on functionality, (9) data on level quantity of intake and precautions, (10) data for checking whether it is the same as or similar to medicine.

The MFDS asks the Health Functional Food Deliberation Committee for advice on the functional ingredient submitted, and the deliberation committee evaluates the standards/specifications and carries out the raw materials approval review.

The Human Body study Evaluation Sub-Committee evaluates reports of human body studies about safety and functionality. This sub-committee consists of experts such as doctors, pharmacists, doctors of Korean medicine and professors in various fields specialising in blood vessels, digestion, nervous system, organ and other physiological activity.

Through the operation of the Good Review Practice (GRP), the MFDS enhanced the expertise of HFF examiners and improved the consistency of approval and evaluation. In order to ensure smooth operation of the GRP, guidelines and training programs have been implemented.

11.4.2 CLASSIFYING FUNCTIONALITIES OF HEALTH FUNCTIONAL FOODS

The functionalities are classified into both the *disease risk reduction function* and the *bioactive function*, depending on the effect. The disease risk reduction function is recognised when the submitted functional data indicates a reduction in the risk of disease occurrence and the level of ensured scientific evidence is high enough to reach a significant scientific agreement. The physiological activity function is recognised if the submitted functional data appears to show a special effect on a body function or a biological activity of a human body.

The functionalities are divided into eight major categories – memory improvement, skin health, liver health, intestinal health, eye health, dental health, circulatory system related, body fat reduction, joint/bone health – so a total of 32 functionalities are recognised.

11.4.3 MANAGEMENT SAFETY OF FUNCTIONAL INGREDIENTS

There are nutritional ingredients (saturated fat, trans fats, sugars and sodium) that could cause nutritional imbalance due to overeating. Thus, it is necessary to set the content standard and comply with them so that consumers can be provided with high-quality HFFs.

As consumer interest in HFF increases, industrial companies are developing various functional ingredients as natural materials. Raw materials that are toxic or have a pharmacological effect are often not suitable for HFF, but there are cases where the industry is studying such materials for commercialisation.

In order to prevent industrial research and development in advance, and to secure the safety of HFFs, some raw materials that are likely to have side effects or toxicity and other raw materials that are not suitable for the health effect of HFFs are listed on and announced as 'raw materials that cannot be used in health functional foods'.

11.4.4 RE-EVALUATION OF FUNCTIONAL INGREDIENTS

In May 2016, the Health Functional Foods Act was amended to introduce a re-evaluation system for the safety and functionality of existing functional ingredients. The re-evaluation is conducted periodically (every 10 years) in accordance with the priorities; it is also conducted on a regular basis in case of urgency. Review of clinical scientific facts opposite to the basis of functional approval, a surge of abnormal case and other social needs are reviewed as well.

11.5 MANUFACTURING MANAGEMENT

11.5.1 ITEM MANUFACTURE REPORT

If a manufacturer licensed by the HFF manufacturing business wants to manufacture HFFs, he/she must report the manufacture of HFFs. The registration of contents includes the location and contact information for the manufacturer, the type of product (e.g. red ginseng product, probiotic product, etc.), form (liquid, capsule, etc.), packaging method, functionality, manufacturing method and reference standard.

11.5.2 INSPECTION OF AUTHENTICITY OF FUNCTIONAL INGREDIENTS

The functional ingredients with components likely to be mixed with similar raw materials should be inspected and confirmed in accordance with the test method prescribed by MFDS and the records should be kept for 2 years. The subjects of the inspection of authenticity of the functional ingredients are as follows: it is difficult to distinguish it from other raw materials with the naked eye, and there is a possible risk of harm caused by the mixture.

11.5.3 SELF-QUALITY INSPECTION

The manufacturer shall inspect whether the manufactured HFF meets the standards and keep the record for 2 years. If it is difficult for the manufacturer who has inspection duty to carry out the inspection directly, the manufacturer can entrust this to a test/inspection organisation. If there is a risk of harm or violation of standards, the manufacturer shall immediately collect all of the HFF in distribution and report it to the MFDS.

11.5.4 GMP Certification

GMP certification was established and operated in order to organically and systematically manage the manufacture of HFFs. A store that has been granted a license to operate an HFF manufacturing business may apply for the GMP-certified designation after applying at least three times. The MFDS will evaluate the factory according to the GMP evaluation standard for the application. If it accomplishes the specified requirements, it can be recognised as a GMP-certified factory. After being recognised as a GMP-certified store, it can be requested as a consigned manufacturer by other HFF industry members.

In February 2016, the Health Functional Food Act was revised and the GMP application was gradually imposed according to the sales volume under obligation. Existing manufacturers have stepped up to 21 per year, and new manufacturers should apply for GMP certification when seeking license approval. In order to facilitate the early settlement and activation of the system, the MFDS is providing on-the-spot technical support consultation for full implementation.

Designation and follow-up management of GMP are carried out by professional workers who are trained as GMP directors through the 'education and training of health functional foods GMP director'. The education and training for the excellent HFF manufacturing standard guideline is aimed at public officials in charge of the field. The education and training courses are carried out through specialised and systematic education programmes, and it appoints excellent manpower as the director.

11.6 DISTRIBUTION MANAGEMENT

11.6.1 Traceability System

The traceability system manages information through each stage from production, distribution and sales to tracking down products in case of problems and taking necessary measures. The Korean traceability system is applied to powdered milk, infant food and HFFs.

11.6.2 Health Functional Food Labelling System

To provide consumers with accurate information on HFFs and to help them make the right choice, the *Health Functional Foods Act* stipulates labelling standards. HFFS are required to be labelled with the phrase 'health functional food', design and nutrition information, approved functional contents and intake standards (daily intake, intake method and caution when taking food). If a manufacturer wants to label and advertise the functionality, it should get a prior review by the 'Functional claim label/Advertisement Review Sub-committee'. The Functionality claim Label/Advertisement Review Subcommittee is composed of various HFF experts such as food science, nutrition, medicine, advertising, academics, law experts, consumer groups and industry.

HFFs contain functional ingredients or nutrients useful for the human body, but there are limitations on functional expression. The citizen surveillance system is currently in operation, so if people report false/exaggerated advertising, they can be paid rewards so the system encourages people's participation.

11.6.3 Abnormal Case Management System

As both the number of HFF products and the consumption rates are increasing, reporting of abnormal cases is continuously expanding. If an abnormal case occurs at the distribution stage, the manufacturer/importer should report the fact and recall all of the products. In order to protect consumers from such cases, if consumers who have suffered from the same damage request collection and inspection, the MFDS conducts an examination of the product. When many consumers (20 or more people) with the same damage request collection and inspection of products from corresponding companies, the system operates as a quick response team composed of public officials and related experts. The quick response team takes charge of the on-site inspection and toxicity data review. The results of analysing the above cases or the contents of the administrative investigation measures would be announced to the concerned consumers over text message or email.

11.6.4 OVERSEAS DIRECT PURCHASE MANAGEMENT

In terms of affordable prices and a variety of products, Korean overseas direct purchases are also steadily increasing. The same applies to healthcare foods, and thus, the MFDS is strengthening collection inspection on overseas Internet sales products.

11.7 OTHER SUPPORTS

11.7.1 EDUCATION AND INFORMATION PROVISION

Consumer education is promoted every year for middle-aged and elderly people, which are the main classes interested in HFFs. Manufacturers, importers and sellers must undergo mandatory education and training to secure safety and improve quality. Various other information such as laws, permits, accreditation and registration related to HFFs is provided through the Food Safety Information Portal (http://www.foodsafetykorea.go.kr) operated by the MFDS. The site provides information in real time, divided into 'Domestic product' – which is manufactured with permission – and 'Imported product' – which is sold after import registration – so that consumers can check information such as product name, manufacturer (import company), functional content, ingestion method, precautions for ingestion, standards and specifications.

11.7.2 MULTIPLE SUPPORT FOR HEALTH FUNCTIONAL FOOD ACTIVATION

With interest in HFFs increasing, interest in the development of HFF ingredients by industry, academia and stakeholders is increasing as well. There is a growing demand for consultation and education on the provision of correct information on HFFs and on regulations as to what can be recognised as functional ingredients of HFFs. To solve these various demands, the necessity of counselling and education for the preparation of materials for sellers preparing approval of functional ingredient for HFF is continuously raised. Since 2011, the 'Health Functional Food Expert Training Course' has been established to promote understanding of the industry. It is conducted by the Korea Human Resources Development Institute for Health and Welfare and seeks to revitalise the industry.

12 Phytopharmaceuticals
Unique Regulatory Category with Immense Potential for Medical Unmet Needs

Chandra Kant Katiyar

CONTENTS

Investment in pharmaceutical research and development has increased substantially over time. However, a corresponding increase in output in terms of new drugs has not appeared (Pammolli et al. 2011). Pammolli et al. (2011) examined the reason for the decline of Research & Development (R&D) productivity in pharmaceuticals over the past 2 decades and found it to be associated with a higher concentration of R&D investment in the areas with a high risk of failure corresponding to unmet therapeutic needs.

The advent of combinatorial chemistry has provided new hope of higher success rates for new chemical entities. However, even this scientific development failed to improve the success rate in new drug discovery (Chandrakant et al. 2012).

Both of the above factors lead to the 'back to nature' approach. The assumption that plants require less research acts as a barrier in this approach. On the contrary because plants contain multiple phytochemical compounds, they need much greater and more sophisticated science and technology inputs compared to synthetic drugs.

Lifestyle diseases normally have multiple factors, so the treatment has to be multi targeted. Plant extracts, therefore, appear to be one of the best options for drug development. With a view to develop plant-based drugs with greater scientific input, the Government of India considered the introduction of a new category of drug called phytopharmaceuticals.

The journey of phytopharmaceuticals began almost a decade ago when the then–drugs controller of India formed a committee under the chairmanship of Dr Nitya Anand and including Dr S.S. Handa, Dr D.B.A. Narayan, Professor R.H. Singh and Dr C.K. Katiyar (author) to prepare and recommend rules for the introduction of phytopharmaceuticals under the category of new drugs. The committee submitted its report, which was later shared with the Department of AYUSH, which raised objections that were further negotiated. Final rules were published on 30 November 2015.

Narayana and Katiyar (2013) have provided a thorough overview of the process behind phytopharmaceuticals. Per the Gazette Notification dated 30 November 2015, phytopharmaceuticals have been defined as:

'Phytopharmaceutical drug' includes purified and standardised fraction with defined minimum four bio-active or phyto-chemical compounds (qualitatively and quantitatively assessed) of an extract of a medicinal plant or its part, for internal or external use of human beings or animals for diagnosis, treatment, mitigation of any disease or disorder but does not include administration by parenteral route.

With introduction of the category of phytopharmaceutical drugs in the Drugs and Cosmetics Act 1940 and rules 1945, India has become the first country in the world to introduce fractions of plant extracts to be developed on the lines of and treated on par with synthetic drugs through the Gazette Notification dated 30 November 2015.

12.1 STAKEHOLDERS

The phytopharmaceutical sector has the following stakeholders:

- Ayurvedic industry
- R&D-based pharmaceutical industry
- Regulators
- Public-funded research lab
- Prescribers from modern medicines
- Prescribers from AYUSH
- Academic institutions
- Consumers/patients

12.1.1 AYURVEDIC INDUSTRY

A look at the current market size of Ayurvedic medicine reveals that the Ayurvedic industry has failed to meet the popularity and expectations of consumers, doctors and patients. One of the reasons is the fact that this industry has always taken shelter behind the concept of traditional use, relying on ancient texts for evidence of efficacy rather than doing high-end science.

A survey of the market most likely would show that cough syrup, menstrual cycle regulators, aphrodisiacs, immunomodulators and digestive aids are some of the categories where almost every company has its products, but the claims are mostly ingredient based. Somehow or other, unfortunately the stakeholders of AYUSH businesses lack the willingness to invest or the patience to wait for 3–5 years before a new product is launched.

At the same time this industry is also not willing to face the competition from the R&D-based pharmaceutical industry and, therefore, is expected to resist the introduction of phytopharmaceuticals that would be hard core science based developmental of herb-based products.

12.1.2 R&D-BASED PHARMACEUTICAL INDUSTRY

Fifteen to 20 years ago, R&D-based pharmaceutical companies forayed into herbal drugs that were mostly based upon Ayurvedic products. Even these companies lacked the zeal to invest in science before the products were launched. They were willing to conduct only as much science as would provide the patent for the product. In parallel, after the turmeric patent case, the Government of India introduced a rule in the Indian Patent Act debarring any product patent emanating from the Indian System of medicines. In addition to that the Supreme Court of India passed a judgment that was interpreted by the Indian Medical Association as meaning that allopathic doctors should not prescribe Ayurvedic medicines. Because all of the pharmaceutical industries have access only to allopathic doctors, this was another big blow for them, and it also acted as a big disincentive for the R&D-based pharmaceutical industry, most of which eventually withdrew from the business of herbals.

Phytopharmaceuticals as a new drug category have been particularly targeted by such R&D-based pharmaceutical companies. This class of drug would take care of both of their concerns:

1. The product would be patentable since it is fraction of the extract and
2. Being licensed as a modern medicine, there would be no bar on their prescription by allopathic doctors

12.1.3 REGULATORS

The R&D-based pharmaceutical industry has been lobbying for patentability and desirability of prescription of products through doctors. Phytopharmaceuticals is a new drug category offers opportunity for both. The category shall be regulated by the Drugs Controller General (India) where they regulate all other allopathic medicines. However, there is a grey area as to whether non-allopathic doctors shall also to be permitted to prescribe phytopharmaceuticals.

Professor R.H. Singh from the faculty of Ayurveda, Banaras Hindu University, in the very first meeting of the Nitya Anand Committee had advised maintaining the provision of phytopharmaceuticals being prescribed by Ayurvedic doctors as well. However, the published Gazette notification does not have any mention of this fact although permissibility of this prescription may be beyond its scope.

12.1.4 PUBLIC-FUNDED RESEARCH LABORATORIES

Public-funded research labs like the Council of Scientific and Industrial Research (CSIR) are important stakeholders for phytopharmaceuticals because they already might have candidates for which regulation was a grey area. Being science-led organisations, several CSIR laboratories like Central Drug Research Institute (CDRI), Lucknow and Indian Institute of Integrative Medicine (IIIM) Jammu have several fractions of extracts that would not see light of day because they could not be treated as Ayurvedic medicines due to regulatory constraints. These products, therefore, faced a crisis of identity. The introduction of phytopharmaceuticals is a boon for such laboratories sitting on the fractions with high level of scientific studies.

12.1.5 PRESCRIBERS FROM MODERN MEDICINE

Practitioners of modern medicine are very selective when it comes to prescribing Ayurvedic medicines. Barring a few eminent companies, they usually prefer not to prescribe Ayurvedic medicines. Advisories from the Indian Medical Association suggesting penal action against doctors found guilty of prescribing non-Ayurvedic medicines also became a deterrent.

The interpretation of the Indian Medical Association that the Supreme Court has barred the prescription of Ayurvedic medicines, coupled with perception of less scientific evidence, has discouraged practitioners from prescribing these products. Phytopharmaceuticals takes care of both of these concerns and, therefore, may be ideal for physicians of modern medicine.

12.1.6 PRESCRIBERS FROM AYUSH

Prescribers from AYUSH would have the opportunity of prescribing scientifically developed products that have been properly evaluated for safety and efficacy through toxicity studies and clinical trials. Introduction of these products would open up a new era for AYUSH practitioners.

12.1.7 ACADEMIC INSTITUTIONS

Most of the research on herbs and their products in terms of pharmacognosy and phytochemistry is currently happening at pharmacy colleges, a few medical colleges and research institutions like the Indian Council of Medical Research, Council of Scientific and Industrial Research. Encouragement of research on Ayurvedic products by successive governments in the past few decades has opened up sources of research funding from multiple government agencies such as the Department of Science and Technology (DST) and Department of Biotechnology (DBT). Many academic institutions have submitted academic research projects for funding to these agencies. Earlier funding agencies were receiving many projects for basic research, but now they are focussing on more product-oriented projects. The introduction of phytopharmaceuticals is expected to create an additional rush of projects to these funding agencies.

12.1.8 CONSUMERS/PATIENTS

The trust of consumers in herbal products has been steadily increasing. The changing preference of consumers has forced companies to innovate to suit them. Phytopharmaceuticals are not likely to be launched as Over The Counter (OTC) products, so they would primarily target patients either as co-therapy or as mainstay therapy providing benefits by both these routes.

12.2 THERAPEUTIC POTENTIAL

By definition, phytopharmaceuticals are fractions of plant extracts and are therefore enriched with multiple phytochemical compounds, meeting the requirement of multi-component drugs for multi-target diseases. Phytopharmaceuticals can be used as:

1. Mainstay therapy
2. Complementary/adjuvant therapy
3. Safer alternative to synthetic drugs

12.2.1 MAINSTAY THERAPY

Following the lead of traditional medicines, phytopharmaceutical can be useful as a mainstay therapy in chronic disorders that include conditions like arthritis, gastroenterological problems, respiratory disorders, psychosomatic problems, stress, anxiety related issues and other disorders.

For example, *Boswellia serrata* has now assumed the status of almost essential component for any product for joint care. It has been subjected to thorough phytochemical studies and a few active principles have also been isolated. However, this does not mean that the resin of this plant does not contain other active compounds. Enough research has not yet been done on the primary metabolites of Boswellia. This may have a major role to play in further enhancing the activity of Boswellia in combinations of such primary and secondary metabolites that may lead to an interesting phytopharmaceutical product. Similarly, *Withania somnifera* is one of the most recognised anti-stress products.

Many chemical studies have been done, but a lot more is required to explore its potential as a phyto-pharmaceutical product. There are other similar examples, too numerous to include here.

12.2.2 COMPLEMENTARY/ADJUVANT USE

It is a well-known fact that there is no cure for lifestyle disorders, and patients end up using a drug for almost their whole life. Most of the time allopathic drugs are consumed that have their own side effects. Phytopharmaceuticals may play a major role in complimentary or adjuvant use to:

1. Delay dose escalation of conventional medicines
2. Delay complications of diseases
3. Alleviate or minimise side effects of drugs
4. Improve efficacy of conventional treatment

12.2.3 SAFER ALTERNATIVE TO SYNTHETIC DRUGS

This is an interesting area of extension for phytopharmaceuticals. There are herbs that provide similar benefits to some of the most effective synthetic compounds like aspirin, statins and alprazolam, as well as for gastric acid regulators like proton pump inhibitors. The development of phytopharmaceutical using the discovery route high-throughput screening (HTS) to identify which fraction is an effective phytopharmaceutical product may be safer than current conventional medicines.

12.3 HOW ARE PHYTOPHARMACEUTICALS DIFFERENT FROM ASU DRUGS?

Several stakeholders such as the pharmaceutical or Ayurvedic industries are still confused as to how phytopharmaceutical drugs differ from Ayurvedic drugs. The characteristic features of both of these categories of drugs are given below to assist in their differentiation.

Sl. No.	Attributes	Products Licensed as Ayurvedic Medicines Made Using Botanicals as Actives	Products Licensed as New Drugs (Phytopharmaceuticals)
1	Manufacturing license and marketing authorisation	As proprietary Ayurvedic medicine issued by licensing authority of the state in which the manufacture is undertaken	As a new drug whose import or marketing is authorised by the Drug Controller General of India (DCGI) Central Drug Standard Control Organisation (CDSCO)
2	Number of herbs or botanicals	Can be single or combination of more than one, with each ingredient being listed in the authoritative texts of the First Schedule, or their processed materials including extracts as permitted under Chapter IV-A of Drugs and Cosmetics Act and Rules (DCAR)	A single botanical to begin with. Combining more than one is not barred, but would need more scientific data on the rationale, interactions and other aspects that are much more difficult to generate
3	Source of the botanical	Has to be mentioned in one of the authoritative texts of Ayurveda as per First Schedule of DCAR	Can be any botanical form any part of globe
4	Combination with mineral or metal	Permitted as per Drugs & Cosmetics Rules	Not permitted
5	Extracts of botanicals	Extracts of herbs as per Chapter IV-A applicable to Ayurveda	Purified/fractionated extracts that meet the definition of phytopharmaceutical and needs to be supported by scientific data. Crude extracts not permitted

(Continued)

Sl. No.	Attributes	Products Licensed as Ayurvedic Medicines Made Using Botanicals as Actives	Products Licensed as New Drugs (Phytopharmaceuticals)
6	Usage of approved medicine	To be sold and used as per Ayurvedic regulations and normally to be taken with advice from Ayurvedic physicians where prescribed	Under the prescription of a Registered Medical Practitioner/ Physician (registered with Medical Council of India, requiring a minimum MBBS degree)
7	Regulatory requirements (RM quality)	As per Ayurvedic Pharmacopeia of India (API) or in-house specifications for extracts or specifications adopted based on monographs in standard books like Indian Council of Medical Research (ICMR)/Indian Pharmacopeia (IP)/British Pharmacopeia (BP)/United States Pharmacopeia (USP)	Adequate testing for the phytopharmaceutical, which includes qualitative/quantitative testing for four compounds that may be either bioactive or analytical markers with other applicable physicochemical parameters
8	Chemistry, manufacturing controls	Information basis authoritative textual process and modifications if any along with in process Quality Control tests	Detailed information describing the process of phytopharmaceutical along with information on the medicinal plants and their passport data from which phyto-compound is manufactured
9	Preclinical requirement	Not mandatory in all cases	Mandatory
10	Clinical trials	Not mandatory in all cases	Mandatory from Phase I to Phase IV in all cases

We believe that, with this notification, a new route for drug development has been opened that can actually be a sunrise sector for the Indian Pharmaceutical industry and the various national research laboratories and academic institutions. This can happen while Ayurvedic medicines also flourish. The authors suggest not only bringing awareness of this regulation to various stakeholders, but also promoting training and discussion around phytopharmaceutical drug development. The regulations provide protection to traditional medicines, but also promote botanical drug development.

12.4   REGULATORY REQUIREMENTS FOR PHYTOPHARMACEUTICAL DRUGS

The Government of India Gazette Notification dated 30 November 2015 has finalised the regulatory requirements for phytopharmaceutical drugs. As per the requirement, information is to be submitted under Part–I and Part–II of Appendix-1B. For convenience Appendix-1B is reproduced below with the comments from author wherever appropriate.

APPENDIX-1B

Data to be submitted along with application to conduct clinical trial or import or manufacture of a phytopharmaceutical drug in the country

PART – I

Author comment:

   This part is related to the information already available in the public domain. A compilation of the same is desired to be provided in as much details as possible under the following headings.

1.1 A brief description or summary of the phytopharmaceutical drug giving the botanical name of the plant (including vernacular or spiritual name, wherever applicable), formulation and route or administration, dosages, therapeutic class for which it is indicated and the claims to be made for the phytopharmaceutical product.

Author's comment:

Summary of the phytopharmaceutical drug along with the complete botanical name, the authority and other vernacular names of the plant, route of administration, dosage, therapeutic class and the claims to be made on phytopharmaceuticals need to be provided under this heading.

1.2 Published literature including information on plant or product or phytopharmaceutical drug, as a traditional medicine or as an ethnomedicine and provide reference to books and other documents, regarding composition, process prescribed, dose or method of usage, proportion of the active ingredients in such traditional preparations per dose or per day's consumption and uses.

Author's comment:

All the published literature including use in traditional ethnomedicine need to be provided under this section. It is recommended that a tabulated summary – including pharmacognostic features, published literature on safety and efficacy – needs to be provided although it may be on the crude drug or on the primary extract (water, alcohol or hydro-alcoholic). This information would be helpful in evaluating the application in terms of safety and claims.

1.3 Information on any contraindications, side effects mentioned in traditional medicine or ethnomedicine literature or reports on current usage of the formulation

Author's comment:

There are not many publications on the side effects of medicinal plants. However, in certain cases traditional medicinal textbooks have mentioned contraindications. There are certain books on the adverse effects of herbal drugs that need to be consulted before providing information in this section. For the past few decades, attention has been drawn to herb–drug interaction studies. Attempts should be made to provide as much comprehensive information as possible under this section.

1.4 Published scientific reports in respect of safety and pharmacological studies relevant for the phytopharmaceutical drug intended to be marketed:

a. Where the process and usages are similar or same to the product known in traditional medicine or ethnomedicine; and

Author's comment:

The references from books or ethnomedical surveys can be provided for support if the process and usage of the herbal ingredients are same. However, it is to be noted that this in no way provides the guarantee of the safety of the phytopharmaceutical because that will be a fraction of the extract and the method of traditional use would not apply.

b. Where process and usages is different from that known in traditional medicine or ethnomedicine.

Author's comment:

Published scientific studies from journals may be sited as support in case the proposed use of the product is different from the one mentioned in traditional medical knowledge.

1.5 Information on any contraindications, side effects mentioned or reported in any of the studies, information on side effects and adverse reactions reported during current usage of the phytopharmaceutical in the last 3 years, wherever applicable.

Author's comment:

This section shall actually apply 3–4 years after the introduction of the first ever phyto-pharmaceutical drug because it is related to information on side and adverse effects during current use of the product. Data need not be submitted at the time of the application of the product because similar phytopharmaceutical products might not exist.

1.6 Present usage of the phytopharmaceutical drug, to establish history of usages, provide details of the product, manufacturer, quantum sold, extent or exposure on human population and number of years for which the product is being sold.

Author's comment:

This section also would not be relevant until at least 3–4 years after the introduction of the first phytopharmaceutical products because it demands data on details of the product manufacturer, sales-related information and exposure of population to the same.

2. Human or clinical pharmacology information:

2.1 Published scientific reports in respect of pharmacological studies including human studies or clinical studies or epidemiological studies, relevant for the phytopharmaceutical drug intended to be marketed:

   a. Where the process and usages are similar or same to the product known in traditional medicine or ethnomedicine; and

Author's comment:

See comment on section 1.4 above.

   b. Where process or usage is different from that known in traditional medicine or ethnomedicine.

Author's comment:

Published scientific studies from journals may be sited as support in case the proposed use of the product is different from the one mentioned in traditional medical knowledge.

2.2 Pharmacodynamic information (if available)

Author's comment:

Because this part is related to the compilation of published information to help the reviewers, published information of any of the bioactive compounds should also be provided. Because there is dearth of pharmacokinetic studies, any information on the pharmacodynamics of the compounds shall be useful.

2.3 Monographs, if any, published on the plant or product or extract or phytopharmaceutical. (Copies of all publications, along with English translation to be attached).

Author's comment:

Monographs on the plants or extracts may be provided under this section. WHO monographs, monographs published by the ICMR or any other detailed monographs would be useful. In addition to that, quality related information from United States Pharmacopeia, Indian Pharmacopeia, British Pharmacopeia and European Pharmacopeia should be provided to support the application.

PART – II
Data generated by applicant

3. Identification, authentication and source of plant used for extraction and fractionation:

3.1 Taxonomical identity of the plant used as a source of the phytopharmaceutical drug giving botanical name of genus, species and family, followed by the authority citation (taxonomist's name who named the species), the variety or the cultivar (if any) needs to be mentioned.

3.2 Morphological and anatomical description giving diagnostic features and a photograph of the plant or plant part for further confirmation of identity and authenticity. (Furnish certificate of confirmation of botanical identity by a qualified taxonomist.)

3.3 Natural habitat and geographical distribution of the plant and also mention whether the part of the plant used is renewable or destructive and the source whether cultivated or wild

3.4 Season or time of collection

3.5 Source of the plant including its geographical location and season or time of collection

3.6 A statement indicating whether the species is any of the following, namely:

a. Determined to be endangered or threatened under the Endangered Species Act or the Convention on International Trade in Endangered species (CITES) of wild Fauna and Flora)

b. Entitled to special protection under the Biological Diversity Act, 2002 (18 of 2003).

c. Any known genotypic, chemotypic and ecotypic variability of species

3.7 A list of growers or suppliers (including names and addresses) and information on the following items for each grower or supplier, if available or identified already, including information of primary processing, namely:

a. Harvest location

b. Growth conditions

c. Stage of plant growth at harvest

d. Harvesting time

e. Collection, washing, drying and storage conditions

f. Handling, garbling and transportation

g. Grinding, pulverising of the plant material; and

h. Sieving for getting uniform particle size of powdered plant material

3.8 Quality specifications, namely:

a. Foreign matter

b. Total ash

c. Acid insoluble ash

d. Pesticide residue

e. Heavy metal contamination

f. Microbial load

g. Chromatographic fingerprint profile with phytochemical reference marker

h. Assay for bioactive or phytochemical compounds; and

i. Chromatographic fingerprint of a sample as per test method given under quality control of the phytopharmaceutical drug (photo documentation)

3.9 An undertaking to supply specimen sample of plant duly labelled and photocopy of the certificate of identify confirmation issued by a qualified taxonomist along with drawings or photographs of the diagnostic morphological and histological features of the botanical raw material used for the confirmation of authenticity.

4. Process for extraction and subsequent fractionation and purification:

4.1 Quality specifications and test methods for starting material

4.2 Steps involved in processing

a. Details of solvent used, extractive values, solvent residue tests or limits, physico-chemical tests, microbial loads, heavy metal contaminants, chromatographic fingerprint profile with phytochemical reference markers, assay for active constituents or characteristic markers, if active constituents are not known

b. Characterisation of final purified fractions

c. Data on bio-active constituent of final purified fraction

d. Information on any excipients or diluents or stabiliser or preservative used, if any

4.3 Details of packaging of the purified and characterised final product, storage conditions and labelling.

5. Formulation of phytopharmaceutical drug applied for:
   5.1 Details of the composition, proportion of the final purified fraction with defined markers of phytopharmaceutical drug per unit dose, name and proportions of all excipients, stabilisers and any other agent used and packaging materials
   5.2 Test for identification for the phytopharmaceutical drug
   5.3 Quality specifications for active and inactive phytopharmaceutical chromatographic fingerprint profile with phytochemical reference marker and assay or active constituent or characteristic chemical marker

6. Manufacturing process of formulation:
   6.1 The outline of the method of manufacture of the dosage form, along with environmental controls, in-process quality control tests and limits for acceptance
   6.2 Details of all packaging materials used, packing steps and description of the final packs
   6.3 Finished product's quality specifications, including tests specific for the dosage form, quality and chromatographic fingerprint profile with phytochemical reference marker and assay for active constituent or characteristic marker, if active constituents are not known

7. Stability data:
   7.1 Stability data of the phytopharmaceutical drug described at 4 above, stored at room temperature at 40+/–2 deg. C and humidity at 75%RH +/–5%RH for 0, 1, 2, 3 and 6 months
   7.2 Stability data of the phytopharmaceutical drug in dosage form or formulation stored at room temperature at 40+/–2 deg. C and humidity at 75%RH+/–5%RH for 0, 1, 2, 3 and 6 months, in the pack intended for marketing

8. Safety and pharmacological information:
   8.1 Data on safety and pharmacological studies to be provided
   8.2 Animal toxicity and safety data:
      a. 28–90 days repeat dose oral toxicity on two species of animals
      b. *In vitro* genotoxicity data (Ames test and chromosomal aberration test as per Schedule Y)
      c. Dermal toxicity tests for topical use products
      d. Teratogenicity study (only if phytopharmaceutical drug is intended for use during pregnancy)

9. Human studies:
   9.1 Clinical trials for phytopharmaceutical drugs to be conducted as per applicable rules and guidelines for new drugs
   9.2 For all phytopharmaceutical drugs data from phase I (to determine maximum tolerated dose and associated toxicities) and the protocols shall be submitted prior to performing the studies
   9.3 Data of results of dose finding studies performed and the protocols shall be submitted prior to performing the studies
      Provided that in the case of phytopharmaceutical drug already marketed for more than 5 years or where there is adequate published evidence regarding the safety of the phytopharmaceutical drug, the studies may be abbreviated, modified or relaxed

10. Confirmatory clinical trials:
   10.1 Submit protocols for approval for any specific or special safety and efficacy study proposed specific to the phytopharmaceutical drug
   10.2 Submit proposed protocol for approval for human clinical studies appropriate to generate or validate safety and efficacy data for the phytopharmaceutical dosage from or product as per applicable rules and guidelines
   10.3 Submit information on how the quality of the formulation would be maintained during the above studies

11. Regulatory status:

    11.1 Status of the phytopharmaceutical drug marketed in any country under any category like functional food or dietary supplement or as traditional medicine or as an approved drug

12. Marketing information:

    12.1 Details of package insert or patient information sheet of the phytopharmaceutical drug to be marketed

    12.2 Draft of the text for label and carton

13. Post marketing surveillance (PMS):

    13.1 The applicant shall furnish periodic safety update reports every 6 months for the first 2 years after approval the drug is granted

    13.2 For subsequent 2 years the periodic safety update reports need to be submitted annually

14. Any other relevant information:

Any other relevant information which the applicant considers that it will help in scientific evaluation of the application.

12.5 CONCLUSION

India has witnessed the development of the thousands of years of a traditional system like Ayurveda into the world's first ever officially recognised category of drug, phytopharmaceuticals.

Introduction of this class of drug would open up new possibilities and potential. Phytopharmaceuticals shall have to undergo the same rigorous level scientific testing as any synthetic drug, and would therefore bear the trust of tradition and the evidence of science in a single product. Phytopharmaceuticals hopefully will offer a silver lining for all struggling R&D organisations with the promise of delivering more products in a shorter time frame with lower investments. Being a new category, most pharmaceutical industries may not even be aware of its importance. It is the duty of the Government as well as of industry associations to create as much awareness about phytopharmaceuticals as possible so that it becomes well established for the benefit of human kind.

REFERENCES

Chandrakant, K., Arun, G., Satyajyoti, K. and Shefali, K. (2012). Drug discovery from plant sources an integrated approach. *AYU*, **33**(1), 10–19.

Gazette Notification no. G.S.R 918(E) dated 30 November 2015, Drugs and Cosmetics Act, 8th Amendment Rules 2015, Ministry of Health and Family Welfare, Government of India.

Narayana, D. B. A. and Katiyar, C. K. (2016). Phytopharmaceutical regulation differentiates from Ayurveda and provides opportunities for future scientific innovation in Botanicals. *IDMA Bulletin*, **47**(17), 45–47.

Narayana, D. B. and Katiyar, C. K. (2013). Discussion kernel: Draft amendment to drugs and cosmetics rules to license science based botanicals, phytopharmaceuticals as drugs in India. *Journal of Ayurveda and Integrative Medicine,* 4(4), 254–256.

Pammolli, F., Magazzini, L. and Riccaboni, M. (2011). The productivity crisis in pharmaceutical R&D. *Natural Review Drug Discovery*, **10**(6), 428–438. doi:10.1038/nrd3405.

Section IV

Clinical Efficacy

13 Cranberry Proanthocyanidins (PACs) in Bacterial Anti-Adhesion

Thomas Brendler and Gunter Haesaerts

CONTENTS

13.1 INTRODUCTION

The primary health-promoting benefit for which cranberry consumption has been used is to maintain urinary tract health. Numerous clinical trials, including meta-analyses, support its use to prevent urinary tract infections (UTIs). Modern herbal practitioners and consumers similarly use cranberry, predominantly as juice products or dietary supplements. Recently, a standardised quantified cranberry juice extract has been registered as a traditional herbal medicine in various countries. It contains 36 mg total PACs, A and B together, measured by the validated DMAC/A2 PAC quantitation method. There is a wealth of clinical data that all support the pharmacological effect of cranberry juice proanthocyanidins (PACs) on *E. coli* bacteria for UTI prevention. Additional work has investigated the use of cranberry as an antioxidant, antiviral, anticancer, anticariogenic, anti-ulcerogenic, cholesterol lowering, and vasorelaxant agent.

To date, medical research on cranberry has focused on observational clinical trials, preclinical trials and some intervention trials. Large RCT clinical studies to confirm the results are still lacking. Nowadays, scientists are actively studying the metabolisation of cranberry PACs to understand the complex pharmacological mechanisms of action in the gut and through cell signalling.

Numerous studies from 1959 to the 1980s support the health benefits of cranberry juice, primarily for the urinary tract, as well as for other indications. One of the earliest formal investigations of cranberry's antibacterial activity occurred in 1959 (Bodel et al. 1959). These researchers suggested that hippuric acid, by lowering the pH of urine to a bacteriostatic level, was the mechanism behind the traditional folkloric use of cranberries in UTIs and reported on the successful prophylactic treatment of chronic pyelonephritis.

In subsequent studies, focus was placed on the antibacterial effects of cranberry in relationship to urinary tract health. A variety of mechanisms were reported, including the ability of cranberry to decrease urinary pH, which both increased the efficacy of other antibacterial agents (Brumfitt and Percival 1962) and was beneficial in preventing and treating some renal problems (Sternlieb 1963); inhibition of growth of *E. coli* (Kraemer 1964); antifungal activity (Ujvary et al. 1961; Swartz and Medrek 1968); reduction of urinary ionised calcium in patients with kidney stones (Light et al. 1973); and antiviral activity (Borukh et al. 1972; Konowalchuk and Speirs 1978; Ibragimov and

Kazanskaia 1981). While many of these reports lacked the methodological strength of formal modern clinical studies, they clearly suggest a trend for benefit and clinical relevance.

Several critical reviews of the cranberry literature, including meta-analyses, have been conducted. Cochrane Reviews of 2007 and 2008 (Jepson and Craig 2007, 2008) supported the efficacy of cranberry for the prevention of UTIs, while later analyses by the same group (Jepson et al. 2012), that included the same studies as the earlier positive review, reported a lack of efficacy. Clearly, the overwhelming trend of the data and individual studies supports efficacy. Numerous other health benefits and actions of cranberry have been investigated including for ulcer prevention, periodontal disease, cancer prevention, viruses, and cardiovascular disease risk factors, among others.

13.2 PROANTHOCYANIDINS

Cranberry PAC oligomers, also referred to as condensed tannins or polyflavan-3-ols, are predominantly made up of epicatechin extender units. PACs or condensed tannins were discovered in 1998 (Howell et al. 1998). The stereochemistry of the flavonoid monomers is predominantly of the 2,3-cis type, with a small proportion of 2,3-trans units (Foo et al. 2000a, 2000b). Some studies also report the presence of epigallocatechin and catechin units in PAC oligomers (Foo et al. 2000a, 2000b; Porter et al. 2001; Howell et al. 2005; Reed et al. 2005; Neto et al. 2006). The structural characterisation of PACs was done for PAC dimers and trimers (Foo et al. 2000a, 2000b), but higher oligomers and polymers have a very complex structure and high molecular weight that could not be characterised until the present time.

There are two common series of PAC dimers. The B-type series are dimers linked either in the C4–C6 or C4–C8 position, whereas the A-type series are dimers linked in the C4–C8 position with an additional C2–O–C7 ether linkage. Cranberry PAC oligomers with a degree of polymerisation (DP) greater than two may incorporate both A-type and B-type interflavan linkages. By extension of this definition, and to discuss differences among oligomers, PACs that contain one or more A-type interflavan bonds in their structure are referred to as A-type PAC, whereas PAC oligomers that contain only B-type interflavan bonds are referred to as B-type PAC (Krueger et al. 2013a). Feliciano et al. (2012) applied a method for the deconvolution of matrix-assisted laser desorption/ionisation time-of-flight mass spectrometry (MALDI-TOF MS) isotope patterns and determined that more than 91% of cranberry PAC molecules had at least one A-type linkage. The ratios of A-type to B-type linkages in PAC are product specific and therefore constitute information that can be used to authenticate cranberry content. PACs in cranberry juice and juice powders are soluble and bioactive, whereas the PACs in the whole berry, whole berry powders and presscake powders are mostly insoluble and show little bioactivity. Insoluble PACs are often bound to complex carbohydrate cell wall components or proteins.

The average degree of polymerisation of PACs differs and is variably reported as 4.7 (Foo et al. 2000a), 8.5–15.3 (Gu et al. 2003) and up to 23 (Reed et al. 2005; Blumberg et al. 2013), in part due to variable findings using different analytical methods that employ thiolysis and pholoroglucinolysis (Karonen et al. 2007; Zhou et al. 2011). The quantity of PACs found in cranberries can vary, partly due to variations in samples and to differences in analytical methodologies. Gu et al. (2004, using HPLC) reported a PAC content of 418.8 ± 75.3 mg/100 mg in fresh fruit and 231 ± 2 mg/L in cranberry juice cocktail, although different values would be detected using other analytical methods. In both matrices, the majority of the PAC had a >10 degrees of polymerisation.

Howell et al. (2001) demonstrated for the first time how cranberry PAC ingestion resulted in urine with bacterial anti-adhesion activity *in vivo*. Urine collected from mice that were fed purified cranberry PACs had bacterial anti-adhesion activity against P-fimbriated *E. coli*. In another study, rats fed 118 mg PACs/animal/day via oral suspension or tablet produced urine that prevented adhesion of *E. coli* by 83% and 52%, respectively (Risco et al. 2010). Very low levels of PAC A2 dimer $(0.541 \pm 0.10$ ng/mL) have been found in rat plasma samples 1 h after cranberry administration (Rajbhandari et al. 2011) and in low levels in human urine (McKay et al. 2015).

While it has generally been assumed that cranberry exerts its effect on UTIs directly through the urine, an alternative and untested hypothesis is that it also works preventatively by affecting the adhesive properties of bacteria in the large intestine and colon (Sobota 1984; Zafriri et al. 1989; Ofek et al. 1996; Kontiokari et al. 2001). Very recent studies have suggested other possible mechanisms of action for cranberry components in the prevention of UTIs (Krueger et al. 2013b; Shanmuganayugari et al. 2013) involving decreases of the relative levels of 8 proteins/peptides in the urine of human subjects post-supplementation with cranberry (Krueger et al. 2003). The functions of these proteins are not fully understood, and the implications of these shifts in UTI are unclear. Recently, it has been shown that exposure of extra-intestinal pathogenic *E. coli* to cranberry PACs inhibits their invasiveness into enterocytes, disrupts surface structures of the *E. coli*, and increases killing of *E. coli* by macrophages (Shanmuganayugari et al. 2013). The action of PACs on prevention of adhesion, invasion and immune function are pharmacologically more complex than previously thought, and require further study to determine more about the metabolism and precisely how these various biological activities exert effects in the urinary tract and gut to maintain urinary tract health.

13.3 EFFECTS OF CRANBERRY PACs ON URINARY TRACT INFECTIONS AND URINARY TRACT HEALTH

Consumption of cranberries and cranberry products has been widely recommended for the maintenance of urinary tract health in general (Bone and Morgan 1999; Kerr 1999; Reid 1999; Henig and Leahy 2000; Patel and Daniels 2000; Wang et al. 2012), as well as for the prevention and prophylactic treatment of UTIs (Rogers 1991; Haverkorn and Mandigers 1994; Walker et al. 1997; Stothers 2002; Hess et al. 2008; Bonetta and Di Pierro 2012). There are an almost equal number of studies with comparable numbers of subjects that report positive and negative outcomes. A variety of preparations have been used in the various studies including cranberry juice, cranberry juice cocktail (~27% juice), and varying cranberry extracts (see review of select studies below and Table 13.1). Some studies do not fully characterise the preparations used, while other studies report low compliance and high dropout rates (see Jepson et al. 2012). Patients with recurrent UTIs appear to prefer 'natural' therapies such as cranberry to avoid prophylactic antibiotic use (Nowack and Schmitt 2008; Mazokopakis et al. 2009), underscoring the importance for healthcare providers to understand the benefits, limitations, dosage and product characterisations to maximise the efficacy of cranberry preparations. The most common dose used in early studies was approximately 300 mL of cranberry juice cocktail that, when calculated, delivers approximately 36 mg of soluble PACs (analysed according to DMAC with an A2 standard).

A variety of mechanisms for cranberry's putative effects have been articulated. For many years, it was assumed that hippuric acid excreted in the urine following cranberry consumption was responsible for the effect on the prevention of UTIs, as hippuric acid can be bacteriostatic against *E. coli* (at concentrations of 1–2 mg/L; Bodel et al. 1959; Hamilton-Miller and Brumfitt 1976). In human trials, urinary pH levels were somewhat reduced following consumption of cranberry juice, but to achieve a bacteriostatic effect, urinary pH must be reduced to at least 5.0, with a minimum hippuric acid concentration of 0.02 M (Blatherwick 1914; Blatherwick and Long 1923; Bodel et al. 1959; Papas et al. 1966; Nickey 1975; Kinney and Blount 1979; Schultz 1984a, 1984b; Jackson and Hicks 1997). To attain these levels, humans would need to consume at least 1500 mL of cranberry juice per day (Kahn et al. 1967). To date, researchers have not yet elucidated an exact *in vivo* mechanism of action, although there is substantial *in vitro* and *ex vivo* evidence indicating that cranberry and cranberry A-type PACs stimulate an activity that results in inhibiting bacteria, particularly *E. coli*, from adhering to uroepithelial cells (Sobota 1984; Zafriri et al. 1989; Howell et al. 1998; Gupta et al. 2007), preventing formation of bacterial biofilms (LaPlante et al. 2012), hindering motility, and downregulating the enzyme urease and the transcription of flagellin, which are important virulence factors (McCall et al. 2013). In addition to other potentially bioactive compounds, cranberries contain a rich and diverse mixture of polyphenolic compounds. More research is needed to determine if

TABLE 13.1

Clinical Trials of Cranberry Preparations in the Prevention of Urinary Tract Infections (UTIs)

References	Study Design	Patient Population	Product and Daily Dosage	Treatment Duration	Outcome
Rogers (1991)	OBS	Children with neuropathic bladders; $n = 17$	CJ, 360–480 mL for 1 week and 540–660 mL for the 2nd week	2 weeks	Observed reduction in red and white cell counts; *E. coli* still present in samples at end of study
Avorn et al. (1994)	DBRPCT	Elderly women; $n = 153$	CJC (27%, saccharin-sweetened), 300 mL	6 months	Lower odds ratio for bacteriuria with pyuria in treatment group ($P = 0.004$)
Haverkorn and Mandigers (1994)	RX, control water	Elderly men and women; $n = 17$	CJ, 30 mL	1 month	Fewer incidences of bacteriuria ($P = 0.004$)
Foda et al. (1995)	PCTX	Children with neuropathic bladders; $n = 21$	CJC, 15 mL/kg	6 months	No reduction in incidence of UTIs
Walker et al. (1997)	DBRPCTX	Women (28–44 years) with history of recurrent UTI; $n = 10$	CE (Cranactin®), 1 capsule equivalent to 400 mg cranberry solids daily	3 months	Significantly fewer UTIs in treatment group ($P = 0.005$)
Dignam et al. (1998)	OBS, cross-sectional	Elderly men/women; $n = 538$	CJ, 120 mL or 6 Azo-cranberry capsules	8 months	Fewer UTIs during the treatment period ($P = 0.008$)
Dignam et al. (1998)	OBS, longitudinal	Elderly men/women; $n = 113$	CJ, 120 mL or 6 Azo-cranberry capsules	16 months	No reduction in incidence of UTIs
Schlager et al. (1999)	DBPCTX	Children with neuropathic bladders; $n = 15$	CC; 60 mL (= 300 mL CJC)	3 months	No reduction in bacteriuria
Kontiokari et al. (2001, 2005)	PRCT, 3 arm, Control *Lactobacillus rhamnosus* drink	Young women suffering from UTI at recruitment; $n = 150$	Cranberry-lingonberry concentrate, 50 mL in 200 mL water	6 months	56% fewer UTIs in cranberry group after 6 months ($P = 0.02$)
McGuinness et al. (2002)	PRCT, control beetroot powder	Multiple sclerosis patients; $n = 126$	Cranberry containing tablet product (NOW Natural Foods): 8000 mg tablet, one tablet/daily	6 months	No significant advantage of cranberry over control
Stothers (2002)	DBRPCT	Women (21–57 years) with history of UTIs; $n = 150$	CJ or CE, brands and dosage unspecified	1 year	Mean number of symptomatic UTIs reduced in both cranberry groups ($P \leq 0.05$)
Linsenmeyer et al. (2004)	PRCTX	Patients with neurogenic bladders secondary to spinal cord injury; $n = 21$	Cranberry tablets: 400 mg standardised tablets	9 weeks	No statistically significant treatment (favourable) effect for cranberry supplement beyond placebo

(Continued)

TABLE 13.1 (Continued)
Clinical Trials of Cranberry Preparations in the Prevention of Urinary Tract Infections (UTIs)

References	Study Design	Patient Population	Product and Daily Dosage	Treatment Duration	Outcome
Waites et al. (2004)	PRCT	Men and women at least 1 year post spinal cord injury; $n = 48$	Concentrated cranberry extract: 2 g in capsule form	6 months	No reduction in bacteriuria and pyuria
McMurdo et al. (2005)	PRCT	Elderly men and women; $n = 376$	Cranberry juice: 300 mL	35 days	Between-group differences not significant
Lee et al. (2007)	PRCT, control methenamine hippurate	Men and women with spinal cord injury; $n = 305$	Treatment group 1 Methenamine hippurate: 2 g; cranberry: 1600 mg Treatment group 2 Methenamine hippurate: 2 g; cranberry placebo Treatment group 3 Cranberry: 1600 mg; methenamine hippurate placebo	6 months	No difference in UTI-free period with either treatment
Bailey et al. (2007)	OBS	Women with a history of recurrent infections of a minimum of 6 UTIs in the preceding year; $n = 12$	One capsule twice daily containing 200 mg of a concentrated cranberry extract standardised to 30% phenolics	3 months	No UTIs during study period
Hess et al. (2008)	RCTX, control rice flour	Men and women with spinal cord injury; $n = 47$	Cranberry tablet: 500 mg twice daily	6 months	Reduction in the likelihood of UTI and symptoms for any month while receiving the cranberry tablet ($P < 0.05$ for all)
Wing et al. (2008)	PRCT, 3 arm	Women <16 weeks gestation; $n = 115$	Treatment group 1 Cranberry juice: 240 mL at breakfast, placebo juice at other meals Treatment group 2 Cranberry drink: 240 mL, 3 times/daily, reducing to twice daily after 52 enrolments because not well tolerated Control group Placebo: 3 daily doses of matched juice product	~5 months	Non-significant trend for reduction in asymptomatic bacteriuria and symptomatic urinary tract infections in pregnancy

(Continued)

TABLE 13.1 (*Continued*)
Clinical Trials of Cranberry Preparations in the Prevention of Urinary Tract Infections (UTIs)

References	Study Design	Patient Population	Product and Daily Dosage	Treatment Duration	Outcome
Ferrara et al. (2009)	PRCT, 3 arm	Girls 3–14 years; $n = 80$	Cranberry-lingonberry concentrate (97.5 and 1.7 g, respectively); *Lactobacillus* GC drink	6 months	Significant reduction in the risk of repeated UTIs in the cranberry group ($P < 0.05$) compared with the *Lactobacillus* group and the control group
Mazokopakis et al. (2009)	OT	Post-menopausal women with recurring UTI; $n = 10$	Four cranberry capsules per day (Natural Cranberry Extract, 400 mg with vitamin C vegetable, capsules, Solgar)	6 months	No symptomatic UTI during trial, almost all urine cultures were sterile
McMurdo et al. (2009)	PRCT	Women >45 years with at least 2 antibiotic treated UTIs in previous 12 months; $n = 120$	Cranberry tablet: 500 mg, 100 mg of trimethoprim	6 months	Study underpowered; trimethoprim had a limited advantage over cranberry, but more adverse effects; cranberry group experienced fewer infections with *E. coli*
Cadkova et al. (2009)	PT	Women during perioperative period leading to gynaecological surgery; $n = 286$	Cranberry extract capsules (equivalent to 17,000 mg of fresh fruit) twice daily, 4 days before and 5 days after the surgery	6 days	No effect on the number of post-surgical UTIs
Vidlar et al. (2009)	RCT	Men, aged 45–70 years; $n = 42$	1500 mg of the dried powdered cranberries or no treatment	6 months	Significant improvement in International Prostate Symptom Score, QOL, urination parameters including voiding parameters, and lower total PSA level for cranberry group
Botto and Neuzillet (2010)	OT	Asymptomatic bacteriuria in patients with an ileal enterocystoplasty; $n = 15$	36 mg/daily PAC A (Urell, Pharmatoka)	32.8 months (median)	Significant decrease in the number of positive urine cultures during cranberry compound treatment
Juthani-Mehta et al. (2010)	PRCT, 3 arm	Elderly men and women >60 years of age with dementia; $n = 56$	Cranberry capsule: 1×650 mg once or twice daily	6 months	No difference between the 3 groups

(*Continued*)

TABLE 13.1 (*Continued*)
Clinical Trials of Cranberry Preparations in the Prevention of Urinary Tract Infections (UTIs)

References	Study Design	Patient Population	Product and Daily Dosage	Treatment Duration	Outcome
Essadi and Elmehashi (2010)	PCT, control water: 250 mL 4 times/daily	Pregnant women; $n = 544$	Cranberry juice: 250 mL 4 times/daily	12 months	To little information to assess
Barbosa-Cesnik et al. (2011)	PRCT, control matched for flavour and colour	Women 18–40 years, with UTI symptoms; $n = 319$	Low calorie cranberry cocktail: 240 mL twice daily	6 months	Among otherwise healthy college women with an acute UTI, drinking cranberry juice did not result in a decrease in the 6-month incidence of a second UTI
Sengupta et al. (2011)	PRCT, 3 arm	Females with a history of recurrent UTIs; $n = 60$	Cranberry: 500 and 1000 mg/daily, 1.5% PAC	3 months	Significant reduction ($P < 0.05$) in the subjects positive for *E. coli* in both the high-dose and low-dose treatment groups
Beerepoot et al. (2011)	PRCT, control trimethoprim-sulfamethoxazole 480 mg	Premenopausal women >18 years with at least 3 symptomatic UTIs in the year prior to enrolment; $n = 221$	Cranberry extract: 500 mg twice daily (9.1 mg/g type A PAC)	12 months	Trimethoprim-sulfamethoxazole is more effective than cranberry capsules to prevent recurrent UTIs; authors suggest that non-antibiotic therapies additionally beneficial to prevent antibiotic resistance
Uberos et al. (2012, 2015); Fernández-Puentes et al. (2015)	PRCT, control trimethoprim 8 mg/kg	Children aged from 1 month to 13 years, with recurrent UTI; $n = 192$	Cranberry syrup: 0.2 mL/kg yielding 36 mg PACs (Urell, Pharmatoka), trimethoprim	12 months	Similar efficacy between trimethoprim and cranberry
Bonetta and Di Pierro (2012)	PCT	Patients with external beam radiotherapy; $n = 370$	200 mg of a highly standardised cranberry extract titre as 30% proanthocyanidins	~7 weeks	Significantly fewer lower urinary tract infections in the verum group
Salo et al. (2012)	PRCT	Children; $n = 255$	Cranberry juice 5 mL/kg up to 300 mL 1–2 doses daily	6 months	No significant reduction in the number of children who experienced a recurrence of UTI; reduction in actual number of recurrences
Afshar et al. (2012)	RCT	Children; $n = 40$	2 cc/kg cranberry juice containing 37% PAC (method not given) Placebo: same volume of juice with no PAC or other cranberry products	12 months	65% reduction in risk of urinary tract infection ($P = 0.045$)

(Continued)

TABLE 13.1 (*Continued*)

Clinical Trials of Cranberry Preparations in the Prevention of Urinary Tract Infections (UTIs)

References	Study Design	Patient Population	Product and Daily Dosage	Treatment Duration	Outcome
Stapleton et al. (2012)	RCT	Premenopausal women with a history of recent UTI; $n = 176$	4 oz. of cranberry juice, 8 oz. of cranberry juice, or placebo	5.6 months (median)	Strong (though not significant) reduction in P-fimbriated *E. coli*; no significant reduction in UTI risk
Bianco et al. (2012)	DBRPCT, 4 arm	Elderly; $n = 80$	108, 72, and 36 mg PAC, placebo	1 month	Dose-dependent trend toward decrease in bacteriuria and pyuria
Cowan et al. (2012)	PRCT, control placebo juice	Adults >18 years with cervical or bladder cancer requiring radiation therapy; $n = 113$	Cranberry juice twice daily (volume and concentration not stated)	6 weeks	Significant decrease of UTI and urinary symptoms ($P = 0.240$)
Mutlu and Ekinci (2012)	RCTX	Children with neurogenic bladder; $n = 20$	One cranberry capsule (no further information given), placebo	12 months	Significant reduction in UTIs ($P = 0.012$); significant decrease in pyuria ($P = 0.000$)
Takahashi et al. (2013)	PRCT	Outpatients aged 20–79 years with acute exacerbation of acute uncomplicated cystitis or chronic complicated cystitis (including self-catheterisation) who had a past history of multiple relapses of UTI; $n = 213$	125 mL cranberry juice or placebo	24 weeks	Significant reduction ($P = 0.0425$) in rate of relapse of UTIs in females 50 years or more
Gallien et al. (2014)	DBRCT	Multiple sclerosis patients; $n = 171$	Cranberry powder 18 mg proanthocyanidins sachets twice daily	12 months	No reduction in incidence of UTIs
Caljouw et al. (2014)	DBPCT	Elderly long-term care facility patients stratified to high or low risk for UTIs; $n = 928$	Undisclosed cranberry preparation and dose given twice daily	12 months	26% reduction in incidence of UTIs in high-risk subjects ($n = 516$); no difference in low-risk subjects
Lin et al. (2014)	OBS; control (catheterised patients)	Elderly long-term care facility; patients with long-term indwelling catheter; $n = 11$	Cranberry juice (300 mL daily; characterisation not disclosed) along with 2200 mL water	6 months	No reduction in asymptomatic bacteriuria or incidence of UTIs

(Continued)

TABLE 13.1 (*Continued*)
Clinical Trials of Cranberry Preparations in the Prevention of Urinary Tract Infections (UTIs)

References	Study Design	Patient Population	Product and Daily Dosage	Treatment Duration	Outcome
Mathison et al. (2014)	DBRCTX	Healthy adults; $n = 12$	Cranberry leaf extract beverage, low-calorie cranberry juice cocktail, or placebo	Single dose	Cranberry showed significant ($P < 0.05$) ex vivo antia-dhesion activity against *P*-fimbriated *E. coli* in urine compared with placebo.
Foxman et al. (2015)	DBRPCT	Female adults post-elective gynaecologic surgery; $n = 160$	TheraCran® cranberry capsules (Theralogix) equivalent to 16 oz. cranberry juice, or placebo	6 weeks after surgery	Incidence of UTI was significantly lower in the cranberry treatment group compared to the placebo group (15/80 (19%) versus 30/80 (38%); OR = 0.38; 95% CI: 0.19, 0.79; $P = 0.008$)
Barnoiu et al. (2015)	OT	Patients with indwelling catheter; $n = 62$	Cranberry preparation (unspecified), 120 mg, or placebo	5 days prophylactic treatment	Reduced incidence of UTI compared to control in patients with indwelling catheters (12.9% versus 38.75%, respectively; $P = 0.04$)
Hamilton et al. (2015)	DBRPCT	Male adults with radiation cystitis; $n = 41$	Cranberry capsules (Naturo Pharm), 72 mg PACs according to UV-VISEP/CN, or placebo	70 days	Incidence of cystitis was lower in men taking cranberry capsules (65%) compared to placebo (90%) ($P = 0.058$); severe cystitis occurred in 30% of men in the cranberry arm and 45% with placebo ($P = 0.30$)
Ledda et al. (2015, 2017)	RCT	Adolescents with history of recurrent UTI, $n = 36$	120 mg of cranberry extract (Anthocran®), standardised to 36 mg PACs	60 days	Number of UTIs in the cranberry group (0.31 ± 0.2) significantly lower than in control (2.3 ± 1.3) and compared to mean number of UTIs at baseline (1.74 ± 1.1), $P = 0.0001$ for both.
Vostalova et al. (2015)	DBRPCT, 2 arm	Female adults with 2 or more UTI episodes over 1 year, $n = 182$	500 mg cranberry fruit powder (NATUREX-DBS), or placebo	6 months	Fewer UTIs in the cranberry group (10.8% vs. 25.8%, $P = 0.04$)

(Continued)

TABLE 13.1 (Continued)

Clinical Trials of Cranberry Preparations in the Prevention of Urinary Tract Infections (UTIs)

References	Study Design	Patient Population	Product and Daily Dosage	Treatment Duration	Outcome
Vidlar et al. (2016)	DBRPCT, 3 arm	Male adults with benign prostate hyperplasia, $n = 124$	250 or 500 mg cranberry powder (Flowens™), or placebo	6 months	Lower international prostate symptoms score (IPSS) in both Flowens™ groups (-3.1 and -4.1 in the 250- and 500-mg groups, $P = 0.05$ and $P < 0.001$, respectively)
Maki et al. (2016)	DBRPCT	Female adults with a history of recurrent UTI, $n = 373$	8 oz. CJC, or placebo	24 weeks	39 UTI episodes in cranberry group vs. 67 in placebo (antibiotic use–adjusted incidence rate ratio: 0.61; 95% CI: 0.41, 0.91; $P = 0.016$
Juthani-Mehta et al. (2016)	DBRPCT	Elderly females in nursing homes, $n = 185$	Two capsules of cranberry dry extract totalling 72 mg PACs (Pharmatoka), or placebo	1 year	No significant difference in the presence of bacteriuria plus pyuria between the treatment group vs. the control group (29.1% vs. 29.0%; OR, 1.01; 95% CI, 0.61–1.66; $P = 0.98$), no significant differences in number of symptomatic UTIs (10 episodes in the treatment group vs. 12 in the control group)
Singh et al. (2016)	RCT	Patients with a history of UTI, $n = 72$	Cranpac™ (containing PAC-A 60 mg per capsule), 2 capsules per day, or placebo	12 weeks	bacterial adhesion scoring decreased (0.28) v. placebo (2.14) ($P < 0.001$); biofilm ($P < 0.01$) and bacterial growth ($p < 0.001$) decreased; microscopic pyuria score was 0.36 vs. 2.0 ($P < 0.001$); UTI decreased to 33.33 vs. 88.89% ($P < 0.001$); mean subjective dysuria score was 0.19 vs. 1.47

(Continued)

TABLE 13.1 (*Continued*)
Clinical Trials of Cranberry Preparations in the Prevention of Urinary Tract Infections (UTIs)

References	Study Design	Patient Population	Product and Daily Dosage	Treatment Duration	Outcome
Lee et al. (2016)	RCT, 3 arm	Circumcised ($n = 12$) and uncircumcised ($n = 55$) boys	4 oz. cranberry juice, or placebo	6 months	Incidence of bacteriuria were 25% (7/28), 37% (10/27), and 33.3% (4/12) in groups 1 (uncircumcised cranberry), 2 (uncircumcised placebo) and 3 (circumcised cranberry), respectively
Thomas et al. (2018)	OT	Males and females with long-term indwelling catheters and recurrent symptomatic UTIs ($n = 22$)	One capsule of cranberry daily (Ellura®, Pharmatoka) containing 36 mg PACs.	6 months	Effective in all patients, with 28% reduction in antibiotic resistance and 58.65% reduction in colony counts
Gunnarsson et al. (2017)	DBRPCT	Females aged 60 and older ($n = 227$) with indwelling urinary catheter post-hip surgery	Two capsules of 550 mg of cranberry powder (NutriCran®) three times a day, or placebo	5 days	No statistically significant difference between treatment and placebo

DB = double blind; R = randomised; CT = controlled trial; PCT = placebo-controlled; PT = prospective trial; X = crossover; OBS = observational; PG parallel group; CJC = Cranberry Juice Cocktail® (Ocean Spray®, CJC ~27% cranberry juice); CJ = cranberry juice of unknown concentration from unknown manufacturer; CE = cranberry extract; CC = cranberry juice concentrate; OT = open trial.

and how these compounds contribute to the anti-adhesion effect and modulate other systems to help prevent UTIs, such as through the immune system or by reducing uropathogenic bacteria invasion in the GI tract (Feliciano et al. 2014). It is likely that a suite of compounds contributes to cranberry's biological activity, although there is a general consensus that PACs may be considered the primary compounds with bacterial anti-adherence activity.

Live bacteria must attach and gain entry to uroepithelial cells in the urinary tract to grow and cause infection, and they do so by binding to certain cell receptors with filamentous appendages called pili or fimbriae. The anti-adhesion activity of cranberry was first recognised by Sobota (1984). A series of experiments using cranberry juice and pure cranberry juice PACs against uropathogenic strains of *E. coli* demonstrated that cranberry juice contains one or more compounds that inhibit *in vitro* bacterial adherence to uroepithelial cells (Zafriri et al. 1989; Howell et al. 1998). It appears that by preventing the *E. coli* from adhering to uroepithelial cells, the bacteria will not grow and cause infection, but be flushed out in the urine stream. Because this mechanism does not kill the bacteria, it is unlikely to result in bacterial resistance to cranberry. The anti-adhesion activity of cranberry has been demonstrated in humans (Howell et al. 2005, 2010; Di Martino et al. 2006; Valentova et al. 2007; Lavigne et al. 2008; Tempera et al. 2010).

13.4 CLINICAL DATA

UTIs are among the most common bacterial infections in the ambulatory setting (Schappert and Rechtsteiner 2011). Although males and females can develop UTIs, infections occur more frequently in women (Foxman and Brown 2003). It is estimated that more than 50% of women will experience at least one UTI in their lifetime (Griebling 2005), and 20%–30% of women who experience a UTI will have two or more recurrent episodes (Foxman 1990). Other populations at risk for developing UTIs include children, pregnant women, the elderly, patients with spinal cord injuries, catheterised patients and those with chronic and/or immune-compromising diseases such as diabetes and HIV/AIDS (Foxman 2002).

Foxman et al. (2015) found that administration of the equivalent of two 8-ounce servings of cranberry daily in solid dosage form (capsule: TheraCran, Theralogix, LLC, Rockville, MD) for 6 weeks significantly ($P = 0.008$) reduced the incidence of UTIs in post-surgical catheterised subjects ($n = 160$) by approximately 50% as compared to placebo controls. Subjects in this study were instructed to take the capsules morning and evening with an 8-ounce glass of water beginning at time of discharge, and were specifically asked to avoid any other cranberry product or vitamin C supplementation for 4–6 weeks or until their post-operative visit. There were no differences in adverse effects, including GI upset in this study.

A recent review of clinical studies (Micali et al. 2014) and evaluation of the cranberry efficacy/safety ratio in the prevention of UTIs supports the use of cranberry in the prevention of recurrent UTIs in young and middle-aged women (Walker et al. 1997; Kontiokari et al. 2001; Stothers 2002; Ferrara et al. 2009; Afshar et al. 2012; Salo et al. 2012; Uberos et al. 2012). However, evidence of its clinical efficacy among other groups remains controversial (Micali et al. 2014). Past clinical reviews have been mixed, with several suggesting that cranberry may help prevent infections, particularly in women with recurrent UTIs (Jepson and Craig 2008; Wang et al. 2012), but with one review finding less benefit for cranberry (Jepson et al. 2012). Risk ratios of <1.0 (calculated relative risk of developing UTIs in the treated versus control groups) were interpreted as positive outcomes by Wang et al. (2012) but not by Jepson et al. (2012) with different confidence intervals reported in each study. Compliance in some studies included in the Cochrane Review (Jepson et al. 2012) was low, but may have been confounded using poor compliance measures. Most of the studies used cranberry products that were not standardised to total PACs and may not have had sufficient amounts of bioactive PAC to achieve clinical efficacy. It is important to note that cranberry is a food that comes in different product forms (juice, powder, dried, etc.) making it difficult to use a meta-analysis to compare results from multiple trials that each used different product forms (Howell 2013). Additionally, the choice of study subjects is particularly important, as the pathogenesis of UTI is specific to different patient groups. Several studies completed since the Cochrane Review (Jepson et al. 2012) had positive outcomes for cranberry in preventing UTI recurrence and are included in the most recent review of Micali et al. (2014). However, more work is needed to determine the optimal dose, frequency of administration, length of consumption, subject characteristics and product form.

Importantly, the Cochrane Review (Jepson et al. 2012) concluded that in studies comparing low-dose antibiotics to cranberry for UTI prevention, there was little difference between cranberry and antibiotic prophylaxes, with both being similarly effective. In fact, in a study conducted by Beerepoot et al. (2011), antibiotic prophylaxis resulted in TMP-SMX resistance in 86.3% of faecal and 90.5% of asymptomatic bacteriuria $E.$ $coli$ isolates after 1 month on low-dose TMP-SMX, while in the cranberry group, 23.7% of faecal and 28.1% of asymptomatic bacteriuria $E.$ $coli$ isolates were TMP-SMX resistant. These same researchers also found increased resistance rates for trimethoprim, amoxicillin and ciprofloxacin in these $E.$ $coli$ isolates after 1 month in the TMP-SMX group. Due to the very low risk of resistant bacterial strain development, cranberry was recommended by these study authors as a viable alternative to low-dose antibiotics to prevent UTI. Since the increasing prevalence of $E.$ $coli$ resistance to first-line antimicrobials in the treatment of acute UTI in women is also a serious problem (Stapleton 2013), use of cranberry to prevent initial infections may help reduce the need for subsequent antibiotic treatments and slow the pace of resistance development. According to the World Health Organization (WHO 2014) Antimicrobial Resistance Global Report on Surveillance, resistance to fluoroquinolones for controlling UTIs is very widespread, and compared to the 1980s, resistance rates have gone from zero to 100% in many parts of the world. Cranberry products, therefore, may be a prudent nutritional-prophylactic therapy that can help maintain urinary tract health (Blumberg et al. 2013). Early 2019 the EMA (European Medicines Agency has limted the use of (fluoro)quinolones to curative treatments of UTI because of the very serious side effects of longer term prophylactic treatment. Well standardized PAC extracts can replace antibiotics for the prophylactic treatment of UTIs.

A pilot study ($n = 5$) suggests that consumption of a single serving of sweetened dried cranberries (Craisins® Ocean Spray) may elicit bacterial anti-adhesion activity in human urine and may be a healthy snack with specific genitourinary benefits (Greenberg et al. 2005).

One of the earliest large, double-blind, placebo-controlled randomised clinical trials evaluated a low-calorie 27% cranberry juice cocktail for its effect on bacteriuria (defined as >10^5 cfu/mL of urine) and pyuria (white blood cells in urine) in 153 elderly women over a 6-month period (Avorn et al. 1994). Participants consumed either 300 mL/day of cranberry juice cocktail or 300 mL/day of a placebo drink. After 48 weeks of treatment, bacteriuria and pyuria were reduced by nearly 50% in the group that consumed cranberry juice cocktail, with their odds of remaining bacteriuric/pyuric at only 27% of the odds of the control group ($P = 0.006$). In another study (randomised, controlled, crossover), Haverkorn and Mandigers (1994) administered 30 mL/day of cranberry juice diluted in water to 17 elderly men and women for 4 weeks. Participants consuming the cranberry treatment had fewer occurrences of bacteriuria compared to those who drank water ($P = 0.004$), confirming Avorn's findings that cranberry juice consumption reduces frequency of bacteriuria in the elderly.

An uncontrolled study of 28 elderly patients in a long-term care facility found that cranberry juice was effective in preventing UTIs (Gibson et al. 1991). Participants drank 120–180 mL of cranberry juice cocktail almost daily for 7 weeks. UTIs were prevented in 19 of the 28 participants. A retrospective cross-sectional study and a longitudinal cohort study (Dignam et al. 1998) were carried out in a long-term care facility in which there was a 20-month pre-intervention period when UTI rates were recorded, and an 8-month intervention period when cranberry juice or cranberry capsules were given to participants (only 4% received the capsules instead of the juice). The cross-sectional study involved 538 elderly people (77% women and 23% men). During the 20-month pre-intervention period, UTIs were reduced significantly between these two periods ($P = 0.008$), with 545 UTIs compared with 164 UTIs during the 8-month intervention period when cranberry juice was consumed. In the longitudinal cohort study, 113 residents participated. There were 103 UTIs during the pre-intervention period and 84 UTIs during the intervention period, which represented a trend toward reduction in UTIs.

A double-blind, randomised, placebo-controlled pilot study aimed at identifying the optimal dose of cranberry capsules that reduced the incidence of bacteriuria plus pyuria was conducted over a 1-month period among elderly nursing home patients (Bianco et al. 2012). Subjects ($n = 80$) were given either 3 cranberry capsules (108 mg PAC determined by DMAC/A2 assay); 2 cranberry capsules (72 mg PAC) plus one placebo; or one cranberry capsule (36 mg PAC) plus 2 placebos; or 3 placebo capsules for 30 days, measuring episodes of bacteriuria and pyuria at days 7, 14, 21 and 28. In those consuming cranberry, a dose-dependent trend towards a reduction in bacteriuria and pyuria (particularly with *E. coli*) was observed, most notably in women. Cranberry did not affect bacteriuria with pathogens other than *E. coli*. The effects of the 2-capsule dose were comparable to those of the 3-capsule dose. Neither the long-term sustainability of the reduction in bacteriuria and pyuria, nor effects on clinical outcomes related to UTI (e.g. hospitalisation, antibiotic therapy) were determined.

A double-blind, randomised, placebo-controlled multicentre trial ($n = 928$) was conducted to determine the efficacy of cranberry (undisclosed characterisation and dose taken twice daily for 12 months) in reducing the incidence of UTIs in residents of long-term care facilities (703 women, median age 84 years) in the Netherlands (Caljouw et al. 2014). Subjects were stratified by low or high UTI-risk (including long-term catheterisation, diabetes mellitus, and ≥ 1 UTI in the preceding year). Of the total subjects, 516 were stratified as having a high risk for UTI; 412 were considered low risk. Compared to placebo, a 26% reduction in UTI was observed in the high-risk group, while no difference was observed in the low-risk group. One limitation of this study is that the actual incidence of UTIs was lower in the cranberry compared to the placebo group.

In a recent study by Barnoiu et al. (2015), prophylactic administration of 120 mg cranberry (preparation not characterised) daily significantly reduced the incidence of UTI as compared to a control group of patients with indwelling catheters (12.9% versus 38.75%, respectively; $n = 31$ in treatment and control groups; $P = 0.04$).

Cranberry products have been evaluated in five clinical trials to determine their efficacy in preventing recurrent UTIs in women. Three of the trials had a successful primary outcome regarding cranberry consumption and the prevention of recurrent UTIs (Walker et al. 1997; Kontiokari et al. 2001; Stothers 2002), while the other studies did not demonstrate a significant effect (Barbosa-Cesnik et al. 2011; Stapleton et al. 2012). Only three trials were randomised, double-blind, placebo-controlled (Walker et al. 1997; Barbosa-Cesnik et al. 2011; Stapleton et al. 2012), but none was adequately powered statistically. All trials recruited healthy women, ages 18–72 years, with a history of at least one UTI within the previous year. Cranberry regimens and dosing varied greatly among these studies.

Walker et al. (1997) in a double-blind, placebo-controlled crossover study, provided participants with 400 mg of encapsulated cranberry solids taken once per day for 3 months (and 3 months of placebo). While taking cranberry pills, 7 out of the 10 women experienced fewer UTIs. Only 6 UTIs occurred among the 10 subjects on cranberry supplementation, while 15 UTIs occurred among the 10 subjects on the placebo. The authors concluded that cranberry extract pills were more effective than the placebo in reducing UTI occurrences ($P < 0.005$).

Kontiokari et al. (2001) used cranberry-lingonberry juice made from concentrates, primarily containing cranberry (7.5 g cranberry concentrate and 1.7 g lingonberry concentrate diluted in 50 mL water) once daily for 6 months. Kontiokari et al. (2001) also compared 100 mL of a probiotic milk drink containing *Lactobacillus* for 5 days/wk for 1 year to 150 women who were recruited with UTIs; an open group served as open controls. After 6 months, the women on the cranberry treatment experienced 56% fewer UTIs (defined as $>10^5$ cfu/mL) than the control group ($P = 0.02$). After 12 months, the cumulative occurrence of the first episode of UTI was still significantly different between the groups ($P = 0.048$), suggesting that the cranberry juice drink was effective in preventing UTI, while the probiotic drink was not.

Stothers (2002) had two cranberry treatment arms, administered as a juice or tablet. Participants in the juice arm consumed 240 mL of 'pure, unsweetened' cranberry juice 3 times/day, and the tablet arm received a 1:30 parts concentrated cranberry juice tablet twice per day for 12 months.

A double-blind, placebo-controlled crossover study by Walker et al. (1997) found that dried cranberry powder was effective in reducing UTI occurrence. Women between the ages of 28 and 44 with a history of recurrent UTIs were recruited to take two 400-mg cranberry extract pills per day for 3 months (and 3 months of placebo). Participants in the Barbosa-Cesnik et al. (2011) study consumed 2–240 mL cranberry beverage per day for 6 months; these subjects entered the trial with acute UTIs.

Participants in the study of Stapleton et al. (2012) consumed the same juice beverage, assigned to one 120 mL/day or 240 mL/day for 6 months. Papas et al. (1966) conducted an uncontrolled study in which 480 mL/day of cranberry juice cocktail was administered for 21 days to 60 patients (44 women and 16 men) diagnosed with acute UTI. After 3 weeks, 53% of the participants experienced fewer UTIs following cranberry juice consumption. Six weeks after discontinuation of cranberry treatment, bacteriuria returned in most subjects. Each study reported total PAC concentration, but used different methods to quantify PACs, thus giving inaccurate and varied results that are inconsistent with current quantification methods.

A recent study in which women with recurrent UTI were given 42 g dried cranberries/day for 2 weeks followed by observations for 6 months showed that women taking dried cranberries had significantly lower incidence of UTI, with a mean UTI rate at 6 months decreasing from 2.4 to 1.1 compared to a historical control group enrolled in a previous vaccine control study (Burleigh et al. 2013). The women in the dried cranberry group also had a significant reduction in *E. coli* in a rectal swab taken post-consumption. Recently, Takahashi et al. (2013) provided 125 mL/day of cranberry juice compared with placebo for 24 weeks to women between 20–79 years with recurrent UTI. In the subgroup of females aged 50 years or more, there was a significant difference in the rate of relapse of UTI between groups A and P (log-rank test; $P = 0.0425$). A study by Sengupta et al. (2011) found symptomatic relief and significant reduction ($P < 0.05$) in subjects positive for *E. coli* in both the high-dose (1000 mg) and low-dose (500 mg) treatment groups given a standardised cranberry powder for 90 days, compared to baseline evaluation in a randomised clinical trial of 60 female subjects between 18–40 years of age.

Asymptomatic bacteriuria (ASB), defined as $>10^5$ CFUs/mL of uropathogenic bacteria in the urine without the traditional symptoms associated with UTIs, is of particular concern in pregnant women due to their association with pre-term delivery and low birth weight (Romero et al. 1989; Sheiner et al. 2009). The first study published to investigate the effect of cranberry on ASB/UTI in pregnant women did not find a statistical difference in ASB, UTI or neonatal outcomes among participants who were compliant with zero, one or two 8-ounce servings of a cranberry beverage per day. The beverage treatments were reduced to 2 servings per day (Wing et al. 2008), and although this study was underpowered and prematurely halted, women compliant with two 8-ounce servings of cranberry per day experienced a 57% reduction in ASB and 41% reduction in UTI, indicating that cranberry may be efficacious in preventing ASB and UTIs in pregnant women. Further studies would help solidify this area of importance for pregnant women and UTI prevention. A recent literature review of pregnant women taking cranberry supplement compared with antibiotics showed no adverse effects on the mother or infants, including no increased risk of malformations nor any of the following pregnancy outcomes: stillbirth/neonatal death, preterm delivery, low birth weight, small for gestational age, low Apgar score or neonatal infections, suggesting that cranberry consumption during pregnancy has no safety concern (Heitmann et al. 2013). Although an association was found between use of cranberry in late pregnancy and vaginal bleeding after pregnancy week 17, further sub-analyses of more severe bleeding outcomes did not support a significant risk.

Recent trials in the paediatric population have demonstrated a benefit from cranberry consumption. The five available trials used a variety of cranberry products: 7.5 g cranberry concentrate plus 1.7 g of lingonberry concentrate diluted in 50 mL of water per day for 6 months (Ferrara et al. 2009); commercially available cranberry juice containing 8.2 g of cranberry concentrate per 200 mL water administered at 5 mL/kg body weight per day for 6 months (Salo et al. 2012); a cranberry syrup containing 36 mg PAC (measured by DMAC with A2 reference standard) administered at 5 mL per day depending on body weight (Uberos et al. 2012); and cranberry juice containing 37% PACs (PAC quantitation method not specified) administered at 2 mL/kg body weight for 1 year (Afshar et al. 2012). The primary outcomes analysed demonstrated that cranberry treatment was efficacious in reducing UTI risk by 65% (Afshar et al. 2012) and preventing UTI recurrences (Ferrara et al. 2009). The primary outcome of reducing the number of children who experienced a recurrent UTI was not statistically significant in the Salo et al. (2012) trial. Cranberry treatment did, however, significantly reduce the number of recurrent UTIs and the number of days on antibiotics.

A further analysis of the study of Uberos et al. (2015) focused on a secondary endpoint of the initial study (Uberos et al. 2012) to determine if there was a correlation between the excretion of phenolic acids (and their metabolites) in urine with bacterial anti-adherent activity of cranberry syrup. One group of subjects had been given a 3% glucose solution of cranberry extract (Urell®, Pharmatoka, Rueil-Maldmaison, France) yielding 4732 µg/mL of PACs at a dose equivalence of 5.6 mg/kg of extract; the other group had been given trimethoprim in a similar syrup base at a concentration of 8 mg/mL and 0.1% CC-1000-WS (E-120) at a dose of 1.6 mg/kg. Subjects included 85 children under 1 year of age, 53 of whom were treated with trimethoprim and 32 with cranberry syrup and 107 children over 1 year of age, 64 of whom were treated with trimethoprim and 43 with cranberry syrup. There were marked differences in efficacy in children under 1 year of age and those over, as well as between treatment groups. In the trimethoprim group, rates of UTI in males and females under 1 year of age were 19% and 43%, respectively. Interestingly, the gender-associated efficacy was reversed in the cranberry group, the UTI rates in male and female children under 1 year of age being 46% and 17%, respectively. When adjusting for gender differences, in those under 1 year of age, the overall rates of UTI recurrence in the trimethoprim group was 28% and in the cranberry group 35%. Similarly, a reversal of the rate of efficacy was observed in children over 1 year of age, the UTI rate being 35% in the trimethoprim group and 26% in the cranberry group. These researchers concluded that overall, cranberry syrup was similar in efficacy and safety to trimethoprim, but that in children under 1 year of age trimethoprim was more effective than cranberry syrup. Conversely, cranberry was slightly more effective than trimethoprim in reducing the incidence of multiresistant bacteria in urine culture, with 22.9% of the cranberry group displaying positive cultures compared to 33.3% in the trimethoprim group. Cranberry intake was correlated with high levels of hydroxycinnamic and hydroxybenzoic acids in urine, both of which have displayed anti-adhesion activity, leading researchers to suggest these active ingredients of cranberry may play a therapeutic role in the UTI preventive effects of cranberry *in vivo*, as suggested in other studies (Uberos et al. 2015).

A recent meta-analysis of the use of cranberry in the prevention of UTIs in children concludes that cranberry products are effective in otherwise healthy children and at least as effective as antibiotics in children with urogenital abnormalities. Dosage and frequency recommendation is confounded by the variability of products and dosages used in the trials included in this analysis (Durham et al. 2015).

13.5 SUMMARY

The accumulative *in vivo* data, including numerous positive clinical studies with almost 3000 subjects, along with strong pharmacological rationale, suggest the efficacy and safety of cranberry and its preparations for maintaining urinary tract health and the potential to help prevent UTIs. Conversely, an almost equal number of studies with more than 1600 subjects failed to show the efficacy in UTI prophylaxis or treatment, perhaps partially due to the use of non-standardised cranberry products that were not administered at an efficacious dose with an unknown soluble PAC content.

The efficacy of cranberry for urinary tract health is likely due to multiple effects that include anti-adhesion activity, modulation of bacterial motility, bactericidal activity and immune modulation by PACs and their metabolites.

This assessment has recently been confirmed by the Committee for Medicinal Products for Human Use of the European Medicines Agency (2016) regarding the mode of action of proanthocyanidins. Based on available data, the committee members opine that metabolites of PACs and other cranberry constituents exhibit pharmacological activity and rule out a purely mechanical mode of action, thus terminating (not challenging) challenging the marketing of cranberry products as medical devices in Europe. Consequently, the European Commission issued a decision that 'the group of products whose principal intended action, depending on proanthocyanidins (PAC) present in cranberry (*Vaccinium macrocarpon*), is to prevent or treat cystitis', does not fall within the definition of medical devices (European Commission 2017).

A-type PACs are predominantly associated with the anti-adhesion activity, with suggestions that 36 mg of total PACs daily, A and B-type together, (measured by DMAC with the A2 reference standard) is the target dose. This 36-mg dose is the amount of total PACs in a typical 300-mL serving of cranberry juice cocktail (27% juice) measured by the same DMAC/A2 method that showed efficacy in prevention of bacteriuria in elderly women (Avorn et al. 1994). Generally, a 240- to 300-mL serving has been recommended for more than 50 years by healthcare providers in the areas where the cranberries are grown.

Efficacy has been demonstrated for a variety of preparations including cranberry juice, cranberry juice cocktail, cranberry juice extracts, dried fruit, solid extracts and a syrup containing a cranberry juice extract. An important aspect of cranberry as a nutritional approach in potential prevention of UTIs is in lessening the need for conventional antibiotic therapy that leads to resistant bacterial strains. The over-consumption of antibiotics worldwide has caused an alarmingly growing resistance of pathogenic bacteria, including *E. coli* bacteria.

In 2017, three meta-analyses with positive conclusions were published.

Luís: A recent meta-analysis of 28 clinical investigations into the effects of cranberry preparations on the reduction of incidence of UTIs found that cranberry significantly reduces the incidence of UTIs (weighted risk ratio 0.6750, 95% CI 0.5516–0.7965, $p < 0.0001$). Additionally, patients at risk for UTI showed more susceptibility to the effect of cranberry treatment (Luís et al. 2017).

Fu: A further meta-analysis (Fu et al. 2017) assessed the efficacy of cranberry on the risk of recurrent UTIs in otherwise healthy women based on seven randomised controlled trials ($n = 1498$). Results showed that cranberry reduced the UTI risk by 26% (pooled risk ratio 0.74; 95% CI: 0.55, 0.98; $I^2 = 54\%$).

Huang: In another review and meta-analysis of randomised controlled trials, Huang et al. (2012) assessed a total of 26 studies with 4709 participants for the efficacy of cranberry in the prevention of UTIs. Through subgroup analysis, the authors found cranberry to be more effective in females (pooled risk ratio 0.73; 95% CI: 0.58, 0.92; $p = 0.002$; $I^2 = 59\%$) with recurrent UTIs (pooled risk ratio 0.71; 95% CI: 0.54, 0.93; $p = 0.002$; $I^2 = 65\%$).

Cranberry is generally recognised as safe (GRAS) and lacks any acute adverse side effects when consumed as a typical part of the diet. Long-term human studies similarly indicate a generally high level of safety for cranberry and its preparations used as foods or dietary supplements.

REFERENCES

Afshar, K., Stothers, L., Scott, H. and MacNeily, A. E. (2012). Cranberry juice for the prevention of pediatric urinary tract infection: A randomized controlled trial. *Journal of Urology*, **188**, 1584–1587.

Avorn, J., Monane, M., Gurwitz, J. H., Glynn, R. J., Choodnovskiy, I. and Lipsitz, L. A. (1994). Reduction of bacteriuria and pyuria after ingestion of cranberry juice. *JAMA*, **271**, 751–754.

Bailey, D. T., Dalton, C., Daugherty, F. J. and Tempesta, M. S. (2007). Can a concentrated cranberry extract prevent recurrent urinary tract infections in women? A pilot study. *Phytomedicine*, **14**, 237–241.

Barbosa-Cesnik, C., Brown, M. B., Buxton, M., Zhang, L., DeBusscher, J. and Foxman, B. (2011). Cranberry juice fails to prevent recurrent urinary tract infection: Results from a randomized placebo-controlled trial. *Clinical Infectious Diseases*, **52**, 23–30.

Barnoiu, O. S., Sequeira, J., del Moral, G., Sanchez-Martinez, N., Diaz-Molina, P., Flores, L. and Baena-Gonzalez, V. (2015). American cranberry (proanthocyanidin 120 mg): Its value for the prevention of urinary tract infections after ureteral catheter placement. *Actas Urológicas Españolas*, **39**, 112–117.

Beerepoot, M. A., ter Riet, G., Nys S., van der, Wal W. M., de Borgie, C. A., de Reijke, T. M., Prins, J. M., et al. (2011). Cranberries vs antibiotics to prevent urinary tract infections: A randomized double-blind noninferiority trial in premenopausal women. *Archives of Internal Medicine*, **171**, 1270–1278.

Bianco, L., Perrelli, E., Towle, V., Van Ness, P. H. and Juthani-Mehta, M. (2012). Pilot randomized controlled dosing study of cranberry capsules for reduction of bacteriuria plus pyuria in female nursing home residents. *Journal of the American Geriatrics Society*, **60**, 1180–1181.

Blatherwick, N. R. (1914). The specific role of foods in relation to the composition of the urine. *Archives of Internal Medicine*, **14**, 409–450.

Blatherwick, N. R. and Long, L. (1923). Studies of urinary acidity. II. The increased acidity produced by eating prunes and cranberries. *Journal of Biological Chemistry*, **57**, 815–819.

Blumberg, J. B., Camesano, T. A., Cassidy, A., Kris-Etherton, P., Howell, A., Manach, C., Ostertag, L. M., Sies, H., Skulas-Ray, A. and Vita, J. A. (2013). Cranberries and their bioactive constituents in human health. *Advances in Nutrition*, **4**, 618–632.

Bodel, P. T., Cotran, R. and Kass, E. H. (1959). Cranberry juice and the antibacterial action of hippuric acid. *Journal of Laboratory and Clinical Medicine*, **54**, 881–888.

Bone, K. and Morgan, M. (1999). Vaccinium macrocarpon-cranberry. *MediHerb Professional Review*, **72**, 1–4.

Bonetta, A, and Di Pierro, F. (2012). Enteric-coated, highly standardized cranberry extract reduces risk of UTIs and urinary symptoms during radiotherapy for prostate carcinoma. *Cancer Management and Research*, **4**, 281–286.

Borukh, I. F., Kirbaba, V. I. and Senchuk, G. V. (1972). [Antimicrobial properties of cranberry]. *Voprosy pitaniia*, **31**, 82.

Botto, H. and Neuzillet, Y. (2010). Effectiveness of a cranberry (*Vaccinium macrocarpon*) preparation in reducing asymptomatic bacteriuria in patients with an ileal enterocystoplasty. *Scandinavian Journal of Urology and Nephrology*, **44**, 165–168.

Brumfitt, W. and Percival, A. (1962). Adjustment of urine pH in the chemotherapy of urinary-tract infections. *Lancet*, **279**, 186–190.

Burleigh, A. E., Benck, S. M., McAchran, S. E., Reed, J. D., Krueger, C. G. and Hopkins, W. J. (2013). Consumption of sweetened, dried cranberries may reduce urinary tract infection incidence in susceptible women—A modified observational study. *Nutrition Journal*, **12**, 139.

Cadkova, I., Doudova, L., Novackova, M. and Chmel, R. (2009). Effect of cranberry extract capsules taken during the perioperative period upon the post-surgical urinary infection in gynecology. *Ceská Gynekologie*, **74**, 454–458.

Caljouw, M. A., van den Hout, W. B., Putter, H., Achterberg, W. P., Cools, H. J. and Gussekloo, J. (2014). Effectiveness of cranberry capsules to prevent urinary tract infections in vulnerable older persons: A double-blind randomized placebo-controlled trial in long-term care facilities. *Journal of the American Geriatrics Society*, **62**, 103–110.

Cowan, C. C., Hutchison, C., Cole, T., Barry, S. J. E., Paul, J., Reed, N. S. and Russell, J. M. (2012). A randomised double-blind placebo-controlled trial to determine the effect of cranberry juice on decreasing the incidence of urinary symptoms and urinary tract infections in patients undergoing radiotherapy for cancer of the bladder or cervix. *Clinical Oncology*, **24**, e31–e38.

Di Martino, P., Agniel, R., David, K., Templer, C., Gaillard, J. L., Denys, P. and Botto, H. (2006). Reduction of *Escherichia coli* adherence to uroepithelial bladder cells after consumption of cranberry juice: A double-blind randomized placebo-controlled cross-over trial. *World Journal of Urology*, **24**, 21–27.

Dignam, R. R., Ahmed, M., Kelly, K. G., Denman, S. J., Zayon, M. and Kleban, M. (1998). The effect of cranberry juice on urinary tract infection rates in a long-term care facility. *Annals of Long-Term Care*, **6**, 163–167.

Durham, S. H., Stamm, P. L. and Eiland, L. S. (2015). Cranberry products for the prophylaxis of urinary tract infections in pediatric patients. *Annals of Pharmacotherapy*, **49**, 1349–1356.

Essadi, F. and Elmehashi, M. O. (2010). Efficacy of cranberry juice for the prevention of urinary tract infections in pregnancy. *Journal of Maternal-Fetal and Neonatal Medicine*, **23**, 378.

European Commission. (2017). *Commission Implementing Decision (EU) 2017/1445 of 8 August 2017 on the group of products whose principal intended action, depending on proanthocyanidins (PAC) present in cranberry (Vaccinium macrocarpon), is to prevent or treat cystitis (notified under document C(2017) 5341)*. [Views 16 November 2017]. Available from: http://data.europa.eu/eli/dec_impl/2017/1445/oj

European Medicines Agency. (2016). *CHMP scientific opinion to DG Internal Market, Industry, Entrepreneurship and SMEs, Unit GROW D.4. 'Health Technology & Cosmetics' on the principal mode of action of proanthocyanidins intended to be used for prevention and treatment of urinary tract infections. EMA/427414/2016*. [Viewed 16 November 2017]. Available from: http://ec.europa.eu/DocsRoom/documents/19961

Feliciano, R. P., Krueger, C. G., Shanmuganayagam, D., Vestling, M. M. and Reed, J. D. (2012). Deconvolution of matrix-assisted laser desorption/ionization time-of-flight mass spectrometry isotope patterns to determine ratios of A-type to B-type interflavan bonds in cranberry proanthocyanidins. *Food Chemistry*, **135**, 1485–1493.

Feliciano, R. P., Meudt, J. J., Shanmuganayagam, D., Krueger, C. G. and Reed, J. D. (2014). Ratio of 'A-type' to 'B-type' proanthocyanidin interflavan bonds affects extra-intestinal pathogenic *Escherichia coli* invasion of gut epithelial cells. *Journal of the American Chemical Society*, **62**, 3919–3925.

Fernández-Puentes, V., Uberos, J., Rodríguez-Belmonte, R., Nogueras-Ocaña, M., Blanca-Jover, E. and Narbona-López, E. (2015). Efficacy and safety profile of cranberry in infants and children with recurrent urinary tract infection. *Anales de Pediatria*, **82**(6), 397–403.

Ferrara, P., Romaniello, L., Vitelli, O., Gatto, A., Serva, M. and Cataldi, L. (2009). Cranberry juice for the prevention of recurrent urinary tract infections: A randomized controlled trial in children. *Scandinavian Journal of Urology and Nephrology*, **43**, 369–372.

Foda, M. M., Middlebrook, P. F., Gatfield, C. T., Potvin, G., Wells, G. and Schillinger, J. F. (1995). Efficacy of cranberry in prevention of urinary tract infection in a susceptible pediatric population. *Canadian Journal of Urology*, **2**, 98–102.

Foo, L. Y., Lu, Y., Howell, A. B. and Vorsa, N. (2000a). The structure of cranberry proanthocyanidins which inhibit adherence of uropathogenic P-fimbriated *Escherichia coli* in vitro. *Phytochemistry*, **54**, 173–181.

Foo, L. Y., Lu, Y., Howell, A. B. and Vorsa, N. (2000b). A-type proanthocyanidin trimers from cranberry that inhibit adherence of uropathogenic P-fimbriated *Escherichia coli*. *Journal of Natural Products*, **63**, 1225–1228.

Foxman, B. (1990). Recurring urinary tract infection: Incidence and risk factors. *American Journal of Public Health*, **80**, 331–333.

Foxman, B. (2002). Epidemiology of urinary tract infections: Incidence, morbidity, and economic costs. *American Journal of Medicine*, **113**(Suppl 1A), 5S–13S.

Foxman, B. and Brown, P. (2003). Epidemiology of urinary tract infections: Transmission and risk factors, incidence, and costs. *Infectious Disease Clinics of North America*, **17**, 227–241.

Foxman, B., Cronenwett, A. E. W., Spino, C., Berger, M. B. and Morgan, D. M. (2015). Cranberry juice capsules and urinary tract infection after surgery: Results of a randomized trial. *American Journal of Obstetrics & Gynecology*, **213**(2), 194ff.

Fu, Z., Liska, D., Talan, D. and Chung, M. (2017). Cranberry reduces the risk of urinary tract infection recurrence in otherwise healthy women: A systematic review and meta-analysis. *Journal of Nutrition*, **18**, jn254961.

Gallien, P., Amarenco, G., Benoit, N., Bonniaud, V., Donzé, C., Kerdraon, J., de Seze, M., et al. (2014). Cranberry versus placebo in the prevention of urinary infections in multiple sclerosis: A multicenter, randomized, placebo-controlled, double-blind trial. *Multiple Sclerosis Journal*, **20**, 1252–1259.

Gibson, L., Pike, L. and Kilbourn, J. P. (1991). Clinical Study: Effectiveness of cranberry juice in preventing urinary tract infections in long-term care facility patients. *Journal of Naturopathic Medicine*, **2**, 45–47.

Greenberg, J. A., Newmann, S. J. and Howell, A. B. (2005). Consumption of sweetened dried cranberries versus unsweetened raisins for inhibition of uropathogenic *Escherichia coli* adhesion in human urine: A pilot study. *Journal of Alternative and Complementary Medicine*, **11**, 875–878.

Griebling, T. L. (2005). Urologic diseases in America project: Trends in resource use for urinary tract infections in women. *Journal of Urology*, **173**, 1281–1287.

Gu, L., Kelm, M. A., Hammerstone, J. F., Beecher, G., Holden, J., Haytowitz, D., Gebhardt, S. and Prior, R. L. (2004). Concentrations of proanthocyanidins in common foods and estimations of normal consumption. *Journal of Nutrition*, **134**, 613–617.

Gu, L., Kelm, M. A., Hammerstone, J. F., Beecher, G., Holden, J., Haytowitz, D. and Prior, R. L. (2003). Screening of foods containing proanthocyanidins and their structural characterization using LC-MS/MS and thiolytic degradation. *Journal of Agricultural and Food Chemistry*, **51**, 7513–7521.

Gunnarsson, A. K., Gunningberg, L., Larsson, S. and Jonsson, K. B. (2017). Cranberry juice concentrate does not significantly decrease the incidence of acquired bacteriuria in female hip fracture patients receiving urine catheter: A double-blind randomized trial. *Clinical Interventions in Aging*, **12**, 137–143.

Gupta, K., Chou, M. Y., Howell, A., Wobbe, C., Grady, R. and Stapleton, A. E. (2007). Cranberry products inhibit adherence of P-fimbriated *Escherichia coli* to primary cultured bladder and vaginal epithelial cells. *Journal of Urology*, **177**, 2357–2360.

Hamilton, K., Bennett, N. C., Purdie, G. and Herst, P. M. (2015). Standardized cranberry capsules for radiation cystitis in prostate cancer patients in New Zealand: A randomized double blinded, placebo controlled pilot study. *Supportive Care in Cancer*, **23**(1), 95–102.

Hamilton-Miller, J. M. T and Brumfitt, W. (1976). Methenamine and its salts as urinary tract antiseptics: Variables affecting the antibacterial activity of formaldehyde, mandelic acid, and hippuric acid in vitro. *Investigative Urology*, **14**, 287–291.

Haverkorn, M. J. and Mandigers, J. (1994). Reduction of bacteriuria and pyuria using cranberry juice. *JAMA*, **272**, 590.

Heitmann, K., Nordeng, H. and Holst, L. (2013). Pregnancy outcome after use of cranberry in pregnancy— The Norwegian mother and child cohort study. *BMC Complementary and Alternative Medicine*, **13**, 345.

Henig, Y. S. and Leahy, M. M. (2000). Cranberry juice and urinary-tract health: Science supports folklore. *Nutrition*, **16**, 684–687.

Hess, M. J., Hess, P. E., Sullivan, M. R., Nee, M. and Yalla, S. V. (2008). Evaluation of cranberry tablets for the prevention of urinary tract infections in spinal cord injured patients with neurogenic bladder. *Spinal Cord*, **46**, 622–626.

Howell, A. (2013). Commentary on: Jepson RG, Williams G and Craig JC. Cranberries for preventing urinary tract infections. *Cochrane Database of Systematic Reviews*, **10**, CD001321.

Howell, A. B., Botto, H., Combescure, C., Blanc-Potard, A. B., Gausa, L., Matsumoto, T., Tenke, P., Sotto, A. and Lavigne, J. P. (2010). Dosage effect on uropathogenic *Escherichia coli* anti-adhesion activity in urine following consumption of cranberry powder standardized for proanthocyanidin content: A multicentric randomized double blind study. *BioMed Central Infectious Diseases*, **10**, 94.

Howell, A. B., Der Marderosian, A. and Foo, L. Y. (1998). Inhibition of the adherence of P-fimbriated *Escherichia coli* to uroepithelial-cell surfaces by proanthocyanidin extracts from cranberries. *New England Journal of Medicine*, **339**, 1085–1086.

Howell, A. B., Leahy, M., Kurowska, E. and Guthrie, N. (2001). In vivo evidence that cranberry proanthocyanidins inhibit adherence of P-fimbriated *E. coli* bacteria to uroepithelial cells. *FASEB Journal*, **15**, A284.

Howell, A. B., Reed, J. D., Krueger, C. G., Winterbottom, R., Cunningham, D. G. and Leahy, M. (2005). A-type cranberry proanthocyanidins and uropathogenic bacterial anti-adhesion activity. *Phytochemistry*, **66**, 2281–2291.

Huang, Y. C., Chen, P. S. and Tung, T. H. (2017). Effectiveness of cranberry ingesting for prevention of urinary tract infection: A systematic review and meta-analysis of randomized controlled trials. *World Academy of Science, Engineering and Technology International Journal of Medical Sciences*, **5**(5).

Ibragimov, D. I. and Kazanskaia, G. B. (1981). Antimicrobial action of cranberry bush, common yarrow and *Achillea biebersteinii*. *Antibiotiki*, **26**, 108–109.

Jackson, B. and Hicks, L. E. (1997). Effect of cranberry juice on urinary pH in older adults. *Home Healthcare Nurse*, **15**, 199–202.

Jepson, R. G. and Craig, J. C. (2007). A systematic review of the evidence for cranberries and blueberries in UTI prevention. *Molecular Nutrition & Food Research*, **51**, 738–745.

Jepson, R. G. and Craig, J. C. (2008). Cranberries for preventing urinary tract infections. *Cochrane Database of Systematic Reviews*, **1**, CD001321.

Jepson, R. G., Williams, G. and Craig, J. C. (2012). Cranberries for preventing urinary tract infections. *Cochrane Database of Systematic Reviews*, **10**, CD001321.

Juthani-Mehta, M., Perley L., Chen, S., Dziura, J. and Gupta, K. (2010). Feasibility of cranberry capsule administration and clean-catch urine collection in long-term care residents. *Journal of the American Geriatrics Society*, **58**, 2028–2030.

Juthani-Mehta, M., Van Ness, P. H., Bianco, L., Rink, A., Rubeck, S., Ginter, S., Argraves, S., et al. (2016). Effect of cranberry capsules on bacteriuria plus pyuria among older women in nursing homes: A randomized clinical trial. *JAMA*, **316**(18), 1879–1887.

Kahn, H. D., Panariello, V. A., Saeli, J., Sampson, J. R. and Schwartz, E. (1967). Implications for therapy of urinary tract infection and calculi: Effect of cranberry juice on urine. *Journal of the American Dietetic Association*, **51**, 251–254.

Karonen, M., Leikas, A., Loponen, J., Sinkkonen, J., Ossipov, V. and Pihlaja, K. (2007). Reversed-phase HPLC–ESI–MS analysis of birch leaf proanthocyanidins after their acidic degradation in the presence of nucleophiles. *Phytochemical Analysis*, **18**, 378–386.

Kerr, K. G. (1999). Cranberry juice and prevention of recurrent urinary tract infection. *Lancet*, **353**, 673.

Kinney, A. B. and Blount, M. (1979). Effect of cranberry juice on urinary pH. *Nursing Research*, **28**, 287–290.

Konowalchuk, J. and Speirs, J. I. (1978). Antiviral effect of commercial juices and beverages. *Applied and Environmental Microbiology*, **35**, 1219–1220.

Kontiokari, T., Salo, J., Eerola, E. and Uhari, M. (2005). Cranberry juice and bacterial colonization in children – A placebo-controlled randomized trial. *Clinical Nutrition*, **24**, 1065–1072.

Kontiokari, T., Sundqvist, K., Nuutinen, M., Pokka, T., Koskela, M. and Uhari, M. (2001). Randomised trial of cranberry-lingonberry juice and *Lactobacillus* GG drink for the prevention of urinary tract infections in women. *British Medical Journal*, **322**, 1571.

Kraemer, R. J. (1964). Cranberry juice and the reduction of ammoniacal odor of urine. *Southwestern Medicine*, **45**, 211–212.

Krueger, C. G., Maudi, J. J., Howell, A. B., Khoo, C., Shanmuganayugari, D. and Reed, J. D. (2013a). Consumption of cranberry powder shifts urinary protein profile in healthy human subjects. *FASEB Journal*, **27**, 637.32.

Krueger, C. G., Reed, J. D., Feliciano, R. and Howell, A. B. (2013b). Quantifying and characterizing proanthocyanidins in cranberries in relation to urinary tract health. *Analytical and Bioanalytical Chemistry*, **405**, 4385–4395.

Krueger, C. G., Vestling, M. M. and Reed, J. D. (2003). Matrix-assisted laser desorption/ionization time-of-flight mass spectrometry of heteropolyflavan-3-ols and glucosylated heteropolyflavans in sorghum (*Sorghum bicolor* (l.) Moench). *Journal of Agricultural and Food Chemistry*, **51**, 538–543.

LaPlante, K. L., Sarkisian, S. A., Woodmansee, S., Rowley, D. C. and Seeram, N. P. (2012). Effects of cranberry extracts on growth and biofilm production of *Escherichia coli* and *Staphylococcus* species. *Phytotherapy Research*, **26**, 1371–1374.

Lavigne, J. P., Bourg, G., Combescure, C., Botto, H. and Sotto, A. (2008). In-vitro and in-vivo evidence of dose-dependent decrease of uropathogenic *Escherichia coli* virulence after consumption of commercial Vaccinium macrocarpon (cranberry) capsules. *Clinical Microbiology and Infection*, **14**, 350–355.

Ledda, A., Belcaro, G., Dugall, M., Riva, A., Togni, S., Eggenhoffner, R. and Giacomelli, L. (2017). Highly standardized cranberry extract supplementation (Anthocran®) as prophylaxis in young healthy subjects with recurrent urinary tract infections. *European Review for Medical and Pharmacological Sciences*, **21**(2), 389–393.

Ledda, A., Bottari, A., Luzzi, R., Belcaro, G., Hu, S., Dugall, M., Hosoi, M., Ippolito, E., Corsi, M., Gizzi G. and Morazzoni, P. (2015). Cranberry supplementation in the prevention of non-severe lower urinary tract infections: A pilot study. *European Review for Medical and Pharmacological Sciences*, **19**(1), 77–80.

Lee, B. B., Haran, M. J., Hunt, L. M., Simpson, J. M., Marial, O., Rutkowski, S. B., Middleton, J. W., Kotsiou, G., Tudehope, M. and Cameron, I. D. (2007). Spinal-injured neuropathic bladder antisepsis (SINBA) trial. *Spinal Cord*, **45**, 542–550.

Lee, W. K., Ko, M. C. and Huang, C. S. (2016). Cranberries for preventing recurrent urinary tract infections in uncircumcised boys. *Alternative Therapies in Health and Medicine*, **22**(6), 20.

Light, I., Gursel, E. and Zinnser, H. H. (1973). Urinary ionized calcium in urolithiasis: Effect of cranberry juice. *Urology*, **1**, 67–70.

Lin, S. C., Wang, C. C., Shih, S. C., Tjung, J. J., Tsou, M. T. and Lin, C. J. (2014). Prevention of asymptomatic bacteriuria with cranberries and Roselle juice in home-care patients with long-term urinary catheterization. *International Journal of Gerontology*, **8**, 152–156.

Linsenmeyer, T. A., Harrison, B., Oakley, A., Kirshblum, S., Stock, J. A. and Millis, S. R. (2004). Evaluation of cranberry supplement for reduction of urinary tract infections in individuals with neurogenic bladders secondary to spinal cord injury. A prospective, double-blinded, placebo-controlled, crossover study. *Journal of Spinal Cord Medicine*, **27**, 29–34.

Luís, Â., Domingues, F. and Pereira, L. (2017). Can cranberries contribute to reduce the incidence of urinary tract infections? A systematic review with meta-analysis and trial sequential analysis of clinical trials. *Journal of Urology*, **198**, 614–621.

Maki, K. C., Kaspar, K. L., Khoo, C., Derrig, L. H., Schild, A. L. and Gupta, K. (2016). Consumption of a cranberry juice beverage lowered the number of clinical urinary tract infection episodes in women with a recent history of urinary tract infection. *American Journal of Clinical Nutrition*, **103**(6), 1434–1442.

Mathison, B. D., Kimble, L. L., Kaspar, K. L., Khoo, C. and Chew, B. P. (2014). Consumption of cranberry beverage improved endogenous antioxidant status and protected against bacteria adhesion in healthy humans: A randomized controlled trial. *Nutrition Research*, **34**, 420–427.

Mazokopakis, E. E., Karefilakis, C. M. and Starakis, I. K. (2009). Efficacy of cranberry capsules in prevention of urinary tract infections in postmenopausal women. *Journal of Alternative and Complementary
Medicine*, **15**, 1155.

McCall, J., Hidalgo, G., Asadishad, B. and Tufenkji, N. (2013). Cranberry impairs selected behaviors essential
for virulence in Proteus mirabilis HI4320. *Canadian Journal of Microbiology*, **59**(6), 430–436.

McGuinness, S. D., Krone, R. and Metz, L. M. (2002). A double-blind, randomized, placebo-controlled trial
of cranberry supplements in multiple sclerosis. *Journal of Neuroscience Nursing*, **34**, 4–7.

McKay, D. L., Chen, C. Y., Zampariello, C. A. and Blumberg, J. B. (2015). Flavonoids and phenolic acids from
cranberry juice are bioavailable and bioactive in healthy older adults. *Food Chemistry*, **168**, 233–240.

McMurdo, M. E., Argo, I., Phillips, G., Daly, F. and Davey, P. (2009). Cranberry or trimethoprim for the prevention of recurrent urinary tract infections? A randomized controlled trial in older women. *Journal of
Antimicrobial Chemotherapy*, **63**, 389–395.

McMurdo, M. E., Bissett, L. Y., Price, R. J., Phillips, G. and Crombie, I. K. (2005). Does ingestion of cranberry juice reduce symptomatic urinary tract infections in older people in hospital? A double-blind,
placebo-controlled trial. *Age and Ageing*, **34**, 256–261.

Micali, S., Isgro, G., Bianchi, G., Miceli, N., Calapai, G. and Navarra, M. (2014). Cranberry and recurrent
cystitis: More than marketing? *Critical Reviews in Food Science and Nutrition*, **54**, 1063–1075.

Mutlu, H. and Ekinci, Z. (2012). Urinary tract infection prophylaxis in children with neurogenic bladder with
cranberry capsules: Randomized controlled trial. *ISRN Pediatrics*, **2012**, 1–4.

Neto, C. C., Krueger, C. G., Lamoureaux, T. L., Kondo, M., Vaisberg, A. J., Hurta, R. A. R., Curtis, S., et al.
(2006). MALDI-TOF MS characterization of proanthocyanidins from cranberry fruit (*Vaccinium
macrocarpon*) that inhibit tumor cell growth and matrix metalloproteinase expression in vitro. *Journal
of the Science of Food and Agriculture*, **86**, 18–25.

Nickey, K. E. (1975). Urinary pH: Effect of prescribed regimes of cranberry juice and ascorbic acid. *Archives
of Physical Medicine and Rehabilitation*, **56**, 556.

Nowack, R. and Schmitt, W. (2008). Cranberry juice for prophylaxis of urinary tract infections – Conclusions
from clinical experience and research. *Phytomedicine*, **15**, 653–667.

Ofek, I., Goldhar, J. and Sharon, N. (1996). Anti-*Escherichia coli* adhesion activity of cranberry and blueberry
juices. In: I. Kahane and I. Ofek, eds. *Toward Anti-adhesion Therapy for Microbial Diseases*. New
York: Plenum. pp. 179–183.

Papas, P. N., Brusch, C. A. and Ceresia, G. C. (1966). Cranberry juice in the treatment of urinary tract infections. *Southwestern Medicine*, **47**, 17–20.

Patel, N. and Daniels, I. R. (2000). Botanical perspectives on health: Of cystitis and cranberries. *Journal of
the Royal Society for the Promotion of Health*, **120**, 52–53.

Porter, M. L., Krueger, C. G., Wiebe, D. A. and Cunningham, D. G. (2001). Cranberry proanthocyanidins
associate with low-density lipoprotein and inhibit in vitro Cu2+-induced oxidation. *Journal of the
Science of Food and Agriculture*, **81**, 1306–1313.

Rajbhandari, R., Peng, N., Moore, R., Arabshahi, A., Wyss, J. M., Barnes, S. and Prasain, J. K. (2011).
Determination of cranberry phenolic metabolites in rats by liquid chromatography-tandem mass spectrometry. *Journal of Agricultural and Food Chemistry*, **59**, 6682–6688.

Reed, J. D., Krueger, C. G. and Vestling, M. M. (2005). MALDI-TOF mass spectrometry of oligomeric food
polyphenols. *Phytochemistry*, **66**, 2248–2263.

Reid, G. (1999). Potential preventive strategies and therapies in urinary tract infection. *World Journal of
Urology*, **17**, 359–363.

Risco, E., Miguelez, C., Sanchez de Badajoz, E. and Rouseaud, A. (2010). Effect of American cranberry
(Cysticlean) on *Escherichia coli* adherence to bladder epithelial cells. In vitro and in vivo study. *Archivos
Españoles de Urología*, **63**, 422–430.

Rogers, J. (1991). Clinical: Pass the cranberry juice. *Nursing Times*, **27**, 36–37.

Romero, R., Oyarzun, E., Mazor, M., Sirtori, M., Hobbins, J. C. and Bracken, M. (1989). Meta-analysis of the
relationship between asymptomatic bacteriuria and preterm delivery/low birth weight. *Obstetrics &
Gynecology*, **73**, 576–582.

Salo, J., Uhari, M., Helminen, M., Korppi, M., Nieminen, T., Pokka, T. and Kontiokari, T. (2012). Cranberry
juice for the prevention of recurrences of urinary tract infections in children: A randomized placebo-
controlled trial. *Clinical Infectious Diseases*, **54**, 340–346.

Schappert, S. M. and Rechtsteiner, E. A. (2011). Ambulatory medical care utilization estimates for 2007. *Vital
and Health Statistics*, **13**, 1–38.

Schlager, T. A., Anderson, S., Trudell, J. and Hendley, J. O. (1999). Effect of cranberry juice on bacteriuria in children with neurogenic bladder receiving intermittent catheterization. *Journal of Pediatrics*, **135**, 698–702.

Schultz, A. S. (1984a). Efficacy of cranberry on urinary pH. *Journal of Community Health Nursing*, **1**, 159–169.

Schultz, A. S. (1984b). Efficacy of cranberry juice and ascorbic acid in acidifying the urine in multiple sclerosis subjects. *Journal of Community Health Nursing*, **1**, 139–169.

Sengupta, K., Alluri, K. V., Golakoti, T., Gottumukkala, G. V., Raavi, J., Kotchrlakota, L., Sigalan, S. C., Dey, D., Gosh, S. and Chatterjee, A. (2011). A randomized, double blind, controlled dose dependent clinical trial to evaluate the efficacy of a standardized whole cranberry (Vaccinium macrocarpon) powder on infections of the urinary tract. *Current Bioactive Compounds*, **7**, 39–46.

Shanmuganayugari, D., Johnson, R. E., Meudt, J. J., Felciano, R. P., Kohlman, K. L., Nechyporenko, A. V., Heinz, J., Krueger, C. G. and Reed, J. D. (2013). A-type proanthocyanidins from cranberry inhibit the ability of extraintestinal pathogenic *E. coli* to invade gut epithelial cells and resist killing by macrophages. *FASEB Journal*, **27**, 637.16.

Sheiner, E., Mazor-Drey, E. and Levy, A. (2009). Asymptomatic bacteriuria during pregnancy. *J Journal of Maternal-Fetal and Neonatal Medicine*, **22**, 423–427.

Singh, I., Gautam, L. K. and Kaur, I. R. (2016). Effect of oral cranberry extract (standardized proanthocyanidin-A) in patients with recurrent UTI by pathogenic *E. coli*: A randomized placebo-controlled clinical research study. *International Urology and Nephrology*, **48**(9), 1379–1386.

Sobota, A. E. (1984). Inhibition of bacterial adherence by cranberry juice: Potential use for the treatment of urinary tract infections. *Journal of Urology*, **131**(5), 1013–1016.

Stapleton, A. E. (2013). Cranberry-containing products are associated with a protective effect against urinary tract infections. *Archives of Internal Medicine*, **172**, 988–996.

Stapleton, A. E., Dziura, J., Hooton, T. M., Cox, M. E., Yarova-Yarovaya, Y., Chen, S. and Gupta, K. (2012). Recurrent urinary tract infection and urinary *Escherichia coli* in women ingesting cranberry juice daily: A randomized controlled trial. *Mayo Clinic Proceedings*, **87**, 143–150.

Sternlieb, P. (1963). Cranberry juice in renal disease. *New England Journal of Medicine*, **268**, 57.

Stothers, L. (2002). A randomized trial to evaluate effectiveness and cost effectiveness of naturopathic cranberry products as prophylaxis against urinary tract infection in women. *Canadian Journal of Urology*, **9**, 1558–1562.

Swartz, J. H. and Medrek, T. F. (1968). Antifungal properties of cranberry juice. *Applied Microbiology*, **16**, 1524.

Takahashi, S., Hamasuna, R., Yasuda, M., Arakawa, S., Tanaka, K., Ishikawa, K., Kiyota, H., et al. (2013). A randomized clinical trial to evaluate the preventive effect of cranberry juice (UR65) for patients with recurrent urinary tract infection. *Journal of Infection and Chemotherapy*, **19**, 112–117.

Tempera, G., Corsello, S., Genovese, C., Caruso, F. E. and Nicolosi, D. (2010). Inhibitory activity of cranberry extract on the bacterial adhesiveness in the urine of women: An ex-vivo study. *International Journal of Immunopathology and Pharmacology*, **23**, 611–618.

Thomas, D., Rutman, M., Cooper, K., Abrams, A., Finkelstein, J. and Chughtai, B. (2018). Does cranberry have a role in catheter-associated urinary tract infections? *Canadian Urological Association Journal*, **11**(11), E421–E424.

Uberos, J., Nogueras-Ocana, M., Fernandez-Puentes, V., Rodriguez-Belmonte, R., Narbona-Lopez, E., Molina-Carballo, A. and Munoz-Hoyos, A. (2012). Cranberry syrup vs trimethoprim in the prophylaxis of recurrent urinary tract infections among children: A controlled trial. *Open Access Journal of Clinical Trials*, **4**, 31–38.

Uberos, J., Rodríguez-Belmonte, R., Rodríguez-Pérez, C., Molina-Oya, M., Blanca-Jover, E., Narbona-Lopez, E. and Muñoz-Hoyos, A. (2015). Phenolic acid content and antiadherence activity in the urine of patients treated with cranberry syrup (*Vaccinium macrocarpon*) vs. trimethoprim for recurrent urinary tract infection. *Journal of Functional Foods*, **18**, 608–616.

Ujvary, I., Orlik, J., Racz, G. and Donath, A. (1961). On the fungistatic effect of the cranberries and cranberry products. Univ Mass Agr Exp (*Vaccinium Vitis* Idaea L.) crop-extract. *Morphologiai és igazságügyi orvosi szemle*, **4**, 406–409.

Upton, R. and Brendler, T., eds., (2016). *American herbal pharmacopoeia and therapeutic compendium: Cranberry fruit: Vaccinium macrocarpon Aiton*. Scotts Valley, CA: American Herbal Pharmacopoeia. Monograph revision.

Valentova, K., Stejskal, D., Bednar, P., Vostalova, J., Cihalik, C., Vecerova, R., Koukalova, D. et al. (2007). Biosafety, antioxidant status, and metabolites in urine after consumption of dried cranberry juice in healthy women: A pilot double-blind placebo-controlled trial. *Journal of Agricultural and Food Chemistry*, **55**, 3217–3224.

Vidlar, A., Student, V., Vostalova, J., Fromentin, E., Roller, M. and Simanek, V. (2016). Cranberry fruit powder (Flowens™) improves lower urinary tract symptoms in men: A double-blind, randomized, placebo-controlled study. *World Journal of Urology*, **34**(3), 419–424.

Vidlar, A., Vostalova, J., Ulrichova, J., Student, V., Stejskal, D., Reichenbach, R., Vrbkova, J., Ruzicka, F. and Simanek, V. (2009). Beneficial effects of cranberries on prostate health: Evidence from a randomized controlled trial. *European Urology Supplements*, **8**, 660.

Vostalova, J., Vidlar, A., Simanek, V., Galandakova, A., Kosina, P., Vacek, J., Vrbkova, J., Zimmermann, B. F., Ulrichova, J. and Student, V. (2015). Are high proanthocyanidins key to cranberry efficacy in the prevention of recurrent urinary tract infection? *Phytotherapy Research*, **29**(10), 1559–1567.

Waites, K. B., Canupp, K. C., Armstrong, S. and DeVivo, M. J. (2004). Effect of cranberry extract on bacteriuria and pyuria in persons with neurogenic bladder secondary to spinal cord injury. *Journal of Spinal Cord Medicine*, **27**, 35–40.

Walker, E. B., Barney, D. P., Mickelsen, J. N., Walton, R. J. and Mickelsen, R. A. (1997). Cranberry concentrate: UTI prophylaxis. *Journal of Family Practice*, **45**, 167–168.

Wang, C. H., Fang, C. C., Chen, N. C., Liu, S. S., Yu, P. H., Wu, T. Y., Chen, W. T., Lee, C. C. and Chen, S. C. (2012). Cranberry-containing products for prevention of urinary tract infections in susceptible populations: A systematic review and meta-analysis of randomized controlled trials. *Archives of Internal Medicine*, **172**, 988–996.

WHO. (2014). Microbial resistance: Global report on surveillance. Available from: www.WHO.INT

Wing, D. A., Rumney, P. J., Preslicka, C. W. and Chung, J. H. (2008). Daily cranberry juice for the prevention of asymptomatic bacteriuria in pregnancy: A randomized, controlled pilot study. *Journal of Urology*, **180**, 1367–1372.

Zafriri, D., Ofek, I., Adar, R., Pocino, M. and Sharon, N. (1989). Inhibitory activity of cranberry juice on adherence of type 1 and type P fimbriated *Escherichia coli* to eucaryotic cells. *Antimicrobial Agents and Chemotherapy*, **33**, 92–98.

Zhou, Y., Zhuang, W., Hu, W., Liu, G. J., Wu, T. X. and Wu, X. T. (2011). Consumption of large amounts of Allium vegetables reduces risk for gastric cancer in a meta-analysis. *Gastroenterology*, **141**, 80–89.

14 The Promise for Alzheimer's Disease Treatment
Bioactive Compounds

Víctor Andrade*, Leonardo Guzmán-Martínez,
Nicole Cortés and Ricardo B. Maccioni

CONTENTS

14.1 INTRODUCTION

14.1.1 ALZHEIMER'S DISEASE

Alzheimer's disease (AD) is the most common type of dementia in the senile population (over 60 years old; Bettens et al. 2010) and gradually affects learning and memory, displaying a prevalence and impact in constant expansion according to the World Health Organization (WHO). Recently, our laboratory has associated this pathology with behavioural disorders prior to cognitive decline (Andrade et al. 2017). This expansive and epidemic brain disorder is of concern to medical and public health opinion, which is focusing efforts on its prevention and treatment. In the biological context, two main aetiological effectors have been reported: (i) neurofibrillary tangles (NFT), derived from the progressive aggregation of hyperphosphorylated protein tau inside the neuron and assembled in oligomeric structures called paired helical filaments (PHF; Maccioni et al. 2001; Farias et al. 2011; Maccioni 2012; Guzman-Martinez et al. 2013); and (ii) senile plaques (SP), composed by deposits of the amyloid-β (Aβ) peptide of 39–42 amino-acid residues that are generated by the proteolytic excision of amyloid precursor protein (APP) by the enzymes β- and γ-secretases in the extracellular space, both promoting loss of synaptic processes and neuronal death (Lambert et al. 2009; Bettens et al. 2010). Among the clinical studies to control progression of this pathology, novel strategies are being implemented to prevent AD based on dietary changes and nutritional supplements, functional foods and natural compounds. We proposed that the onset of AD is a consequence of the response of microglial cells to 'damage signals' or tau oligomers, which trigger a

---

* Corresponding author.

neuroinflammatory response, promoting the misfolding of the cytoskeleton structure (Fernandez et al. 2008; Maccioni et al. 2009; Farias et al. 2011). Innovative treatments, such as we are going to review here, are essential to improve life quality and ameliorate the symptoms of affected subjects. However, the pharmaceutical industry has failed in developing new, effective drugs to control AD. In this context, major attention has been given to nutraceuticals and novel bioactive compounds, such as the Andean compound, obtained from areas in the north of Chilean desert mountains and, its new formulation, BrainUp-10®, supplemented with a complex of B vitamins (Carrasco-Gallardo et al. 2012a,b). Preliminary studies suggest that this compound is effective in controlling the disease or serving as a co-adjuvant for effective treatment (Carrasco-Gallardo et al. 2012a,b). Intensive work toward the elucidation of the molecular mechanisms of action of this compound is being carried out. In addition, an advanced second phase clinical trial is actually being developed.

14.1.2 Neuroinflammation and Neurological Diseases

Neuroinflammation is defined as the response of the central nervous system (CNS) against exogenous and/or endogenous agents that can interfere with the normal homeostatic processes in the cell. This inflammatory response is usually triggered from a secondary signalling cascade after a trauma or infection. Nevertheless, this mechanism has been characterised as a central axis during the progression of neurodegeneration. During this secondary response there is probably an important loss of neurons, in contrast with the first damage (Akiyama et al. 2000). The previous effect is also involved in every neurological disease, including developmental pathologies, traumatic, ischaemic, metabolic, infectious, toxics, neoplasic and neurodegenerative disorders. Inflammation plays a key main role in triggering a number of different neuropathologies, such as AD, Parkinson's or amyotrophic lateral sclerosis, among others (Morales et al. 2017b). In AD, a continuously active inflammatory condition could promote neural damage and, consequently, neuronal cells death, which then induces the release of pathological forms of tau protein to the extracellular environment. Because it has been reported that certain tau oligomers are able to activate microglial cells, they subsequently trigger a positive feedback mechanism, generating constant damage to cells (Maccioni et al. 2009; Morales et al. 2013, 2014). An overexpression of inflammatory mediators has also been reported in the vicinity of Aβ and the paired helical filaments (PHF) in AD, which, in the meantime, are associated with highly affected zones in the pathology (Morales et al. 2010).

Chronic metabolic diseases as hypertension, diabetes, clinical depression, dementia or traumatic lesions in the brain, are considered silent contributors to neuroinflammation (Chen et al. 2016). In the same context, other risk factors causing impairment or even death in the CNS tissue are stroke and atherosclerosis. Moreover, during normal ageing, there is a natural chronic activation of pro-inflammatory signals in the same areas, contributing to an even higher vulnerability for neuropsychiatric disorders (Capuron et al. 2008). Finally, pro-inflammatory agents such as interleukin 6 (IL-6), interleukin 8 (IL-8), tumour necrosis factor alpha (TNF-α), C-reactive protein and adipokines are correlated with clinical depression and anxiety symptoms (Ouchi et al. 2011; Chen et al. 2016).

Over-activation of the immune response in the CNS compromises the generation of neurotrophic factors and the release of cytotoxic agents to the microglial cell (Maccioni et al. 2009). The microglia has an important role in the immune system of the brain, and it is widely distributed in every region of the CNS, especially in the hippocampal region and the substantia nigra (Venneti et al. 2009). The effect of this positive feedback of microglial activation gives insight on the genesis and progression of neurodegenerative diseases.

14.1.3 Microglial Cells Role on Neuroinflammation

Microglial cells have an irregular morphology, with an enlarged nucleus and represent between 5% and 20% of the total glial cell population in the CNS. They are able to produce phagocytosis, releasing cytotoxic factors and behaving as an antigen presentation cell (Perry 1998). These cells are derived from macrophages produced during the haematopoietic processes in the primitive yolk sac (Alliot et al. 1999) and migrate to the neural tube during development (Ginhoux et al. 2013). Their physiological functions are essential for the control of normal homeostasis in the CNS, even in altered conditions such as the presence of disease (Morales et al. 2010). They are capable of sensing different damage signals that could represent a possible impairment for the CNS, and include (i) microorganisms, (ii) abnormal endogenous proteins, (iii) complement factors, (iv) antibodies, and (v) cytokines, chemokines, among others. These impairment agents are able to interact with receptors such as the toll-like receptor (TLR), inducing the cellular activation of the microglia (Streit et al. 2008; Venneti et al. 2009). Under the previous conditions, microglial cells control the expression of different surface markers, such as major histocompatibility complex II (CMH-II) and the pattern of molecular recognition receptors (PRRs). After these interactions, the production of pro-inflammatory cytokines is triggered, which include interleukin I beta (IL-1β), IL-6, interleukin 12 (IL-12), interferon gamma (IFN-γ) and TNF-α (Morales et al. 2010). In the meantime, there is synthesis and release of cytotoxic factors with a low biological half-life as superoxide radicals (O_2^-), nitric oxide (NO) and other reactive oxygen species (ROS) (Meda et al. 2001; Colton and Wilcock 2010). During brain development, microglial cells play a specific role in apoptotic cell elimination. In the cerebellum, however, they regulate phagocytosis of Purkinje neurons after cell death mediated by caspase-3. Therefore, microglia has been implicated in synapse pruning during development after birth (Kettenmann et al. 2011). Finally, the activation process for these cells is related with the intensity, context and kind of stimulus generated and, depending on these factors, the microglia could trigger a neuroprotective or neuroinflammatory effect. The equilibrium between neurotoxicity and neuroprotection is what determines the microglia functional effect in neurological diseases and/or specific condition (Morales et al. 2010).

As mentioned, microglial cells mediate the immune response in the CNS. To accomplish this task, the microglia turn into a functional polarised state, being able to carry out a specific effector program. This brain cellular type exhibits two polarised forms, one of which develops the classical pro-inflammatory response and this is the most common phenotype. The alternative form generates an anti-inflammatory effect directed to heal a zone affected by an acute injury (Jha et al. 2016).

Additionally, microglial cells are characterised by the expression of several receptors in the membrane surface and also, by the release of different soluble factors. The activated cell, with the pro-inflammatory phenotype, promotes the regulation of Fc receptors such as CD16, CD32, CD64, CD86, IL-1b, IL-6, IL-12, IL-23, TNF-α, inducible nitric oxide synthase (iNOS) and chemokines, while the alternative anti-inflammatory phenotype regulates positively arginase-1 (Arg-1), the mannose receptor (CD206), insulin growth factor-1 (IGF-1), the triggering receptor expressed in myeloid cells 2 (TREM1) and chitinase-3-like 1 (Ym-1), among others. All these proteins contribute, with the active microglia, to produce additional cytokines and inflammatory mediators that could direct the neurons to apoptotic mechanisms in multiple neurodegenerative pathologies (Morales et al. 2017b). Although microorganisms and their related secreted proteins (LPS, others) are recognised by the Toll-receptor family, neurons suffering apoptosis are sensed by different receptor systems, such as those mediated by asialoglycoproteins, vitronectin and phosphatidylserine (Witting et al. 2000).

Recent reports have demonstrated that after the microglial cells are activated, they overexpress several receptors and ligands belonging to the main chemokine families (CC, CXC and CX3C). Some of these are also expressed in astrocytes, which suggests that chemokines may serve as communication signals between them and microglia. It has been proposed that CX3CR1 and its ligand, fraktalkine (CX3CL1), which are expressed in neurons, also play a paramount role in neuronal signalling with the microglial cells (Rock et al. 2004). There are diverse factors regulating the phagocytic activity of microglial cells, one of which is the chloride intracellular channel (CLIC1). Pharmacological inhibition of this channel or negative regulation of its expression at the transcriptional level by an interference RNA alters the normal phagocytic activity of the microglia. On the other hand, it has been reported that the ciliary neurotrophic factor (CNTF) promotes phagocytosis in a way mediated by Ca^{2+} (Lee et al. 2009). In conclusion, microglial cells can receive stimulus from environmental agents or endogenous proteins, which triggers an over-activated state, releasing pro-inflammatory factors, ROS, reactive nitrogen species (RNS) and evoking toxicity in the vicinity of neuronal population (Innamorato et al. 2009).

14.2 NEW PROPOSALS: INNOVATIVE APPROACHES TO TACKLE AD

New compounds are currently being proposed to treat AD effectively, most of them, without success in clinical trials. Here, we are reviewing some of the alternatives, focusing in their molecular mechanisms, whether they are obtained from natural or synthetic sources and, if they are being tested at preclinical or clinical levels.

14.2.1 Synthetic Compounds

Concerning synthetic compounds, efforts have been directed to the most characterised aetiological agents in AD, mainly to Aβ and plaques. However, after several clinical trials, the medical community has reached the conclusion that tau-directed agents seem to be more promising in the improvement of cognitive decline in comparison to Aβ approaches (Bondi et al. 2017). At the preclinical level, functional and molecular assays have evaluated the response of cellular models *in vitro* or even *in vivo*, aiming to decrease the amount of Aβ or SP and sometimes tau, PHF or NFT. Furthermore, the use of their cryostructure – because the vast majority of the synthetic targets are tested after being compared to natural structures – has been used to determine the possible interaction of these new alternatives by docking *in silico* assays, with less than 1% of success when the clinical trials are reached (Lahlou 2013; Vlachogianni et al. 2014). Nonetheless, considering the difficulty of assessing these possible interactions, because of the powerful equipment necessary, the use of predictors for clinical trials presents an attractive option to determine the success rate for new pharmacological therapies, because the evaluation of efficacy for 5 or more years on each patient presents an enormous variability and has a high cost (Anderson et al. 2017).

Several new targets attempt to control AD by modulation of inflammatory signals (Table 14.1); among them, some are based on inhibitors of acetylcholinesterase like rivastigmine to improve cholinergic synapses which are severely diminished in AD, and inhibitors of *N*-Methyl-D-Aspartate receptor, which is hyperactivated in AD and exerts excitotoxicity, however these drugs only delay the progress of disease (Tan et al. 2014). As mentioned, neuroinflammation is an early event of AD, even earlier than NFT and Aβ plaque formation, which makes *the modulation of inflammation an attractive target for the development of new drugs for the treatment* and prevention of AD. An alternative was nonsteroidal anti-inflammatory drugs (NSAIDs) – such as ibuprofen, paracetamol, aspirin and sulindac – that are commonly used for treatment of other illnesses whose symptoms are inflammation (e.g. infections, headache) and that appear to reduce the risk of AD onset in patients that

TABLE 14.1
Drugs or Active Synthetic Compounds for AD Therapy

Drug/Active Agent	Mechanism	References
Rivastigmine	Inhibition of AchE	Tan et al. (2014)
Memantine	Inhibition of NMDAr	
Nonsteroidal anti-inflammatories	Inhibition of NF-κB signalling pathway	Ajmone-Cat et al. (2010)
	Inhibition of Cyclooxygenase enzymatic activity	
	Activation of PPAR-γ receptor	
Dihydropyridines	Reduce all type of tau levels	Huang and Mucke (2012)
Galantamine	Inhibition of AchE	Heinrich (2004)
Cilostazol	Reduce altered tau levels	Schaler and Myeku (2017)

have been in treatment for a long period (Gupta et al. 2010). One of the mechanisms of action that has been proposed to explain their preventive capability for AD is the inhibition of the NF-κB signalling pathway by inhibiting the phosphorylation of the IκBα subunit of the inhibitor of kappa beta kinases complex, thus impairing NF-κB release for its translocation to the nucleus and so the induction of expression of pro-inflammatory cytokines (Giannakopoulos et al. 2003). Another mechanism consists of the inhibition of enzymatic activity of cyclooxygenases, preventing the production of prostaglandins (Ajmone-Cat et al. 2010). NSAIDs also activate peroxisome proliferator-activated receptor gamma (PPAR-γ) signalling, which induces expression of anti-inflammatory substances, and reduction of Aβ release, impairing the formation of plaques. These anti-inflammatory drugs also act by inhibiting microglial activation, thus impairing NFT and AP formation mediated by chronic inflammation (Imbimbo et al. 2010). However, these drugs have failed in patients who are already suffering from AD with cognitive impairment, so for the effective use of NSAIDs, early diagnosis is necessary – that is, when the inflammatory process is developing but prior to inflammation-induced formation of NFT (Breitner et al. 2011). Another approach is the use of biological-active molecules of polyunsaturated fatty acids as agonists of the PPAR-γ transcription factor, which inhibits the expression of pro-inflammatory cytokines and turns the response of immune cells to an anti-inflammatory response (Martin 2010). Another challenge to overcome for these approaches is tissue specificity, because these compounds inhibit signalling pathways that are ubiquitously expressed, which means that their use as therapy for AD would be detrimental for immune response against pathogen aggressions. A recent study has targeted the ionic hemi-channels of astrocytes by using cannabinoids to impair the aperture of astrocytic hemi-channels triggered by cytokines released upon Aβ stimulation, thus impairing the activation of astrocytes (Gajardo-Gomez et al. 2017). The use of stem cells has been proposed as treatment for AD, because administration of mesenchymal stem cells reduces plaque formation, promotes Aβ degradation and reduces levels of pro-inflammatory cytokines. This reduces microglial proliferation and general neuroinflammation (Harach et al. 2017). However, clinical studies have shown their lack of efficiency in AD treatment. Taking the above context into account, no successful results were obtained for the treatment for AD with these synthetic compounds.

14.2.2 Natural Compounds

In this confusing clinical scenario, important efforts have been made to find natural compounds for effective and non-invasive treatment against AD. These include quercetin, a flavonoid able to reduce astrocyte activation and thus reduce neuroinflammation and improving memory in SAMP8-accelerated senescence mice. The animals were treated with an oral formulation of quercetin encapsulated as nanoparticles (Moreno et al. 2017). Another flavonoid compound with AD treatment potential is apigenin, which can be found, among other sources, in chamomile and grapefruit. This compound is able to inhibit microglia-mediated release of IL-6 and TNF-α, the prostaglandin and NO production by inhibiting COX-2 and iNOS enzymatic activities respectively, and also inhibits the NF-κB signalling pathway (Venigalla et al. 2015). However, the most promising natural compound for anti-inflammatory treatment of AD is curcumin (Morales et al. 2017a), a polyphenol isolated from rhizomes of curcuma, which reduces the expression of COX-2 and iNOS, impairs IL-6, NF-κB and MAPK signalling pathways, reduces astroglial activation and also prevents and reverts tau aggregation *in vitro* (Morales et al. 2017a). These data suggest that this compound could be used in AD patients with cognitive impairment. Moreover, it has the same effects in animal models and humans, which suggests this compound as an attractive alternative for further studies and also to develop new natural or synthetic anti-inflammatory and anti-aggregative formulations to treat AD (Venigalla et al. 2015).

Natural alternatives have thus emerged as possible solutions, supported by clinical research. Nowadays, there are 105 trials to evaluate potential treatments for AD and among them are a few number of natural compounds accepted by the US Food and Drug Administration (FDA; Cummings et al. 2017). Most of these are enhanced by antioxidant, anti-inflammatory or

TABLE 14.2

Active Natural Compounds or Nutraceuticals for AD Therapy

Drug/Active Agent	Mechanism	References
Cannabinoids	Impairment of aperture of ion channels of astrocytes	Gajardo-Gomez et al. (2017)
	Inhibits tau hyperphosphorylation and inflammation	Bedse et al. (2015)
Apigenin	Reduction of expression of COX and iNOS	Venigalla et al. (2015)
Curcumin	Reduction of the expression of COX-2, iNOS	Venigalla et al. (2015); Morales et al.
	Impairment of IL-6, NF-κB and MAPK signalling pathways	(2017a)
Quercetin	Reduction of levels of IL-6 and TNF-α	Rinwa and Kumar (2013)
Magnesium	Inhibits GSK3-β	Xu et al. (2014)
Lithium	Inhibits GSK3-β	Klein and Melton, (1996)
Nobiletin	Reduce tau hyperphosphorylation and oxidative stress	Nakajima et al. (2014)
AXONA AC-1200®	Increase ketone bodies	Henderson et al. (2009)
Perceptiv®	Antioxidant and transformation of homocysteine to methionine	Chan et al. (2010)
Cognitex®	Promotes production of acetylcholine, antioxidant, anti-inflammatory, reversible inhibition of acetylcholinesterase	Richter et al. (2011)
Ginkgo biloba	Increases production of nitric oxide in blood vessels; Inhibits the platelet-activating factor	Vellas et al. (2012); DeKosky et al. (2008)
Souvenaid®	Antioxidant and anti-inflammatory; Promotes synapses	Scheltens et al. (2010)
Oxaloacetate	Mitochondria metabolism	Wilkins et al. (2014); Swerdlow et al. (2016)
S-quol	Mitochondria metabolism	Hirai et al. (2001); Swerdlow, (2012)
L-serine	Neuroprotective	Cox et al. (2016)
MCL901	Neuroprotective	Pasinetti and Ho, (2010); Lee et al. (2017)
Meganatural	Tau anti-aggregative	Ho et al. (2009); Pasinetti and Ho, (2010)
Resveratrol®	SIRT1 activator	Li et al. (2012)
Omega-3	Antioxidant and anti-inflammatory	Yehuda et al. (2005)
BrainUp-10®	Reduces tau aggregation and increases neuritogenesis	Carrasco-Gallardo et al. (2012a, 2012b)

metabolic properties (Pasinetti and Ho 2010; Rege et al. 2014), and have diverse natural origins (Table 14.2). They are at different stages in trials and present high potential to continue scaling in the cure or treatment of AD.

Oxaloacetate (*3-carboxy-3-oxopropanoic acid*, OAA) is a natural chemical that participates in Krebs cycle and acts as a glutamate scavenger (Zlotnik et al. 2012). It is found in blueberries, blackberries, tangerines and plums, and in vegetables as spinach, beets and quinoa (Simpson et al. 2009; Ghosh Das and Savage 2013; Lin et al. 2016; Siener et al. 2016). Legumes and nuts also have high OAA content (Chai and Liebman 2005). Due to its bioenergetic, anti-inflammatory and neurogenetic properties, OAA has been postulated as a possible treatment for AD (Wilkins et al. 2014). An incipient phase 1, non-randomised clinical trial is now recruiting subjects with diagnosis of probable AD to verify safety and tolerance (Table 14.2). In a previous study, a very modest cohort of 6 participants showed that twice daily treatment of 100 mg of OAA for 4 weeks was safe and well-tolerated (Swerdlow et al. 2016). Another natural compound related to mitochondria metabolism is S-equol (7-hydroxy-3-(4′-hydroxyphenyl)-chroman). It is an oestrogen receptor β (ERβ) agonist, present predominantly in soy (Setchell et al. 2005; Jackson et al. 2011). It has been found in the brains of AD patients, evidence of a decrease in mitochondria activity by dysfunction (Hirai et al. 2001; Swerdlow 2012). S-equol has been proposed as a potential treatment for this pathology. A phase 2, randomised, double-blind trial is recruiting AD subjects to evaluate safety and tolerability in addition to mitochondrial activity and cognitive functions (Table 14.2).

Several other natural compounds have already overcome the first stage of clinical trials, researching the efficacy and side effects on AD subjects. Among them, L-serine (2-amino-3-hydroxypropanoic acid) is a naturally occurring non-essential amino acid with diverse biological functions that is key in cellular metabolism and maintenance of the CNS, enhancing its role by phosphorylation (Verleysdonk and Hamprecht 2000; Humphrey et al. 2015). It is present in eggs, soy and its derivates, as well as in meat, fish and cheese. Moreover, the FDA considers that it is generally regarded as a safe (GRAS) product. L-serine is synthesised by astrocytes and neurons in the CNS (Wolosker and Radzishevsky 2013) and has been shown to be neuroprotective in amyotrophic lateral sclerosis (ALS; Cox et al. 2016; Levine et al. 2017). L-serine was also capable of attenuating the density of NFT and SP in the brains of primates that exhibit these traits (Cox et al. 2016). Based on the previous data and its importance in the CNS, a phase 2, randomised, double-blind, placebo-controlled study is recruiting AD patients at early stages of disease to assay the effects of L-serine over tolerability and cognitive skills of subjects (Table 14.2). MLC901 is a group of natural herbs used in traditional Chinese medicine (Heurteaux et al. 2010). It is the simplified version of MLC601, which contains animal substances in addition to the plant-based components (Heurteaux et al. 2010, 2013). MLC901 has been previously used for recovery after stroke (Navarro et al. 2012; Chen et al. 2013; Quintard et al. 2014) and has shown protective properties in cognitive tasks in mouse models, improving neurogenesis (Lorivel et al. 2015). MLC901 is also capable of a significant decrease in tau phosphorylation levels in a cellular model of tauopathies (Pasinetti and Ho 2010; Lee et al. 2017). On this basis, a randomised, double-blind, placebo-controlled trial is recruiting subjects with mild to moderate AD to assay the safety and efficacy of MLC901, as well as its effect on cognitive and functional skills (Table 14.2).

Meganatural-az (MN) corresponds to a group of polyphenolic extracts derived from grape seeds (Pasinetti and Ho 2010). It is a blood pressure stabiliser (Sivaprakasapillai et al. 2009). MN ameliorates the cognitive damage and decrease in Aβ oligomerisation in brains of a mouse model of AD (Wang et al. 2008). There is also evidence of its neuroprotective properties, through its disassembly of tau protein aggregates (Ho et al. 2009; Pasinetti and Ho 2010). A phase 2, randomised clinical trial is recruiting AD subjects to assess its safety and pharmacokinetics.

Resveratrol (3,5,4'-trihydroxy-trans-stilbene) is a natural polyphenol, capable of penetrating the blood–brain barrier efficiently (Barber et al. 2009). It is present in multiple plants, mainly in grape seed, and is abundant in red wine (Harikumar and Aggarwal 2008; Markus and Morris 2008). It has beneficial properties in different pathological contexts, such as diabetes, cancer and cardiovascular diseases (Berman et al. 2017). Its mechanism appears to act through regulation of sirtuin 1 (SIRT), a protein involved in cell cycle, metabolic and inflammatory function (Chung et al. 2011). In regard to AD, preclinical research presents this compound as a potential treatment because it has the capacity to ameliorate amyloid beta (Aβ) in cellular lines and to decrease the levels of Aβ and p-tau in serum of induced AD rats (Marambaud et al. 2005; Al-Bishri et al. 2017). In addition, due to its antioxidant power, it has shown to be protective in diverse neurodegenerative disease models, both in cell lines and animals (Karuppagounder et al. 2009; Rege et al. 2014). In humans, resveratrol has been beneficial in these disorders (Albani et al. 2010), and recently it has been shown to be a regulator of inflammation in subjects with mild to moderate AD, reducing the expression of pro-inflammatory agents and improving cognitive skills in comparison to placebo patients, in a randomised, phase 2, double-blind trial (Moussa et al. 2017). These results do not show a decrease of modified tau levels.

Omega-3 is predominant in fish and algae. In the same context of oxidative stress and inflammation, polyunsaturated fatty acids, such as Omega-3, are essential for proper brain and neuronal function. These compounds are key components of the plasma membrane and modulate important processes such as inflammation and oxidative stress (Chen et al. 2013). Omega-3 are classified mainly into 3 fatty acids, alpha-linolenic acid, docosahexaenoic acid (DHA) and eicosapentaenoic acid (EPA). Although DHA and EPA can be synthesised endogenously from α-linolenic acid (18: 3n-3), the conversion rate in humans is very low; so the main source of both fatty acids is the diet (Quintard et al. 2014; Lorivel et al. 2015). Studies have reported that in the brain DHA protects against oxidative and inflammatory processes, which are involved in the aetiopathogenesis of AD (Ho et al. 2009). In fact, healthy adults who receive a supplement of this fatty acid have decreased serum levels of pro-inflammatory cytokines after 4 years of treatment (Silva et al. 2017). It is known that a DHA derivative, neuroprotectin D1, represses the activation of the pro-inflammatory gene triggered by Aβ42 in human neuronal cells. It has been shown that the levels of DHA and neuro-protectin D1 in the hippocampus are low in the brains of patients with AD (Ho et al. 2009; Pietrini et al. 2009). DHA also increases the activity of glutathione reductase and decreases the levels of ROS and pro-apoptotic components in the cortex and hippocampus (Goedert et al. 1996). A series of longitudinal studies have been conducted in the general population that have shown that a higher intake of these fatty acids in the diet is associated with a lower risk of suffering dementia (Anderson et al. 2017; Bondi et al. 2017). In addition, the risk of developing MCI may be lower with a high dietary intake of Omega-3 (Cummings et al. 2017).

Ginkgo biloba is among the most widely used natural compounds worldwide for the prevention and treatment of neurodegenerative diseases such as AD (Sivaprakasapillai et al. 2009). Extract from the leaves of this tree contains mainly terpenoids, flavonol glycosides and proanthocyanidins. It is thought that the active components of ginkgo act mainly at the brain level by increasing cerebral blood flow, inhibiting the platelet activating factor and increasing the production of nitric oxide in the blood vessels. In turn, it produces a modification of the monoamine neurotransmitter systems; it also shows a free radical scavenger activity and has neuroprotective and anti-apoptotic properties, as well as potentiating neurogenesis (Schneider 2012; Brondino et al. 2013). In clinical trials that seek the prevention of dementia in participants without cognitive impairment, they have used a stan-dardised extract of Ginkgo EGb761 during 4–6 years of follow-up at a dose of 240 mg/day. Despite all the beneficial effects of the extracts, no decrease in the incidence of dementia was observed in the participants treated with the active compound versus the placebo group in the GuidAge trial (2854 participants; Vellas et al. 2012). In summary, at present there is no concrete evidence that *Ginkgo biloba* extract reduces the incidence of dementia, and there are inconsistent data on its effects on cognition (Farias et al. 2014).

Vitamins. In the neuroimmunomodulatory context, ROS are intrinsically associated with microg-lial activation, by stimulating the inflammatory cascade. This activation of the microglia is strongly associated with neuronal damage in AD during neuroinflammatory processes. Several studies have investigated the possible therapeutic and/or protective effects of the antioxidant agents present in some foods and also in supplements in relation to AD. Among the antioxidants investigated are (i) α-tocopherol (vitamin E), (ii) ascorbic acid (vitamin C) and (iii) carotenes (vitamin A). In *in vitro* studies, it has been observed that α-tocopherol decreases lipid peroxidation induced by Aβ and oxi-dative stress and also suppresses the cascade of inflammation signalling. Ascorbic acid, by reducing nitrites, blocks the creation of and may also affect the synthesis of catecholamines, while carotenes affect lipid peroxidation (Markus and Morris 2008).

At present, there are a growing number of studies with different methodological approaches related to antioxidant consumption and cognitive deterioration (Chai and Liebman 2005); most controlled clinical trials include observational cross-sectional design studies and some prospec-tive community cohorts (Marambaud et al. 2005; Karuppagounder et al. 2009; Chung et al. 2011; Al-Bishri et al. 2017; Berman et al. 2017). In turn, there is variability in the source of vitamin administered, where some studies assess the daily consumption of vitamins through diet, while other studies use vitamin supplements. Finally, other approaches consider their results only at plasma vitamin levels (Chai and Liebman 2005). In observational studies there is some evidence of an association between the dietary intake of antioxidants and a reduced risk of stroke, how-ever, controlled clinical trials with antioxidant supplements have not shown this decrease (Li et al. 2012; Ghosh Das and Savage 2013; Quintard et al. 2014). A recent meta-analysis evaluated the effect of dietary intake of α-tocopherol, ascorbic acid and β-carotene on the risk of developing AD. Li and co-workers found that the relative risk reduction for cognitive impairment was similar for the three vitamins, concluding that the dietary intakes of the three antioxidants can reduce the risk of AD, and vitamin E exhibits the most pronounced protective effect (Ghosh Das and Savage 2013). Controlled trials have shown contradictory results (Marambaud et al. 2005; Simpson et al. 2009; Chung et al. 2011; Berman et al. 2017). According to the history of these vitamins, it is believed that ascorbic acid is the most effective antioxidant in plasma, partly due to its solubility in water and the wide range of ROS that it can eliminate. This is because ROS and oxidative stress trigger the neuroimmune response, which is related to the pathophysiology of AD (Fernandez et al. 2008; Jackson et al. 2011). In studies conducted by Kennard in 2014, it is showed that in an animal model of AD (AβPP/PSEN1 mice), a single dose of intravenous vitamin C (125 mg/kg, iv) improved short-term spatial memory in middle-aged mice (9 months) (Setchell et al. 2005).

In turn, vitamins may also have a neuroprotective function by eliminating toxic compounds such as homocysteine, which is has been related to an increased risk of cerebrovascular events (Quintard et al. 2014). Lack of vitamins has been associated with poor cognitive performance in addition to the factors that promote vascular risk (Swerdlow 2012), which are also associated with increased cognitive impairment and AD (Hirai et al. 2001). Homocysteine is active in the brain tissue and could contribute to the AD pathway through vascular mechanisms or as a neurotoxin (Markus and Morris 2008). Vitamins B_6, B_9 (folic acid) and B_{12} can safely reduce homocysteine by daily intake (Quintard et al. 2014). Folate and vitamin B_{12} are necessary for the conversion of homocysteine to methionine, and vitamin B_6 for the conversion of homocysteine to cysteine. There is contradictory evidence about the benefits of daily consumption of these three vitamins (B_6, B_9 and B_{12}). A recent meta-analysis evaluates the effects of supplementation with vitamins B_{12}, B_6 and folic acid in cognitive deterioration, concluding there is insufficient evidence of its reduction (Navarro et al. 2012) in patients with or without previous cognitive impairment or who have suffered some type of trauma. However, there are studies that reported an improvement in cognitive abilities with the administration of B_9 and B_{12}, but only in patients with high total homocysteine. There is significant progress in a VITACOG trial, evaluating patients with mild cognitive impairment and high homocysteine levels. The treatment is a combination of 0.8 mg/day of folic acid, 0.5 mg/day of vitamin B_{12} and 20 mg/day of vitamin B_6 for 24 months. The dose of vitamin B_{12} was up to 300 times higher than the recommended daily amount in most countries, to try to counteract poorer absorption older people. The results showed that the rate of brain atrophy is significantly lower in those who received treatment, and that there is a significant interaction of treatment with basal levels of homocysteine. Among patients with a basal homocysteine level greater than 13 μmol/L, brain atrophy decreased by 53% with treatment (Wolosker and Radzishevsky 2013). In the FACIT trial, subjects (55–70 years old) with elevated levels of plasma homocysteine and normal levels of vitamin B_{12} received a folic acid supplement for 3 years and showed significantly improved memory and information processing speed (Heurteaux et al. 2013). All previous reports suggest the incredible potential of these supplements to the daily diet, proposing new formulas or dietary regimes to improve cognitive performance.

14.2.3 BrainUp-10: A Novel Formula with a Novel Focus

Our laboratory has developed an in-depth study on the effects of the *Andean compound* and proposed a formulation containing the compound and the vitamins B_6, B_9 and B_{12}, called BrainUp-10. The Andean compound derives from a natural peat moss extracted in a desert area from the Andes Mountains in the north of Chile. It is an endemic product of this area. Its composition corresponds to a fossilised product that results from the millenary degradation of plants by the action of several types of microbial agents. This compound is rich in humins, including fulvic acids (FA), humic acids (HA) and some inorganic molecules such as selenium, magnesium and other minerals. Interestingly, our findings indicate the safety of this formulation in cell murine lines at increasing concentrations, showing also that the Andean compound is nontoxic in neuronal cell cultures. The safety and absence of adverse and side effects of this compound was corroborated by a

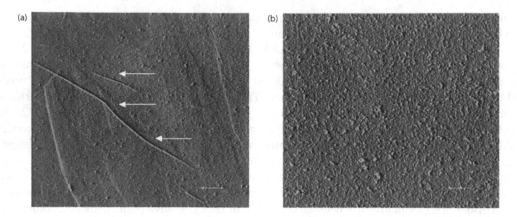

FIGURE 14.1   **(See color insert.)** Atomic force microscopy. BrainUp-10 disassembles pathological tau filaments. Recombinant human tau hTAU40 was allowed to self-assemble in the presence of arachidonic acid, and samples were withdrawn before (a) and after (b) the addition of 10 μg/mL of water-solubilised formula BrainUp-10. (a) Tau control without BrainUp-10. (b) The effects of BrainUp-10 on tau aggregates. Disassembly of tau filaments.

phase 1 study. Moreover, functional studies were carried out showing that the formulation promotes neuritogenesis in hippocampal cells in primary cultures (Carrasco-Gallardo et al. 2012a) and neuroblastoma N2a murine cells (Andrade et al. unpublished results). These results indicate that the Andean compound and the formulation BrainUp-10, can increase the outgrowth of neurites and other cell prolongations in hippocampal and N2a cells in culture. Additionally, increasing concentrations of FA show evidence of neuritogenesis as revealed by immunofluorescence microscopy in N2a cell line cultures. These findings suggest that FA contained in the Andean compound may have neurotrophic effects in cells in culture. This effect seems to be intensified in the presence of other known neuroprotective compounds such as B complex vitamins. Other studies performed with FA *in vitro* show that this compound not only exerts an antioxidant action, but also binds specifically to tau and prevents pathological self-association (Cornejo et al. 2011). Furthermore, the neuroprotective role of BrainUp-10 has also been evidenced in studies that show that the formula prevents tau aggregation in an *in vitro* system. Moreover, addition of BrainUp-10 to aggregated polymers obtained from recombinant hTAU40 results in the disassembly of already generated polymers (Figure 14.1) (Andrade et al. unpublished results). Finally, the BrainUp-10 nutraceutical formulation is already in an advanced second-phase clinical trial for the elucidation of its molecular, functional and pharmacological effects in cognition and empathy of AD subjects.

14.3   CONCLUSION

Cases of Alzheimer's disease are increasing faster every year, not just in the senile population but also with early onset cases. We have studied different issues related to the beginning and progression of neurodegenerative pathologies. In a biological context, the neuroimmune inflammatory response theory could be a new focus for possible treatments, and the research efforts to follow up should be focused in the control of neuroinflammatory processes.

Microglia seem to be the main brain cells in the pathological pathway of damage signals in the neuronal population of neurodegenerative diseases. The positive feedback cycle between microglia and neurons is started by tau oligomers released in the extracellular space after neuron degeneration, triggering activation of the microglia. Different clinical trials on pharmacological agents have attempted to stop the progress of AD or revert its consequences, but only a few are promising. Natural compounds have received special attention, however, because of their benefits in promoting

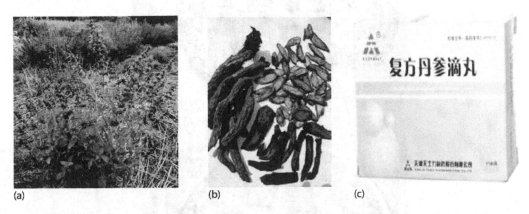

FIGURE 4.12 (a) *Salvia miltiorrhiza* (*Danshen* or *Tanshen*), (b) root or rhizomes and (c) manufactured by Tasly Pharmaceuticals (http://www.tasly.com/) has completed phase II clinical trials in the United States (No. NCT00797953).

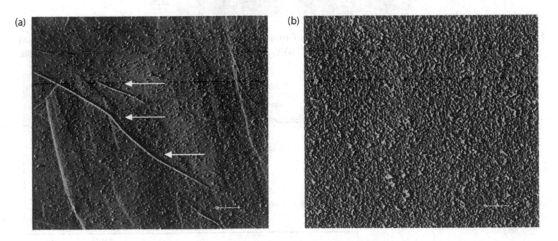

FIGURE 14.1 Atomic force microscopy. BrainUp-10 disassembles pathological tau filaments. Recombinant human tau hTAU40 was allowed to self-assemble in the presence of arachidonic acid, and samples were withdrawn before (a) and after (b) the addition of 10 µg/mL of water-solubilised formula BrainUp-10. (a) Tau control without BrainUp-10. (b) The effects of BrainUp-10 on tau aggregates. Disassembly of tau filaments.

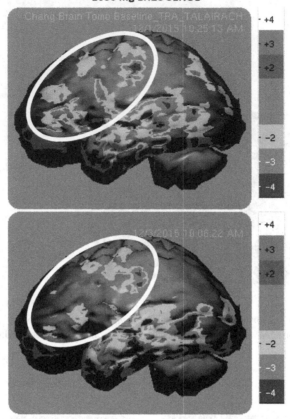

Improvements in brain perfusion in an individual with concussion history after three doses of 1000 mg ENZOGENOL

FIGURE 15.8 Talairach comparison of high-resolution SPECT scans of an individual with a concussion history before (top) and after (bottom) three doses of 1000 mg ENZOGENOL, showing reduced hypoperfusion.

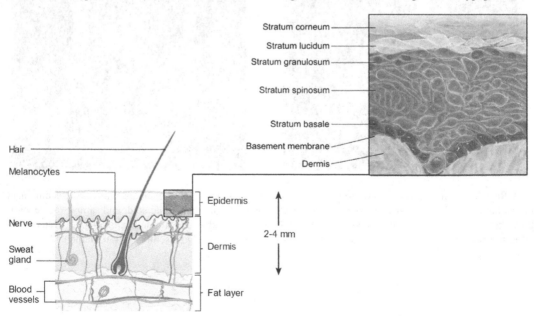

Stratum corneum
Stratum lucidum
Stratum granulosum
Stratum spinosum
Stratum basale
Basement membrane
Dermis

Hair
Melanocytes
Epidermis
2-4 mm
Nerve
Dermis
Sweat gland
Blood vessels
Fat layer

FIGURE 21.1 The three main layers of skin, namely the epidermis, dermis and subcutaneous or fat layer. (Courtesy of Cancer Research UK, 2014.)

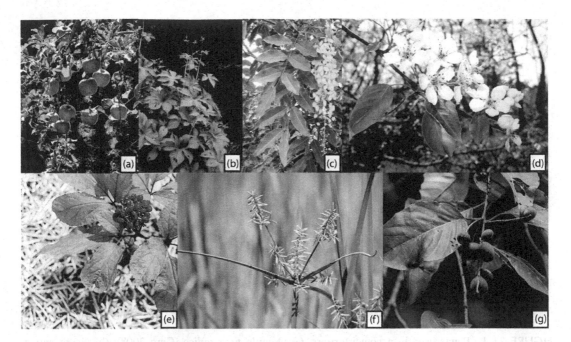

FIGURE 21.2 Plants used in anti-ageing skin care therapies: (a) *Malus pumila* (Aomorikuma 2007), (b) *Humulus japonicus* (United States Department of Agriculture 2012); (c) *Cassia fistula* (Conrad 2008), (d) *Pyrus pyrifolia* (Quert 2010); (e) *Panax ginseng* (Lohrie 2006); (f) *Cyperus rotundus* (Jose 2009); and (g) *Terminalia chebula* (Zhangzhugang 2013).

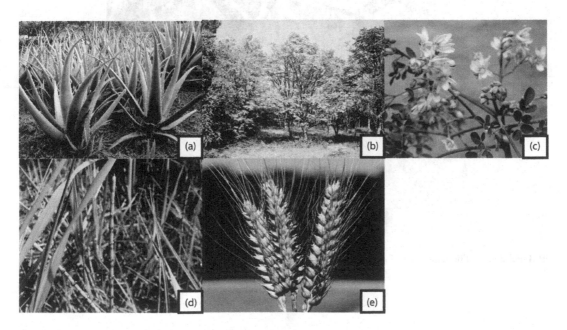

FIGURE 21.3 Plants for skin moisturising therapies: (a) *Aloe barbadensis* (Maari 2012); (b) *Cedrela sinensis* (Willow 2007); (c) *Moringa oleifera* (Garg 2008); (d) *Equisetum palustre* (Peters 2006); and (e) *Triticum vulgare* (Dist 2008).

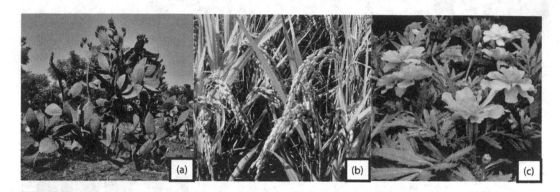

FIGURE 21.4 Plants used in nanomoisturisers. (a) *Opuntia ficus-indica* (Garg 2008); (b) *Oryza sativa* (Green, 2006); and (c) *Tagetes erecta* (Starr and Starr 2007).

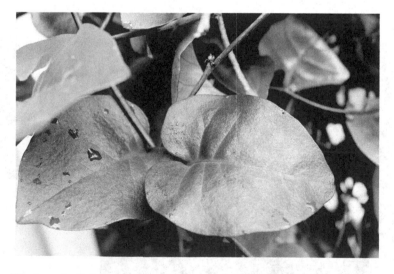

FIGURE 22.1 The heart leaf of *Anredera cordifolia*.

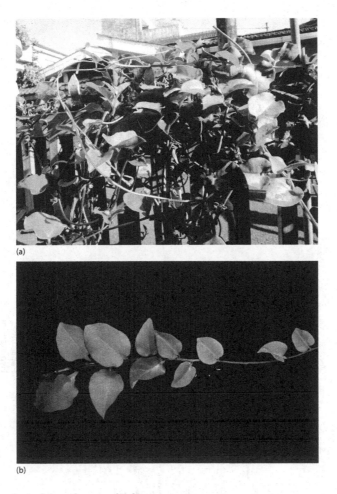

(a)

(b)

FIGURE 22.2   The plant of *Anredera cordifolia*.

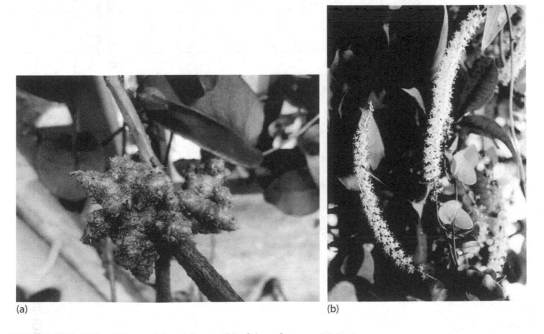

(a)

(b)

FIGURE 22.3   The rhizome (a) and flower (b) of *Anredera cordifolia*.

Traditional Use of *Anredera cordifolia* (Ten.) Steenis

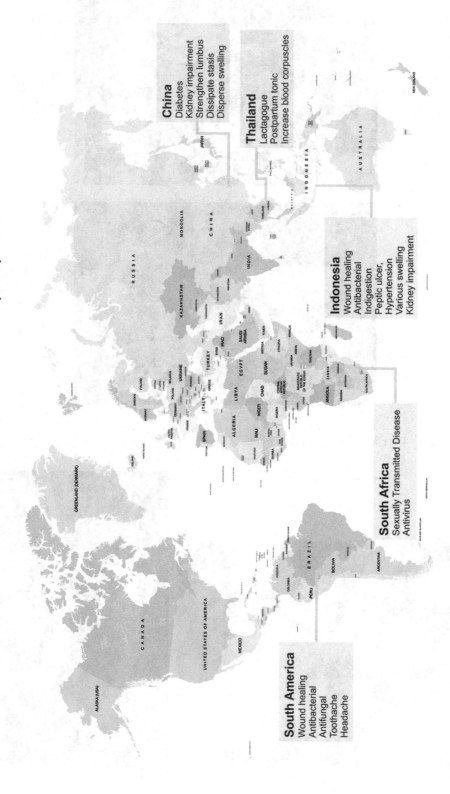

China
Diabetes
Kidney impairment
Strengthen lumbus
Dissipate stasis
Disperse swelling

Thailand
Lactagogue
Postpartum tonic
Increase blood corpuscles

Indonesia
Wound healing
Antibacterial
Indigestion
Peptic ulcer,
Hypertension
Various swelling
Kidney impairment

South Africa
Sexually Transmitted Disease
Antivirus

South America
Wound healing
Antibacterial
Antifungal
Toothache
Headache

FIGURE 22.4 Traditional use of *Anredera cordifolia* in various countries.

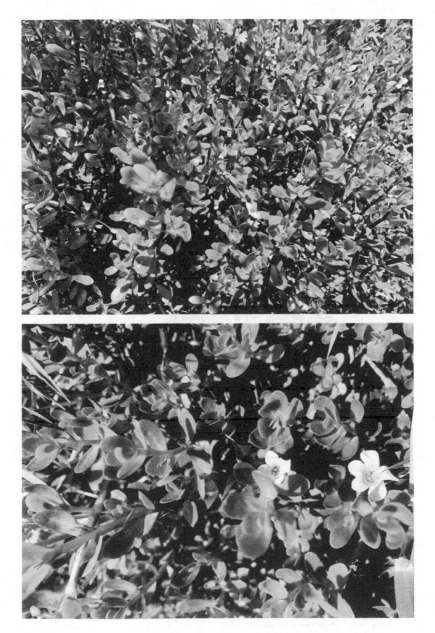

FIGURE 25.1 *Bacopa monnieri* in its natural habitat. (Courtesy of Muhammad Shahid, Margalla Hills near Quaid-i-Azam University, Islamabad, Pakistan.)

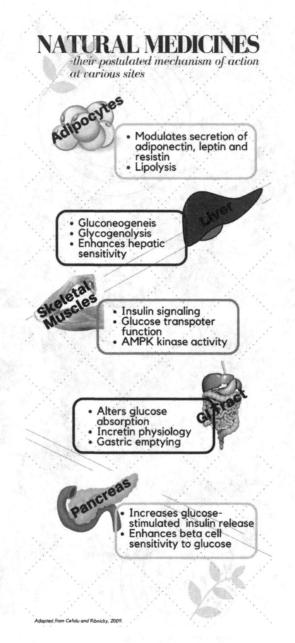

FIGURE 27.1   Natural medicines and their postulated mechanism of action.

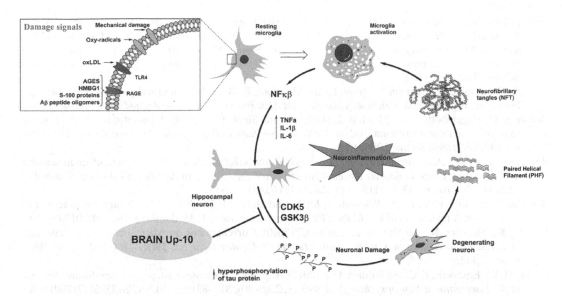

FIGURE 14.2 Model of neuroinflammation and neurodegeneration cycle modulated by BrainUp-10. Non-activated microglial cells are susceptible to different damage signals, including the aggregated forms of the tau protein, leading to its activation. After activation, several pro-inflammatory agents are released into the extracellular media, being able to promote neuronal damage and degeneration. While neurons are degraded, different tau forms are released, causing a positive feedback in this neurodegenerative pro-inflammatory cycle and triggering the onset and progression of pathologies such as AD. BrainUp-10 displays an anti-aggregation effect on tau oligomers, diminishing damage signals. In the meantime, it promotes neuritogenesis. Tau assembly is an excellent target for the treatment of AD.

neuritogenesis and their possible neuroprotective applications to control the progression of the inflammatory process in AD. Such is the case with BrainUp-10, which we present as an alternative treatment for this pathology (Figures 14.1 and 14.2).

We encourage researchers to focus on new neuroprotective and anti-neuroinflammatory drugs or nutraceuticals, projecting the answers for neurodegenerative diseases on the basis of the neuroimmunomodulation theory as the most valuable and useful tools for AD treatment.

ACKNOWLEDGEMENTS

We are grateful to the Corfo Project on High Technology and to the International Center for Biomedicine (ICC) for their generous financial support to carry out this research. We also acknowledge José Pablo Tapia, Romina Lehmann and Constanza Maccioni for their assistance and data organisation in this research process.

REFERENCES

Ajmone-Cat, M. A., Bernardo, A., Greco, A. and Minghetti, L. (2010). Non-steroidal anti-inflammatory drugs and brain inflammation: Effects on microglial functions. *Pharmaceuticals (Basel)*, **3**(6), 1949–1965.

Akiyama, H., Barger, S., Barnum, S., Bradt, B., Bauer, J., Cole, G. M., Cooper, N. R., et al. (2000). Inflammation and Alzheimer's disease. *Neurobiology of Aging*, **21**(3), 383–421.

Al-Bishri, W. M., Hamza, A. H. and Farran, S. K. (2017). Resveratrol treatment attenuates amyloid beta, Tau protein and markers of oxidative stress, and inflammation in Alzheimer's disease rat model. *International Journal of Pharmaceutical Research and Allied Sciences*, **6**(3), 71–78.

Albani, D., Polito, L., Signorini, A. and Forloni, G. (2010). Neuroprotective properties of resveratrol in different neurodegenerative disorders. *Biofactors*, **36**(5), 370–376. doi:10.1002/biof.118.

Alliot, F., Godin, I. and Pessac, B. (1999). Microglia derive from progenitors, originating from the yolk sac, and which proliferate in the brain. *Brain Research. Developmental Brain Research*, **117**(2), 145–152.

Anderson, R. M., Hadjichrysanthou, C., Evans, S. and Wong, M. M. (2017). Why do so many clinical trials of therapies for Alzheimer's disease fail? *Lancet*, **390**(10110), 2327–2329. doi:10.1016/S0140-6736(17)32399-1.

Andrade, V., Cortes, N., Guzman-Martinez, L. and Maccioni, R. B. (2017). An overview of the links between behavioral disorders and Alzheimer's disease. *JSM Alzheimer's Disease and Related Dementia*, **4**(1), 103.

Barber, S. C., Higginbottom, A., Mead, R. J., Barber, S. and Shaw, P. J. (2009). An in vitro screening cascade to identify neuroprotective antioxidants in ALS. *Free Radical Biology and Medicine*, **46**(8), 1127–1138. doi:10.1016/j.freeradbiomed.2009.01.019.

Bedse, G., Romano, A., Lavecchia, A. M., Cassano, T. and Gaetani, S. (2015). The role of endocannabinoid signaling in the molecular mechanisms of neurodegeneration in Alzheimer's disease. *Journal of Alzheimer's Disease*, **43**(4), 1115–1136. doi:10.3233/JAD-141635.

Berman, A. Y., Motechin, R. A., Wiesenfeld, M. Y. and Holz, M. K. (2017). The therapeutic potential of resveratrol: A review of clinical trials. *NPJ Precision Oncology*, **1**, 35. doi:10.1038/s41698-017-0038-6.

Bettens, K., Sleegers, K. and Van Broeckhoven, C. (2010). Current status on Alzheimer disease molecular genetics: From past, to present, to future. *Human Molecular Genetics*, **19**(R1), R4–R11. doi:10.1093/hmg/ddq142.

Bondi, M. W., Edmonds, E. C. and Salmon, D. P. (2017). Alzheimer's disease: Past, present, and future. *Journal of the International Neuropsychological Society*, **23**(9–10), 818–831. doi:10.1017/S135561771700100X.

Breitner, J. C., Baker, L. D., Montine, T. J., Meinert, C. L., Lyketsos, C. G., Ashe, K. H., Brandt, J., et al. (2011). Extended results of the Alzheimer's disease anti-inflammatory prevention trial. *Alzheimer's & Dementia*, **7**(4), 402–411. doi:10.1016/j.jalz.2010.12.014.

Brondino, N., De Silvestri, A., Re, S., Lanati, N., Thiemann, P., Verna, A., Emanuele, E. et al. (2013). A systematic review and meta-analysis of *Ginkgo biloba* in neuropsychiatric disorders: From ancient tradition to modern-day medicine. *Evidence-Based Complementary and Alternative Medicine*, **2013**, 915691. doi:10.1155/2013/915691.

Capuron, L., Su, S., Miller, A. H., Bremner, J. D., Goldberg, J., Vogt, G. J. Maisano, G. et al. (2008). Depressive symptoms and metabolic syndrome: Is inflammation the underlying link? *Biological Psychiatry*, **64**(10), 896–900. doi:10.1016/j.biopsych.2008.05.019.

Carrasco-Gallardo, C., Farias, G. A., Fuentes, P., Crespo, F. and Maccioni, R. B. (2012a). Can nutraceuticals prevent Alzheimer's disease? Potential therapeutic role of a formulation containing shilajit and complex B vitamins. *Archives of Medical Research*, **43**(8), 699–704. doi:10.1016/j.arcmed.2012.10.010.

Carrasco-Gallardo, C., Guzman, L. and Maccioni, R. B. (2012b). Shilajit: A natural phytocomplex with potential procognitive activity. *International Journal of Alzheimer's Disease*, **2012**, 674142. doi:10.1155/2012/674142.

Chai, W. and Liebman, M. (2005). Effect of different cooking methods on vegetable oxalate content. *Journal of Agricultural and Food Chemistry*, **53**(8), 3027–3030. doi:10.1021/jf048128d.

Chan, A., Remington, R., Kotyla, E., Lepore, A., Zemianek, J. and Shea, T. B. (2010). A vitamin/nutriceutical formulation improves memory and cognitive performance in community-dwelling adults without dementia. *Journal of Nutrition Health and Aging*, **14**(3), 224–230.

Chen, C. L., Ikram, K., Anqi, Q., Yin, W. T., Chen, A.and Venketasubramanian, N. (2013). The NeuroAiD II (MLC901) in vascular cognitive impairment study (NEURITES). *Cerebrovascular Diseases*, **35**(Suppl 1), 23–29. doi:10.1159/000346234.

Chen, W. W., Zhang, X. and Huang, W. J. (2016). Role of neuroinflammation in neurodegenerative diseases (Review). *Molecular Medicine Reports*, **13**(4), 3391–3396. doi:10.3892/mmr.2016.4948.

Chung, I. M., Yeo, M. A., Kim, S. J. and Moon, H. I. (2011). Neuroprotective effects of resveratrol derivatives from the roots of *Vitis thunbergii* var. sinuate against glutamate-induced neurotoxicity in primary cultured rat cortical cells. *Human & Experimental Toxicology*, **30**(9), 1404–1408. doi:10.1177/0960327110390065.

Colton, C. and Wilcock, D. M. (2010). Assessing activation states in microglia. *CNS & Neurological Disorders–Drug Targets*, **9**(2), 174–191.

Cornejo, A., Jimenez, J. M., Caballero, L., Melo, F. and Maccioni, R. B. (2011). Fulvic acid inhibits aggregation and promotes disassembly of tau fibrils associated with Alzheimer's disease. *Journal of Alzheimer's Disease*, **27**(1), 143–153. doi:10.3233/JAD-2011-110623.

Cox, P. A., Davis, D. A., Mash, D. C., Metcalf, J. S. and Banack, S. A. (2016). Dietary exposure to an environmental toxin triggers neurofibrillary tangles and amyloid deposits in the brain. *Proceedings of the Royal Society B: Biological Sciences*, **283**(1823). doi:10.1098/rspb.2015.2397.

Cummings, J., Lee, G., Mortsdorf, T., Ritter, A.and Zhong, K. (2017). Alzheimer's disease drug development pipeline: 2017. *Alzheimer's & Dementia*, **3**(3), 367–384. doi:10.1016/j.trci.2017.05.002.

DeKosky, S. T., Williamson, J. D., Fitzpatrick, A. L., Kronmal, R. A., Ives, D. G., Saxton, J. A., Lopez, O. L., et al. (2008). Ginkgo biloba for prevention of dementia: A randomized controlled trial. *JAMA*, **300**(19), 2253–2262. doi:10.1001/jama.2008.683.

Farias, G., Cornejo, A., Jimenez, J., Guzman, L. and Maccioni, R. B. (2011). Mechanisms of tau self-aggregation and neurotoxicity. *Current Alzheimer Research*, **8**(6), 608–614.

Farias, G. A., Guzman-Martinez, L., Delgado, C. and Maccioni, R. B. (2014). Nutraceuticals: A novel concept in prevention and treatment of Alzheimer's disease and related disorders. *Journal of Alzheimer's Disease*, **42**(2), 357–367. doi:10.3233/JAD-132741.

Fernandez, J. A., Rojo, L., Kuljis, R. O. and Maccioni, R. B. (2008). The damage signals hypothesis of Alzheimer's disease pathogenesis. *Journal of Alzheimer's Disease*, **14**(3), 329–333.

Gajardo-Gomez, R., Labra, V. C., Maturana, C. J., Shoji, K. F., Santibanez, C. A., Saez, J. C., Giaume, C. and Orellana, J. A. (2017). Cannabinoids prevent the amyloid beta-induced activation of astroglial hemichannels: A neuroprotective mechanism. *Glia*, **65**(1), 122–137. doi:10.1002/glia.23080.

Ghosh Das, S. and Savage, G. P. (2013). Oxalate content of Indian spinach dishes cooked in a wok. *Journal of Food Composition and Analysis*, **30**(2), 125–129. doi:10.1016/j.jfca.2013.03.001.

Giannakopoulos, P., Herrmann, F. R., Bussiere, T., Bouras, C., Kovari, E., Perl, D. P., Morrison, J. H., et al. (2003). Tangle and neuron numbers, but not amyloid load, predict cognitive status in Alzheimer's disease. *Neurology*, **60**(9), 1495–1500.

Ginhoux, F., Lim, S., Hoeffel, G., Low, D. and Huber, T. (2013). Origin and differentiation of microglia. *Frontiers in Cellular Neuroscience*, **7**, 45. doi:10.3389/fncel.2013.00045.

Goedert, M., Jakes, R., Spillantini, M. G., Hasegawa, M., Smith, M. J. and Crowther, R. A. (1996). Assembly of microtubule-associated protein tau into Alzheimer-like filaments induced by sulphated glycosaminoglycans. *Nature*, **383**(6600), 550–553. doi:10.1038/383550a0.

Gupta, S. C., Sundaram, C., Reuter, S. and Aggarwal, B. B. (2010). Inhibiting NF-kappaB activation by small molecules as a therapeutic strategy. *Biochimica et Biophysica Acta*, **1799**(10–12), 775–787. doi:10.1016/j.bbagrm.2010.05.004.

Guzman-Martinez, L., Farias, G. A. and Maccioni, R. B. (2013). Tau oligomers as potential targets for Alzheimer's diagnosis and novel drugs. *Frontiers in Neurology*, **4**, 167. doi:10.3389/fneur.2013.00167.

Harach, T., Jammes, F., Muller, C., Duthilleul, N., Cheatham, V., Zufferey, V., Cheatham, D. et al. (2017). Administrations of human adult ischemia-tolerant mesenchymal stem cells and factors reduce amyloid beta pathology in a mouse model of Alzheimer's disease. *Neurobiology of Aging*, **51**, 83–96. doi:10.1016/j.neurobiolaging.2016.11.009.

Harikumar, K. B. and Aggarwal, B. B. (2008). Resveratrol: A multitargeted agent for age-associated chronic diseases. *Cell Cycle*, **7**(8), 1020–1035. doi:10.4161/cc.7.8.5740.

Heinrich, M. (2004). Snowdrops: The heralds of spring and a modern drug for Alzheimer's disease. *Pharmaceutical Journal*, **273**(7330), 905–906.

Henderson, S. T., Vogel, J. L., Barr, L. J., Garvin, F., Jones, J. J. and Costantini, L. C. (2009). Study of the ketogenic agent AC-1202 in mild to moderate Alzheimer's disease: A randomized, double-blind, placebo-controlled, multicenter trial. *Nutrition & Metabolism*, **6**, 31. doi:10.1186/1743-7075-6-31.

Heurteaux, C., Gandin, C., Borsotto, M., Widmann, C., Brau, F., Lhuillier, M., Onteniente, B., et al. (2010). Neuroprotective and neuroproliferative activities of NeuroAid (MLC601, MLC901), a Chinese medicine, in vitro and in vivo. *Neuropharmacology*, **58**(7), 987–1001. doi:10.1016/j.neuropharm.2010.01.001.

Heurteaux, C., Widmann, C., Moha ou Maati, H., Quintard, H., Gandin, C., Borsotto, M., Veyssiere, J., et al. (2013). NeuroAiD: Properties for neuroprotection and neurorepair. *Cerebrovascular Diseases*, **35**(Suppl 1), 1–7. doi:10.1159/000346228.

Hirai, K., G. Aliev, Nunomura, A., Fujioka, H., Russell, R. L., Atwood, C. S., Johnson, A. B., et al. (2001). Mitochondrial abnormalities in Alzheimer's disease. *Journal of Neuroscience*, **21**(9), 3017–3023.

Ho, L., Yemul, S.m Wang, J. and Pasinetti, G. M. (2009). Grape seed polyphenolic extract as a potential novel therapeutic agent in tauopathies. *Journal of Alzheimer's Disease*, **16**(2), 433–439. doi:10.3233/JAD-2009-0969.

Huang, Y. and L. Mucke, L. (2012). Alzheimer mechanisms and therapeutic strategies. *Cell*, **148**(6), 1204–1222. doi:10.1016/j.cell.2012.02.040.

Humphrey, S. J., James, D. E. and Mann, M. (2015). Protein phosphorylation: A major switch mechanism for metabolic regulation. *Trends in Endocrinology and Metabolism*, **26**(12), 676–687. doi:10.1016/j.tem.2015.09.013.

Imbimbo, B. P., Solfrizzi, V. and Panza, F. (2010). Are NSAIDs useful to treat Alzheimer's disease or mild cognitive impairment? *Frontiers in Aging Neuroscience*, **2**. doi:10.3389/fnagi.2010.00019.

Innamorato, N. G., Lastres-Becker, I. and Cuadrado, A. (2009). Role of microglial redox balance in modulation of neuroinflammation. *Current Opinion in Neurology*, **22**(3), 308–314. doi:10.1097/WCO.0b013e32832a3225.

Jackson, R. L., Greiwe, J. S. and Schwen, R. J. (2011). Emerging evidence of the health benefits of S-equol, an estrogen receptor beta agonist. *Nutrition Reviews*, **69**(8), 432–448. doi:10.1111/j.1753-4887.2011.00400.x.

Jha, M. K., Lee, W. H. and Suk, K. (2016). Functional polarization of neuroglia: Implications in neuroinflammation and neurological disorders. *Biochemical Pharmacology*, **103**, 1–16. doi:10.1016/j.bcp.2015.11.003.

Karuppagounder, S. S., Pinto, J. T., Xu, H., Chen, H. L., Beal, M. F. and Gibson, G. E. (2009). Dietary supplementation with resveratrol reduces plaque pathology in a transgenic model of Alzheimer's disease. *Neurochemistry International*, **54**(2), 111–118. doi:10.1016/j.neuint.2008.10.008.

Kettenmann, H., Hanisch, U. K., Noda, M. and Verkhratsky, A. (2011). Physiology of microglia. *Physiological Reviews*, **91**(2), 461–553. doi:10.1152/physrev.00011.2010.

Klein, P. S. and Melton, D. A. (1996). A molecular mechanism for the effect of lithium on development. *Proceedings of the National Academy of Sciences of the United States of America*, **93**(16), 8455–8459.

Lahlou, M. (2013). The success of natural products in drug discovery. *Pharmacology & Pharmacy*, **4**(3A), 17–31. doi:10.4236/pp.2013.43A003.

Lambert, J. C., Schraen-Maschke, S., Richard, F., Fievet, N., Rouaud, O., Berr, C., Dartigues, J. F., et al. (2009). Association of plasma amyloid beta with risk of dementia: The prospective three-city study. *Neurology*, **73**(11), 847–853. doi:10.1212/WNL.0b013e3181b78448.

Lee, T. I., Yang, C. S., Fang, K. M. and Tzeng, S. F. (2009). Role of ciliary neurotrophic factor in microglial phagocytosis. *Neurochemical Research*, **34**(1), 109–117. doi:10.1007/s11064-008-9682-0.

Lee, W. T., Hsian, C. C. L. and Lim, Y. A. (2017). The effects of MLC901 on tau phosphorylation. *NeuroReport*, **28**(16), 1043–1048. doi:10.1097/WNR.0000000000000884.

Levine, T. D., Miller, R. G., Bradley, W. G., Moore, D. H., Saperstein, D. S., Flynn, L. E., Katz, J. S., et al. (2017). Phase I clinical trial of safety of L-serine for ALS patients. *Amyotrophic Lateral Sclerosis and Frontotemporal Degeneration*, **18**(1–2), 107–111. doi:10.1080/21678421.2016.1221971.

Li, F., Gong, Q., Dong, H. and Shi, J. (2012). Resveratrol, a neuroprotective supplement for Alzheimer's disease. *Current Pharmaceutical Design*, **18**(1), 27–33.

Lin, Z., Zhao, C., Luo, Q., Xia, X., Yu, X. and Huang, F. (2016). Prevalence of restless legs syndrome in chronic kidney disease: A systematic review and meta-analysis of observational studies. *Renal Failure*, **38**(9), 1335–1346. doi:10.1080/0886022X.2016.1227564.

Lorivel, T., Gandin, C., Veyssiere, J., Lazdunski, M. and Heurteaux, C. (2015). Positive effects of the traditional Chinese medicine MLC901 in cognitive tasks. *Journal of Neuroscience Research*, **93**(11), 1648–1663. doi:10.1002/jnr.23591.

Maccioni, R. B. (2012). Introductory remarks. Molecular, biological and clinical aspects of Alzheimer's disease. *Archives of Medical Research*, **43**(8), 593–594. doi:10.1016/j.arcmed.2012.11.001.

Maccioni, R. B., Munoz, J. P. and Barbeito, L. (2001). The molecular bases of Alzheimer's disease and other neurodegenerative disorders. *Archives of Medical Research*, **32**(5), 367–381.

Maccioni, R. B., Rojo, L. E., Fernandez, J. A. and Kuljis, R. O. (2009). The role of neuroimmunomodulation in Alzheimer's disease. *Annals of the New York Academy of Sciences*, **1153**, 240–246. doi:10.1111/j.1749-6632.2008.03972.x.

Marambaud, P., Zhao, H. and Davies, P. (2005). Resveratrol promotes clearance of Alzheimer's disease amyloid-beta peptides. *Journal of Biological Chemistry*, **280**(45), 37377–37382. doi:10.1074/jbc.M508246200.

Markus, M. A., and Morris, B. J. (2008). Resveratrol in prevention and treatment of common clinical conditions of aging. *Clinical Interventions in Aging*, **3**(2), 331–339.

Martin, H. (2010). Role of PPAR-gamma in inflammation. Prospects for therapeutic intervention by food components. *Mutation Research*, **690**(1–2), 57–63.

Meda, L., Baron, P. and Scarlato, G. (2001). Glial activation in Alzheimer's disease: The role of Abeta and its associated proteins. *Neurobiology of Aging*, **22**(6), 885–893.

Morales, I., Cerda-Troncoso, C., Andrade, V. and Maccioni, R. B. (2017a). The natural product curcumin as a potential coadjuvant in Alzheimer's treatment. *Journal of Alzheimer's Disease*, **60**(2), 451–460. doi:10.3233/JAD-170354.

Morales, I., Farias, G. and Maccioni, R. B. (2010). Neuroimmunomodulation in the pathogenesis of Alzheimer's disease. *Neuroimmunomodulation*, **17**(3), 202–204. doi:10.1159/000258724.

Morales, I., G. A. Farias, N. Cortes, and Maccioni, R. B. (2017b). Neuroinflammation and Neurodegeneration. In D. Moretti, ed., *Update on Dementia.* Rijeka: InTech. Ch. 2

Morales, I., Guzman-Martinez, L., Cerda-Troncoso, C., Farias, G. A. and Maccioni, R. B. (2014). Neuroinflammation in the pathogenesis of Alzheimer's disease. A rational framework for the search of novel therapeutic approaches. *Frontiers in Cellular Neuroscience,* **8**, 112. doi:10.3389/fncel.2014.00112.

Morales, I., Jimenez, J. M., Mancilla, M. and Maccioni, R. B. (2013). Tau oligomers and fibrils induce activation of microglial cells. *Journal of Alzheimer's Disease,* **37**(4), 849–856. doi:10.3233/JAD-131843.

Moreno, L. C., Puerta, E., Suarez-Santiago, J. E., Santos-Magalhaes, N. S., MRamirez, . J. and Irache, J. M. (2017). Effect of the oral administration of nanoencapsulated quercetin on a mouse model of Alzheimer's disease. *International Journal of Pharmaceutics,* **517**(1–2), 50–57. doi:10.1016/j.ijpharm.2016.11.061.

Moussa, C., Hebron, M., Huang, X., Ahn, J., Rissman, R. A., Aisen, P. S. and Turner, R. S. (2017). Resveratrol regulates neuro-inflammation and induces adaptive immunity in Alzheimer's disease. *Journal of Neuroinflammation,* **14**(1), 1. doi:10.1186/s12974-016-0779-0.

Nakajima, A., Ohizumi, Y. and Yamada, K. (2014). Anti-dementia activity of nobiletin, a citrus flavonoid: A review of animal studies. *Clinical Psychopharmacology and Neuroscience,* **12**(2), 75–82. doi:10.9758/cpn.2014.12.2.75.

Navarro, J. C., Molina, M. C., Baroque II, A. C. and Lokin, J. K. (2012). The use of NeuroAiD (MLC601) in post-ischemic stroke patients. *Rehabilitation Research and Practice,* **2012**, 506387. doi:10.1155/2012/506387.

Ouchi, N., Parker, J. L., Lugus, J. J. and Walsh, K. (2011). Adipokines in inflammation and metabolic disease. *Nature Reviews Immunology,* **11**(2), 85–97. doi:10.1038/nri2921.

Pasinetti, G. M., and Ho, L. (2010). Role of grape seed polyphenols in Alzheimer's disease neuropathology. *Nutrition and Dietary Supplements,* **2010**(2), 97–103. doi:10.2147/NDS.S6898.

Perry, V. H. (1998). A revised view of the central nervous system microenvironment and major histocompatibility complex class II antigen presentation. *Journal of Neuroimmunology,* **90**(2), 113–121.

Pietrini, P., Salmon, E. and Nichelli, P. (2009). Consciousness and dementia: How the brain loses its self. In S. Laureys and G. Tononi, eds., *The Neurology of Consciousness.* San Diego, CA: Academic Press. pp. 204–216.

Quintard, H., Lorivel, T., Gandin, C., Lazdunski, M. and Heurteaux, C. (2014). MLC901, a traditional Chinese medicine induces neuroprotective and neuroregenerative benefits after traumatic brain injury in rats. *Neuroscience,* **277**, 72–86. doi:10.1016/j.neuroscience.2014.06.047.

Rege, S. D., Geetha, T., Griffin, G. D., Broderick, T. L. and Babu, J. R. (2014). Neuroprotective effects of resveratrol in Alzheimer disease pathology. *Frontiers in Aging Neuroscience,* **6**, 218. doi:10.3389/fnagi.2014.00218.

Richter, Y., Herzog, Y., Eyal, I. and Cohen, T. (2011). Cognitex supplementation in elderly adults with memory complaints: An uncontrolled open label trial. *Journal of Dietary Supplements,* **8**(2), 158–168. doi:10.3109/19390211.2011.569514.

Rinwa, P. and Kumar, A. (2013). Quercetin suppress microglial neuroinflammatory response and induce antidepressent-like effect in olfactory bulbectomized rats. *Neuroscience,* **255**, 86–98. doi:10.1016/j.neuroscience.2013.09.044.

Rock, R. B., Gekker, G., Hu, S., Sheng, W. S., Cheeran, M., Lokensgard, J. R. and Peterson, P. K. (2004). Role of microglia in central nervous system infections. *Clinical Microbiology Reviews,* **17**(4), 942–964, table of contents. doi:10.1128/CMR.17.4.942-964.2004.

Schaler, A. W. and Myeku, N. (2017). Cilostazol, a phosphodiesterase 3 inhibitor, activates proteasome-mediated proteolysis and attenuates tauopathy and cognitive decline. *Translational Research,* **193**, 31–41. doi:10.1016/j.trsl.2017.11.004.

Scheltens, P., Kamphuis, P. J., Verhey, F. R., Olde Rikkert, M. G., Wurtman, R. J., Wilkinson, D., Twisk, J. W., et al. (2010). Efficacy of a medical food in mild Alzheimer's disease: A randomized, controlled trial. *Alzheimer's & Dementia,* **6**(1), 1–10 e1. doi:10.1016/j.jalz.2009.10.003.

Schneider, L. S. (2012). Ginkgo and AD: Key negatives and lessons from GuidAge. *Lancet Neurology,* **11**(10), 836–837. doi:10.1016/S1474-4422(12)70212-0.

Setchell, K. D., Clerici, C., Lephart, E. D., Cole, S. J., Heenan, C., Castellani, D., Wolfe, B. E., et al. (2005). S-equol, a potent ligand for estrogen receptor beta, is the exclusive enantiomeric form of the soy isoflavone metabolite produced by human intestinal bacterial flora. *American Journal of Clinical Nutrition,* **8**(5), 1072–1079.

Siener, R., Seidler, A., Voss, S. and Hesse, A. (2016). The oxalate content of fruit and vegetable juices, nectars and drinks. *Journal of Food Composition and Analysis,* **45**(Suppl C), 108–112. doi:10.1016/j.jfca.2015.10.004.

Silva, G., Andrade, V. G., Paixao, V. N., Pardini, M. I., Grotto, R., Braz, A. M., Golim, M.et al. (2017). Waiting list mortality impact in Hcv cirrhotic patients. *Value in Health*, **20**(9), A882–A882.

Simpson, T. S., Savage, G. P., Sherlock, R. and Vanhanen, L. P. (2009). Oxalate content of silver beet leaves (*Beta vulgaris* var. cicla) at different stages of maturation and the effect of cooking with different milk sources. *Journal of Agricultural and Food Chemistry*, **57**(22), 10804–10808. doi:10.1021/jf902124w.

Sivaprakasapillai, B., Edirisinghe, I., Randolph, J., Steinberg, F. and Kappagoda, T. (2009). Effect of grape seed extract on blood pressure in subjects with the metabolic syndrome. *Metabolism*, **58**(12), 1743–1746. doi:10.1016/j.metabol.2009.05.030.

Streit, W. J., Miller, K. R., Lopes, K. O. and Njie, E. (2008). Microglial degeneration in the aging brain – bad news for neurons? *Frontiers in Bioscience*, **13**, 3423–3438.

Swerdlow, R. H. (2012). Mitochondria and cell bioenergetics: increasingly recognized components and a possible etiologic cause of Alzheimer's disease. *Antioxidants & Redox Signaling*, **16**(12), 1434–1455. doi:10.1089/ars.2011.4149.

Swerdlow, R. H., Bothwell, R., Hutfles, L., Burns, J. M. and Reed, G. A. (2016). Tolerability and pharmacokinetics of oxaloacetate 100 mg capsules in Alzheimer's subjects. *BBA Clinical*, **5**, 120–123. doi:10.1016/j.bbacli.2016.03.005.

Tan, C. C., Yu, J. T., Wang, H. F., Tan, M. S., Meng, X. F., Wang, C., Jiang, T., et al. (2014). Efficacy and safety of donepezil, galantamine, rivastigmine, and memantine for the treatment of Alzheimer's disease: A systematic review and meta-analysis. *Journal of Alzheimer's Disease*, **41**(2), 615–631. doi:10.3233/JAD-132690.

Vellas, B., Coley, N., Ousset, P. J., Berrut, G., Dartigues, J. F., Dubois, B., Grandjean, H., et al. (2012). Long-term use of standardised *Ginkgo biloba* extract for the prevention of Alzheimer's disease (GuidAge): A randomised placebo-controlled trial. *Lancet Neurology*, **11**(10), 851–859. doi:10.1016/S1474-4422(12)70206-5.

Venigalla, M., Gyengesi, E. and Munch, G. (2015). Curcumin and apigenin–novel and promising therapeutics against chronic neuroinflammation in Alzheimer's disease. *Neural Regeneration Research*, **10**(8), 1181–1185. doi:10.4103/1673-5374.162686.

Venneti, S., Wiley, C. A. and Kofler, J. (2009). Imaging microglial activation during neuroinflammation and Alzheimer's disease. *Journal of Neuroimmune Pharmacology*, **4**(2), 227–243. doi:10.1007/s11481-008-9142-2.

Verleysdonk, S. and Hamprecht, B. (2000). Synthesis and release of L-serine by rat astroglia-rich primary cultures. *Glia*, **30**(1), 19–26.

Vlachogianni, T., Loridas, S. Fiotakis, K. and Valavanidis, A. (2014). From traditional medicine to the modern era of synthetic pharmaceuticals. Natural products and reverse pharmacology approaches have expedited new Drug Discovery. *Pharmakeftiki*, **26**, 17–31.

Wang, J., L. Ho, Zhao, W., Ono, K., Rosensweig, C., Chen, L., Humala, N., et al. (2008). Grape-derived polyphenolics prevent Abeta oligomerization and attenuate cognitive deterioration in a mouse model of Alzheimer's disease. *Journal of Neuroscience*, **28**(25), 6388–6392. doi:10.1523/JNEUROSCI.0364-08.2008.

Wilkins, H. M., Harris, J. L., Carl, S. M., E, L., Lu, J., Selfridge, J. Eva, Roy, N., et al. (2014). Oxaloacetate activates brain mitochondrial biogenesis, enhances the insulin pathway, reduces inflammation and stimulates neurogenesis. *Human Molecular Genetics*, **23**(24), 6528–6541. doi:10.1093/hmg/ddu371.

Witting, A., Muller, P., Herrmann, A., Kettenmann, H. and Nolte, C. (2000). Phagocytic clearance of apoptotic neurons by microglia/brain macrophages in vitro: Involvement of lectin-, integrin-, and phosphatidylserine-mediated recognition. *Journal of Neurochemistry*, **75**(3), 1060–1070.

Wolosker, H. and Radzishevsky, I. (2013). The serine shuttle between glia and neurons: Implications for neurotransmission and neurodegeneration. *Biochemical Society Transactions*, **41**(6), 1546–1550. doi:10.1042/BST20130220.

Xu, Z. P., Li, L., Bao, J., Wang, Z. H., Zeng, J., Liu, E. J., Li, X. G., et al. (2014). Magnesium protects cognitive functions and synaptic plasticity in streptozotocin-induced sporadic Alzheimer's model. *PLoS One*, **9**(9), e108645. doi:10.1371/journal.pone.0108645.

Yehuda, S., Rabinovitz, S. and Mostofsky, D. I. (2005). Essential fatty acids and the brain: From infancy to aging. *Neurobiology of Aging*, **26**(Suppl 1), 98–102. doi:10.1016/j.neurobiolaging.2005.09.013.

Zlotnik, A., Sinelnikov, I., Gruenbaum, B. F., Gruenbaum, S. E., Dubilet, M., Dubilet, E., Leibowitz, A., et al. (2012). Effect of glutamate and blood glutamate scavengers oxaloacetate and pyruvate on neurological outcome and pathohistology of the hippocampus after traumatic brain injury in rats. *Anesthesiology*, **116**(1), 73–83. doi:10.1097/ALN.0b013e31823d7731.

15 ENZOGENOL Pine Bark Extract

From an Ancient Remedy to a Natural Neurotherapeutic

M. Frevel

CONTENTS

15.1 INTRODUCTION

Humankind is facing increasing global health challenges due to ageing populations in many Western countries, and through the expanding Westernisation of lifestyles and loss of traditional ways of living and eating. Chronic disease is on the rise in many Western societies like the United States, Great Britain, Australia and New Zealand, but also in Eastern societies like China and India. Chronic diseases and conditions – such as heart disease, stroke, cancer, type 2 diabetes, obesity, arthritis, Alzheimer's disease and other dementias – are among the most common, costly and preventable of all health problems. Modern mainstream medical practice that concentrates on using pharmaceutical and surgical interventions to treat or suppress symptoms of diseases often struggles to achieve healing outcomes in patients with chronic conditions. Traditional 'whole-body' healing systems, such as Indian Ayurvedic medicine, traditional Chinese medicine and dietary and nutritional interventions, can be used in combination with modern medicine to improve outcomes in many chronic conditions. Practicing this combined approach of integrative medicine is becoming more common, and in part is driven by demand from patients seeking more holistic treatments and better outcomes. From a modern scientific perspective there is a great need for more research into nutritional and traditional treatments to increase the evidence base for the effectiveness of these treatments so they will penetrate mainstream medicine.

15.2 HISTORY OF CONIFER BARK AS AN ANCIENT REMEDY

The bark of a tree is the outer skin that functions to protect the inner tissues from disease, invasion by pathogens and UV radiation. Part of the tree's defence system is an abundance of phytochemicals in the bark, including many polyphenol-type compounds that, upon consumption, can work as antioxidants and protect our health.

The first historic account of using conifer bark to cure human disease stems from the French explorer Jacques Cartier who, in May 1535, set out on his second voyage of discovery to the new 'Western lands'. His ship made landfall in what is now Quebec, Canada, and he stayed there for 1 year. During the winter of 1535, many of the crew on Cartier's ships fell ill with scurvy. The local Iroquois had a traditional remedy that could cure the illness – a tea prepared from the bark and leaves of a local conifer. Despite some reluctance from the crew to consume the beverage, a few tried it and it turned out to help. The remedy allowed many of the crew to survive the winter, and the expedition sailed home to France in May 1536.

15.3 DISCOVERY, DEVELOPMENT AND COMPOSITION OF ENZOGENOL

In the 1990s, a multidisciplinary research team at the University of Canterbury in Christchurch, New Zealand, led by Dr Kelvin Duncan and Dr Ian Gilmour, sought to identify plant-based materials best suited for the extraction of highly active antioxidant fractions that could be useful in medical, nutritional and cosmetic applications. This project identified the bark of *Pinus radiata*, also known as Monterey pine or radiata pine, to be an excellent raw material for the extraction of polyphenols, and in particular proanthocyanidins (PAC) and other flavonoids. PACs have very high antioxidant activity and are regularly consumed in the diet as they are present in a wide range of plant foods; they are non-toxic, and therefore ideal for health applications. New Zealand has a substantial forestry industry and is home to large sustainably managed *Pinus radiata* plantations, so radiata pine bark is a readily available resource in New Zealand. With the ongoing discovery of its health benefits, the tree bark may in future become a highly valuable product for the industry.

The University of Canterbury research team developed an extraction method that was ecologically sound and effectively purified the polyphenol compounds from the pine bark. The water-based extraction method did not rely on solvents or chemicals and delivered a high antioxidant pine bark extract in dry powder form that was named ENZOGENOL. The production method was later

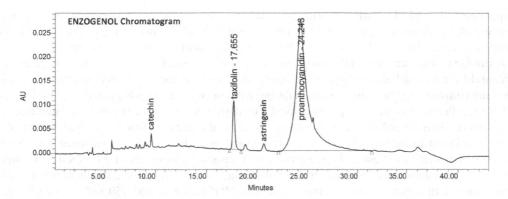

FIGURE 15.1 C18-reverse phase HPLC of ENZOGENOL.

patented in several countries with patent text being available online from the respective patent offices (e.g. New Zealand patent no. NZ329658, or US patent no. US5968517).

Frevel (2012) described the production and compositional analyses of ENZOGENOL. In summary, the starting material, New Zealand–grown *P. radiata* bark, is cleaned and visually inspected. Impurities like wood chips or stones and bark contaminated with mould, moss or other growth are removed. The extraction process is a closed continuous flow system involving grinding, washing, extraction with de-ionised hot water, removal of extracted solids, cooling of the raw liquor by heat exchanger and concentration of the raw liquor by reverse osmosis with removal of the undissolved solids. Subsequent freeze-drying, milling, blending and quality control steps deliver the final extract. Only pine bark and deionised water are used in the process. Quality controls include physical, chemical, microbiological, heavy metal, herbicide and pesticide testing to ensure the final product conforms to specifications.

Compositional analyses of ENZOGENOL have shown that the extract has a very high batch-to-batch consistency, with approximately 84% PAC content (specifications >80%) and 1.5% taxifolin content (specification >1%; Frevel 2012). Other polyphenols found in the extract include catechin, astringenin (= piceatannol), quercetin and several phenolic acids. Co-extracted carbohydrates are present at approximately 8.6%. Figure 15.1 shows a characteristic C18-reverse-phase HPLC profile of ENZOGENOL.

15.4 SAFETY AND TOXICOLOGY OF ENZOGENOL

A label such as *Natural* or *Traditional* does not make a medicinal product safe. In today's marketplace, such labels are often used to suggest to the consumer that a product is safe and there are no risks in consuming it. In reality the companies producing or marketing dietary products with medicinal properties are responsible for ensuring their products are fit for purpose and have no ill effects on people's health.

The safety profile of ENZOGENOL has been well established through mutagenicity testing, toxicological studies in animals and in human clinical trials, as well as through in-market monitoring of adverse events over many years. The studies outlined below were published in Frevel (2012). Mutagenicity of ENZOGENOL was tested by the bacterial reverse mutation (Ames) test (Frevel 2012). There was no increase in the number of revertant colonies in the five bacterial strains tested at any concentrations of ENZOGENOL in two assay series in the presence or absence of S-9 mix, establishing the extract is non-mutagenic in the Ames test.

Acute oral toxicity and maximum tolerated dose (MTD) for ENZOGENOL was investigated in Sprague Dawley rats at escalating dose levels in acute single-dose administration and 14-day repeat-dose administration (Frevel 2012). ENZOGENOL did not cause any adverse effects, and did not influence food intake or body weight. No treatment-related alterations in any haematological, coagulation, clinical chemistry or urine parameters were found, and no pathological changes observed. A MTD was not reached in this study, even at 2500 mg/kg body weight. The NOAEL (no observed adverse effect level) in rats was 2500 mg/kg/day under the 14-day treatment.

A similar oral toxicity and MTD study was carried out in dogs (Frevel 2012). There were no significant differences in haematology, coagulation, urine analysis and ECG. Inconsistent changes in blood urea nitrogen appeared in some animals, but without any liver pathology, and were toxicologically insignificant. No other changes in clinical chemistry occurred. One treatment-related clinical sign observed in male and female dogs was soft faeces and diarrhoea, which occurred mostly after administration in fasted animals and very rarely in fed animals. The total occurrence was 18.6%. Toxicokinetic analyses showed that catechin and taxifolin constituents of ENZOGENOL were found in the blood for up to 2 hours after administration. There was no accumulation of the analytes in the animals. In summary, oral administration of ENZOGENOL at 300, 750 and 1250 mg/kg/day had no effect on the general health of male and female dogs. Adverse digestive symptoms occurred primarily in the fasted state in the dogs, suggesting that ENZOGENOL may better be consumed with food. The MTD for ENZOGENOL in fed dogs is considered to be 1250 mg/kg/day, and the NOAEL on repeated oral administration (14 days) to fed dogs is 750 mg/kg/day.

Safety relevant data on consumption of ENZOGENOL is available from six human clinical trials. In two trials, a total of 46 individuals, 50–75 years old, consumed 480 mg ENZOGENOL daily as part of an ENZOGENOL–vitamin C dietary supplement formula for 12 weeks. No adverse events were reported in these studies, and there were no changes in any biochemical or haematological safety indices. ENZOGENOL was judged to be safe and well tolerated (Shand 2003; Young 2006). In a 6-month randomised, placebo-controlled trial (RCT) 30 retirement village residents over the age of 70 were given ENZOGENOL. Consumption of 480 mg ENZOGENOL per day for 6 months appeared to be safe and well tolerated by the elderly population without any adverse influence on blood parameters or causing any other adverse effects. In fact, there were significantly fewer adverse effects in the treatment group compared to the placebo group, indicating some general beneficial effects of ENZOGENOL in this elderly group (Frevel 2012). In another RCT, supplementation with 960 mg ENZOGENOL daily for 5 weeks in men 50–65 years of age caused no changes in blood parameters, urea and electrolytes, liver function and lipid profiles. There were no adverse events reported by any participant (Pipingas 2008). One RCT investigated a population of people with mild traumatic brain injury (mTBI). In this 12-week study of 60 individuals, 1000 mg ENZOGENOL as a single daily dose was shown to be safe and well tolerated (Theadom 2013). In a further study, 42 student athletes aged 18–24 with history of concussion received 1000 mg ENZOGENOL daily for 6 weeks. Again, ENZOGENOL was well tolerated and no adverse events reported by Walter (2017).

In-market safety monitoring has confirmed the safety of ENZOGENOL for human consumption. Since 1998, approximately 68 tons of ENZOGENOL have entered the world market in the form of various dietary supplement products with different dosages ranging from 25 to 240 mg per capsule. Most of these products are combination formulas combining ENZOGENOL with other nutritional actives. Depending on the target application, commonly consumed daily doses range from 50 to 1000 mg. Assuming an average daily dose of 480 mg, equivalent to two capsules of a high dosage formulation called ENZO Professional (available since 2003), 142 million daily doses of ENZOGENOL have been consumed. No reports of any serious adverse events have been received by the manufacturer or any regulatory authorities as a result of consuming ENZOGENOL.

15.5   RESEARCH OF ANTIOXIDANT PROPERTIES

Research into the potential health benefits of ENZOGENOL started with testing the free radical scavenging abilities using *in vitro* antioxidant assays. ENZOGENOL was compared to other well-known polyphenol extracts and antioxidants including *Pinus pinaster (maritima)* bark extract, grape seed and grape skin extracts, catechin and ascorbic acid (Wood 2002). Antioxidant activities were measured at different pH values to represent the different pH environments that these extracts

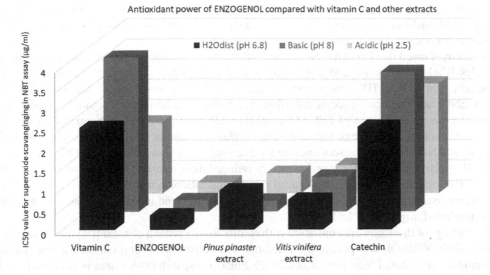

FIGURE 15.2 Comparison of antioxidant activity of ENZOGENOL, vitamin C and other plant extracts measured by NBT assay given as IC_{50} values (concentrations required for 50% reduction in superoxide radical concentration).

would encounter within the human body while moving through the digestive tract and into the blood stream. Results showed that ENZOGENOL had the strongest antioxidant activity across the range of pH values. Antioxidant activities were measured as superoxide radical scavenging ability using NBT (Figure 15.2) and WST-1 assays, and reported as IC_{50}-values.

Antioxidant activity in ENZOGENOL was also tested using the popular and widely used Oxygen Radical Absorbance Capacity (ORAC) assay (Ou 2001). This assay measures the scavenging capacity of antioxidants against peroxyl radicals, which are one of the most common reactive oxygen species in the body. The ORAC value of ENZOGENOL was determined to be 8974 µmol Trolox equivalents per 1 g of extract (independently tested by Brunswick Laboratories, USA, April 2004). By comparison, blueberries, which are commonly regarded to be a high antioxidant 'superfood' have an ORAC value of 4669 µmol Trolox equivalents per 100 g of fresh fruit according to the USDA database for ORAC of selected foods (Release 2). These tests confirm that ENZOGENOL pine bark extract is a concentrated source of highly active antioxidants.

15.6 *IN VITRO* STUDIES

Atherosclerosis is the process of hardening of arterial blood vessel walls and narrowing of the arteries, which may eventually result in cardiovascular diseases (CVD) such as coronary thrombosis, myocardial infarction and stroke. Many complex steps have to occur for this progressive disease to initiate and develop to the stage were atherosclerotic changes of the blood vessels can be diagnosed. These steps involve inflammatory mediators and the immune system, and begin with the interaction of vascular endothelial cells and circulating leukocytes. Leukocytes adhere to the inside of the inflamed vessel wall and transmigrate through the endothelial cell layer into the extracellular matrix. These processes involve several key molecules including the pro-inflammatory cytokine tumour necrosis factor alpha (TNF-α), adhesion factors vascular cell adhesion molecule-1 (VCAM-1), intercellular cell adhesion molecule-1 (ICAM-1) and E-selectin, and the matrix-degrading metalloproteinase 9 (MMP-9) required for monocyte penetration into the vessel wall.

Polyphenol-rich plant extracts containing different types of flavonoids and proanthocyanidins have been reported to possess various anti-inflammatory properties in different cellular and animal based tests. Kim et al. (2010) investigated the anti-atherogenic properties of ENZOGENOL in a leukocyte endothelium interaction system with human umbilical vein endothelial cells (HUVEC) and human monocytic THP-1 cells.

This study showed that ENZOGENOL could substantially reduce the expression of the adhesion molecules ICAM-1, VCAM-1 and E-selectin in TNF-α stimulated endothelial cells and greatly reduce adhesion of the THP-1 monocytes to activated HUVEC cells. These results suggest that ENZOGENOL may reduce leukocyte adhesion in response to inflammatory signals from the endothelium. Increased expression of PECAM-1, another adhesion molecule concentrated in the tight junctions of endothelial cells and induced on the surfaces of monocytes and neutrophils, was also inhibited by ENZOGENOL, as was integrinβ2. The study also showed that ENZOGENOL inhibited MMP-9 activity in monocytes and markedly reduced their transmigration abilities. In the process of inflammation, MMP-9 plays a crucial role for migration, extravasation and infiltration into surrounding tissue. Hence, ENZOGENOL may, in addition to the initial adhesion, also attenuate trans-endothelial migration of leukocytes.

The findings of this study are consistent with results from a human clinical trial discussed below in which ENZOGENOL was part of a formulation that improved several cardiovascular risk factors including endothelial function (Shand 2003). Further research in this area is necessary, and it appears that ENZOGENOL would be an excellent candidate for nutritional intervention trials in people with atherosclerosis.

15.7   ANIMAL STUDIES

15.7.1   MOUSE LONGEVITY TRIALS

The strong antioxidant properties of ENZOGENOL seen in the *in vitro* assays led to further research investigating possible effects on lifespan in laboratory mice. The free radical theory of ageing first formulated by Harman (1956) suggests that free radicals produced internally by respiratory energy production and pathological disorders and externally through environmental factors play a crucial role in initiating and driving the ageing processes in our body.

Two small animal feeding trials were carried out at the University of Canterbury, Christchurch, New Zealand (previously unpublished data), to investigate whether ENZOGENOL has an effect on lifespan. Results showed a significant increase in mean lifespan of 18.4% from 84.7 weeks in the control group to 100.3 weeks in the ENZOGENOL group ($p < 0.05$). There were 24 mice in each group, with treatment starting at 52 weeks of age receiving either 21 mg/kg ENZOGENOL in the drinking water or receiving water without ENZOGENOL. This increase in mean lifespan was remarkable considering that the feeding started at 52 weeks when the mice were already middle age. An earlier trial with younger mice also trended toward an increase in mean lifespan, but this did not reach significance, perhaps due to the low numbers of mice used in this trial (10 mice in each of five feeding groups received 0, 1, 5, 21 and 100 mg/kg body weight of ENZOGENOL). Neither trial showed an increase in maximum lifespan. These findings suggest that ENZOGENOL may not slow the rate of ageing, which would have resulted in increasing the maximum lifespan, but rather reduced the susceptibility to disease leading to a greater number of mice living longer and apparently healthier lives.

15.7.2   RAT TELOMERE TRIAL

To further investigate the anti-ageing properties of ENZOGENOL, another animal feeding trial was carried out that analysed telomere length in leukocytes. Telomeres are the end sequences of chromosomes in all vertebrates composed of the six nucleotides TTAGGG repeated a few hundred to several thousand times. During DNA replication in mitotic cell division, the very ends of the telomeres are not replicated leading to a progressive shortening of the telomere sequence through cell divisions. This shortening is thought to contribute to cellular senescence. The length of telomeres can therefore be used as a proxy of how well somatic cells age. In this trial, three groups of Sprague Dawley rats (20 males and 18 females per group) received either 21 mg/kg body weight of ENZOGENOL, 9 mg/kg of vitamin C, or nothing with the drinking water. Telomere length was measured in leukocytes using a fluorescent telomere-specific peptide nucleic acid hybridisation probe. Signals detected in flow cytometry analyses gave a measure of the total amount of telomeric sequence in the cellular DNA, corresponding to the length of the telomeres.

As a positive control, telomeres from untreated young (3 months) and old (22 months) rats were analysed and compared, and the results from this showed an approximately 50% reduction in telomere length over this period of the animals' life.

Comparing the three trial groups after 9 months of treatment (Figure 15.3), the ENZOGENOL group had significantly longer telomeres than both the control and the vitamin C groups. These results suggest that ENZOGENOL may help preserve telomeres, possibly indicating a slowing of the age-related telomere shortening process.

15.7.3 MOUSE DIABETES TRIAL

In 2014, a research group in Korea published initial investigations of ENZOGENOL's antidiabetic effects in a mouse model of type 2 diabetes mellitus (Bang 2014). The researchers found that ENZOGENOL improved diabetes-related metabolic changes, including improved glucose tolerance, reduced glycosylated haemoglobin levels, as well as lower insulin and glucagon levels in the blood, and improved liver lipid profiles. In this study the diabetic mice received ENZOGENOL at 12.5, 25 and 50 mg/kg body weight, equivalent to 1, 2.1 and 4.2 mg/kg body weight in humans. Both, medium- and high-dose treatments were effective at improving glucose and lipid metabolism. In detail, the ENZOGENOL medium-dose treatment (equivalent to ≈210 mg for a 100 kg human) decreased fasting blood glucose levels by 27% at 4 weeks and 20% at 6 weeks. The high-dose treatment (≈420 mg for a 100 kg human) decreased fasting blood glucose levels by 37% and 41%

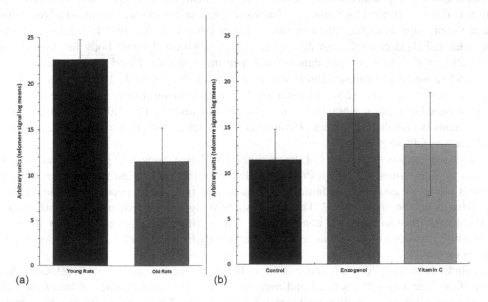

FIGURE 15.3 Telomere length in rat leukocytes. Flow cytometry measurements used the DAKO Telomere DNA Kit. The means of the raw log telomere signal were used as a measure of telomere length: (a) Telomere length in young versus old rats and (b) telomere length after 9 months of treatment.

at 4 and 6 weeks, respectively. A 2-hour oral glucose tolerance test showed that ENZOGENOL significantly improved glucose clearance from the blood, indicating a significant decrease in insulin resistance. In untreated diabetic controls HbA1C, serum insulin and glucagon levels were elevated. ENZOGENOL at 25 and 50 mg/kg significantly reduced HbA1c by 35.2% and 57.8%, serum insulin by 60.1% and 70% and glucagon levels by 46.1% and 66.8%, respectively. Investigating the parameters of lipid metabolism showed that ENZOGENOL increased activation of AMPK (AMP activated protein kinase). This liver enzyme stimulates hepatic lipid oxidation, and inhibits cholesterol and triglyceride synthesis. Reduced AMPK activity in diabetes leads to a negative liver fatty acid profile. Yet, ENZOGENOL treatment was able to normalise triglycerides, total cholesterol and HDL cholesterol to non-diabetic levels in the mice. Further effects on liver enzymes included increased amounts of glucokinase and glycogen synthase, thereby improving glucose clearance from the blood, and reduced glucose-6-phosphatase and phosphoenolpyruvate-carboxykinase levels, which reduced unnecessary glucose synthesis.

In conclusion, using a mouse model of type 2 diabetes, this study showed that ENZOGENOL has potential hypoglycaemic effects by modulating the expression of hepatic glucose-regulating enzymes and enzymatic activity of AMPK in the liver. These potential benefits require further confirmation in clinical studies.

15.8 CLINICAL TRIALS

15.8.1 AN OPEN-LABEL PILOT TRIAL ON CARDIOVASCULAR AND ANTIOXIDANT BENEFITS OF ENZOGENOL

The first clinical study using ENZOGENOL was an open-label trial investigating cardiovascular (Shand 2003) and antioxidant (Senthilmohan 2003) health benefits of an established capsule product containing 120 mg ENZOGENOL and 60 mg vitamin C per capsule. Twenty-four generally healthy subjects (14 males, 10 females) aged between 55 and 75 years took two capsules twice daily for 12 weeks. Assessments at baseline, 6 and 12 weeks included routine biochemical and haematological indices, and anthropometric, blood pressure, forearm blood flow and haemorheological measurements. Supplementation at a dosage of 480 mg/day of ENZOGENOL and 240 mg/day vitamin C did not change biochemical or haematological safety measures and no adverse effects were reported, supporting the safety of the treatment (Shand 2003). Over 12 weeks, mean body mass index (BMI) decreased from 26.1 to 25.7 ($p \leq 0.001$), and mean body fat decrease from 30.9 to 29.3 ($p \leq 0.001$). A significant reduction in mean systolic blood pressure was observed after 6 and 12 weeks of treatment [mean decrease = 7 mmHg, $p \leq 0.01$]. Diastolic blood pressure remained unchanged. After 12 weeks basal and hyperaemic blood flow in forearm resistance vessels as measured by plethysmography had increased significantly by 17%–20% ($p \leq 0.01$), indicating improvements in endothelial function. Plasma viscosity showed a small but physiologically significant decrease of 4% ($p \leq 0.001$).

To assess the antioxidant effects of the treatment, oxidative damage to proteins and DNA were analysed by Senthilmohan (2003). Protein oxidation in the blood plasma was measured using a protein carbonyl assay. DNA damage was measured in isolated peripheral blood mononuclear cells using the comet assay. This study showed significant reductions in both oxidative stress markers. Protein carbonyl concentration fell significantly after 6 weeks by about 50% ($p \leq 0.0001$), and DNA damage was reduced significantly by about 40% after 12 weeks ($p \leq 0.01$) of supplementation.

The findings of this pilot study indicated that dietary supplementation with ENZOGENOL and vitamin C is safe and well tolerated and may be associated with a number of beneficial effects on a range of established cardiovascular risk factors (Shand 2003) and oxidative stress markers (Senthilmohan 2003). P-values above indicate significance of change over time within the treatment group. Randomised controlled trials are required to verify these findings.

15.8.2   An RCT on the Cardiovascular and Antioxidant Benefits of ENZOGENOL in Smokers

Young et al. (2006) investigated the effects of ENZOGENOL on cardiovascular, inflammatory and oxidative stress markers in an RCT in chronic smokers, as smoking has been shown to increase systemic inflammation and oxidative stress in the body. Forty-four chronic smokers without cardiovascular symptoms received either 480 mg ENZOGENOL and 60 mg vitamin C, or 60 mg vitamin C alone daily for 12 weeks. Endothelial function in the brachial artery was assessed as flow-mediated vasodilation (FMD) using ultrasound measurements. FMD improved in both treatment groups, with the ENZOGENOL group showing greater improvement after 12 weeks compared to the vitamin C only controls. However, the difference between the two groups did not reach statistical significance likely due to the small sample size. A larger trial in individuals with established atherosclerosis or CVD comparing ENZOGENOL alone to placebo is recommended. Protein carbonyl content in the blood plasma was reduced by 35% after 12 weeks in the ENZOGENOL group, whereas vitamin C alone had no effect on protein oxidation, indicating a significant reduction in oxidative stress with ENZOGENOL over the control ($p = 0.03$). This finding confirmed the results obtained by Senthilmohan (2003) in the previous open-label pilot trial. Another interesting finding was the significant reduction of fibrinogen levels in the sub-group of heavy smokers. Smokers with a long history of smoking or particularly heavy cigarette consumption had higher fibrinogen levels compared to lighter smoking subjects. In the heavy smokers, the ENZOGENOL formulation significantly reduced fibrinogen levels by approximately 0.6 g/L compared to controls ($p = 0.009$) to reach the level found in the lighter smoking individuals. Elevated fibrinogen levels in the plasma can signal inflammation, hence this reduction may indicate an anti-inflammatory action of the ENZOGENOL formula.

15.8.3   An RCT on Brain Function Benefits of ENZOGENOL in Older Men

Age-related cognitive decline, including mild cognitive impairment and dementias, are of great concern to many people and may become a major socioeconomic challenge for many countries with ageing populations. Lifestyle choices including quality of diet and nutrition are important determinants of our individual capacity to maintain optimal brain health and function as we age. Dietary intake of flavonoid antioxidants has been shown in a prospective cohort study to be inversely correlated with cognitive decline (Letenneur 2007). In this study, 1640 subjects aged 65 and older without dementia were followed for 10 years with regular psychometric and reliable dietary assessments. Individuals with higher flavonoid intake, comparing the two highest quartiles to the lowest quartile, showed lesser cognitive decline over 10 years. After 10 years, participants with the lowest flavonoid intake showed twice the decline in cognitive function assessed by the Mini-Mental State Examination (MMSE) compared to those with the highest quartile flavonoid intake, losing 2.1 versus 1.2 points on the MMSE scale.

Our brain has the propensity to suffer oxidative damage given its particular biochemical characteristics. One, the brain uses the greatest amount of oxygen in the body, being solely dependent on glycolytic energy production; two, it is especially rich in peroxidisable fatty acids; and three, brain tissue has a high content of both Fe and ascorbate, key ingredients in causing membrane lipid peroxidation.

Given the brain's susceptibility to oxidative damage and the fact that increased dietary flavonoid intake is associated with better cognitive function as we age, an intervention with a flavonoid-based antioxidant product may have potential to reduce cognitive decline or improve cognitive functioning. With this premise, researchers Pipingas and Silberstein at the Brain Sciences Institute of Swinburne University in Melbourne, Australia, set out to test ENZOGENOL's effects on brain function in individuals that are at risk of cognitive decline with age due to their negative cardiovascular risk profile (Pipingas 2008). Hence, this RCT recruited

42 overweight males (BMI > 25) that were 50–65 years old, had a sedentary occupation and did not exercise regularly. Eleven participants were taking anti-hypertensive medications. The treatment group ($n = 22$) received a daily dose of 960 mg ENZOGENOL and 120 mg vitamin C, whereas the control group ($n = 20$) received 120 mg vitamin C only. Cognitive performance on verified computer-based cognitive tests, coherence analyses of brain electrical measurements, blood pressure and standard haematological safety parameters were assessed before and after 5 weeks of treatment. The study hypothesis was that performance on cognitive tasks that are most sensitive to age-related cognitive impairment may improve with the treatment containing ENZOGENOL. Primary outcome measures were performance on spatial working memory (SWM) and immediate recognition memory (IRM) tasks, as these have been shown to be the most sensitive measures of age-related cognitive decline.

Study results showed that there were significant improvements in response times (RT) on SWM and IRM tasks in the ENZOGENOL group over the controls ($p < 0.05$) (Figure 15.4). SWM RT improved by 64 ms (6.4%) and IRM RT by 60 ms (5.4%) after 5 weeks of treatment. These improvements can be put into clinical perspective on the basis of normal age-related decline. RT on the SWM task slows down with age from an average of about 700 ms for a 20 year old to approximately 1300 ms for a 90 year old. Roughly, this amounts to a decline in reaction time of 8.6 ms per year. The improvement seen with ENZOGENOL on the SWM task of 64 ms after only 5 weeks was therefore equivalent to 7.4 years recovery in brain performance (Figure 15.4). The improvement in RT of 60 ms on the IRM task was equivalent to 12 years of brain age recovery. In other words, there is a possibility that a 60-year-old person may improve their speed of memory to that of a 48- to 52-year-old person. This could obviously have considerable benefits for things like ability to safely operate a car or for performance in the work place, and so on.

Pipingas (2008) also presents a combined statistical analyses of systolic blood pressure data from two RCTs, including the data from the study by Young et al. (2006), showing a significant reduction in systolic blood pressure of 5 mmHg in the ENZOGENOL groups ($n = 39$) compared to controls. ($n = 35$) ($p < 0.05$). The positive safety results from this study were discussed above in the safety and toxicology section.

To investigate whether ENZOGENOL may influence brain activities directly, the study also examined effects on brain functional connectivity during the performance of a recognition memory task (Pipingas and Silberstein 2007). Functional connectivity is a term that describes how different

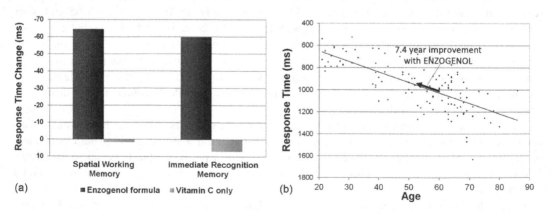

FIGURE 15.4 Improvement of brain performance after 5 weeks of ENZOGENOL treatment: (a) The bar graph shows improved response times on two computer-based cognitive tests. (b) The scatter plot shows the normal age related decline on Spatial Working Memory performance and indicates the magnitude of improvement seen with ENZOGENOL.

brain regions interact or interfere with each other. The hypothesis was that the ENZOGENOL formula would improve functional connectivity by reducing cortical coupling between certain neural regions. In this test, a constant 50 Hz light flicker is projected onto the retina, which results in a constant EEG signal that was detected over 64 electrodes across the scalp, referred to as steady-state visually evoked potential (SSVEP). This signal is influenced and modified by the brain's own electrical activities during task performance. Measuring this signal over the course of the task allows the calculation of event-related partial coherence (ERPC), which is a measure of functional connections between brain regions. These functional connections are referred to as cortical couplings. One could think of this as more coupling equates to more noise across the brain and less coupling indicates less noise.

Studies by Silberstein have shown that reduced long-range cortical coupling between frontal and posterior sites are a prominent feature of increased individual proficiency on this task. Other brain-active drugs such as an acute dose methylphenidate – used as a medication for ADHD and as a brain function enhancer – cause a robust reduction in long range cortical coupling associated with improved task performance (Silberstein 2005).

SSVEP-ERPC measures were calculated and compared before and after supplementation for each group. Supplementation with the ENZOGENOL formula, but not vitamin C, was associated with a frontal to posterior decrease in SSVEP-ERPC that is characteristic for correct responses in this task. This finding was similar to the effects seen with methylphenidate in ADHD and indicates that ENZOGENOL may enhance brain mechanisms mediating memory processes.

15.8.4 Effects of an ENZOGENOL Vitamin Antioxidant Formula in Patients with Severe Migraine

Two open-label trials have investigated the use of ENZOGENOL antioxidant formulas in migraine prevention (Chayasirisobhon 2006, 2013). These studies were carried out in an outpatient clinic setting by Dr Chayasirisobhon, Department of Neurology, Kaiser Permanente Medical Center, Anaheim, California.

In the first trial, 12 patients with a long-term history of migraines with and without aura were enrolled (Chayasirisobhon 2006). All patients had failed to respond to multiple treatments with β-blockers, antidepressants, anticonvulsants and 5-hydroxytryptamine receptor agonists. They received a once daily oral dose of 1200 mg ENZOGENOL, 600 mg vitamin C and 300 IU vitamin E for the duration of 3 months, in addition to any pharmacological medication. At baseline, before beginning the antioxidant treatment, patients completed a migraine disability assessment (MIDAS) questionnaire that measured the migraine impact on work, school, domestic and social activities over the previous 3 months. After the 3-month treatment, patients completed the MIDAS questionnaire again.

The study results showed a highly significant mean improvement in MIDAS score of 50.6% for the 3-month treatment period compared with the 3 months prior to baseline ($p < 0.005$). Patients also experienced a significant reduction in the number of days they suffered a migraine attack, and the severity of the migraine headaches that did occur was significantly reduced. The mean number of headache days fell from 44.4 days during the previous 3 months to 26.0 days during the 3-month therapy ($p < 0.005$). The mean headache severity score was reduced from 7.5 to 5.5 out of 10 ($p < 0.005$). These results suggested that the antioxidant therapy combining high dose ENZOGENOL with vitamins C and E as used in this study may be beneficial as a migraine preventative treatment, and possibly reduce headache frequency and severity.

In the second study, Dr Chayasirisobhon used the commercially available antioxidant formula called ENZO Professional, giving five capsules once daily for 3 months, with some patients continuing treatment for 12 months (Chayasirisobhon 2013). With this formula, patients received the same amount of ENZOGENOL with 1200 mg, but much less vitamin C, which was reduced from 600 to only 150 mg, and no vitamin E. This again was an open-label uncontrolled study. Fifty-five outpatients with chronic migraine that had failed to respond to at least two prophylactic pharmaceutical medications were enrolled. Five patients dropped out early in the study and were not analysed. Among the 50 patients completing the 3-month treatment there were 44 women and 6 men aged 14–68 years, average age 41.6. Patients exhibited various different headache presentations, including right or left sides or bilateral and frontal, parietal or temporal or diffuse, with and without aura. The age of onset varied widely from 6 to 57 (mean 23.3) years; headache frequency varied from 2 to 30 (mean 15.7) per month and duration varied from 0.25 to 4 days (mean 1.4 days). As in the previous study, patients completed the MIDAS questionnaire at the beginning and end of the study to compare migraine impact over the 3 months prior to enrolment with the 3-month treatment period. Patients continued on existing pharmacologic medications during the study. Twenty-nine patients (58.0%) showed a significant reduction in MIDAS score, and reduced number of headache days and headache severity ($p < 0.0001$). It took on average 25 days for headache relief to be noticed, ranging from 3 to 80 days.

Patients were graded according to their MIDAS scores indicating the overall level of disability: grade I, little or no disability (score of 0–5); grade II, mild disability (score of 6–10); grade III, moderate disability (score of 11–20); and grade IV, severe disability (score of $\geq$ 21). After 3 months of treatment, 19 patients had no change in their disability grade, whereas 31 patients were downgraded (see details in Figure 15.5.). The mean MIDAS score for all patients was significantly reduced from 30.3 to 14.4 – a mean improvement of 52.3% ($p < 0.0001$). The average number of headache days for the 3 months before treatment for all patients was 47.9 days, and this reduced significantly during the 3-month treatment period to 25.9 days ($p < 0.0001$). Headache severity over the same period was reduced from an average score of 8.1 to 5.6 out of 10 ($p < 0.0001$). When looking at the patients that had responded to the treatment, the results were even more impressive, with average reductions in MIDAS score by 25.8 points (91%), number of days with headaches down by 39.7 (82%), and headache severity down by 4.1 points (51%).

Sixteen patients that had responded continued the treatment for a further 9 months. Assessments were repeated at 6, 9 and 12 months. The average MIDAS score, number of headaches for each 3-month period and headache severity are shown in Figure 15.6.

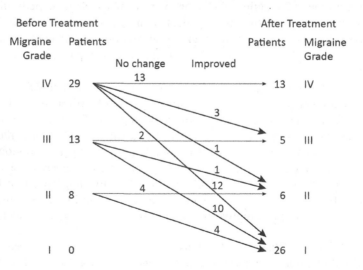

FIGURE 15.5 Changes in grades of migraine disability before and after 3 months of ENZOGENOL treatment.

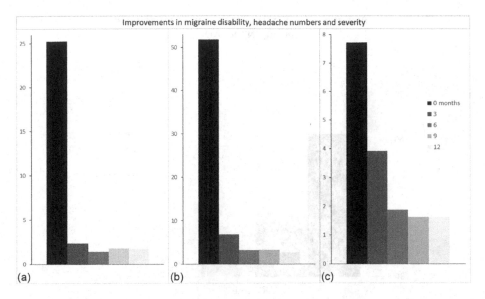

FIGURE 15.6 Improvements in (a) MIDAS score, (b) number of headache days and (c) headache severity in 16 responders that continued ENZOGENOL treatment for 12 months.

In conclusion, both of these open-label trials have shown great promise for the use of ENZOGENOL with vitamin C in the treatment of migraine. A well-designed controlled clinical study is now needed to confirm these findings and allow ENZOGENOL to be accepted as a general medical treatment for migraine.

15.8.5 EFFECTS OF ENZOGENOL ON BRAIN FUNCTION IN PATIENTS WITH MILD TRAUMATIC BRAIN INJURY

Drs Feigin and Theadom of the National Institute for Stroke and Applied Neurosciences, Auckland University of Technology, investigated the effects of ENZOGENOL in 60 people with persistent cognitive deficits after sustaining a mild traumatic brain injury (mTBI; Theadom 2013). This RCT found that ENZOGENOL helped patients steadily improve recovery of brain function over a 3-month period without regression of cognitive functioning after discontinuation of treatment. Participants, aged between 21 and 64 years (average 44.5), had suffered mTBIs 3–12 months prior to enrolling in the study. The causes of brain injuries were included motor vehicle accidents (33.3%), falls (33.3%), assaults (15.0%), sports-related injuries (10.0%), and being hit by objects (8.3%). Patients were recruited through concussion clinics that specialise in brain injury rehabilitation. An important inclusion criteria was a minimum level of cognitive dysfunction assessed by using the cognitive failures questionnaire (CFQ), a common measure of everyday cognitive functioning. This questionnaire measures how often minor cognitive mistakes, which everyone makes from time to time, happened to participants during the past week. Eligibility criteria included a CFQ score > 38 = 0.5-times the standard deviation above the mean for healthy individuals. The CFQ average for all participants at baseline was a score of 60, indicating a considerable level of everyday cognitive difficulties in these patients.

Participants were randomised to receive ENZOGENOL, 1000 mg per day in two 500 mg capsules taken together in the morning before breakfast, or matching placebo capsules for 6 weeks. Subsequently, all participants received ENZOGENOL for a further 6 weeks, followed by placebo for all patients for 4 weeks. Compliance, side effects, cognitive failures, working and episodic memory, post-concussive symptoms, and mood were assessed at baseline, 6, 12 and 16 weeks.

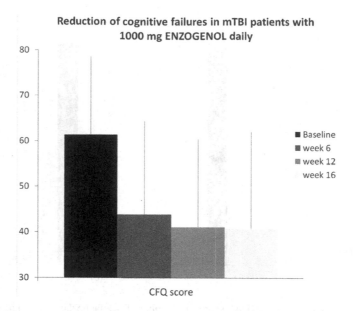

FIGURE 15.7 Cognitive failure questionnaire (CFQ) results in patients with mild traumatic brain injury (mTBI).

The treatment was found to be safe and well tolerated. Non-treatment related events of headache, sleep disturbance and blurred vision were reported by participants in both treatment and placebo groups.

Analyses of CFQ scores showed a significant reduction in cognitive failures with ENZOGENOL versus placebo after 6 weeks [mean CFQ score −6.9 (95% confidence interval −10.8 to −4.1)]. The reduction in cognitive failures continued over the 12 weeks of treatment, and stayed at their reduced level at the end of the 4-week washout period (Figure 15.7). Other outcome measures also showed positive trends, but did not reach statistical significance, among these were anxiety and depression often associated with TBI. More patients in the ENZOGENOL group showed improvements on the Hospital Anxiety and Depression Scale (HADS) compared to the placebo group.

15.8.6 EFFECTS OF ENZOGENOL ON BRAIN FUNCTION IN STUDENT-ATHLETES WITH A CONCUSSION HISTORY

Dr Slobounov at Penn State Center for Sport Concussion, Pennsylvania State University, tested the feasibility of dietary supplementation with 1000 mg ENZOGENOL daily as a treatment modality in college-age athletes with a history of sports-related concussions (Walter 2017). The participants were in a chronic phase of concussion, 6–36 months post-injury and still experiencing residual symptoms that impacted their ability to study and perform in training. Twenty male and 22 female student athletes, 18–24 years old, were enrolled. Equal numbers of participants were randomly assigned to receive ENZOGENOL as 2 × 500 mg capsules taken approximately 15 min before breakfast or identical looking placebo capsules. The students underwent testing sessions at baseline and after 6 weeks of treatment. Brain activities were measured by electroencephalography (EEG) during neuropsychological tasks used to induce cognitive challenges.

The EEG analyses revealed that after 6 weeks of treatment, the ENZOGENOL group showed enhanced frontal-midline theta, and decreased parietal theta power during the brain loading with the psychological tests. These findings indicated reduced mental fatigue when performing the brain challenging tasks. In contrast to the controls, the student athletes receiving ENZOGENOL also reported experiencing lesser mental fatigue and reduced sleep problems. This suggested that ENZOGENOL can reduce brain fatigue during cognitive loading and has the potential to improve brain functioning in the chronic phase of concussion. Further studies are needed to confirm these findings.

15.8.7 Effects of ENZOGENOL on Cerebral Circulation in a Patient with a History of Concussions

In an attempt to elucidate the mechanism of action, a feasibility study was undertaken to see if ENZOGENOL could impact blood circulation in the brain in an individual that had suffered several sports-related concussions over previous years. The participant was a 47-year-old, right-handed male, practicing martial arts for 25 years. During this time he had experienced several hits to the head, sometimes severe. In 2012, 3 years before this experimental study, he was hit in the middle of his face, leading to severe nosebleed and some headaches. In a second incident 10 days later, he experienced another blow to the back of his head and neck. In the following months, he experienced severe headaches, fatigue while looking at screens, mental fatigue and greatly reduced mental stamina. Those symptoms slowly improved over several months before becoming asymptomatic.

To investigate the impact the concussive injuries had, and the potential effect ENZOGENOL may have on brain perfusion, the individual underwent two high-resolution brain SPECT (Single Photon Emission Computed Tomography) imaging scans at CereScan in Denver, Colorado. The two scans were performed under equal conditions 48 hours apart at 9 a.m. on day 1 and day 3 of the experiment. The individual had refrained from taking any medications or supplements for 2 weeks prior to the first scan. This first scan on day 1 established the baseline brain perfusion pattern. Immediately following the scan on day 1, the individual took the first dose of 1000 mg ENZOGENOL, a second dose on the morning of day 2 and a third dose on day 3 exactly 1 hour before the second scan. This second scan established the impact of three doses of ENZOGENOL on brain perfusion.

Analyses showed the high-resolution brain SPECT images at baseline and after treatment were of good quality. No abnormal motion or artefacts were detected. The overall cortical activity was within normal limits to slightly reduced. At baseline, focal areas of abnormal cortical hypoperfusion were noted in the frontal, temporal, occipital and cerebellar lobes. Focal areas of abnormal subcortical hypoperfusion were noted in the bilateral lentiform and right caudate areas. Talairach comparisons of the baseline data to an age-match normal sample, as well as the 3D/isocontour and surface-rendered images, revealed hypoperfusion abnormalities consistent with those seen on the tomographic images. The nature, location and pattern of these abnormalities was primarily consistent with the scientific literature pertaining to traumatic brain injury and the individual's history of repeated concussive injury.

In the second scan, a generalised cortical activation was noted after the ENZOGENOL treatment, and Talairach comparison of baseline and post-treatment scans showed increases in cortical activity with the intervention (Figure 15.8). Table 15.1 shows the increases in blood circulation to those regions that were found hypoperfused in the baseline scan.

Another interesting finding was a small reduction in perfusion of the left and right amygdala of approximately −4% post-treatment. This reduction in activity appears unusual given that the

Improvements in brain perfusion in an individual with concussion history after three doses of 1000 mg ENZOGENOL

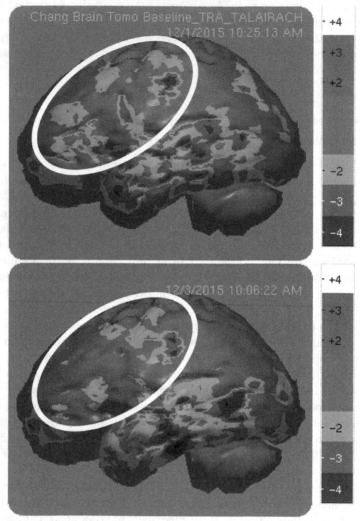

FIGURE 15.8 **(See color insert.)** Talairach comparison of high-resolution SPECT scans of an individual with a concussion history before (top) and after (bottom) three doses of 1000 mg ENZOGENOL, showing reduced hypoperfusion.

treatment led to a generalised activation across the brain averaging +11%. This is particularly interesting in view of the function of the amygdala in behaviour traits and neuropsychological disorders including anxiety and depression. Reduced activity of the amygdala following ENZOGENOL treatment would be consistent with the trend of reduced anxiety and depression seen previously in the study of mTBI patients.

In summary, clinical research has shown that ENZOGENOL improves brain functions that ordinarily decline with age, assists in recovery of brain functions after concussion/TBI, may be used as a migraine preventative, supports cardiovascular health and reduces oxidative stress.

TABLE 15.1

Increase in Blood Circulation in Hypoperfused Brain Regions

14%	R Olfactory Cortex
13%	R Inferior Frontal Gyrus, Pars Opercularis
16%	R Parahippocampal Gyrus
13%	R Medial Temporal Lobe
16%	L Insula
13%	L Cuneus
5%	R Inferior Occipital Gyrus
17%	L Inferior Frontal Gyrus, Pars Triangularis
16%	L Inferior Frontal Gyrus
6%	L Parahippocampal Gyrus
20%	L Temporal Operculum
7%	L Middle Occipital Gyrus
14%	L Inferior Frontal Gyrus, Pars Opercularis
6%	R Hippocampus
5%	R Insula
7%	L Medial Temporal Lobe
9%	R Inferior Medial Frontal Gyrus
9%	L Superior Occipital Gyrus
6%	R Inferior Frontal Gyrus
8%	L Occipital Lobe
7%	R Supramarginal Gyrus
13%	R Heschl Gyrus
7%	R Middle Occipital Gyrus
13%	L Rolandic Operculum
8%	R Occipital Lobe
9%	L Heschl Gyrus
11%	**Average Increase**
	p-value = 0.000000000005

15.9 DISCUSSION ON POTENTIAL MECHANISMS OF ACTION AND BIOAVAILABILITY

Mechanisms of action of plant extracts are often difficult to determine due to complex composition and lack of knowledge on bioavailability and metabolism of the different constituents in the human body. As discussed above, ENZOGENOL consists of a mixture of polyphenols with approximately 80% or more of proanthocyanidins, 1.5% taxifolin (dihydroquercetin), 0.2%–1% each of catechin, quercetin and piceatannol, and several other minor polyphenols. Only the antioxidant actions as described earlier have been studied for the whole ENZOGENOL extract *in vitro* and in the human body. Significant reductions of oxidative stress markers provide a strong evidence that the ENZOGENOL polyphenol mixture exerts antioxidant actions *in vivo*. Hence, these antioxidation effects likely contribute as one mechanism to the clinical effects on cardiovascular and brain functions described above. For example, improvements in endothelial function may be a direct consequence of reductions in oxidation in the arterial environment, which may improve nitric-oxide production from the endothelium (Cannon 1998) and lead to the improvements in blood flow seen by Shand et al. Similarly, a systemic reduction in oxidation levels in the body may also contribute mechanistically to the prevention of migraine attacks seen with the ENZOGENOL antioxidant formula as elevated levels of oxidation have been found in migraine patient compared to healthy controls (Tuncel 2008). Regarding the benefits for brain function described in older people by Pipingas et al. and in recovery from mTBI by Theadom et al., antioxidative effects may again contribute as one mechanism of action. Brain ageing is associated with increased lipid peroxidation, protein and DNA oxidation indicating progressive age-related antioxidant imbalances. Increased oxidative conditions can cause structural damage and change redox-sensitive signaling processes including insulin receptor signaling, sirtuin pathway, and autophagy. Impaired autophagic activity has been associated with neurodegeneration (Dröge and Schipper 2007). Hence, reducing oxidative stress levels may counteract neurodegenerative processes, but may also influence redox-sensitive signaling directly. Oxidative damage to mitochondrial DNA and the electron transport chain, perturbations in brain iron and calcium homeostasis, and changes in plasma cysteine homeostasis may all be consequences of increased oxidative stress. Direct or indirect effects of ENZOGENOL consumption on these parameters should be investigated in future studies to advance our understanding on its mechanisms of action.

Bioactivities of the compounds present in ENZOGENOL have been studied from different plant sources and in many different model systems, offering a number of mechanisms, other than antioxidant effects, by which ENZOGENOL may be influencing human physiology. Only a few particularly interesting studies are mentioned here. Proanthocyanidins (PACs) from grape-seeds were shown in healthy rats to significantly increase hepatic nicotinamide adenine dinucleotide (NAD+) content in a dose-dependent manner by specifically modulating hepatic concentrations of the major NAD+ precursors as well as the mRNA levels of the genes encoding the enzymes involved in the cellular metabolism of NAD+. Sirtuin 1 (Sirt1) gene expression was also significantly upregulated. The increase in both the NAD+ availability and Sirt1 mRNA levels, in turn, resulted in the hepatic activation of SIRT1, which was significantly associated with improved protection against hepatic triglyceride accumulation. This data indicates that PAC consumption may benefit liver lipid profiles via modulation of NAD+ levels and SIRT1 activity (Aragonès et al. 2016). These may be another part of the mechanisms by which ENZOGENOL normalizes hepatic liver profiles in diabetic rats as described above (*mouse diabetes trial*).

An excellent study on bioavailability of monomeric epicatechin, procyanidin dimer B1, and oligo/polymeric PACs (mean degree of polymerization 5.9) in humans has been published by Wiese and colleagues (Wiese et al. 2015). Epicatechin monomers and glucoronidated, sulphated and methylated forms were present in plasma. Procyanidin B1 was present in plasma in very low amounts and also in mono-methylated form. PACs were absent in plasma, hence not absorbable as intact oligo- and polymers. The major microbial metabolite, 5-(3′,4′-dihydroxyphenyl)-valerolactone (DHPVL) was the dominant metabolite in blood and urine from all parent compounds; yet amounts varied largely between individuals as well as with the degree of polymerization of flavan-3-ols. Monomer units were not detectable in plasma or urine after procyanidin B1 and PAC intake.

This study has highlighted the importance of investigating the clinical effects of this microbial metabolite DHPVL in humans, as it appears to be the main molecule to be absorbed after consumption of PACs. Initial evidence for cognitive-enhancing effects of DHPVL was recently provided in a mouse-model of Alzheimer's disease (AD) (Dal-Pan et al. 2017). In this study, feeding of a PAC-rich fruit extract from blueberries and grapes prevented decrease in brain-derived neurotropic factor (BDNF) in the cortex of the 3TG-AD mice and led to improved performance on a novel object recognition task that declined in the untreated control mice. Plasma concentrations of DHPVL correlated with memory performance in the supplemented mice. Interestingly, the polyphenol supplementation did not reduce beta-ameloid and tau pathologies in the mice. The authors note that rescuing the decline in active BDNF in the cortex of the 3TG-AD mice is possibly the mechanism of action responsible for the improvements on the cognitive task. Intracerebral application of active

BDNF has previously been shown to improve cognitive task performance in this mouse model, and other flavonoids have also been shown to increase BDNF levels.

The effects of ENZOGENOL on BDNF are not known and need to be investigated, but given the similarity of high PAC concentration with the above polyphenol extract it appears likely that ENZOGENOL would give a similar result.

15.10   IN-MARKET EXPERIENCES AND PRODUCT DEVELOPMENT

Research on ENZOGENOL has led to the development of numerous dietary supplement products in the market, most prominently the brands *ENZO Professional* and *ENZO Brain Recovery* marketed by the New Zealand manufacturer of the extract, ENZO Nutraceuticals Limited. Many other brands exist internationally that use ENZOGENOL in combination with other active ingredients for various different health applications.

In the product development phase, ENZO Professional (240 mg ENZOGENOL and 30 mg vitamin C per capsule) was first tested in a small open-label trial of 42 mostly older participants, 26 female and 16 male (average age 63), that took two capsules every morning for 5 weeks. Assessment was by General Health Questionnaire (GHQ). Results (Figure 15.9) were promising, as 64% of participants showed improvements in their general health perception.

ENZO Professional has now become a well known nutritional therapeutic among health professionals and is used in many integrative medical practices in New Zealand and Australia. It is frequently recommended for use in children – but also adults – with ADHD and other patients with atypical behaviour. The similarities to methylphenidate, with respect to improving brain cortical coupling and raising levels of attention and concentration, qualify ENZOGENOL as a first choice nutritional support in ADHD. In a series of case studies, ENZO Professional has shown success in approximately 50% of children, improving behaviour in several ways including better attention and focus, less hyperactivity, less aggression and improved school performance and socialisation with other children. ENZO Professional is also used by many doctors and naturopaths to support cardiovascular and brain health in patients with diabetes, atherosclerosis, high blood pressure and post stroke,

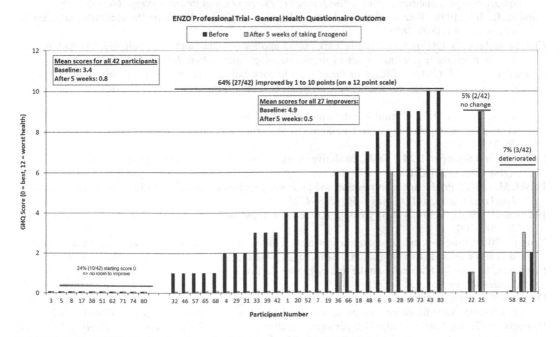

FIGURE 15.9   ENZO Professional product development open-label trial.

and in neurological conditions including dementias, Parkinson's disease, obsessive compulsive disorder and other chronic conditions.

ENZO Brain Recovery, a combination of ENZOGENOL 200 mg with 166 mg Docosahexaenoic acid and 33 mg Eicosapentaenoic acid per capsule, has become a much used nutritional therapeutic for people with brain injury and cognitive dysfunction. At 5 capsules per day, this formula delivers the 1000 mg dose of ENZOGENOL shown to be clinically effective in supporting brain function recovery and reduced fatigue after TBI and concussion.

Although ENZOGENOL has not been clinically tested in some of the above conditions, the antioxidant action in itself and the likely cardiovascular and certain brain benefits justify further trials of the product by patients.

15.11   CONCLUSION

Research has demonstrated that ENZOGENOL is very safe and well tolerated. No serious adverse events have surfaced in any clinical study or during the 18 years it has been in the market as a dietary supplement. The excellent safety profile qualifies ENZOGENOL for use as a natural support agent in any of the applications for which it has been studied.

The body of research to date shows ENZOGENOL has great potential as a natural neurotherapeutic with applications in brain injury rehabilitation, migraine prevention and as a nootropic that may be used in prevention or treatment of cognitive decline with age. Other applications include the use as a support agent for maintenance of cardiovascular, oxidative and metabolic health. Further research is necessary to promote ENZOGENOL for use in all of these areas and to fully penetrate mainstream medical practice.

REFERENCES

Aragonès, G. et al. (2016). Dietary proanthocyanidins boost hepatic NAD(+) metabolism and SIRT1 expression and activity in a dose-dependent manner in healthy rats. *Scientific Reports*, **6**, 24977.

Bang, C.-Y. (2014). Enzogenol improves diabetes-related metabolic change in C57BL/KsJ-db/db mice, a model of type 2 diabetes mellitus. *The Journal of Pharmacy and Pharmacology*, **66**, 875–885.

Cannon, R. 3rd. (1998). Role of nitric oxide in cardiovascular disease: Focus on the endothelium. *Clinical Chemistry*, **44**, 1809–1819.

Chayasirisobhon, S. (2006). Use of a pine bark extract and antioxidant vitamin combination product as therapy for migraine in patients refractory to pharmacologic medication. *Headache*, **46**, 788–793.

Chayasirisobhon, S. (2013). Efficacy of *Pinus radiata* bark extract and vitamin C combination product as a prophylactic therapy for recalcitrant migraine and long-term results. *Acta Neurologica Taiwanica*, **22**, 13–21.

Dal-Pan, A. et al. (2017). Cognitive-enhancing effects of a polyphenols-rich extract from fruits without changes in neuropathology in an animal model of Alzheimer's disease. *Journal of Alzheimers Disease*, **55**, 115–135.

Dröge, W. and Schipper, H.M. (2007). Oxidative stress and aberrant signaling in aging and cognitive decline. *Aging Cell*, **6**, 361–370.

Frevel, M. (2012). Production, composition and toxicology studies of Enzogenol *Pinus radiata* bark extract. *Food and Chemical Toxicology*, **50**, 4316–4324.

Harman, D. (1956). Aging: A theory based on free radical and radiation chemistry. *Journal of Gerontology*, **11**, 298–300.

Kim, D. (2010). Pine bark extract enzogenol attenuated tumor necrosis factor-r-induced endothelial cell adhesion and monocyte transmigration. *Journal of Agricultural and Food Chemistry*, **58**, 7088–7095.

Letenneur, L. (2007). Flavonoid intake and cognitive decline over a 10-year period. *American Journal of Epidemiology*, **165**, 1364–1371.

Ou, B. (2001). Development and validation of an improved oxygen radical absorbance capacity assay using fluorescein as the fluorescent probe. *Journal of Agricultural and Food Chemistry*, **49**, 4619–4626.

Pipingas, A. (2008). Improved cognitive performance after dietary supplementation with a *Pinus radiata* bark extract formulation. *Phytotherapy Research*, **22**, 1168–1174.

Pipingas, A. and Silberstein, R. (2007). Effects of flavonoids on brain functional connectivity during a recognition memory task. *Journal of Clinical EEG & Neuroscience; 16th Annual Conference of the Australasian Society for Psychophysiology.*

Senthilmohan, S. (2003). Effects of flavonoid extract Enzogenol® with vitamin C on protein oxidation and DNA damage in older human subjects. *Nutrition Research,* **23**, 1199–1210.

Shand, B. (2003). Pilot study on the clinical effects of dietary supplementation with Enzogenol®, a flavonoid extract of pine bark and vitamin C. *Phytotherapy Research,* **17**, 490–494.

Silberstein, R. (2005). Effects of methylphenidate on cortical connectivity during an attention task in children diagnosed with attention deficit hyperactivity disorder (ADHD). *Australian Journal of Psychology,* **57**, 36.

Theadom, A. (2013). Enzogenol for cognitive functioning in traumatic brain injury: A pilot placebo-controlled RCT. *European Journal of Neurology,* **20**, 1135–1144.

Tuncel, D. (2008). Oxidative stress in migraine with and without aura. *Biological Trace Element Research,* **126**, 92–97.

Walter, A. (2017). Effect of Enzogenol® supplementation on cognitive, executive, and vestibular/balance functioning in chronic phase of concussion. *Developmental Neuropsychology,* **42**, 93–103.

Wiese, S. et al. (2015). Comparative biokinetics and metabolism of pure monomeric, dimeric, and polymeric flavan-3-ols: A randomized cross-over study in humans. *Molecular Nutrition and Food Research,* **59**, 610–621.

Wood, J. (2002). Antioxidant activity of procyanidin-containing plant extracts at different pHs. *Food Chemistry,* **77**, 155–161.

Young, J. (2006). Comparative effects of enzogenol and vitamin C supplementation versus vitamin C alone on endothelial function and biochemical markers of oxidative stress and inflammation in chronic smokers. *Free Radical Research,* **40**, 85–94.

16 Current State of Clinical Translation of Natural Cardioprotective Agents

Asim K. Duttaroy

CONTENTS

16.1 INTRODUCTION

The importance of natural compounds in health and disease has been well recognised for a long time, although naturally derived compounds have taken a secondary role in drug development during the last few decades. Recently, there has been renewed interest in the use of these compounds as a basis for drug development. Recent advances in the modern tools of chemistry and biology have allowed us to investigate the mechanisms of the effects of naturally derived compounds on the human body, which can be used in the development of new therapies against many diseases, including cardiovascular disease (CVD), dementia and cancer.

CVD involves two main pathophysiological processes such as atherosclerosis and thrombotic events. CVD is the foremost cause of morbidity and mortality in the Western world. Atherosclerosis followed by thrombosis (atherothrombosis) is the pathological process underlying most myocardial, cerebral, and peripheral vascular events. Human blood platelets play a major role in both these processes as outlined in Figure 16.1. Their importance in CVD is indirectly confirmed by the benefit of antiplatelet agents such as aspirin, clopidogrel and glycoprotein IIb/IIIa inhibitors (Muller et al. 2002). Human blood platelets are not only involved in the thrombotic events but are also involved in the initiation and progression of atherosclerotic plaque. Consequently, platelets act as bridge between the processes characteristic of atherosclerosis and thrombosis (Dutta-Roy 1994; Kaplan and Jackson 2011). Platelets in individuals with diabetes, sedentary life style, obesity and insulin resistance show increased activity at baseline and in response to agonists, ultimately leading to increased aggregation and plaque development (Massberg et al. 2002; Natarajan et al. 2008). However, aspirin therapy cannot be used in such cases because it is responsible for a number of serious side effects, rendering it unsuitable for use in primary prevention of CVD (Hennekens and Dalen 2014; Cai et al. 2016). Very few new antithrombotics are currently progressing beyond Phase II trials, and those that have been developed are similarly unsuitable for use in primary prevention (Hennekens and Dalen 2014). Hyperactive platelets as observed in diabetes mellitus, insulin resistance, obesity, sedentary life and smoking, therefore contribute to the development of CVD (Ferroni et al. 2004, 2008; Davi and Patrono 2007; Pamukcu et al. 2011; Huang et al. 2012; Shimodaira et al. 2013), so there is great concern to find the naturally occurring compound(s) that might lack such

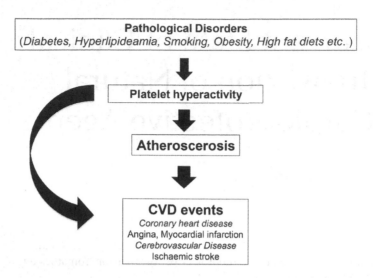

FIGURE 16.1 Platelet hyperactivity and cardiovascular disease. Hyperactivity of platelets and impact on health. Platelets play an important role in CVD both in the pathogenesis of atherosclerosis and in the development of acute thrombotic events. Hyperactive platelets are involved in the development of atherosclerosis by different mechanisms such as membrane shedding, growth factor secretion and expression of several adhesive factors. In addition, hyperactive platelets are involved in the well-known penultimate thrombotic events. (Adapted from O'Kennedy, N. et al., *Eur. J. Nutr.*, 56, 461–462, 2017. With permission.)

side effects and could be used as primary preventives. Various research laboratories are involved in identifying bioactive compounds in fruits and vegetables that modulate human blood platelet function and have utilised the findings to characterise the mechanisms involved in this process, in the hope of identifying potential dietary antiplatelet components (Dutta-Roy et al. 2001; Dutta-Roy 2002; O'Kennedy et al. 2006a–c; Grice et al. 2011; O'Kennedy et al. 2017a). Flavonoids present in fruits and vegetables are inhibitors of cyclic nucleotide phosphodiesterase and TxA$_2$ synthesis, two of the main mechanisms responsible for the inhibition of platelet activation/aggregation. Consequently, these bioactive components of fruits and vegetables may reduce more than one CVD risk factors (Obarzanek et al. 2001; Dutta-Roy 2002).

Epidemiological studies have suggested an association between the consumption of fruits and vegetables and the prevention of several diseases, including CVD. The beneficial effects of fruits and vegetables are thought to be associated mostly with their polyphenol content. Polyphenols, usually antioxidants, are thought to prevent various diseases associated with oxidative stress such as CVD, cancer and neurological degenerative diseases (Fernandes et al. 2017). To date, an increasing number of *in vitro* and *ex vivo* studies strongly suggest that polyphenols in plants may exert a beneficial effect by reducing platelet hyper-reactivity and lowering blood pressure and oxidative stress, which play a major role in the development of CVD (Nieswandt et al. 2005). Major research is currently underway to identify the mechanisms responsible for the effect of polyphenols on CVD development such as blood platelet function, blood pressure, oxidative stress and hyperlipidaemia (Pignatelli et al. 2000; Dutta-Roy 2002; Bucki et al. 2003, Hubbard et al. 2003; Pearson et al. 2005; Guerrero et al. 2007).

During the last 50 years, the tomato (*Lycopersicon esculentum*) has become a highly consumed healthy food (Canene-Adams et al. 2005). Tomatoes contain several components that are beneficial to overall health, including vitamin E, polyphenols, carotenoids, and several water-soluble vitamins and minerals (Agarwal and Rao 2000; Weisburger 2002; Jacques et al. 2013). Because oxidative stress triggers inflammatory disorders, the basis for the development of several diseases such as immune disorders, CVD and rupture of plaque (Willcox et al. 2003), antioxidants present in tomato are therefore believed to slow the progression of many diseases including CVD (Garcia-Alonso et al. 2012).

Epidemiologic studies focused on tomato and tomato products have associated their intake with a reduced risk of CVD. Tomatoes contain several known and unknown compounds that might affect platelet function, lipid metabolism, blood pressure and endothelial function, all of which are important determinants of CVD. There are several excellent reviews available on the overall health benefits of tomatoes (Giovannucci 1999a,b; Agarwal and Rao 2000; Weisburger 2002; Willcox et al. 2003; Canene-Adams et al. 2005).

Kiwi fruit also contains very significant amounts of vitamin C, vitamin E, folic acid and various phytochemicals, such as anthocyanidins and flavonols (Fiorentino et al. 2009; Ferguson 2013). Kiwi fruit is the best-known crop in the genus *Actinidia*. There is a large and diverse range of species and cultivars of *Actinidia* with different characteristics and attributes, of which the *Actinidia deliciosa* 'Hayward' (green kiwi fruit) and *Actinidia chinensis* 'Hort 16A', ZESPRI® (gold kiwi fruit) are the most popular commercially available cultivars (Ferguson 2013). The common green kiwi fruit, *Actinidia deliciosa* cv. 'Hayward', has been used in several human trials to examine effects on biomarkers relevant to both cancer and CVD (Duttaroy and Jorgensen 2004; Chang and Liu 2009; Brevik et al. 2011). The common green kiwi fruit, *Actinidia deliciosa*, has been used in several human trials to examine effects on biomarkers relevant to CVD (Duttaroy and Jorgensen 2004; Chang and Liu 2009; Brevik et al. 2011). The bioactive compounds present in fruits and vegetables, although not yet well characterised, individually or in concert may protect the cardiovascular system by favourably modulating oxidative stress, plasma lipid levels, hypertension, platelet hyperactivity and other CVD risk factors (Dutta-Roy et al. 2001; Duttaroy and Jorgensen 2004). Hyperlipidaemia, hypertension and hyperactivity of blood platelets are the critical contributors to pathogenesis of CVD (Grundy et al. 2005). In fact, the presence of diverse activities such as antiplatelet and anti-angiotensin converting enzyme (ACE) was also demonstrated in aqueous extract of kiwi fruit and tomatoes (Dutta-Roy et al. 2001; Duttaroy and Jorgensen 2004; Jung et al. 2005; O'Kennedy et al. 2017a). This chapter will discuss the development of cardioprotective factors, and the clinical trials and efficacy of the antiplatelet factors isolated from tomatoes and kiwi fruit.

16.2 IDENTIFICATION AND ISOLATION OF CARDIOPROTECTIVE AGENTS FROM TOMATOES AND KIWI FRUIT: MECHANISMS OF ACTION

In a variety of studies, it was demonstrated that water soluble components of tomatoes and kiwi fruit are capable of inhibiting platelet aggregation both *in vitro* and *in vivo* (Dutta-Roy et al. 2001; Dutta-Roy 2002; O'Kennedy et al. 2006a–c; Grice et al. 2011; O'Kennedy et al. 2017a). The maximum inhibitory effect (70%–75%) was found to be with tomato and kiwi fruit extracts whereas, apple and pear had very little activity (2%–5%). Grapefruit, melon and strawberry had intermediate activity on platelet aggregation (33%–44%). The antiplatelet potential of the fruits tested appeared to have no relationship with their antioxidant activity (Dutta-Roy et al. 2001). The antiplatelet activity of several fruits showed that kiwi fruit and tomato extract had maximum antiplatelet activity and this activity was not related to the antioxidants potential of fruits (Dutta-Roy et al. 2001). Among all fruits tested for their *in vitro* antiplatelet activity, tomato and kiwi fruit had the highest activity followed by grapefruit, melon and strawberry, whereas pear and apple had little or no activity (Table 16.1). The antiplatelet compounds in tomatoes had a molecular mass less than 1000 Da, were highly water soluble and stable to boiling. These bioactive compounds were concentrated into an aqueous extract produced by homogenising the fruit and removing particulate matter. The aqueous extract was then further fractioned by gel filtration (Dutta-Roy et al. 2001; Dizdarevic et al. 2014). Further work has shown that the aqueous extract of both tomato and kiwi fruit consisted largely of soluble sugars (85%–90% of dry matter), which showed no *in vitro* antiplatelet activity (O'Kennedy et al. 2006a, 2017a). These water-soluble components were also found to inhibit angiotensin converting enzyme (ACE) (Dizdarevic et al. 2014; Biswas et al. 2014) and to

TABLE 16.1

Inhibition of Platelet Aggregation Expressed as the Decrease in the Area under the Curve Compared with Control

Fruit	% Inhibition of ADP-Induced Platelet Aggregation
Kiwi	89
Tomato	72
Grapefruit	44
Melon	42
Strawberry	33
Orange	18
Grape	16
Plum	16
Cranberry	9
Apple	5
Pear	2

Source: Dutta-Roy, A.K. et al., *Platelets*, 12, 218–227, 2017; Dizdarevic, L.L. et al., *Platelets*, 25, 567–575, 2014.

relax the vascular endothelium, the other important limbs of the cardiovascular system. A water-soluble tomato extract containing all the bioactive components was developed, and later given the trade name Fruitflow (O'Kennedy et al. 2017a). Fruitflow is now an established naturally derived functional food ingredient. Since its discovery in 1999, several mechanistic studies and human trials with Fruitflow have been carried out. Studies included localisation of the antiplatelet activity within the tomato fruit, its modes of action, its stability under various conditions and identification of the compounds with antiplatelet activity.

The non-sugar material that was isolated accounted for 4% of the aqueous tomato extract dry matter and showed strong inhibition of platelet aggregation *in vitro*. Isolation of many individual components from this sugar free fraction followed, and it was found that most fell into one of three categories – nucleosides, simple phenolic derivatives and flavonoid derivatives. All showed anti-platelet activities consistent with their compound categories. Proteomic experiments carried out to examine the effects of sugar-free tomato extract on platelet signalling pathways showed that these components altered a range of platelet functions. One of the most strongly affected proteins was the protein disulphide isomerase (PDI), an oxidoreductase that catalyses the formation and isomerisation of disulphide bonds. In platelets, blocking PDI with inhibitory antibodies inhibits a number of platelet activation pathways, including aggregation, secretion and fibrinogen binding (Manickam et al. 2008; Cho 2013). Other investigators (Jordan et al. 2005) have reported similar functional effects after blockage of cell-surface thiol isomerases. Glycosides related to quercetin, of which several are present in this tomato fraction, have been shown to interact with PDI in this way (Jasuja et al. 2012; Sheu et al. 2004). Interaction of polyphenols with PDI suggested a possible mechanism by which tomato extract components could inhibit different pathways of platelet aggregation. The sugar-free tomato extract and its sub-fractions prepared by semi-preparative reversed-phase HPLC as described by O'Kennedy et al. (2006a), were observed to prevent activation of integrin αIIbβ3 (i.e. GPIIb/IIIa). Inhibition of the GPIIb/IIIa activation step – which is common to multiple aggregation pathways – could underlie the wide-ranging effects of tomato extract (O'Kennedy et al. 2006a). This is consistent with the observation that basal platelet cyclic AMP concentrations (controlled by phospholipase C enzyme family-mediated cascade reactions) are unaltered by tomato extract active components *in vitro*. In addition, tomato extract reduced the expression of P-selectin (CD62P) on the platelet surface in response to ADP-induced platelet activation in whole blood (O'Kennedy et al. 2006a). In resting platelets, P-selectin is localised in the membranes of platelet α-granules. On platelet activation, it is redistributed to the platelet surface, where it initiates adhesion to leukocytes. Under conditions of blood flow and shear stress, this glycoprotein promotes platelet cohesion and stabilises newly formed aggregates. Thus, the tomato components can potentially affect the size and longevity of platelet aggregates. Tomato components were also found to affect the binding of tissue factor to activated platelets, at least in part due to effects on P-selectin. These results demonstrating the actions of tomato extract on different platelet functions were all consistent with potential effects mediated partly through polyphenols and PDI, and partly through nucleosides elevating cAMP and cGMP levels in platelets (Fuentes et al. 2012b; Dutta-Roy et al. 2001).

Initially, 100% kiwi fruit extract (KFE; w/v) was prepared to study its inhibitory effect on platelet aggregation (Duttaroy and Jorgensen 2004). The KFE extract inhibited both collagen- and ADP-induced platelet aggregation extent, whereas it had very little inhibitory effects on ARA-induced aggregation, indicating that the inhibition of platelet aggregation by kiwi fruit extract may not involve the thromboxane pathway. This is quite different than that of aspirin's mode of action in platelets. Aspirin's antiplatelet action involves inhibition of the COX-1 in platelets, leading to a decreased formation of PGG_2, a precursor of TxA_2.

The compounds responsible for the observed antiplatelet activity in KFE were isolated. These compounds in kiwi fruit are water soluble and heat stable, and their molecular mass is less than 1000 Da (Duttaroy and Jorgensen 2004). Delipidation followed by ultrafiltration of the KFE indicated that the active factors in KFE were water-soluble, heat-stable and with a molecular mass >1000 Da. KFE contained glucose (8.9 ± 0.4 mg/ml), fructose (9.9 ± 0.5 mg/ml) and sucrose (2.3 ± 0.2 mg/ml). Soluble sugars were removed using SPE column chromatography. Typically, 100 g of kiwi fruit produced 66.3 ± 5.8 mg of sugar-free KFE containing both antiplatelet and anti-ACE activities. An aqueous KFE contained compounds (Mw <1000 Da) that strongly inhibited both platelet aggregation and plasma ACE activity. The amount of total phenolic content in sugar free KFE was 1.2 ± 0.10 mg per 100 g of kiwi fruit. The polar compounds were eluted earlier than the nonpolar compounds under the experimental conditions. The molecular mechanisms of actions are not yet well known; however, the platelet inhibitory action of the extract may be mediated in part by reducing TxA_2 synthesis. The dose-dependent inhibition of ADP-induced platelet aggregation by sugar-free KFE was observed. ADP-induced aggregation was inhibited by 11% with 0.30 mg/ml, 71% inhibition with 0.90 mg/ml and 80% with 1.44 mg/ml of KFE. KFE also inhibited collagen-induced platelet aggregation; however, the level of inhibition was lower with 1.47 and 2.0 mg/ml incubations. The sugar fraction isolated from kiwi fruit was effective against all three platelet-aggregating agents – collagen, ADP and arachidonic acid. The IC_{50} for ADP-induced platelet aggregation was 1.52 ± 0.mg/ml KFE and for collagen–induced aggregation, the value was 1.83 ± 0.21 mg/ml. The presence of increasing amounts of KFE inhibited ADP-induced PF4 release in a dose-dependent manner. The inhibition of platelet aggregation by sugar-free KFE was concomitantly associated with inhibition of TxB_2 synthesis. KFE dose-dependently inhibited TxB_2 synthesis in the platelets. KFE at 1.68 mg/ml inhibited ADP- and collagen-induced TxB_2 synthesis by 91% and 81%. KFE at this concentration inhibited 54% and 45% platelet aggregation induced by ADP and collagen, respectively. Basal cAMP levels were not significantly different in the presence of the KFE as compared with control levels, and so cAMP may not be involved in the process. cAMP is a signalling molecule produced by the enzyme adenylyl cyclase in resting platelets to help maintain platelet quiescence (Kroll and Schafer 1989).

16.3 HUMAN TRIALS

After standardisation of the ingredients of Fruitflow, a unified set of studies was carried out to establish the efficacy of these ingredients *ex vivo*. Studies that established the onset time of an acute antiplatelet effect after oral ingestion of a dose of Fruitflow 1 have been published elsewhere (O'Kennedy et al. 2006a). These studies showed that in all subjects, an acute lowering of platelet aggregability to ADP and collagen was observed 3 hours after consuming Fruitflow. The range of onset times was from 1½ to 3 hours after consumption. In contrast, the normal diurnal increases in platelet aggregability were illustrated in subjects consuming the control supplement over the time course measured. The persistence of this acute effect varied between individuals, but in all cases platelet aggregability returned to baseline 18 hours after consumption of a single dose of Fruitflow. On average, these studies have shown an inhibition of the platelet response to ADP agonist of approximately 17%–25%, and an inhibition of the response to collagen of approximately 10%–18%. Platelet aggregation induced by arachidonic acid and thrombin receptor-activating peptide (TRAP) has also been shown to fall after Fruitflow administration. A study in which Fruitflow 1 was administered to 93 healthy men and women (O'Kennedy et al. 2006c) showed that some variability in response may occur, with men responding more than women, and subjects with higher risk factors for CVD responding more highly than others. A dose response was established in studies administering different amounts of Fruitflow 1. This dose-response work established that a dose of Fruitflow equivalent to 65 mg sugar-free tomato extract or approximately 3 average bowls of tinned tomato soup already caused close to the maximum level of platelet inhibition achievable by this extract, and that no significant gain would be obtained in an acute setting from increasing the dose. The antiplatelet effects observed in all matrices were similar to those seen in previous studies. Studies examining the effects of daily consumption of Fruitflow showed that the size of the antiplatelet effect observed after consuming a single dose of Fruitflow daily for 2 or for 4 weeks was not significantly different from the size of effect observed after a single dose – that is, the observed effects were not cumulative. Suppression of platelet function achieved through chronic consumption was continuous – measurements of platelet function were made in fasted subjects in the morning, approximately 24 hours after consumption of their last Fruitflow dose, and suppression of original baseline platelet function was observed after 2 and 4 weeks. Compounds found in Fruitflow have been shown to affect many aspects of platelet function, including thrombin generation. However in all intervention studies undertaken, clotting time measurements showed no significant increases from baseline levels. Fruitflow does not directly affect blood coagulation at any dose tested. Even without affecting blood coagulation directly, many antiplatelet drugs, taken on a chronic basis, give rise to excessive platelet inhibition, and are associated with internal bleeding. These potentially serious side effects mean that antiplatelet therapy, a fundamental aspect of CVD secondary prevention, is contraindicated for primary prevention as the benefit conferred (lowering risk of a first CVD event in relatively low-risk groups) is outweighed by the increased risk of gastric or intracranial bleeding (Sarbacker et al. 2016). This judgement was recently revisited by the US FDA, in the context of increasing levels of obesity and type 2 diabetes mellitus in relatively young populations, but was upheld (George and Copeland 2013). The known side effects of existing antiplatelet drugs related to internal bleeding were clearly pertinent for consideration during Fruitflow development. However, Fruitflow differs fundamentally from antiplatelet drugs in the reversibility of its action. The widely used antiplatelet drugs have irreversible mechanisms of action. Over the course of 10 days, approximately 90% of the circulating platelet population can be irreversibly affected for the lifetime of those platelets. This level of platelet inhibition is then maintained by daily drug treatment. Conversely, the antiplatelet effects of Fruitflow are neither irreversible nor cumulative and can be overcome by increased agonist concentrations. This very significant difference in mode of action renders Fruitflow suitable for use by the general population as a dietary functional ingredient, while antiplatelet drugs cannot be used. An intervention study comparing with aspirin was also carried out (O'Kennedy et al. 2017). The trial followed in 47 healthy subjects showed that the effects of a single dose of Fruitflow were similar – in terms of antiplatelet action, effects on thromboxane synthesis, and time to form a primary haemostatic clot (PFA-100 closure time) – to those of a single 75 mg dose of aspirin. When aspirin was taken daily for 7 days, the associated increase in PFA-100 closure time was three times higher than that associated with a single aspirin dose. The cumulative antiplatelet effect of aspirin when taken daily is well known, and reflects its irreversible disabling of platelet COX-1 and associated signalling. Fruitflow's effects are not cumulative in this way, as its effects do not irreversibly disable platelet signalling pathways. Thus, taking the results for the study population as a whole, daily aspirin supplementation may be viewed as approximately three times as efficacious as daily Fruitflow supplementation, due to the irreversibility of its action. This overall result seemed to echo the proteomic data, but further examination showed that it masked some interesting behaviour in study subgroups. The antiplatelet effects of aspirin in healthy subjects are extremely heterogeneous, with some subjects experiencing a very large increase in time to form a primary haemostatic clot, while others respond poorly (O'Kennedy et al. 2017). Approximately 50% of aspirin responders had a response to the drug that was lower than the average response for the treatment group, in terms of time to form a primary haemostatic clot. This group of subjects had a residually strong response to collagen after 7 days of aspirin treatment, and over one third of the group responded better to Fruitflow supplementation than to 7-day aspirin supplementation. At the other end of the spectrum, for 18% of the study population, taking aspirin for 7 days more than tripled the time to clot. This underlines the reasons behind the known internal bleeding risks associated with aspirin, and its unsuitability for use in primary prevention. While the response to Fruitflow, in terms of time to clot data, was also heterogeneous, it was markedly less so than the response to aspirin. The majority of the subject group experienced increases in time to form a primary haemostatic clot of up to two-fold, with fewer subjects at either extreme. It would appear that the proteomic predictions of stronger aspirin-led effects on platelet signalling may not be observed *ex vivo*, possibly due to wide variability in the extent of aspirin metabolism, but also possibly due to differences in the relative importance of platelet collagen signalling pathways between individuals. Fruitflow, with its wider range of antiplatelet compounds, may have a less variable metabolism and thus achieve its more moderate effects more widely. These more moderate effects, which can be related to the reversibility its antiplatelet action rather than its mode of action *per se*, render it a possible option for use in primary prevention of CVD, in contrast to aspirin at any dosage (O'Kennedy et al. 2017).

Several human intervention trials have been carried out to investigate the *ex vivo* effects of platelet aggregation using kiwi fruit (Duttaroy and Jorgensen 2004; Karlsen et al. 2013). In one human trial, 30 healthy volunteers aged 20–51 years were included (Duttaroy and Jorgensen 2004). Exclusion criteria were the presence of overt vascular, haematological or respiratory disease; hypertension; infection; and frequent consumption of drugs that affect platelet function (e.g., aspirin, paracetamol, ibuprofen, steroids or habitual consumption of n-3 fatty acid supplements). Subjects were allocated randomly to two groups ($n = 15$), each of which was given green kiwi fruit doses in different orders. One group took two kiwi fruit per day in the first period and three kiwi fruit per day in the second period, whereas the second group took three and two kiwi fruit. Each volunteer consumed two and three kiwi fruit per day for successive 28 day periods separated by at least 2 weeks washout periods. During the supplementation period, no statistically significant change in their mean BMI was observed. The kiwi fruit was well tolerated, without any adverse effect. Plasma vitamin C levels in these volunteers increased significantly. Platelet aggregation response to different concentrations of ADP and collagen were tested at day 0 and at 28 days after consuming two or three kiwi fruit per day. Platelet response to both low and high concentrations of ADP or collagen was inhibited by kiwi fruit consumption. Consuming two kiwi fruits daily inhibited platelet aggregation induced by ADP significantly (18% in case of 4 μM ADP and 15% in case of 8 μM ADP) compared with those at day 0 ($p < 0.05$). A similar reduction in platelet aggregation was observed in response to collagen when volunteers consumed two or three kiwi fruit per day for 28 days. Mean total plasma levels of cholesterol, LDL and HDL were unchanged from days 0 to 28 in both groups, whereas triglyceride concentrations were significantly lowered on day 28. After the washout period (minimum 2 weeks), plasma triglyceride concentrations returned to the baseline level (Duttaroy and Jorgensen 2004).

In another human intervention trial, it was demonstrated that consuming one gold kiwi fruit per day for 4 weeks reduced whole-blood platelet aggregation in healthy volunteers. Consumption of gold kiwi fruit reduced plasma triglyceride levels without affecting cholesterol levels: original levels were restored after the washout period. Lowering of plasma triglycerides by kiwi fruit was observed despite the fact that the volunteers maintained their regular diet during the supplementation period.

In a randomised, controlled trial in male smokers aged 44–74 years, the effects of green kiwi fruit and an antioxidant-rich diet on CVD risk factors (such as blood pressure, plasma lipids and whole-blood platelet aggregation) were compared with a control group after 8 weeks (Karlsen et al. 2013). The kiwi fruit group received three green kiwi fruit per day, whereas the antioxidant-rich diet group received a comprehensive combination of antioxidant-rich foods. In the kiwi fruit group, reductions of 10 mmHg in systolic blood pressure and 9 mmHg in diastolic blood pressure were observed. In the antioxidant-rich diet group, a reduction of 10 mmHg in systolic blood pressure was observed among hypertensives. Additionally, a 15% reduction in whole-blood aggregation and an 11% reduction in angiotensin-converting enzyme activity were observed in the kiwi fruit group. No effects on these parameters were observed in the antioxidant-rich diet group. This study suggests that intake of kiwi fruit may have beneficial effects on blood pressure and platelet aggregation in male smokers.

The presence of these diverse activities such as antiplatelet and anti-ACE was also demonstrated in differently processed extracts of kiwi fruit (Duttaroy and Jorgensen 2004; Jung et al. 2005). In conclusion, consuming kiwi fruit is an effective way of inhibiting platelet aggregation induced by collagen and ADP in human volunteers. Our data thus provide evidence that consuming kiwi fruit has the potential to increase the effectiveness of thrombosis prophylaxis. Modulation of platelet reactivity towards collagen, ADP and plasma triglyceride levels by kiwi fruit could be potentially prophylactic for CVD. Platelets are involved in atherosclerosis disease development, and the reduction of platelet activity by medications reduces the incidence and severity of disease. Consumption of kiwi fruit lowered the platelet aggregation response in human volunteers (Duttaroy and Jorgensen 2004). Consuming two or three kiwi fruit reduced platelet aggregation to a similar extent. There were no correlations between individual changes in plasma vitamin C and platelet aggregation response and plasma lipids values. The inhibitory effects on platelet aggregation response and the lowering effects on plasma triglyceride of kiwi fruit disappeared during the washout period. This indicates that the effects of kiwi fruit on platelets and plasma lipids are reversible.

16.4   CLINICAL AND SAFETY ISSUES OF THESE FRUIT EXTRACTS

Consumption of fruit or fruit extracts is responsible for several health-promoting properties. Both tomatoes and kiwi fruit are widely consumed worldwide. Both tomato and kiwi fruit extracts have shown outstanding preclinical antiplatelet effects through various mechanisms (Dizdarevic et al. 2014; O'Kennedy et al. 2017a; Uddin et al. 2017). These extracts could provide an ideal approach as templates for new, clinically effective and safe antiplatelet agents due to their inherent safety and efficiency. As far as the safety of tomatoes is concerned, they are generally recognised as safe, owing to the long history of use and consumption of these fruits as extracts, soups and other formats. Comprehensive and independent data on the nutritional composition of kiwi fruit can be found in the USDA National Nutrient Database for Standard Reference (Richardson et al. 2018). A study published in 2007 in the journal *Food Chemistry and Toxicology* showed that a daily intake of 68 mg of total flavonoids present in the fruits is not correlated to the lung, breast or gastrointestinal cancer onset. However, safety studies of each and every component are a basic requirement as part of the discovery process for new potential drugs from natural sources. The potential toxicity of flavonoids depends on their type, dose, bioavailability and vulnerability of subject, which occurs especially among elderly subjects. However, the flavonoid content in these fruit extracts is too low to cause any health problems.

In 2006, the European Union (EU) adopted a regulation on the use of nutrition and health claims for foods, which set down harmonised EU-wide rules for the use of health or nutritional claims on foodstuffs (Regulation [EC] No 1924/2006). One of the key objectives of this regulation is to ensure that any claim made on a food label in the EU is clear and substantiated by scientific evidence. The first Article 13 claim based on newly developed evidence or proprietary data (a special category under Article 13[5]) to be achieved, in December 2009, was for Fruitflow, when the EU Commission authorised the health claim 'water-soluble tomato concentrate (WSTC) I and II helps maintain normal platelet aggregation, which contributes to healthy blood flow'. The authorised claim was based on the eight human studies (seven proprietary), and seven non-human studies (three proprietary), conducted with Fruitflow. Thus, Fruitflow is now authorised by EFSA for daily consumption. As the amount of Fruitflow in any one food product serving is low, equivalent to approximately three bowls of tinned tomato soup, and as dose-response studies had shown that increasing the dose significantly would not result in a much bigger acute effect on platelets, no significant dangers were anticipated. The known side effects of existing antiplatelet drugs related to internal bleeding were clearly pertinent for consideration during Fruitflow development. However, Fruitflow differs fundamentally from antiplatelet drugs in the reversibility of its action. The widely used antiplatelet drugs have irreversible mechanisms of action. Over the course of 10 days, approximately 90% of the circulating platelet population can be irreversibly affected for the lifetime of those platelets. This level of platelet inhibition is then maintained by daily drug treatment. Conversely, the antiplatelet effects of Fruitflow are neither irreversible nor cumulative and can be overcome by increased agonist concentrations. This very significant difference in mode of action renders Fruitflow suitable for use by the general population, unlike standard antiplatelet drugs. Three kiwi fruit consumed per day had no negative effects in humans (Karlsen et al. 2011).

16.5 CONCLUSIONS

Antiplatelet agents are emerging as some of the newest agents that seem to have cardioprotective capabilities by modulating platelet function, blood flow and vascular integrity. Hyperactive platelets interact with vessel walls by shedding macroparticles, secreting several adhesive growth factors, and inflammatory agents interrupt the blood flow and produce a pro-thrombotic state in people with obesity, diabetes, a sedentary life style or hypertension and in people who smoke. It has long been known that disturbances in blood flow, changes in platelet reactivity and enhanced coagulation reactions facilitate pathological thrombus formation, and the maintenance of normal platelet activity is critical to overall haemostasis. Fruitflow – developed from tomato and KFE containing bioavailable cardioprotective compounds – can be of benefit to people who are vulnerable to develop CVD. An array of extensive basic, mechanistic, compositional and several human trials are testimony to its cardioprotective benefits. Through modulation of platelet reactivity towards collagen, ADP could be of potentially prophylactic and therapeutic benefit in preventing and halting pathologic processes that lead to CVD. The active components were found to be primarily associated with, or extractable from, the juice and the flesh surrounding the pips of these fruits. The bioactive compounds are not only polyphenols but could be of diverse nature, as adenosine was shown to be an important antiplatelet compound in tomato extract (Dutta-Roy et al. 2001; Duttaroy and Jorgensen 2004; Fuentes et al. 2012a,b). Platelet-endothelial interactions promote expression of adhesion molecules on the endothelium and the recruitment of inflammatory cells, and stimulate the activation of circulating platelets. Platelets are involved in the atherosclerosis process and therefore reduction of platelet activity decreases the incidence of CVD in diabetes, smokers and in metabolic syndromes (Dutta-Roy 2002; Ferroni et al. 2007, 2008). It is now recognised that 20%–30% of persons experience the so-called aspirin-resistance syndrome, in which the expected antiplatelet effects are not observed (Hankey and Eikelboom 2006). This finding indicates an advantage of broad antiplatelet activity profile over single-target drugs such as aspirin. The greater benefits of combined antiplatelet therapies that target more than one mode of platelet aggregation, as compared with single-drug therapeutic strategies, have been shown both *in vitro* and *ex vivo*. The scientific evidence for the health benefits of these fruit extracts needs to be expanded through well-designed and executed human intervention studies that clearly define the study populations and the specific beneficial physiological effects. A greater understanding of the mechanisms of action of these extracts and their bioactive constituents in promoting health in different populations also needs to be fully elucidated.

REFERENCES

Agarwal, S., and Rao, A. V. (2000). Tomato lycopene and its role in human health and chronic diseases. *Canadian Medical Association Journal*, **163**(6), 739–744.

Biswas, D., Uddin, M. M., Dizdarevic, L. L., Jorgensen, A. and Duttaroy, A. K. (2014). Inhibition of angiotensin-converting enzyme by aqueous extract of tomato. *European Journal of Nutrition*, **53**(8), 1699–1706. doi:10.1007/s00394-014-0676-1.

Brevik, A., Gaivao, I., Medin, T., Jorgenesen, A., Piasek, A., Elilasson, J., Karlsen, A., et al. (2011). Supplementation of a western diet with golden kiwifruits (*Actinidia chinensis* var. 'Hort 16A'): Effects on biomarkers of oxidation damage and antioxidant protection. *Nutrition Journal*, **10**, 54. doi:10.1186/1475-2891-10-54.

Bucki, R., Pastore, J. J., Giraud, F., Sulpice, J. C. and Janmey, P. A. (2003). Flavonoid inhibition of platelet procoagulant activity and phosphoinositide synthesis. *Journal of Thrombosis and Haemostasis*, **1**(8), 1820–1828.

Cai, G., Zhou, W., Lu, Y., Chen, P., Lu, Z. and Fu, Y. (2016). Aspirin resistance and other aspirin-related concerns. *Neurological Sciences*, **37**(2), 181–189. doi:10.1007/s10072-015-2412-x.

Canene-Adams, K., Campbell, J. K., Zaripheh, S., Jeffery, E. H. and Erdman, J. W. Jr. (2005). The tomato as a functional food. *Journal of Nutrition*, **135**(5), 1226–1230.

Chang, W. H. and Liu, J. F. (2009). Effects of kiwifruit consumption on serum lipid profiles and antioxidative status in hyperlipidemic subjects. *International Journal of Food Sciences and Nutrition*, **60**(8), 709–716. doi:10.3109/09637480802063517.

Cho, J. (2013). Protein disulfide isomerase in thrombosis and vascular inflammation. *Journal of Thrombosis and Haemostasis*, **11**(12), 2084–2091. doi:10.1111/jth.12413.

Davi, G. and Patrono, C. (2007). Platelet activation and atherothrombosis. *New England Journal of Medicine*, **357**(24), 2482–2494. doi:10.1056/NEJMra071014.

Dizdarevic, L. L., Biswas, D., Uddin, M. D., Jorgenesen, A., Falch, E., Bastani, N. E. and Duttaroy, A. K. (2014). Inhibitory effects of kiwifruit extract on human platelet aggregation and plasma angiotensin-converting enzyme activity. *Platelets*, **25**(8), 567–575. doi:10.3109/09537104.2013.852658.

Dutta-Roy, A. K. (1994). Insulin mediated processes in platelets, erythrocytes and monocytes/macrophages: Effects of essential fatty acid metabolism. *Prostaglandins, Leukotrienes and Essential Fatty Acids*, **51**(6), 385–399.

Dutta-Roy, A. K. (2002). Dietary components and human platelet activity. *Platelets*, **13**(2), 67–75. doi:10.1080/09537100120111540.

Duttaroy, A. K. and Jorgensen, A. (2004). Effects of kiwi fruit consumption on platelet aggregation and plasma lipids in healthy human volunteers. *Platelets*, **15**(5), 287–292. doi:10.1080/09537100410001710290.

Dutta-Roy, A. K., Crosbie, L. and Gordon, M. J. (2001). Effects of tomato extract on human platelet aggregation *in vitro*. *Platelets*, **12**(4), 218–227. doi:10.1080/09537100120058757.

Ferguson, A. R. (2013). Kiwifruit: The wild and the cultivated plants. *Advances in Food and Nutrition Research*, **68**, 15–32. doi:10.1016/B978-0-12-394294-4.00002-X.

Fernandes, I., Perez-Gregorio, R., Soares, S., Mateus, N. and de Freitas, V. (2017). Wine flavonoids in health and disease prevention. *Molecules*, **22**(2), 292. doi:10.3390/molecules22020292.

Ferroni, P., Martini, F., D'Alessandro, R., Magnapera, A., Raparelli, V., Scarno, A., Davi, G., Basili, S. and Guadagni, F. (2008). *In vivo* platelet activation is responsible for enhanced vascular endothelial growth factor levels in hypertensive patients. *Clinica Chimica Acta*, **388**(1–2), 33–37. doi:10.1016/j.cca.2007.09.026.

Ferroni, P., Santilli, F., Guadagni, F., Basili, S. and Davi, G. (2007). Contribution of platelet-derived CD40 ligand to inflammation, thrombosis and neoangiogenesis. *Current Medicinal Chemistry*, **14**(20), 2170–2180.

Ferroni, P., Basili, S., Falco, A. and Davi, G. (2004). Platelet activation in type 2 diabetes mellitus. *Journal of Thrombosis and Haemostasis*, **2**(8), 1282–1291. doi:10.1111/j.1538-7836.2004.00836.x.

Fiorentino, A., D'Abrosca, B., Pacifico, S., Mastellone, C., Scognamiglio, M. and Monaco, P. (2009). Identification and assessment of antioxidant capacity of phytochemicals from kiwi fruits. *Journal of Agricultural and Food Chemistry*, **57**(10), 4148–4155. doi:10.1021/jf900210z.

Fuentes, E. J., Astudillo, L. A., Gutierrez, M. I., Contreras, S. O., Bustamante, L. O., Rubio, P. I., Moore-Carrasco, R. et al. (2012a). Fractions of aqueous and methanolic extracts from tomato (*Solanum lycopersicum* L.) present platelet antiaggregant activity. *Blood Coagulation & Fibrinolysis*, **23**(2), 109–117. doi:10.1097/MBC.0b013e32834d78dd.

Fuentes, E., Castro, R., Astudillo, L., Carrasco, G., Alarcon, M., Gutierrez, M. and Palomo, I. (2012b). Bioassay-guided isolation and HPLC determination of bioactive compound that relate to the antiplatelet activity (Adhesion, Secretion, and Aggregation) from Solanum lycopersicum. *Evidence-Based Complementary and Alternative Medicine*, **2012**, 147031. doi:10.1155/2012/147031.

Garcia-Alonso, F. J., Jorge-Vidal, V., Ros, G. and Periago, M. J. (2012). Effect of consumption of tomato juice enriched with n-3 polyunsaturated fatty acids on the lipid profile, antioxidant biomarker status, and cardiovascular disease risk in healthy women. *European Journal of Nutrition*, **51**(4), 415–424. doi:10.1007/s00394-011-0225-0.

George, M. M. and Copeland, K. C. (2013). Current treatment options for type 2 diabetes mellitus in youth: Today's realities and lessons from the TODAY study. *Current Diabetes Reports*, **13**(1), 72–80. doi:10.1007/s11892-012-0334-z.

Giovannucci, E. (1999a). Tomatoes, tomato-based products, lycopene, and prostate cancer: Review of the epidemiologic literature. *Journal of the National Cancer Institute*, **91**(15), 1331A–1331.

Giovannucci, E. (1999b). Tomatoes, tomato-based products, lycopene, and cancer: Review of the epidemiologic literature. *Journal of the National Cancer Institute*, **91**(4), 317–331.

Grice, I. D., Rogers, K. L. and Griffiths, L. R. (2011). Isolation of bioactive compounds that relate to the anti-platelet activity of cymbopogon ambiguus. *Evidence-Based Complementary and Alternative Medicine*, **2011**, 467134. doi:10.1093/ecam/nep213.

Grundy, S. M., Cleeman, J. I., Daniels, S. R., Donato, K. A., Eckel, R. H., Franklin, B. A., Gordon, D. J., et al. (2005). Diagnosis and management of the metabolic syndrome: An American Heart Association/National Heart, Lung, and Blood Institute Scientific Statement. *Circulation*, **112**(17), 2735–2752. doi:10.1161/CIRCULATIONAHA.105.169404.

Guerrero, J. A., L. Navarro-Nunez, M. L. Lozano, C. Martinez, V. Vicente, J. M. Gibbins, and J. Rivera. (2007). Flavonoids inhibit the platelet TxA(2) signalling pathway and antagonize TxA(2) receptors (TP) in platelets and smooth muscle cells. *British Journal of Clinical Pharmacology*, **64**(2), 133–144. doi:10.1111/j.1365-2125.2007.02881.x.

Hankey, G. J. and Eikelboom, J. W. (2006). Aspirin resistance. *Lancet*, **367**(9510), 606–617. doi:10.1016/S0140-6736(06)68040-9.

Hennekens, C. H. and Dalen, J. E. (2014). Aspirin in the primary prevention of cardiovascular disease: Current knowledge and future research needs. *Trends in Cardiovascular Medicine*, **24**(8), 360–366. doi:10.1016/j.tcm.2014.08.006.

Huang, Y., Yang, Z., Ye, Z., Li, Q., Wen, J., Tao, X., Chen, L., et al. (2012). Lipocalin-2, glucose metabolism and chronic low-grade systemic inflammation in Chinese people. *Cardiovascular Diabetology*, **11**, 11. doi:10.1186/1475-2840-11-11.

Hubbard, G. P., Stevens, J. M., Cicmil, M., Sage, T., Jordan, P. A., Williams, C. M., Lovegrove, J. A. and Gibbins, J. M. (2003). Quercetin inhibits collagen-stimulated platelet activation through inhibition of multiple components of the glycoprotein VI signaling pathway. *Journal of Thrombosis and Haemostasis*, **1**(5), 1079–1088.

Jacques, P. F., Lyass, A., Massaro, J. M., Vasan, R. S. and D'Agostino, R. B. Sr. (2013). Relationship of lycopene intake and consumption of tomato products to incident CVD. *British Journal of Nutrition*, **110**(3), 545–551. doi:10.1017/S0007114512005417.

Jasuja, R., Passam, F. H., Kennedy, D. R., Kim, S. H., van Hessem, L., Lin, L., Bowley, S. R., et al. (2012). Protein disulfide isomerase inhibitors constitute a new class of antithrombotic agents. *Journal of Clinical Investigations*, **122**(6), 2104–2113. doi:10.1172/JCI61228.

Jordan, P. A., Stevens, J. M., Hubbard, G. P., Barrett, N. E., Sage, T., Authi, K. S. and Gibbins, J. M. (2005). A role for the thiol isomerase protein ERP5 in platelet function. *Blood*, **105**(4), 1500–1507. doi:10.1182/blood-2004-02-0608.

Jung, K. A., Song, T. C., Han, D., Kim, I. H., Kim, Y. E. and Lee, C. H. (2005). Cardiovascular protective properties of kiwifruit extracts *in vitro*. *Biological and Pharmaceutical Bulletin*, **28**(9), 1782–1785.

Kaplan, Z. S. and Jackson, S. P. (2011). The role of platelets in atherothrombosis. *Hematology*, **2011**, 51–61. doi:10.1182/asheducation-2011.1.51.

Karlsen, A., Svendsen, M., Seljeflot, I., Sommernes, M. A., Sexton, J., Brevik, A., Erlund, I., et al. (2011). Compliance, tolerability and safety of two antioxidant-rich diets: A randomised controlled trial in male smokers. *British Journal of Nutrition*, **106**(4), 557–571. doi:10.1017/S0007114511000353.

Karlsen, A., Svendsen, M., Seljeflot, I., Laake, P., Duttaroy, A. K., Drevon, C. A., Arnesen, H., Tonstad, S. and Blomhoff, R. (2013). Kiwifruit decreases blood pressure and whole-blood platelet aggregation in male smokers. *Journal of Human Hypertension*, **27**(2), 126–130. doi:10.1038/jhh.2011.116.

Kroll, M. H. and Schafer, A. I. (1989). Biochemical mechanisms of platelet activation. *Blood*, **74**(4), 1181–1195.

Manickam, N., Sun, X., Li, M., Gazitt, Y. and Essex, D. W. (2008). Protein disulphide isomerase in platelet function. *British Journal of Haematology*, **140**(2), 223–229. doi:10.1111/j.1365-2141.2007.06898.x.

Massberg, S., Brand, K., Gruner, S., Page, S., Muller, E., Muller, I., Bergmeier, W., et al. (2002). A critical role of platelet adhesion in the initiation of atherosclerotic lesion formation. *Journal of Experimental Medicine*, **196**(7), 887–896.

Muller, I., Massberg, S., Zierhut, W., Binz, C., Schuster, A., Rudiger-von Hoch, S., Braun, S. and Gawaz, M. (2002). Effects of aspirin and clopidogrel versus oral anticoagulation on platelet function and on coagulation in patients with nonvalvular atrial fibrillation (CLAFIB). *Pathophysiology of Haemostasis and Thrombosis*, **32**(1), 16–24.

Natarajan, A., Zaman, A. G. and Marshall, S. M. (2008). Platelet hyperactivity in type 2 diabetes: Role of antiplatelet agents. *Diabetes and Vascular Disease Research*, **5**(2), 138–144. doi:10.3132/dvdr.2008.023.

Nieswandt, B., Aktas, B., Moers, A. and Sachs, U. J. (2005). Platelets in atherothrombosis: Lessons from mouse models. *Journal of Thrombosis and Haemostasis*, **3**(8), 1725–1736. doi:10.1111/j.1538-7836.2005.01488.x.

O'Kennedy, N., Crosbie, L., Song, H. J., Zhang, X., Horgan, G. and Duttaroy, A. K. (2017a). A randomised controlled trial comparing a dietary antiplatelet, the water-soluble tomato extract Fruitflow, with 75 mg aspirin in healthy subjects. *European Journal of Clinical Nutrition*, **71**(6), 723–730. doi:10.1038/ejcn.2016.222.

O'Kennedy, N., Crosbie, L., van Lieshout, M., Broom, J. I., Webb, D. J. and Duttaroy, A. K. (2006a). Effects of antiplatelet components of tomato extract on platelet function *in vitro* and *ex vivo*: A time-course cannulation study in healthy humans. *American Journal of Clinical Nutrition*, **84**(3), 570–579.

O'Kennedy, N., Crosbie, L.Song, V., Broom, J. I., Webb, D. J. and Duttaroy, A. K. (2006b). Potential for use of lycopene-free tomato extracts as dietary antiplatelet agents. *Atherosclerosis*, **188**(1), S9–S9.

O'Kennedy, N., Crosbie, L., Whelan, S., Luther, V., Horgan, G., Broom, J. I., Webb, D. J. and Duttaroy, A. K. (2006c). Effects of tomato extract on platelet function: A double-blinded crossover study in healthy humans. *American Journal of Clinical Nutrition*, **84**(3), 561–569.

O'Kennedy, N., Raederstorff, D. and Duttaroy, A. K. (2017b). Fruitflow(R): The first European food safety authority-approved natural cardio-protective functional ingredient. *European Journal of Nutrition*, **56**, 461–482. doi:10.1007/s00394-016-1265-2.

Obarzanek, E., Sacks, F. M., Vollmer, W. M., Bray, G. A., Miller, 3rd, E. R., Lin, P. H., Karanja, N. M., et al. (2001). Effects on blood lipids of a blood pressure-lowering diet: The dietary approaches to stop hypertension (DASH) trial. *American Journal of Clinical Nutrition*, **74**(1), 80–89.

Pamukcu, B., Lip, G. Y., Snezhitskiy, V. and Shantsila, E. (2011). The CD40-CD40L system in cardiovascular disease. *Annals of Medicine*, **43**(5), 331–340. doi:10.3109/07853890.2010.546362.

Pearson, D. A., Holt, R. R., Rein, D., Paglieroni, T., Schmitz, H. H. and Keen, C. L. (2005). Flavanols and platelet reactivity. *Clinical and Developmental Immunology*, **12**(1), 1–9.

Pignatelli, P., Pulcinelli, F. M., Celestini, A., Lenti, L., Ghiselli, A., Gazzaniga, P. P. and Violi, F. (2000). The flavonoids quercetin and catechin synergistically inhibit platelet function by antagonizing the intracellular production of hydrogen peroxide. *American Journal of Clinical Nutrition*, **72**(5), 1150–1155.

Richardson, D. P., Ansell, J. and Drummond, L. N. (2018). The nutritional and health attributes of kiwifruit: A review. *European Journal of Nutrition*, **57**(8), 2659–2676. doi:10.1007/s00394-018-1627-z.

Sarbacker, G. B., Lusk, K. A., Flieller, L. A. and Van Liew, J. R. (2016). Aspirin use for the primary prevention of cardiovascular disease in the elderly. *Consultant Pharmacist*, **31**(1), 24–32. doi:10.4140/TCP.n.2016.24.

Sheu, J. R., Hsiao, G., Chou, P. H., Shen, M. Y. and Chou, D. S. (2004). Mechanisms involved in the antiplatelet activity of rutin, a glycoside of the flavonol quercetin, in human platelets. *Journal of Agricultural and Food Chemistry*, **52**(14), 4414–4418. doi:10.1021/jf040059f.

Shimodaira, M., Niwa, T., Nakajima, K., Kobayashi, M., Hanyu, N. and Nakayama, T. (2013). Correlation between mean platelet volume and fasting plasma glucose levels in prediabetic and normoglycemic individuals. *Cardiovascular Diabetology*, **12**, 14. doi:10.1186/1475-2840-12-14.

Uddin, M., D. Biswas, Ghosh, A., O'Kennedy, N. and Duttaroy, A. K. (2017). Consumption of Fruitflow((R)) lowers blood pressure in pre-hypertensive males: A randomised, placebo controlled, double blind, cross-over study. *International Journal of Food Sciences and Nutrition*, **69**(4), 494–502. doi:10.1080/09637486.2017.1376621.

Weisburger, J. H. (2002). Lycopene and tomato products in health promotion. *Experimental Biology and Medicine*, **227**(10), 924–927.

Willcox, J. K., Catignani, G. L. and Lazarus, S. (2003). Tomatoes and cardiovascular health. *Critical Reviews in Food Science and Nutrition*, **43**(1), 1–18. doi:10.1080/10408690390826437.

17 Herbal Products in Antihypertensive Therapy
Potentialities and Challenges – A Brazilian Perspective

Fernão C. Braga and Steyner F. Côrtes

CONTENTS

17.1 INTRODUCTION

Cardiovascular diseases (CVDs) are the leading cause of premature death worldwide and a major public health problem due to the high morbimortality rates and cost of treatment (WHO 2013). Systemic arterial hypertension (SAH) is the main risk factor for the development of CVD, with over 1 billion cases diagnosed in 2008 and the annual death toll estimated to reach 23.5 million people by 2030 (WHO 2013). The therapeutic approach for SAH management takes into account the risk factors associated with the patient and the effects on the cardiovascular system (Mancia et al. 2007). It is estimated that high blood pressure is managed in only 34% of hypertensive patients (Wang and Xiong 2012). The low adherence to treatment results from high costs of antihypertensive drugs and undesired side effects, as well as to failure in restoring the blood pressure and to difficulties in defining the appropriate drugs and/or doses, demanding the search for alternative antihypertensive agents (Wagner 2011).

Herbal medicine is currently used worldwide to treat several conditions, hypertension included, and its use has increased substantially in the last decade both in developed and developing nations (WHO 2008; Frishman et al. 2009). Secondary metabolites of different classes, found in various medicinal plants and spices, have been demonstrated to possess antihypertensive properties.

17.2 HERBAL PRODUCTS CURRENTLY USED IN ANTIHYPERTENSIVE THERAPY

Herein we present some examples of plants species largely used for their alleged antihypertensive properties, for which scientific evidence seems to support their benefits in hypertension therapy, although there are some contradictory results. This section does not intend to make an exhaustive review of antihypertensive plants used globally, but to pick some examples of well-studied active plants and, in counterpart, to demonstrate the potential of the underexplored Brazilian plant species, reported in Section 4 of this chapter. Several reviews recently published cover globally used antihypertensive plants, such as *Astragalus membranaceus* (astragalus), *Allium sativum* (garlic), *Camellia sinensis* (green tea), *Crataegus* spp. (hawthorn), *Gingko biloba* (gingko), *Glycine max* (soy), *Hibiscus sabdariffa* (roselle), *Panax ginseng* (Asian ginseng), *Salvia miltiorrhiza* (Chinese sage) and *Vitis vinifera* (grapes, particularly the seeds), among others, showing their active compounds, preclinical and clinical data. For further reading, see the revisions of Li et al. (2015), Al Disi et al. (2016), Anwar et al. (2016), Rastogi et al. (2016) and Liperoti et al. (2017).

Interestingly, several of the above mentioned species contain the same classes of bioactive compounds such as flavones, triterpenic acids and phenol carboxylic acids, which have shown positive effects on CVD (Li et al. 2015). For those readers interested in the chemical structures of natural compounds with antihypertensive activity, including alkaloids, coumarins, diterpenes, flavonoids and peptides, along with their mechanisms of action, the review published by Bai et al. (2015) is a good source of information.

17.2.1 CRATAEGUS SPP. (HAWTHORN)

The genus *Crataegus* (Rosaceae) comprises almost 300 species of trees and shrubs. Preparations from the leaves and flowers of some *Crataegus* species (hawthorn) have been used for treating CVD since the late 1800s (Hobbs and Foster 1990). Over 20 species of *Crataegus* are used as medicinal plants worldwide, and based on their efficacy and safety the species *Crataegus oxyacantha* L. and *Crataegus monogyna* Jacq. are listed in the pharmacopoeias of France (1998), England (2000), Germany (DAB, 1997) and Switzerland (1997), as well as in the European Pharmacopoeia (1998; Rastogi et al. 2016).

C. oxyacantha, popularly known as hawthorn, haw, maybush, or whitehorn, is traditionally used to treat CVD in addition to a plethora of conditions like diarrhoea, gallbladder, insomnia, asthma, digestive problems and hyperlipidaemia, among others (Wang et al. 2013). Hawthorn-derived products include tinctures, tablets, teas and extracts (hydroethanolic, hydromethanolic, or aqueous) prepared with the berries or leaves and flowers from the species (Wang et al. 2013).

The chemistry of *C. oxyacantha* has been thoroughly investigated, and the bioactive constituents identified so far include flavonoids, triterpenic acids and phenol carboxylic acids (Chang and Zuo 2002; Verma et al. 2007; Edwards et al. 2012; Wang et al. 2013; Rastogi et al. 2016). Flavonoids like vitexin, hyperoside, rutin and vitexin-2″-O-α-L-rhamnoside together with oligomeric procyanidins from catechin/epicatechin are considered the most important cardioactive constituents (Figure 17.1). Other constituents like triterpenic acids (ursolic, oleanolic and crataegolic acids) and phenol carboxylic acids (chlorogenic and caffeic acids and various amines) have been also identified.

The hawthorn dry extracts coded WS 1442 (45% ethanol extract from leaves with flowers) and LI 132 (70% methanol extract from leaves, flowers and berries) are currently the most studied, and their efficacy and safety have been extensively evaluated (Koch and Malek 2011; Wang et al. 2013). The first one is standardised to contain 18.75% of oligomeric procyanidins and the second one 2.2% of flavonoids (European Scientific Cooperative on Phytotherapy 1999; WHO 2002).

Hawthorn is considered an alternative therapy to treat several CVD, such as angina, hypertension, hyperlipidaemia, arrhythmia, and New York Heart Association (NYHA) functional class II congestive heart failure (Chang et al. 2005).

There is a large volume of preclinical pharmacological data published for hawthorn, demonstrating its antioxidant and anti-inflammatory activities, positive inotropic effect, antiarrhythmic

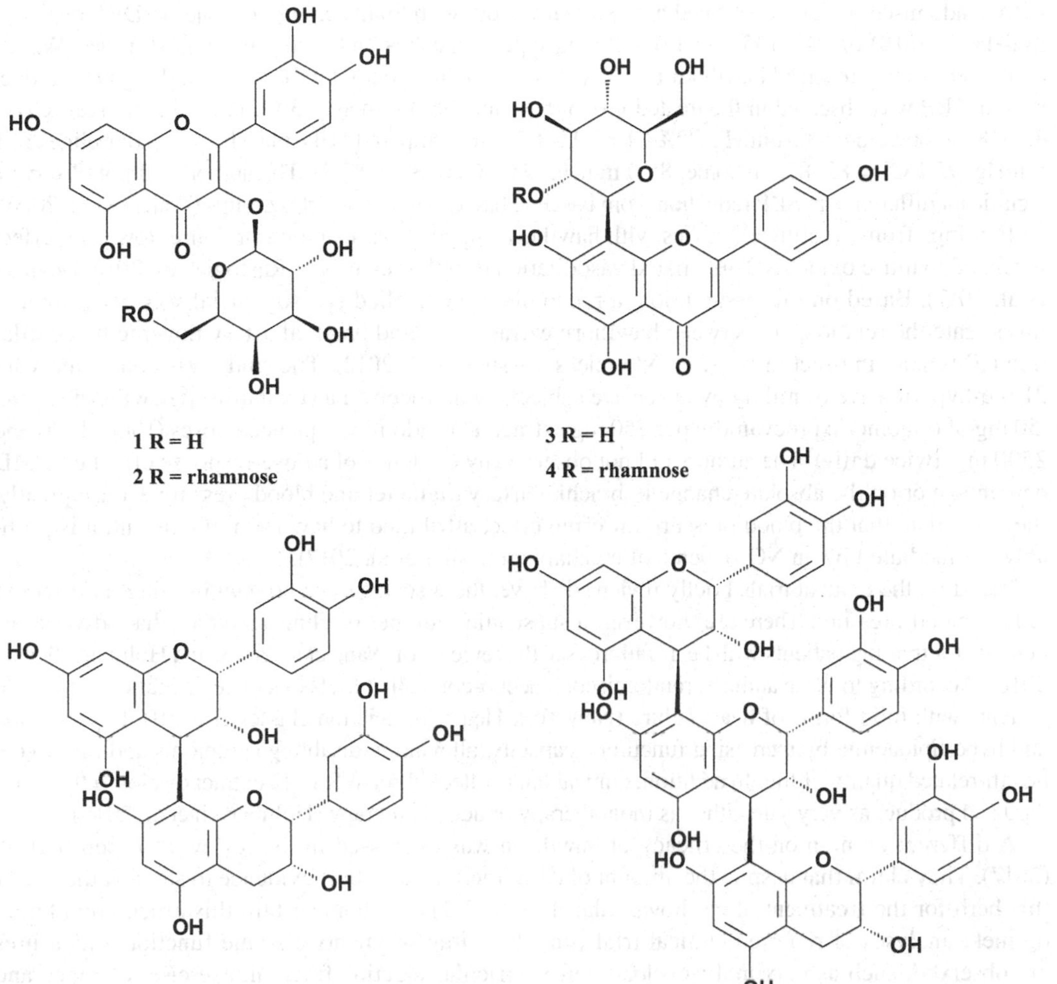

FIGURE 17.1 Chemical structures of *Crataegus* constituents. (1) Hyperoside, (2) rutin, (3) vitexin, (4) vitexin-2″-*O*-α-L-rhamnoside, (5) procyanidin B1, (6) procyanidin C1.

effects, anti-cardiac remodelling effect, endothelial protective effect, antiplatelet aggregation effect, vasodilating activity in coronary and peripheral vessels, anti-atherosclerotic effect, inhibition of cholesterol synthesis in the liver and lipid absorption in the intestine, protective effect against ischemia/reperfusion injury, and decrease of arterial blood pressure (Rastogi et al. 2016; Liperoti et al. 2017).

The potential benefits of hawthorn in antihypertensive therapy have been evaluated by a few clinical studies, and the outcomes are contradictory and not solid enough to corroborate its use for controlling blood pressure. Hence, a randomised, double-blind, placebo-controlled pilot study performed with mildly hypertensive subjects treated with hawthorn extract (500 mg, 10 weeks) showed a tendency for reducing diastolic blood pressure (DBP), although no statistically significant results were observed (Walker et al. 2002). In another randomised, double-blind, placebo-controlled clinical trial, 92 patients with primary mild hypertension were treated with a hydroethanolic extract from the leaves and flowers of *Crataegus curvisepala* Lind, an Iranian species, standardised based on the flavonoid and procyanidin content (Asgary et al. 2004). After 3 months of treatment (20 drops of extract, three times daily), a decrease in systolic blood pressure (SBP) and DBP by about 13 and 8 mmHg, respectively, was observed.

A randomised placebo-controlled trial was carried out with 80 hypertensive subjects (DBP of 85–95 mmHg and SBP of 145–165 mmHg) suffering type 2 diabetes and taking prescribed drugs (Walker et al. 2006). They received hawthorn LI 132 extract (1200 mg) daily for 16 weeks and a greater reduction in DBP was observed in the treated group (baseline: 85.6 mmHg, 95% confidence interval [CI] = 83.3–87.8; outcome: 83.0 mmHg, 95% CI = 80.5–85.7) as compared to the placebo group (baseline: 84.5 mmHg, 95% CI = 82–87; outcome: 85.0 mmHg, 95% CI = 82.2–87.8). The authors did not observe a significant difference in SBP reduction from baseline hawthorn and placebo groups (Walker et al. 2006).

Findings from preclinical studies with hawthorn suggest that its blood pressure–lowering effect is related to nitric oxide (NO)-mediated vasodilation (see the reviews of Rastogi et al. 2016; Liperoti et al. 2017). Based on this assumption, a randomised, controlled crossover trial was performed to investigate the relationship between hawthorn extract dose and brachial artery flow mediated dilation (FMD), an indirect measure of NO release (Asher et al. 2012). The study was conducted with 21 pre-hypertensive or mildly hypertensive subjects, who received a standardised hawthorn extract (50 mg of oligomeric procyanidin per 250 mg extract) at randomly sequenced doses (1000, 1500 and 2500 mg, twice daily). The authors did not observe any evidence of a dose-response effect on FMD percentage or on the absolute change in brachial artery diameter and blood pressure. Consequently, they postulate that the blood pressure lowering effect attributed to hawthorn, if existent, it is probably not mediated by an NO-dependent mechanism (Asher et al. 2012).

Based on the clinical trials briefly reviewed above, there seems to be no gain in using hawthorn to reduce blood pressure. There are, however, a substantial number of clinical studies that advocate its benefits for treating patients with heart failure (see the reviews of Wang et al. 2013, and Holubarsch et al. 2018). According to these authors, randomised, placebo-controlled trials evidenced beneficial effects to patients with mild forms of heart failure (New York Heart Association classes II or III), hypertension and hyperlipidaemia by increasing functional capacity, alleviating disabling symptoms and improving health-related quality of life. In addition, clinical data collected for WS 1442 extract disclosed this standardised product as very safe either as monotherapy or add-on therapy (Holubarsch et al. 2018).

A different opinion on the efficacy of hawthorn was expressed in the review of Liperoti et al. (2017). They claim that despite the amount of data 'there is no robust evidence to support the use of this herb for the treatment of cardiovascular diseases.' The authors sustain this affirmation based on meta-analyses of reported clinical trials, in which improvements of some functional measures are observed, such as maximal workload, left ventricular ejection fraction, exercise tolerance and pressure heart rate product in patients with chronic heart failure. However, according to them, data to assess the effect of hawthorn on hard cardiac outcomes are still lacking.

17.2.2 *ALLIUM SATIVUM* (GARLIC)

Garlic (*Allium sativum* L.; Amaryllidaceae) has different traditional uses worldwide, due to its alleged therapeutic benefits for infectious diseases, gastrointestinal problems, cancer and CVD (Al Disi et al. 2016; Liperoti et al. 2017). The effect of garlic on CVD is credited to three major activities: lowering effect on blood pressure, reduction of plasmatic cholesterol and triglycerides and inhibition of platelet aggregation (Breithaupt-Grögler et al. 1997; Rahman and Lowe 2006; Ried and Fakler 2014). Besides the antihypertensive effect, other biological activities related to the traditional uses of garlic have been demonstrated, such as anti-inflammatory, antioxidant, antibacterial, hypocholesterolaemic and cytotoxic (Banerjee et al. 2002; Mousa and Mousa 2007; Frishman et al. 2009; Qidwai and Ashfaq 2013).

Garlic is consumed in different forms for its hypotensive effect: raw, aged, aqueous extract, oil, in powder form and in capsules (Banerjee et al. 2002; Frishman et al. 2009; Ried et al. 2013). Allicin (Figure 17.2) is considered the bioactive constituent of garlic, along with other sulphur-containing compounds. Allicin is found in freshly crushed gloves, but degrades into several allyl sulphides and polysulphides commonly termed garlic organosulphides (Figure 17.2). These organosulphides are also constituents of fresh garlic, but their concentrations increase in aged preparations (Schäfer and Kaschula

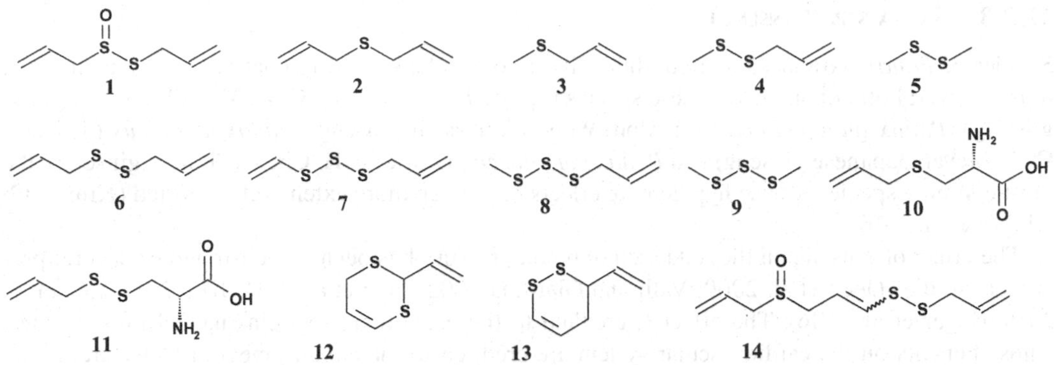

FIGURE 17.2 Chemical structure of garlic constituent allicin and products formed thereof: (1) Allicin, (2) diallyl sulphide (DAS), (3) allyl methyl sulphide (AMS), (4) allyl methyl disulphide (AMDS), (5) dimethyl disulphide (DMDS), (6) diallyl disulphide (DADS), (7) diallyl trisulphide (DATS), (8) allyl methyl trisulphide (AMTS), (9) dimethyl trisulphide (DMTS), (10) S-allyl cysteine (SAC), (11) S-allyl mercaptocysteine (SAMC), (12) 2-vinyl-4H-1,3-dithiin, (13) 3-vinyl-3,4-dihydro-1,2-dithiin, (14) E/Z-4,5,9-trithiadodeca-1,6,11-triene 9-oxide (E/Z-ajoene). (From Schäfer, G. and Kaschula, C.H., *Anticancer Agents Med. Chem.*, **4**, 233–240, 2014.)

2014). Outcomes from meta-analysis studies suggest that aged garlic extract (AGE) produces a consistent lowering of blood pressure in comparison to other forms (Al Disi et al. 2016). Additionally, AGEs exhibit higher antioxidant potency than other types of garlic clove derivatives (Mathew and Biju 2008).

Several clinical trials have been performed to evaluate the hypotensive effect of garlic and the results are conflicting. A recent meta-analysis covering 20 trials with 970 participants showed a decrease (mean ± SE) in SBP of 5.1 ± 2.2 mmHg, whereas DBP was reduced by 2.5 ± 1.6 mmHg in comparison to placebo (Ried 2016). The author also performed a meta-analysis of clinical trials reported with hypertensive subjects (SBP/DBP ≥ 140/90 mmHg), which evidenced larger significant reductions both in SBP (8.7 ± 2.2 mmHg) and DBP (6.1 ± 1.3 mmHg). In the same direction, another meta-analysis performed with randomised controlled trials, evidenced that garlic supplements induce a significant reduction in both SBP (3.75 mmHg) and DBP (3.39 mmHg; Wang et al. 2015). Moreover, a randomised, parallel, placebo-controlled trial demonstrated the reduction of SBP (9.2 mmHg) and DBP (6.27 mmHg) in hypertensive patients treated with garlic tablets (300–1500 mg/day, 24 weeks; Ashraf et al. 2013).

The positive effect of garlic on reducing cardiovascular morbidity and mortality in hypertensive subjects could not be confirmed by a previous Cochrane review (Stabler et al. 2012). Conversely, a significant reduction of SBP was evidenced by a previous meta-analysis (Ried et al. 2008), as well as by a double-blind, parallel-randomised, placebo-controlled study carried out with hypertensive subjects treated with aged garlic extracts (960 mg/day, 12 weeks) (Ried et al. 2010).

The hypotensive effect induced by garlic is related to an increase in bioavailability of the vasodilating gases NO and H_2S, as well to the upregulation of endothelial NO synthase (eNOS) (Banerjee et al. 2002; Mousa and Mousa 2007; Vazquez-Prieto et al. 2011; Ried et al. 2013), in addition to the angiotensin-converting enzyme (ACE) inhibition elicited by gamma-glutamyl-cysteines (Sendl et al. 1992). Besides the hypotensive effect, the positive effects of garlic on CVD by reducing blood lipids have been demonstrated by various clinical trials, including a decrease in LDL cholesterol (Gardner et al. 2001; Ried et al. 2013).

Although there is a substantial amount of clinical data reporting the effects of garlic on CVD, Liperoti et al. (2017) have doubts on the efficacy of this plant. In spite of some positive data, the authors claim that there are several methodological limitations in the randomised clinical trials published so far with garlic, including sample sizes, duration of treatments, statistical analyses, randomisation, quality of the tested preparations and dosages.

17.2.3 PANAX SPP. (GINSENG)

Species of *Panax* (Araliaceae) are traditionally used as adaptogens, to control blood pressure and to treat several other conditions; these species include *Panax ginseng* C. A. Mey (Asian or Korean ginseng), *Panax quinquefolius* (L.) Alph. Wood (American ginseng), *Panax japonicus* (T. Nees) C. A. Meyer (Japanese ginseng) and *Panax notoginseng* (Burk.) F. H. Chen. (Chinese ginseng), the most common species, whose hypotensive effects have been more extensively reported (Kim 2012; Al Disi et al. 2016).

The effect of ginseng on the reduction of blood pressure has been demonstrated by several pre-clinical studies (Jeon et al. 2000; Valli and Giardina 2002; Jang et al. 2011; Kim 2012; Lee et al. 2016; Nagar et al. 2016). The effect is credited to the constituent saponins named ginsenosides, whose benefits on the cardiovascular system are credited to the enhancement of NO secretion by endothelial cells, modulation of calcium ions channels in myocardial cells, antioxidant activity, reduction of platelet adhesion and stabilisation of glucose homeostasis cells (Kim 2012). However, low doses of ginseng increase the blood pressure and this conflicting effect was credited to the actions of different ginsenosides (Valli and Giardina 2002).

The antihypertensive effect of ginseng has been investigated by several clinical trials. In a recent study, red Korean ginseng was given to pre-hypertensive subjects (5 g divided into 10 capsules, daily). After 12 weeks, the treated group showed reductions of 6.5 and 5.0 mmHg in systolic and diastolic blood pressure, respectively, in comparison to control. The reduction in blood pressure was associated with decreased lipoprotein-associated phospholipase A2 and lysophosphatidylcho-lines levels and increased dihydrobiopterin concentration in the treated subjects (Cha et al. 2016). In another study performed with mild hypertensive patients, a *P. ginseng* extract enriched in gin-senoside protopanaxatriol (300 mg/day) induced a significant decrease of 3.1 and 2.3 mmHg in SBP and DBP, respectively (Rhee et al. 2014). In turn, a *P. ginseng* extract enriched in ginsenoside Rg3 (400 mg) given to healthy subjects induced a significant reduction in SBP and DBP respectively by 4.8 ± 6.8 and 3.6 ± 6.4 mmHg hours after ingestion (Jovanovski et al. 2014). A clinical trial carried out with hypertensive patients treated with *P. quinquefolius* (3 g/day, 12 weeks) showed a decrease in SBP by 17.4 mmHg (Mucalo et al. 2013).

Although the results from the above mentioned clinical trials seem to corroborate the benefits of ginseng in hypertension, the clinical evidence evaluating repeated ginseng exposure is still con-troversial. Komishon et al. (2016) conducted a systematic review and meta-analysis of randomised controlled trials (performed over at least 4 weeks) to compare the effect of ginseng on SBP, DBP and/or mean arterial blood pressure (MAP). After analysing 17 clinical trials ($n = 1381$), the authors found no significant effect of ginseng on SBP, DBP and MAP. Although statistical significance was not found by the authors, ginseng treatment seems to favour systolic blood pressure improvement in diabetes, metabolic syndrome and obesity. Moreover, the authors concluded that there is no concern of increasing blood pressure by ginseng consumption because it apparently has no vascular effects.

To better evaluate and understand the cardiovascular benefits of ginseng, it is mandatory to have more robust randomised controlled trials assessing the effect on blood pressure, performed with high-quality standardised extracts/formulations (Komishon et al. 2016).

17.3 REGULATION OF HERBAL MEDICINES IN BRAZIL

The regulation of herbal medicines varies from country to country and as a result distinct sani-tary requirements are demanded to release a new product into the market, which may explain the concerns associated with the prescription or use of such products by clinicians and patients. In the United States, herbal products are categorised as dietary supplements and regulated by the Food and Drug Administration (FDA 2018). Unlike conventional medicines, herbal products do not require previous approval by the FDA before they are launched and, therefore, their safety and efficacy do not have to be proven by clinical trials. Only after an herbal product reaches the market, the FDA is responsible for monitoring its safety by following adverse effects reported by the manufacturer, consumers or healthcare professionals through the Safety Reporting Portal (Liperoti et al. 2017).

The situation is distinct in the European Union, where each member country has its own legislation, but the general regulatory pathways for marketing authorisation or registration of herbal medicinal products are established by the European Medicines Agency (EMA). According to EMA guidelines, products registered based on their traditional use, that is, those used in the European Union for at least 15 years, do not require clinical trials to prove their safety and efficacy, while all other herbal products do have to present results from such studies (EMA 2004).

In Brazil, herbal medicinal products (HMP) are regulated by the Brazilian Health Regulatory Agency (ANVISA), which defines HMP as a medicine obtained from plant, fungal or algae sources, except for isolated compounds, used for prophylactic, curative or palliative purposes. Since 2014, Brazil (2014) has a new regulatory framework for the regulation of HMP. The current regulation (RDC n° 26/2014) establishes two categories of plant-based products for registration: herbal medicines (HM), which have to prove their safety and efficacy through non-clinical and clinical trials; and traditional herbal products (THP), which are registered based on traditional use and preclude safety and efficacy studies (Brazil 2014). In spite of these differences, both products follow the same quality requirements established by ANVISA (Brazil 2014).

The preclusion of safety and efficacy trials for THP in Brazil is aligned with the regulations of countries like Canada, Australia and the European Union. To be included in this category, the product must follow some requirements, such as continued use for at least 30 years and be consistent with traditional use. For readers interested in more details on the registration of herbal products in Brazil, Bezerra Carvalho et al. (2014) is a useful reference.

The provisions of ANVISA to perform preclinical toxicological assays for HM registration are aligned with the guidelines of the OECD (Organisation for Economic Cooperation and Development), ICH (International Conference on Harmonisation), FDA and EMA, as well as with other institutions like the National Cancer Institute (USA) and the World Health Organization (WHO). ANVISA guidelines establish toxicological tests with different levels of complexity, including single-dose toxicity studies and genotoxicity studies, repeated dose, reproductive toxicity studies, local tolerance studies, studies of carcinogenicity, studies of interest to evaluate the pharmacological safety and toxicokinetic studies (Brazil 2013).

The main differences in the preclinical and clinical evaluation of the efficacy and safety of a pure compound (natural, synthetic or semi-synthetic derivatives) and a mixture (extract or fraction), as found in HM, are inherent to their complexity. The production of HM presents technological challenges to ensure reproducibility in the chemical composition of different lots and requires the development of reliable analytical methods to access the chemical composition of intermediate and final products. In addition, the pharmacological/toxicological trials of HM demand the selection of vehicles and routes for administration of the product, along with the definition of markers for pharmacokinetic studies (Braga et al. 2017).

According to ANVISA, a marker is a compound or class of compounds (e.g. alkaloids, flavonoids, fatty acids, etc.) used as a reference in the quality control of the raw material and HM, preferably having correlation with the therapeutic effect. The marker can be active, when related to the therapeutic activity of the HM, or analytical, when this relationship has not been demonstrated so far (Brazil 2014). Therefore, one of the first challenges in HM development is to define a suitable marker for study, whether active or analytical, and perform its isolation and purification at the purity required for using it as a reference compound, in case the compound is not commercially available. It is important to notice that markers not related to the pharmacological activity of HMs are not appropriate for pharmacokinetic studies and their value to predict the therapeutic effect or clinical outcome is questionable (Braga et al. 2017).

In addition to the complexity of the matrix, herbal derivatives (extracts and fractions) have some peculiarities that can affect their effectiveness and safety. The herbal raw material used for HM production can contain various contaminants, and ANVISA regulates the accepted levels of heavy metals, pesticides, radioactivity and mycotoxins, among other contaminants (Brazil 2014). Another variable that may directly impact the efficacy and safety of HM is the presence of residues of solvents used in the extraction of an herbal raw material to produce the extract/fraction. It is therefore also mandatory to investigate the presence of residues of solvents and establish analytical methods for their determination. A joint publication of WHO and ANVISA establishes the quality requirements for herbal materials and final products needed to conduct clinical trials for registration of herbal medicines in Brazil (2008).

In conclusion, Brazil has a rigid framework for registering and launching a new herbal medicine in the market, in which the safety, efficacy and quality of the new product have to be proven by consistent pharmacological and toxicological preclinical and clinical data, as similarly required for a new synthetic drug.

17.4 BRAZILIAN PLANTS WITH ANTIHYPERTENSIVE ACTIVITY

Brazil is a megadiverse country and is considered to host the largest plant biodiversity on earth, with 46,096 plant species registered in different ecosystems (Rio de Janeiro Botanical Garden 2015). The Brazilian population has a broad tradition of the use of medicinal plants to treat different acute and chronic diseases. Despite these two favourable features – rich biodiversity and broad ethnomedical knowledge – the number of HM registered in the country is still limited and the herbal medicine market is very modest, totalling around US$261 million, which represents less than 5% of the global market of medicines in Brazil (Dutra et al. 2016). However, the country also has a solid scientific basis for the investigation of medicinal plants, as demonstrated by the publication of over 10,000 papers on this subject in the years 2011–2013 (Dutra et al. 2016).

Several plant species are traditionally used in Brazil for their antihypertensive effect. Some of them have been investigated by preclinical pharmacological and toxicological studies, but only a few have been evaluated so far in clinical trials. We selected two promising plant species with antihypertensive potential – *Euterpe oleracea* and *Hancornia speciosa* – and discuss their chemical composition and major preclinical and clinical findings in the following sections. We also discuss the pharmacological potential of some less-studied vasodilating plants.

17.4.1 *EUTERPE OLERACEA* (AÇAÍ)

Euterpe oleracea Mart. (Arecaceae) is a palm species popularly called açaí, found in the Amazonas region of Brazil, in the states of Maranhão, Tocantins, and Amapá. The açaí fruits are widely consumed as food by indigenous populations and Amazonian communities and are also used to treat fever, pain and tiredness, among other medicinal uses (Plotkin and Balick 1984). In recent years, the consumption of açaí has spread along the country and has reached Europe, the United States, Japan and China.

The chemical composition of açaí has been thoroughly investigated. Cyanidin 3-glucoside and cyanidin 3-rutinoside were found to be the main constituents of the pulp from the berries (Figure 17.3), which account for its violet colour, in addition to significant amounts of flavonoids and its minor protocatechuic acid and epicatechin contents (Del Pozo-Insfran et al. 2004; Schauss et al. 2006a). In turn, the hydroethanolic extract of açaí seeds is primarily composed of catechin and epicatechin, along with polymeric and oligomeric proanthocyanidins (Rodrigues et al. 2006, Moura et al. 2012).

Recent reviews cover the chemical composition and pharmacological activities reported for extracts of açaí pulp and/or seeds, mainly focused on the cardiovascular, renal, metabolic and antioxidant effects (Ulbricht et al. 2012; Yamaguchi et al. 2015; Moura and Resende 2016).

Prospective studies suggest an inverse correlation between the intake of polyphenols found in fruits and vegetables and the incidence of CVD and cancer (Manach et al. 2005; Wang et al. 2014). The consumption of polyphenols is associated with enhanced antioxidant potential in plasma and generally results in vascular protection. Therefore, keeping in mind the high contents of cyanidins

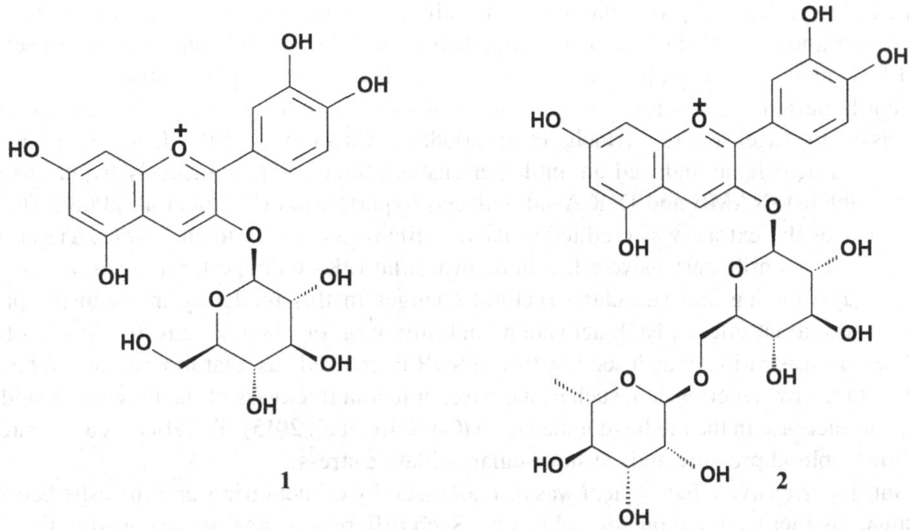

FIGURE 17.3 Chemical structures of cyanidin 3-glucoside (1) and cyanidin 3-rutinoside (2), the main constituents of the pulp from *Euterpe oleracea* (açaí).

and other polyphenols found in açaí, the pulp and seeds of this berry were initially evaluated for their antioxidant potential. The antioxidant capacity of açaí has been demonstrated using different antioxidant assays against peroxyl, peroxynitrite and hydroxyl radicals (see Moura and Resende 2016). In addition, açaí was reported to inhibit the generation of reactive oxygen species and the activity of cyclooxygenases 1 and 2 (Schauss et al. 2006b).

The antioxidant effect of a juice blend containing açaí as the predominant ingredient was demonstrated by a randomised, double-blinded, placebo-controlled, crossover trial with 12 healthy subjects (Jensen et al. 2008). The authors measured the antioxidant capacity of blood samples after the juice consumption (baseline, 1 h, and 2 h) using several antioxidant assays and the thiobarbituric acid reactive substances (TBARS) assay – a measure of lipid peroxidation. The results showed an increase in serum antioxidants and inhibition of lipid peroxidation post-consumption. Moreover, another acute clinical trial was performed with 12 healthy volunteers treated with açaí pulp and juice (Mertens-Talcott et al. 2008). The subjects receiving açaí juice and pulp presented individual increases in plasma antioxidant capacity of up to 2.3- and 3-fold, respectively. However, the antioxidant capacity in urine, generation of reactive oxygen species, and uric acid concentrations in plasma were not significantly altered by the treatments.

Another randomised, placebo-controlled clinical trial was performed with 12 healthy volunteers, who received a blended juice of açaí and *Myrciaria dubia* (H.B.K.) McVaugh, an anthocyanin-rich species (Ellinger et al. 2012). Markers of antioxidant capacity and oxidative stress were measured in the blood before and after juice ingestion. The plasma of juice-treated subjects presented enhanced ascorbic acid, and maintained total oxidant scavenging capacity and partly Folin–Ciocalteu reducing capacity in comparison to the placebo group. These findings led the authors to conclude that the juice may stabilise the pro-/antioxidant balance in healthy volunteers without affecting markers of oxidative stress (Ellinger et al. 2012).

Polyphenols are also known to present vasodilating activity, so extracts from açaí pulp and seeds were evaluated for this activity. Extracts prepared with the skin and seeds of açaí berries induced a complete, dose-dependent, long-lasting vasodilating effect in isolated mesenteric vascular bed of rats (Rocha et al. 2007). The authors observed a higher potency for the seed extract and credited this effect to differences in the polyphenol composition. The endothelial-dependent vasodilator response induced by açaí seed extract was characterised as dependent on the synthesis of NO, but is not related to the release of prostaglandins or the stimulation of muscarinic, histaminergic, alpha-2 adrenoceptors and bradykinin receptors in endothelial cells. The endothelium-derived hyperpolarisation (EDH) may be also involved in the vasodilator effect induced by the extract.

The antihypertensive potential of açaí was investigated *in vivo*, using different experimental models of hypertensive rats (Rocha et al. 2008; da Costa et al. 2012; Cordeiro et al. 2015). The extract of açaí fruits induced an antihypertensive effect on spontaneously hypertensive rats (SHR), Goldblatt L-NAME and DOCA-salt-induced hypertension (Rocha et al. 2008). The hypotensive effect of the extract was credited to its vasodilator and antioxidant actions. The açaí seed extract showed an antihypertensive effect in renovascular (2K-1C) hypertensive rats and prevented endothelial dysfunction and vascular structural changes in this model by mechanisms probably involving antioxidant effects, NOS activation, and inhibition of MMP-2 activation (da Costa et al. 2012). The administration of açaí seed extract to SHR decreased vascular morphological structural changes induced by hypertension, such as increase on media thickness of the mesenteric and aortic arteries, and increase in the media to lumen ratio (Cordeiro et al. 2015). The effect is associated with a reduction of blood pressure and cardiovascular oxidative stress.

The antihypertensive effect of açaí was also assessed by clinical trials and furnished contradictory results, distinct from the preclinical results. Such differences may be attributed to the composition of the tested matrices: while the majority of *in vivo* assays were performed with açaí seed extracts, the clinical trials were mostly conducted with açaí pulp or derivatives. Hence, açaí pulp (100 g twice daily, 30 days) was given to 10 overweight adults in an open-label pilot study (Udani et al. 2011). After 30 days of treatment, the authors observed no effect on blood pressure, NO metabolites and plasma levels of high sensitivity C-reactive protein, whereas the levels of fasting glucose and insulin were decreased, as well as total cholesterol. Another randomised, double-blind, placebo-controlled crossover study was carried out with 18 healthy subjects (Gale et al. 2014). The group receiving açaí (500 mg gel capsule, twice daily) did not show significant differences in baseline ECG or blood pressure variables as compared to the placebo group. The only exception was a significantly lower standing SBP observed 6 h after açaí administration in comparison to the placebo group (-4.6 ± 9.3 mmHg vs. 2.2 ± 8.5 mmHg).

More recently, a double-blind, crossover, acute dietary intervention trial was conducted with 23 overweight healthy volunteers receiving an açaí-based smoothie, containing 694 mg total phenolics (Alqurashi et al. 2016). No significant changes were observed in blood pressure, heart rate or postprandial glucose response of the group consuming the açaí-based smoothie in comparison to the control group. On the other hand, improvements in vascular function were visible in the açaí-treated group, with postprandial increases in the brachial artery by flow-mediated dilatation after 2 and 6 h of treatment, as well as reduction of total peroxide oxidative status.

In addition to the studies here reviewed, there are several reports of preclinical data showing the benefits of açaí on myocardial ischemia, renal failure, dyslipidaemia and diabetes (see Ulbricht et al. 2012; Moura and Resende 2016). Although the existing clinical trials could not prove the antihypertensive properties of açaí that were demonstrated in different preclinical models, the conflicting results seem to be related to differences in the products employed for testing. Therefore, it is mandatory to undertake more robust clinical trials, with a larger number of subjects, and to employ standardised extracts based on the contents of cyanidins, regarded as the active markers.

17.4.2 *Hancornia speciosa* (Mangaba)

To investigate the potential antihypertensive activity of Brazilian plants, we initially developed and validated a low-cost simple *in vitro* assay for extract screening, based on the inhibition of ACE (Serra et al. 2005). ACE is part of the renin-angiotensin system and plays a key role in the homeostatic mechanism of mammals, contributing to the maintenance of the normal blood pressure, and for electrolyte balance, being involved in the regulation and control of the arterial pressure. ACE inhibitors are well established in antihypertensive therapy and natural products of different classes are known to inhibit this enzyme. It is noteworthy that some vasoactive peptides isolated from the venom of the Brazilian viper *Bothrops jararaca* were the template for the development of captopril and other synthetic antihypertensive drugs currently used in therapy (Newman 2017).

The screening of 60 plant extracts prepared from 48 plants species indicated ACE-inhibiting activity for about 20% of them (ACE inhibition $\geq$ 50%), including the ethanol extract from mangaba leaves (Serra et al. 2005; Braga et al. 2007). Mangaba or mangabeira is the vulgar name of *Hancornia speciosa* Gomes (Apocynaceae), a plant species found in *cerrado*, a savannah-like eco-region in Brazil (Rodrigues and Carvalho 2001). The species is traditionally employed to treat hypertension and inflammatory processes, among several other uses, and its fruits are consumed *in natura* or employed in the preparation of juices, ice creams and jams (Hirschmann and Arias 1990).

We evaluated the vasodilator effect induced by an ethanolic extract from mangaba leaves in *ex vivo* preparations. In rat aortic rings, the extract produced a concentration-dependent vasodilatation (pIC$_{50}$ = 5.6 $\pm$ 0.1), which was completely abolished in endothelium-denuded vessels (Ferreira et al. 2007a). The effect was abolished by L-NAME, but not by atropine or indomethacin. The vasodilator effect was dramatically reduced in the presence of wortmannin, an inhibitor of phosphatidylinositol 3-kinase (PI3K). Based on these findings, we could conclude that the ethanolic extract from mangaba leaves induces a NO- and endothelium-dependent vasodilatation in rat aortic preparations, likely by a mechanism dependent on the activation of PI3K.

The same leaf extract produced a concentration-dependent vasodilation (pIC$_{50}$ = 4.97 $\pm$ 0.36) in superior mesenteric artery rings pre-contracted with phenylephrine, an effect that was completely abolished in endothelium-denuded vessels (Ferreira et al. 2007b). The mechanism of the vasodilator effect in mesenteric rings was characterised as dependent on NO, on the activation of potassium channels and EDH. Rutin, identified as the major peak in the HPLC fingerprint obtained for the extract, was postulated as one of the vasodilator active constituents, because it was able to induce an endothelium-dependent vasodilation in rat superior mesenteric arteries.

Fractionation of the mangaba leaf extract bioguided by the ACE inhibition assay led to the identification of the cyclitol L-(+)-bornesitol (IC$_{50}$ = 41.4 μM) and the flavonoid rutin (IC$_{50}$ = 453.9 μM) as the major ACE-inhibiting compounds (Endringer 2007; Endringer et al. 2014). Other constituents isolated from the mangaba leaf extract include kaempferol-*O*-3-rutinoside, 5-*O*-caffeoyl-quinic acid, *trans*-4-hydroxy-cinnamic acid, *cis*-4-hydroxy-cinnamic acid, α-amyrin, lupeol and a long-chain fatty acid ester derivative from lupeol (Endringer 2007). The chemical structures of some bioactive constituents of *H. speciosa* leaves are depicted in Figure 17.4.

The phenolic compounds of *H. speciosa* leaves were recently investigated by ultra-high-performance liquid chromatography (UHPLC) coupled to Orbitrap high-resolution mass spectrometry (HRMS; Bastos et al. 2017). According to the authors, 14 compounds were identified, including protocatechuic acid, catechin and quercetin, along with 14 putatively identified compounds, comprising B- and C-type procyanidins.

The identification of L-(+)-bornesitol as the main ACE-inhibiting constituent of *H. speciosa* disclosed cyclitols as a new class of ACE inhibitors. Therefore, we assayed several structure-related compounds (4 cyclitols and 15 sugars) for *in vitro* ACE inhibition, aiming to identify some structural

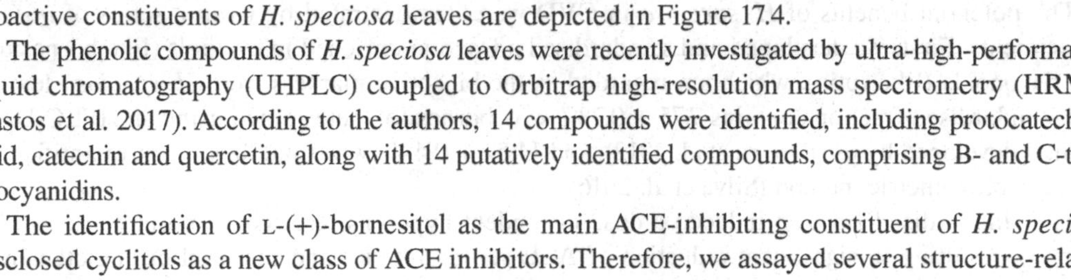

FIGURE 17.4 Chemical structures of L-(+)-bornesitol (1) and rutin (2), the active markers of *Hancornia speciosa* (mangaba) leaves.

features required for activity (Endringer et al. 2014). The presence of an axial-located hydroxyl group vicinal to either a carbon bearing hydroxyl-methylene or a methoxyl group as substituent, as found in L-(+)-bornesitol ($IC_{50} = 41.4$ µM) and D-galactose ($IC_{50} = 35.7$ µM), seems to be relevant for ACE inhibition. The lack of this group at C6 might explain the considerably lower potency of *myo*-inositol ($CI_{50} = 449.2$ µM). The presence of hydroxyl groups appears to be also essential for ACE inhibition, because peracetylation of bornesitol abolished the biological activity.

In addition, we performed molecular docking studies to investigate interactions between the active compounds and human ACE (Endringer et al. 2014). As the result of several calculations, we demonstrated that L-(+)-bornesitol and all active sugars bind to the same enzyme region, which is a tunnel directed towards the active site, distinct from the binding site of the classical ACE-inhibitors like captopril. In agreement with the experimental data, D-galactose ($Ki = 19.6$ µM, $IC_{50} = 35.7$ µM) and L-(+)-bornesitol ($Ki = 25.3$ µM, $IC_{50} = 41.4$ µM) were the most active compounds, followed by D-glucose ($Ki = 32.9$ µM, $IC_{50} = 85.7$ µM). Therefore, we identified a new binding region for sugar-like molecules, which may be explored for the development of new ACE inhibitors.

Several studies have shown the involvement of inflammatory process in CVD, whereas the ability of angiotensin II to modulate inflammation has also been established. Based on the assumption that an antihypertensive herbal product should combine both ACE-inhibitory effect and anti-inflammatory activity, we investigated *in vitro* the effect of mangaba leaf extract and constituents on NF-κB inhibition (Endringer et al. 2009, 2010). The study disclosed the potential anti-inflammatory activity of the crude ethanolic extract from mangaba leaves ($IC_{50} = 17.4 \pm 5.8$ µg/mL) and the constituents thereof quinic acid ($IC_{50} = 85.0 \pm 12.3$ µM), L-(+)-bornesitol ($IC_{50} = 27.5 \pm 3.8$ µM) and rutin ($IC_{50} = 26.8 \pm 6.3$ µM). Interestingly, a fraction derived from the crude extract, enriched in cyclitols and flavonoids, exhibited a significantly higher NF-κB inhibitory activity ($IC_{50} = 1.0 \pm 0.0$ µg/mL) than the above-mentioned constituents, suggesting synergistic effects.

The potential anti-inflammatory activity of *H. speciosa* has also been shown by other experiments. The release of the pro-inflammatory cytokine tumour necrosis factor (TNF-α) by lipopolysaccharide (LPS)-stimulated human acute monocytic (THP-1) cells was significantly reduced by the ethanol extract from *H. speciosa* leaves ($62.9 \pm 8.2\%$, at 10 µg/mL), as well as by its constituents L-bornesitol ($48.9 \pm 0.9\%$, at 50 µM), quinic acid ($90.2 \pm 3.4\%$, at 10 µM) and rutin ($82.4 \pm 5.6\%$, at 10 µM; Geller et al. 2015).

The potential benefits of *H. speciosa* in CVD were demonstrated by us in a series of *in vivo* experiments. First, we developed and standardised a fraction enriched in cyclitols (like bornesitol) and flavonoids (like rutin), which are regarded as the bioactive markers from *H. speciosa* leaves. The standardised fraction contains $7.75 \pm 0.78\%$ w/w bornesitol, determined using an HPLC-DAD method developed by us (Pereira et al. 2012), and $14.52 \pm 0.44\%$ w/w total flavonoids, quantified by a spectrophotometric method (Silva et al. 2016).

The standardised fraction induced a dose-dependent hypotensive effect in normotensive mice (*per os*), resulting in significant reduction of ACE serum activity and the level of angiotensin II (Silva et al. 2011). Treatment with *H. speciosa* fraction also induced a significant increase on plasmatic level of nitrites and the systemic inhibition of eNOS by L-NAME reduced the hypotensive effect of the fraction. In the sequence, the standardised fraction of *H. speciosa* leaves was evaluated in DOCA-salt hypertensive mice (Silva et al. 2016). Administration of the fraction orally (0.03, 0.1 or 1 mg/kg) induced a dose-dependent, long-lasting reduction in SBP of the animals and resulted in increased plasmatic level of nitrites. The antihypertensive effect was reduced by administration of L-NAME. The standardised fraction also induced a concentration-dependent vasodilatation of mesenteric resistance arteries contracted with phenylephrine, which was more potent in arteries from DOCA mice. Removal of the endothelium or pretreatment with L-NAME or catalase reduced the vasodilator response for the fraction. The nitrite production induced by the fraction was significantly bigger in mesenteric arteries from DOCA than in SHAM mice, whereas H_2O_2 production resulting from fraction treatment was twice as high in DOCA mice.

H. *speciosa* is also traditionally used to treat diabetes in Brazil. Because hypertension and diabetes share common risk factors and frequently co-occur, we investigated the potential antidiabetic effect of the ethanol extract from mangaba leaves and fractions thereof (Pereira et al. 2015). Although the extract and fractions significantly inhibited α-glycosidase *in vitro*, only the crude extract and its dichloromethane fraction inhibited the hyperglycaemic effect induced by starch or glucose on mice. Both the extract and dichloromethane fraction were also able to increase glucose uptake in adipocytes. Therefore, the antidiabetic constituents of *H. speciosa* seem to be concentrated in the lipophilic fraction, which was shown to be composed by esters of lupeol and/or α/β-amyrin.

Another potential benefit of the ethanol extract from *H. speciosa* leaves on CVD is related to its antioxidant activity (Santos et al. 2016). Experimental data indicate that reactive oxygen species and oxidative stress play an important rule on CVD, including hypertension. The antioxidant activity of *H. speciosa* leaf extract was demonstrated via the sequestration of 2,2-diphenyl-1-picrylhydrazyl free radicals, inhibition of haemolysis, and inhibition of lipid peroxidation induced by 2,2'-azobis (2-amidinopropane) in human erythrocytes. The authors attributed these effects to the presence of phenolic constituents identified in the extract, namely chlorogenic acid, catechin, rutin, isoquercitrin, kaempferol-rutinoside, and catechin-pentoside, along with quinic acid.

The publications here reviewed indicate a considerable volume of preclinical data that supports the hypotensive effects ascribed to *H. speciosa* leaves, especially the *in vivo* data reported for the standardised fraction enriched in flavonoids and cyclitols. Furthermore, this fraction was subjected to acute, subchronic and chronic toxicological studies, carried out according to OECD guidelines, and no sign of toxicity was observed (data not published). In view of the favourable preclinical pharmacological and toxicological data demonstrated for the standardised fraction of mangaba, in addition to the existence of reliable analytical methods to assure its quality, this fraction represents a good candidate for the development of a HMP and shall undergo clinical trials in the near future.

17.4.3 Vasodilating Plants

Vasodilator drugs represent the main therapeutic option for the treatment of hypertension. They are considered direct or indirect vasodilators, classified accordingly to their mechanism of action. In this category, the main drugs act in the renin-angiotensin system, calcium channel blockers, and potassium channels activators (Mancia et al. 2007). In this section, we have chosen to depict some native Brazilian species, or adapted plants, traditionally used to treat hypertension, where the vasodilator effects were well characterised.

17.4.3.1 *Dicksonia sellowiana* (Xaxim)

Dicksonia sellowiana Presl. Hook (Dicksoniaceae) is a fern popularly known in Brazil as xaxim or samambaiaçu and is distributed in Central and South America (Tryon and Tryon 1982). In Brazil, this fern is found in Atlantic forests in the south and southwest regions (Fernandes 2000). It is used by the indigenous population for the treatment of parasitic diseases and asthma (Marquesini 1995). The chemical composition of a standardised extract from *D. sellowiana* leaves was investigated by UPLC-PDA-MS and disclosed the presence of kaempferol, quercetin, quinic acid and chlorogenic acid (Rattmann et al. 2011). The hydroalcoholic extract of the leaves presented an endothelium- and NO-dependent vasodilator effect (pIC_{50} = 4.6) in rat aorta by a mechanism involving the activation of muscarinic receptors (Rattmann et al. 2009). Interestingly, the extract of *D. sellowiana* leaves also induced relaxation in porcine coronary arteries, by a mechanism dependent on an intact endothelium and on the production of NO (Rattmann et al. 2012). In this last report, a more detailed mechanism of action was described, showing that *D. sellowiana* activated eNOS through a redox-sensitive Src- and Akt-dependent mechanism. However, in porcine coronary arteries the muscarinic receptors did not participate in the effect of this plant. Although the preclinical results for the acute treatment are promising, no chronic preclinical study was carried out with *D. sellowiana* for the treatment of hypertension.

17.4.3.2 *Alpinia zerumbet* (Colonia)

Alpinia zerumbet (Pers) B. L. Burtt and Smith (syn. *Alpinia speciosa* K. Schum) is a medicinal plant that belongs to the Zingiberaceae family, originating from East Asia and accidentally brought to Brazil by Portuguese caravels (Victório 2011). *A. zerumbet* is known in Brazil as colonia and is traditionally used to treat rheumatism, heart diseases, as a diuretic and antihypertensive (Carlini 1972; Medeiros et al. 2004). Early studies demonstrated that the hydroalcoholic extract from *A. zerumbet* leaves reduced the blood pressure and the heart rate in normotensive rats and dogs (Mendonça et al. 1991). Phytochemical analysis of the aqueous extract from *A. zerumbet* leaves led to the identification of the flavonoids rutin, kaempferol-3-*O*-rutinoside, kaempferol-3-*O*-glucuronide, (+)-catechin, and (−)-epicatechin (Mpalantinos et al. 1998). The diuretic and antihypertensive effects elicited by the extract were credited to these compounds. The hydroalcoholic extract of *A. zerumbet* leaves induced an endothelium- and NO-dependent vasodilator effect in mesenteric arteries from normotensive rats, by a mechanism independent of the activation of muscarinic, histaminic and adrenergic receptors, but it appeared to be partially dependent on the activation of bradykinin B_2 receptors (Soares de Moura et al. 2005). The same study suggested an antihypertensive effect of a subchronic treatment with *A. zerumbet* in DOCA-salt hypertensive rats (50 mg/kg; orally, 28 days). In addition to the polyphenol compounds, the essential oil from the aerial parts of *A. zerumbet* and its main constituents, 1,8-cineole and terpinen-4-ol, are able to induce an endothelium- and NO-dependent, as well as an endothelium-independent vasodilator effect in rat aorta, and to induce an antihypertensive effect in rats (Lahlou et al. 2002; Maia-Joca et al. 2014; Pinto et al. 2009).

17.4.3.3 *Cuphea carthagenensis* (Sete-Sangrias)

Cuphea carthagenensis (Jacq.) J. F. Macbride (Lythraceae) is popularly known as sete-sangrias in Brazil. It is an herbaceous species natural from Central and South America, including Brazil (Graham et al. 2006). The aerial parts of *C. carthagenensis* are traditionally used to treat hypertension, varicose and to activate the circulation (de Lima et al. 2007; Lorenzi and Matos 2008). Based on the traditional use of the aerial parts this plant, Braga et al. (2000) described its ACE inhibitory activity and, in the same time, the endothelium- and NO-dependent vasodilator effect of the hydroalcoholic extract, buthanolic and ethyl acetate fractions were described in rat aorta (Schuldt et al. 2000). The phytochemical study of the ethanolic extract from *C. carthagenensis* aerial parts led to the isolation of the flavonoids quercetin-5-*O*-β-glucopyranoside, quercetin-3-*O*-α-arabinofuranoside and quercetin-3-sulphate, the last one being considered as the chemical marker of the species (Krepsky et al. 2010, 2012). In addition, the total content of proanthocyanidins, tannins and phenolic compounds were quantified and positively correlated with the vasodilator effect of the total extract and fractions of *C. carthagenensis* (Krepsky et al. 2012). Although promising, these results did not lead to any study on the effects of the chronic treatment with the extract or fractions of *C. carthagenensis* in animal models of hypertension. Such studies would give a better view on the potential use of this plant for the treatment of hypertension, which could result in the future development of an HM.

17.5 CONCLUSIONS AND PERSPECTIVES

Brazil possesses two relevant features that could foster drug development in the country: rich plant biodiversity and a broad tradition on the use of medicinal plants. Furthermore, in 2014 the Brazilian Health Regulatory Agency (ANVISA) established a rigid framework to regulate the approval of new herbal medicines, based on consistent pharmacological and toxicological preclinical and clinical data, in addition to strict quality requirements. In spite of these favourable aspects, the development of medicinal herbal products in the country is still incipient, although there is a considerable volume of pharmacological preclinical data to corroborate the use of the Brazilian plants *Euterpe oleracea* (açaí) and *Hancornia speciosa* (mangaba) as an antihypertensive.

However, the clinical data reported for açaí did not evidence the antihypertensive properties demonstrated by various preclinical studies, and the apparent discrepancy could be related to differences in the products employed for testing. In the case of mangaba, no clinical trial has been performed so far to investigate the potent hypotensive effect demonstrated by preclinical studies for a standardised fraction. It is therefore mandatory to undertake well-planned robust clinical trials with both species employing an adequate number of subjects and using high-quality herbal products, standardised based on the contents of their bioactive markers.

In view of the complex composition of herbal medicines, their clinical trials present some challenges that should be overcome to generate consistent data. Even for the three globally-used well-studied plants reviewed in this chapter – hawthorn, garlic and ginseng – the existing clinical data are somewhat contradictory and do not confirm the preclinical findings. Thus, there is a common demand for reliable clinical trials, accurately designed in terms of sample sizes, duration of treatments, statistical analyses, randomisation, quality of the tested preparations and dosages.

REFERENCES

Al Disi, S. S., Anwar, M. A. and Eid, A. H. (2016). Anti-hypertensive herbs and their mechanisms of action: Part I. *Frontiers in Pharmacology*, **6**, 323.

Alqurashi, R. M., Galante, L. A., Rowland, I. R., Spencer, J. P. and Commane, D. M. (2016). Consumption of a flavonoid-rich açaí meal is associated with acute improvements in vascular function and a reduction in total oxidative status in healthy overweight men. *American Journal of Clinical Nutrition*, **104**, 1227–1235.

Anwar, M. A., Al Disi, S. S. and Eid, A. H. (2016). Anti-hypertensive herbs and their mechanisms of action: Part II. *Frontiers in Pharmacology*, **7**, 50.

Asgary, S., Naderi, G. H., Sadeghi, M., Kelishadi, R. and Amiri, M. (2004). Antihypertensive effect of Iranian *Crataegus curvisepala* Lind: A randomized, double-blind study. *Drugs under Experimental and Clinical Research*, **30**(5–6), 221–225.

Asher, G. N., Viera, A. J., Weaver, M. A., Dominik, R., Caughey, M. and Hinderliter, A. L. (2012). Effect of hawthorn standardized extract on flow mediated dilation in prehypertensive and mildly hypertensive adults: A randomized, controlled cross-over trial. *BMC Complementary and Alternative Medicine*, **12**, 26.

Ashraf, R., Khan, R. A., Ashraf, I. and Qureshi, A. A. (2013). Effects of *Allium sativum* (garlic) on systolic and diastolic blood pressure in patients with essential hypertension. *Pakistan Journal of Pharmaceutical Sciences*, **26**, 859–863.

Bai, R. R., Wu, X. M. and Xu, J. Y. (2015). Current natural products with antihypertensive activity. *Chinese Journal of Natural Medicines*, **13**, 721–729.

Banerjee, S. K., Maulik, M., Mancahanda, S. C., Dinda, A. K., Gupta, S. K. and Maulik, S. K. (2002). Dose-dependent induction of endogenous antioxidants in rat heart by chronic administration of garlic. *Life Sciences*, **70**, 1509–1518.

Bastos, K. X., Dias, C. N., Nascimento, Y. M., da Silva, M. S., Langassner, S. M., Wessjohann, L. A. and Tavares, J. F. (2017). Identification of phenolic compounds from *Hancornia speciosa* (Apocynaceae) leaves by UHPLC Orbitrap-HRMS. *Molecules*, **22**, E143.

Braga, F. C., Rates, S. M. K. and Simões, C. M. O. (2017). Avaliação da eficácia e segurança de produtos naturais candidatos a fármacos e medicamentos. In C. M. O. Simões, E. P. Schenkel, J. C. P. de Mello, L. A. Mentz and P. R. Petrovick, eds., *Farmacognosia: do produto natural ao medicamento*. 1st ed. Porto Alegre, Brazil: ArtMed. pp. 53–68.

Braga, F. C., Serra, C. P., Viana, N. S. Jr, Oliveira, A. B., Côrtes, S. F. and Lombardi, J. A. (2007). Angiotensin-converting enzyme inhibition by Brazilian plants. *Fitoterapia*, **78**, 353–358.

Braga, F. C., Wagner, H., Lombardi, J. A. and de Oliveira, A. B. (2000). Screening the Brazilian flora for antihypertensive plant species for *in vitro* angiotensin-I-converting enzyme inhibiting activity. *Phytomedicine*, **7**, 245–250.

Brazil. Agência Nacional de Vigilância Sanitária (ANVISA). (2013). *Guia para a condução de estudos não clínicos de toxicologia e segurança farmacológica necessários ao desenvolvimento de medicamentos*. Available from: http://portal.anvisa.gov.br/documents/33836/2492465/Guia+para+a+Condu%C3%A7%C3%A3o+de+Estudos+N%C3%A3o+Cl%C3%ADnicos+de+Toxicologia+e+Segura

n%C3%A7a+Farmacol%C3%B3gica+Necess%C3%A1rios+ao+Desenvolvimento+de+Medic
amentos+-+Vers%C3%A3o+2/a8cad67c-14c8-4722-bf0f-058a3a284f75.

Brazil. Agência Nacional de Vigilância Sanitária (ANVISA). (2014). *Resolução da Diretoria Colegiada—RDC N° 26. Dispõe sobre o registro de medicamentos fitoterápicos e o registro e a notificação de produtos tradicionais fitoterápicos.* Available from: http://bvsms.saude.gov.br/bvs/saudelegis/anvisa/2014/rdc0026_13_05_2014.pdf.

Brazil. Ministry of Health. (2008). *Instruções operacionais: informações necessárias para a condução de ensaios clínicos com fitoterápicos.* Brasília, Brazil: Ministério da Saúde.

Breithaupt-Grögler, K., Ling, M., Boudoulas, H. and Belz, G. G. (1997). Protective effect of chronic garlic intake on elastic properties of aorta in the elderly. *Circulation*, **96**, 2649–55.

Carlini, E. A. (1972). 'Screening' farmacológico de plantas brasileiras. *Revista Brasileira de Biologia*, **32**, 265–274.

Carvalho, A. C., Ramalho, L. S., Marques, R. F. and Perfeito, J. P. (2014). Regulation of herbal medicines in Brazil. *Journal of Ethnopharmacology*, **158**, 503–506.

Cha, T. W., Kim, M., Kim, M., Chae, J. S. and Lee, J. H. (2016). Blood pressure-lowering effect of Korean red ginseng associated with decreased circulating Lp-PLA$_2$ activity and lysophosphatidylcholines and increased dihydrobiopterin level in prehypertensive subjects. *Hypertension Research*, **39**, 449–456.

Chang, Q. and Zuo, Z. (2002). Hawthorn. *Journal of Clinical Pharmacology*, **42**, 605–612.

Chang, W. T., Dao, J. and Shao, Z. H. (2005). Hawthorn: Potential roles in cardiovascular disease. *American Journal of Chinese Medicine*, **33**, 1–10.

Cordeiro, V. S., Carvalho, L. R. and de Bem, G. F. (2015). *Euterpe oleracea* Mart. Extract prevents vascular remodeling and endothelial dysfunction in spontaneously hypertensive rats. *International Journal of Applied Research in Natural Products*, **8**, 6–16.

da Costa, C. A., de Oliveira, P. R., de Bem, G. F., de Cavalho, L. C., Ognibene, D. T., da Silva, A. F., dos Santos Valença, S., et al. (2012). *Euterpe oleracea* Mart.-derived polyphenols prevent endothelial dysfunction and vascular structural changes in renovascular hypertensive rats: Role of oxidative stress. *Naunyn Schmiedebergs Archives of Pharmacology*, **385**, 1199–1209.

de Lima, C. B., Bellettini, N. M. T., da Silva, A. S., Cheirubim, A. P., Janani, J. K., Vieira, M. A. V. and Amador, T. S. (2007). Uso de plantas medicinais pela população da zona urbana de Bandeirantes-PR. *Revista Brasileira de Biociências*, **5**, 600–602.

Del Pozo-Insfran, D., Brenes, C. H. and Talcott, S. T. (2004). Phytochemical composition and pigment stability of açaí (*Euterpe oleracea* Mart.). *Journal of Agricultural and Food Chemistry*, **52**, 1539–1545.

Dutra, R. C., Campos, M. M., Santos, A. R. and Calixto, J. B. (2016). Medicinal plants in Brazil: Pharmacological studies, drug discovery, challenges and perspectives. *Pharmacology Research*, **112**, 4–29.

Edwards, J. E., Paula, N., Brown, N. T., Dickinson, T. A. and Shipley, P. R. (2012). A review of the chemistry of the genus *Crataegus*. *Phytochemistry*, **79**, 5–26.

Ellinger, S., Gordon, A., Kürten, M., Jungfer, E., Zimmermann, B. F., Zur, B., Ellinger, J., Marx, F. and Stehle, P. (2012). Bolus consumption of a specifically designed fruit juice rich in anthocyanins and ascorbic acid did not influence markers of antioxidative defense in healthy humans. *Journal of Agricultural and Food Chemistry*, **60**, 11292–11300.

EMA (European Medicines Agency). (2004). Herbal Medicinal Products. Available from: https://ec.europa.eu/health//sites/health/files/files/eudralex/vol-1/dir_2004_24/dir_2004_24_en.pdf.

Endringer, D. C. (2007). *Química e atividades biológicas de Hancornia speciosa Gomes (Apocynaceae): Inibição da enzima conversora de angiotensina (ECA) e efeito na quimioprevenção de câncer.* Belo Horizonte, Brazil: Faculdade de Farmácia da Universidade Federal de Minas Gerais.

Endringer, D. C., Oliveira, O. V. and Braga, F. C. (2014). *In vitro* and *in silico* inhibition of angiotensin-converting enzyme by carbohydrates and cyclitols. *Chemical Papers*, **68**, 37–45.

Endringer, D. C., Pezzuto, J. M. and Braga, F. C. (2009). NF-kappaB inhibitory activity of cyclitols isolated from *Hancornia speciosa*. *Phytomedicine*, **16**, 1064–1069.

Endringer, D. C., Valadares, Y. M., Campana, P. R., Campos, J. J., Guimarães, K. G., Pezzuto, J. M. and Braga, F. C. (2010). Evaluation of Brazilian plants on cancer chemoprevention targets *in vitro*. *Phytotherapy Research*, **24**, 928–933.

ESCOP (European Scientific Cooperative on Phytotherapy). (1999). *Hawthorn Leaf and Flower*. Exeter, UK: ESCOP Monographs on the Medicinal Uses of Plant Drugs.

Fernandes, I. (2000). Taxonomia dos representantes de Dicksoniaceae no Brasil. *Pesquisas Botanica*, **50**, 5–26.

Ferreira, H. C., Serra, C. P., Endringer, D. C., Lemos, V. S., Braga, F. C. and Cortes, S. F. (2007b). Endothelium-dependent vasodilation induced by *Hancornia speciosa* in rat superior mesenteric artery. *Phytomedicine*, **14**, 473–478.

Ferreira, H. C., Serra, C. P., Lemos, V. S., Braga, F. C. and Cortes, S. F. (2007a). Nitric oxide-dependent vasodilatation by ethanolic extract of *Hancornia speciosa* via phosphatidyl-inositol 3-kinase. *Journal of Ethnopharmacology*, **109**, 161–164.

Frishman, W. H., Beravol, P. and Carosella, C. (2009). Alternative and complementary medicine for preventing and treating cardiovascular disease. *Disease-a-Month*, **55**, 121–192.

Gale, A. M., Kaur, R. and Baker, W. L. (2014). Hemodynamic and electrocardiographic effects of açaí berry in healthy volunteers: A randomized controlled trial. *International Journal of Cardiology*, **174**, 421–423.

Gardner, C. D., Chatterjee, L. M. and Carlson, J. J. (2001). The effect of garlic preparation on plasma lipid levels in moderately hypercholesterolemic adults. *Atherosclerosis*, **154**, 213–220.

Geller, F. C., Teixeira, M. R., Pereira, A. B., Dourado, L. P., Souza, D. G., Braga, F. C. and Simões, C. M. (2015). Evaluation of the wound healing properties of *Hancornia speciosa* leaves. *Phytotherapy Research*, **29**, 1887–1893.

Graham, S. A., Freudenstein, J. and Luker, M. (2006). A phylogenetic study of *Cuphea* (Lythraceae) based on morphology and nuclear rDNA ITS sequences. *Systematic Botany*, **31**, 764–778.

Hirschmann, G. S. and Arias, A. R. A. (1990). Survey of medicinal plants of Minas Gerais, Brazil. *Journal of Ethnopharmacology*, **29**, 159–172.

Hobbs, C. and Foster, S. (1990). Hawthorn: A literature review. *HerbalGram*, **22**, 19–33.

Holubarsch, C. J. F., Colucci, W. S. and Eha, J. (2018). Benefit-risk assessment of *Crataegus* extract WS 1442: An evidence-based review. *American Journal Cardiovascular Drugs*, **18**, 25–36.

Jang, S. J., Lim, H. J. and Lim, D. Y. (2011). Inhibitory effects of total Ginseng saponin on catecholamine secretion from the perfused adrenal medulla of SHRs. *Journal of Ginseng Research*, **35**, 176–190.

Jensen, G. S., Wu, X., Patterson, K. M., Barnes, J., Carter, S. G., Scherwitz, L., Beaman, R., Endres, J. R. and Schauss, A. G. (2008). *In vitro* and *in vivo* antioxidant and anti-inflammatory capacities of an antioxidant-rich fruit and berry juice blend. Results of a pilot and randomized, double-blinded, placebo-controlled, crossover study. *Journal of Agricultural and Food Chemistry*, **56**, 8326–8333.

Jeon, B. H., Kim, C. S., Park, K. S., Lee, J. W., Park, J. B., Kim, K. J., Kim, S. H., Chang, S. J. and Nam, K. Y. (2000). Effect of Korea red ginseng on the blood pressure in conscious hypertensive rats. *General Pharmacology*, **35**, 135–141.

Jovanovski, E., Bateman, E. A., Bhardwaj, J., Fairgrieve, C., Mucalo, I., Jenkins, A. L. and Vuksan, V. (2014). Effect of Rg3-enriched Korean red ginseng (*Panax ginseng*) on arterial stiffness and blood pressure in healthy individuals: A randomized controlled trial. *Journal of the American Society of Hypertension*, **8**, 537–541.

Kim, J. H. (2012). Cardiovascular diseases and *Panax ginseng*: A review on molecular mechanisms and medical applications. *Journal of Ginseng Research*, **36**, 16–26.

Koch, E. and Malek, F. A. (2011). Standardized extracts from hawthorn leaves and flowers in the treatment of cardiovascular disorders—Preclinical and clinical studies. *Planta Medica*, **77**, 1123–1128.

Komishon, A. M., Shishtar, E., Ha, V., Sievenpiper, J. L., de Souza, R. J., Jovanovski, E., Ho, H. V., Duvnjak, L. S. and Vuksan, V. (2016). The effect of ginseng (genus *Panax*) on blood pressure: A systematic review and meta-analysis of randomized controlled clinical trials. *Journal of Human Hypertension*, **30**, 619–626.

Krepsky, P. B., Farias, M. R., Côrtes, S. F. and Braga, F. C. (2010). Quercetin-3-sulfate: A chemical marker for *Cuphea carthagenensis*. *Biochemical Systematics and Ecology*, **38**, 125–127.

Krepsky, P. B., Isidório, R. G., de Souza, Filho, J. D., Côrtes, S. F., Braga, F. C. (2012). Chemical composition and vasodilatation induced by *Cuphea carthagenensis* preparations. *Phytomedicine*, **19**, 953–957.

Lahlou, S., Galindo, C. A. B., Leal-Cardoso, J. H., Fonteles, M. C. and Duarte, G. P. (2002). Cardiovascular effects of the essential oil of *Alpinia zerumbet* leaves and its main constituent, terpinen-4-ol, in rats: Role of the autonomic nervous system. *Planta Medica*, **68**, 1097–1102.

Lee, K. H., Bae, I. Y., Park, S. I., Park, J. D. and Lee, H. G. (2016). Antihypertensive effect of Korean Red Ginseng by enrichment of ginsenoside Rg3 and arginine-fructose. *Journal of Ginseng Research*, **40**, 237–244.

Li, L., Zhou, X., Li, N., Sun, M., Lv, J. and Xu, Z. (2015). Herbal drugs against cardiovascular disease: Traditional medicine and modern development. *Drug Discovery Today*, **20**, 1074–1086.

Liperoti, R., Vetrano, D. L., Bernabei, R. and Onder, G. (2017). Herbal medications in cardiovascular medicine. *Journal of the American College of Cardiology*, **69**, 1188–1199.

Lorenzi, H. and Matos, F. J. A. (2008). *Plantas Medicinais no Brasil: Nativas e exóticas*, 2nd ed. São Paulo, Brazil: Instituto Plantarum. pp. 348–349.

Maia-Joca, R. P., Joca, H. C., Ribeiro, F. J., do Nascimento, R. V., Silva-Alves, K. S., Cruz, J. S., Coelho-de-Souza, A. N. and Leal-Cardoso J. H. (2014). Investigation of terpinen-4-ol effects on vascular smooth muscle relaxation. *Life Sciences*, **115**, 52–58.

Manach, C., Mazur, A. and Scalbert, A. (2005). Polyphenols and prevention of cardiovascular diseases. *Current Opinion in Lipidology*, **16**, 77–84.

Mancia, G., Backer, G., Dominiczak, A., Cifkova, R., Fagard, R., Germano, G., Grassi, G., et al. (2007). Guidelines for the management of arterial hypertension. The task force for the management of arterial hypertension of the European Society of Hypertension (ESH) and of the European Society of Cardiology (ESC). *Journal of Hypertension*, **25**, 1105–1187.

Marquesini, N. R. (1995). *Plantas usadas como medicinais pelos índios do Paraná e Santa Catarina, Sul do Brasil: Guarani, Kaingãng, Xokleng, Ava-Guarani, Kraô e Cayua*. Curitiba, Brazil: Universidade Federal do Paraná.

Mathew, B. and Biju, R. (2008). Neuroprotective effects of garlic a review. *Libyan Journal of Medicine*, **3**, 23–33.

Medeiros, M. F. T., Fonseca, V. S. and Andreata, R. H. P. (2004). Medicinal plants and its uses by the ranchers from the Rio das Pedras Reserve, Mangaratiba, RJ, Brazil. *Acta Botanica Brasilica*, **18**, 391–399.

Mendonça,V. L. M., Oliveira, C. L. A., Craveiro, A. A., Rao, V. S. and Fontenele, M. C. (1991). Pharmacological and toxicological evaluation of *Alpinia speciosa*. *Memórias do Instituto Oswaldo Cruz*, **86**, 93–97.

Mertens-Talcott, S. U., Rios, J., Jilma-Stohlawetz, P., Pacheco-Palencia, L. A., Meibohm, B., Talcott, S. T. and Derendorf, H. (2008). Pharmacokinetics of anthocyanins and antioxidant effects after the consumption of anthocyanin-rich acai juice and pulp (Euterpe oleracea Mart.) in human healthy volunteers. *Journal of Agricultural and Food Chemistry*, **56**, 7796–7802.

Moura, R. S., Ferreira, T. S., Lopes, A. A., Pires, K. M., Nesi, R. T., Resende, A. C., Souza, P. J., et al. (2012). Effects of *Euterpe oleracea* Mart. (Açaí) extract in acute lung inflammation induced by cigarette smoke in the mouse. *Phytomedicine*, **19**, 262–269.

Moura, R. S. and Resende, A. C. (2016). Cardiovascular and metabolic effects of açaí, an Amazon plant. *Journal of Cardiovascular Pharmacology*, **68**, 19–26.

Mousa, A. S. and Mousa, S. A. (2007). Cellular effects of garlic supplements and antioxidant vitamins in lowering marginally high blood pressure in humans: Pilot study. *Nutrition Research*, **27**, 119–123.

Mpalantinos, M. A., Soares de Moura, R., Parente, J. P. and Kuste, R. M. (1998). Biologically active flavonoids and kava pyrones from the aqueous extract of *Alpinia zerumbet*. *Phytotherapy Research*, **12**, 442–444.

Mucalo, I., Jovanovski, E., Rahelić, D., Božikov, V., Romić, Z. and Vuksan V. (2013). Effect of American ginseng (*Panax quinquefolius* L.) on arterial stiffness in subjects with type2 diabetes and concomitant hypertension. *Journal of Ethnopharmacology*, **150**, 148–153.

Nagar, H., Choi, S., Jung, S. B., Jeon, B. H. and Kim, C. S. (2016). Rg3-enriched Korean red ginseng enhances blood pressure stability in spontaneously hypertensive rats. *Integrative Medicine Research*, **5**, 223–229.

Newman, D. J. (2017). The influence of Brazilian biodiversity on searching for human use pharmaceuticals. *Journal of the Brazilian Chemical Society*, **28**, 402–414.

Pereira, A. B., Veríssimo, T. M., Oliveira, M. A., Araujo, I. A., Alves, R. J. and Braga, F. C. (2012). Development and validation of an HPLC-DAD method for quantification of bornesitol in extracts from *Hancornia speciosa* leaves after derivatization with *p*-toluenesulfonyl chloride. *Journal of Chromatography B*, **887–888**, 133–137.

Pereira, A. C., Pereira, A. B., Moreira, C. C., Botion, L. M., Lemos, V. S., Braga, F. C. and Cortes S. F. (2015). *Hancornia speciosa* Gomes (Apocynaceae) as a potential anti-diabetic drug. *Journal of Ethnopharmacology*, **161**, 30–35.

Pinto, N. V., Assreuy, A. M., Coelho-de-Souza, A. N., Ceccatto, V. M., Magalhaes, P. J., Lahlou, S. and Leal-Cardoso, J. H. (2009). Endothelium-dependent vasorelaxant effects of the essential oil from aerial parts of *Alpinia zerumbet* and its main constituent 1,8-cineole in rats. *Phytomedicine*, **16**, 1151–1155.

Plotkin, M. J. and Balick, M. J. (1984). Medicinal uses of South American palms. *Journal of Ethnopharmacology*, **10**, 157–179.

Qidwai, W. and Ashfaq, T. (2013). Role of garlic usage in cardiovascular disease prevention: An evidence-based approach. *Evidence-Based Complementary and Alternative Medicine*, **2013**, 125649.

Rahman, K. and Lowe, G. M. (2006). Garlic and cardiovascular disease: A critical review. *Journal of Nutrition*, **136**, 736S–740S.

Rastogi, S., Pandey, M. M. and Rawat, A. K. (2016). Traditional herbs: A remedy for cardiovascular disorders. *Phytomedicine*, **23**, 1082–1089.

Rattmann, Y. D., Anselm, E., Kim, J. H., Dal-Ros, S., Auger, C., Miguel, O. G., Santos, A. R. S., Chataigneau, T. and Schini-Kerth V. B. (2012). Natural product extract of *Dicksonia sellowiana* induces endothelium-dependent relaxations by a redox-sensitive Src- and Akt-dependent activation of eNOS in porcine coronary arteries. *Journal of Vascular Research*, **49**, 284–298.

Rattmann, Y. D., Crestani, S., Lapa, F. R., Miguel, O. G., Marques, M. C. A., da Silva-Santos, J. E. and Santos, A. R. S. (2009). Activation of muscarinic receptors by a hydroalcoholic extract of *Dicksonia sellowiana* Presl. HooK (Dicksoniaceae) induces vascular relaxation and hypotension in rats. *Vascular Pharmacology*, **50**, 27–33.

Rattmann, Y. D., Mendéz-Sánchez, S. C., Furian, A. F., Paludo, K. S., de Souza, L. M., Dartora, N., Oliveira, M. S., et al. (2011). Standardized extract of *Dicksonia sellowiana* Presl. Hook (Dicksoniaceae) decreases oxidative damage in cultured endothelial cells and in rats. *Journal of Ethnopharmacology*, **133**, 999–1007.

Rhee, M. Y., Cho, B., Kim, K. I., Kim, J., Kim, M. K., Lee, E. K., Kim, H. J. and Kim, C. H. (2014). Blood pressure lowering effect of Korea ginseng derived ginseol K-g1. *American Journal of Chinese Medicine*, **42**, 605–618.

Ried, K. (2016). Garlic lowers blood pressure in hypertensive individuals, regulates serum cholesterol, and stimulates immunity: An updated meta-analysis and review. *Journal of Nutrition*, **146**, 389S–396S.

Ried, K. and Fakler, P. (2014). Potential of garlic (*Allium sativum*) in lowering high blood pressure: Mechanisms of action and clinical relevance. *Integrated Blood Pressure Control*, **7**, 71–82.

Ried, K., Frank, O. R. and Stocks, N. P. (2010). Aged garlic extract lowers blood pressure in patients with treated but uncontrolled hypertension: A randomized controlled trial. *Maturitas*, **67**, 144–150.

Ried, K., Frank, O. R., Stocks, N. P., Fakler, P. and Sullivan, T. (2008). Effect of garlic on blood pressure: A systematic review and meta-analysis. *BMC Cardiovascular Disorders*, **8**, 13.

Ried, K., Toben, C. and Fakler, P. (2013). Effect of garlic on serum lipids: An updated meta-analysis. *Nutrition Reviews*, **71**, 282–299.

Rio de Janeiro Botanical Garden. (2015). *Flora do Brasil*. Available from: http://floradobrasil.jbrj.gov.br/.

Rocha, A. P., Carvalho, L. C., Sousa, M. A., Madeira, S. V., Sousa, P. J., Tano, T., Schini-Kerth, V. B., Resende, A. C. and Soares de Moura, R. (2007). Endothelium-dependent vasodilator effect of *Euterpe oleracea* Mart. (Açaí) extracts in mesenteric vascular bed of the rat. *Vascular Pharmacology*, **46**, 97–104.

Rocha, A. P., Resende, A. C., Souza, M.A., Carvalho, L. C., Sousa, P. J., Tano, T., Criddle, D. N., et al. (2008). Antihypertensive effects and antioxidant action of a hydro-alcoholic extract obtained from fruits of *Euterpe oleracea* Mart. (açaí). *Journal of Pharmacology and Toxicology*, **3**, 435–448.

Rodrigues, R. B., Lichtenthäler, R., Zimmermann, B. F., Papagiannopoulos, M., Fabricius, H., Marx, F., Maia, J. G. and Almeida, O. (2006). Total oxidant scavenging capacity of *Euterpe oleracea* Mart. (acai) seeds and identification of their polyphenolic compounds. *Journal of Agricultural and Food Chemistry*, **54**, 4162–4167.

Rodrigues, V. E. G. and Carvalho, D. A. (2001). Levantamento etnobotânico de plantas medicinais no domínio Cerrado na região do Alto Rio Grande—Minas Gerais. *Ciência e Agrotecnologia*, **25**, 102–123.

Santos, U. P., Campos, J. F., Torquato, H. F., Paredes-Gamero, E. J., Carollo, C. A., Estevinho, L. M., de Picoli Souza, K. and dos Santos, E. L. (2016). Antioxidant, antimicrobial and cytotoxic properties as well as the phenolic content of the extract from *Hancornia speciosa* Gomes. *PLoS One*, **11**, e0167531.

Schäfer, G. and Kaschula, C. H. (2014). The immunomodulation and anti-inflammatory effects of garlic organosulfur compounds in cancer chemoprevention. *Anti-Cancer Agents in Medicinal Chemistry*, **4**, 233–240.

Schauss, A. G., Wu, X., Prior, R. L., Ou, B., Huang, D., Owens, J., Agarwal, A., Jensen, G. S., Hart, A. N. and Shanbrom, E. (2006b). Antioxidant capacity and other bioactivities of the freeze-dried Amazonian palm berry, *Euterpe oleraceae* Mart. (açaí). *Journal of Agricultural and Food Chemistry*, **54**, 8604–8610.

Schauss, A. G., Wu, X., Prior, R. L., Ou, B., Patel, D., Huang, D. and Kababick, J. P. (2006a). Phytochemical and nutrient composition of the freeze-dried Amazonian palm berry, *Euterpe oleraceae* Mart. (açaí). *Journal of Agricultural and Food Chemistry*, **54**, 8598–8603.

Schuldt, E. Z., Ckless, K., Simas, M. E., Farias, M. R. and Ribeiro-Do-Valle, R. M. (2000). Butanolic fraction from *Cuphea carthagenensis* Jacq McBride relaxes rat thoracic aorta through endothelium-dependent and endothelium-independent mechanisms. *Journal of Cardiovascular Pharmacology*, **35**, 234–239.

Sendl, A., Elbl, G., Steinke, B., Redl, K., Breu, W. and Wagner, H. (1992). Comparative pharmacological investigations of *Allium ursinum* and *Allium sativum*. *Planta Medica*, **58**, 1–7.

Serra, C .P., Côrtes, S. F., Lombardi, J. A., Braga de Oliveira, A. and Braga, F. C. (2005). Validation of a colorimetric assay for the *in vitro* screening of inhibitors of angiotensin-converting enzyme (ACE) from plant extracts. *Phytomedicine*, **12**, 424–432.

Silva, G. C., Braga, F. C., Lemos, V. S. and Cortes, S. F. (2016). Potent antihypertensive effect of *Hancornia speciosa* leaves extract. *Phytomedicine*, **23**, 214–219.

Silva, G. C., Braga, F. C., Lima, M. P., Pesquero, J. L., Lemos, V. S. and Cortes, S. F. (2011). *Hancornia speciosa* Gomes induces hypotensive effect through inhibition of ACE and increase on NO. *Journal of Ethnopharmacology*, **137**, 709–713

Soares de Moura, R., Emiliano, A. F., de Carvalho, L. C., Souza, M. A., Guedes, D. C., Tano, T. and Resende, A. C. (2005). Antihypertensive and endothelium-dependent vasodilator effects of *Alpinia zerumbet*, a medicinal plant. *Journal of Cardiovascular Pharmacology*, **46**, 288–294.

Stabler, S. N., Tejani, A. M., Huynh, F. and Fowkes, C. (2012). Garlic for the prevention of cardiovascular morbidity and mortality in hypertensive patients. *Cochrane Database of Systematic Reviews*, **8**, CD007653.

Tryon, R. M. and Tryon, A. F. (1982). *Ferns and Allied Plants With Special Reference to Tropical America*. 1st ed. New York: Springer Verlag. pp. 129–133.

Udani, J. K., Singh, B. B., Singh, V. J. and Barrett, M. L. (2011). Effects of açaí (*Euterpe oleracea* Mart.) berry preparation on metabolic parameters in a healthy overweight population: A pilot study. *Nutrition Journal*, **10**, 45.

Ulbricht, C., Brigham, A., Burke, D., Costa, D., Giese, N., Iovin, R., Grimes Serrano, J. M., Tanguay-Colucci, S., Weissner, W. and Windsor, R. (2012). An evidence-based systematic review of açaí (*Euterpe oleracea*) by the Natural Standard Research Collaboration. *Journal of Dietary Supplements*, **9**, 128–147.

US Food and Drug Administration (2018). Dietary Supplements. *U.S. Food and Drug Administration*. Available from: http://www.fda.gov/Food/DietarySupplements.

Valli, G. and Giardina, E. G. (2002). Benefits, adverse effects and drug interactions of herbal therapies with cardiovascular effects. *Journal of the American College of Cardiology*, **39**, 1083–1095.

Vazquez-Prieto, M. A., Rodriguez Lanzi, C., Lembo, C., Galmarini, C. R. and Miatello, R. M. (2011). Garlic and onion attenuates vascular inflammation and oxidative stress in fructose-fed rats. *Journal of Nutrition and Metabolism*, **2011**, 475216.

Verma, S. K., Jain, V., Verma, D. and Khamesra, R. (2007). *Crataegus oxyacantha*—A cardioprotective herb. *Journal of Herbal Medicine and Toxicology*, **1**, 65–71.

Victório, C. P. (2011).Therapeutic value of the genus *Alpinia*, Zingiberaceae. *Revista Brasileira de Farmacognosia*, **21**, 194–201.

Wagner, H. (2011). Synergy research: Approaching a new generation of phytopharmaceuticals. *Fitoterapia*, **82**, 34–37.

Walker, A. F., Marakis, G., Morris, A. P., Robinson, P. A. (2002). Promising hypotensive effect of hawthorn extract: A randomized double-blind pilot study of mild, essential hypertension. *Phytotherapy Research*, **16**, 48–54.

Walker, A. F., Marakis, G., Simpson, E., Hope, J. L., Robinson, P. A., Hassanein, M. and Simpson, H. C. (2006). Hypotensive effects of hawthorn for patients with diabetes taking prescription drugs: A randomised controlled trial. *British Journal of General Practice*, **56**, 437–443.

Wang, H. P., Yang, J., Qin, L. Q. and Yang, X. J. (2015). Effect of garlic on blood pressure: A meta-analysis. *Journal of Clinical Hypertension*, **17**, 223–231.

Wang, J. and Xiong, X. (2012). Outcome measures of Chinese herbal medicine for hypertension: An overview of systematic reviews. *Evidence-Based Complementary and Alternative Medicine*, **2012**, 697237.

Wang, J., Xiong, X. and Feng, B. (2013). Effect of *Crataegus* usage in cardiovascular disease prevention: An evidence-based approach. *Evidence-Based Complementary and Alternative Medicine*, **2013**, 149363.

Wang, X., Ouyang, Y., Liu, J., Zhu, M., Zhao, G., Bao, W. and Hu, F. B. (2014). Fruit and vegetable consumption and mortality from all causes, cardiovascular disease, and cancer: Systematic review and dose-response meta-analysis of prospective cohort studies. *BMJ*, **349**, g4490.

WHO. (2002) Folium cum flore crataegi. In *WHO Monographs on Selected Medicinal Plants*, Vol. 2. World Health Organization, Geneva, Switzerland. pp. 66–82.

WHO. (2008). Traditional medicine. Geneva, Switzerland: World Health Organization. Fact Sheet No. 134.

WHO. (2013). Cardiovascular Diseases (CVDs). Geneva, Switzerland: World Health Organization. Fact sheet No. 317.

Yamaguchi, K. K., Pereira, L. F. R., Lamarão, C. V., Lima, E. S. and da Veiga-Junior, V. F. (2015). Amazon açaí: Chemistry and biological activities: A review. *Food Chemistry*, **179**, 137–151.

18 Role of the Ayurvedic Medicinal Herb *Bacopa monnieri* in Child and Adolescent Populations

James Kean and Con Stough

CONTENTS

18.1 INTRODUCTION

As children develop, parents become increasingly aware of how their child is doing socially, academically, mentally and physically. Children are weighed and measured from birth, with regular updates as to their progress towards what is perceived to be *normal development*. A *disorder* describes the state a person is in that is not in *order* with what is perceived to be normal human functioning. When people speak about *developmental disorders*, it conveys the message that this child has deviated from the typical *order* of mental or physical functioning for a child of that age. In these circumstances, it is natural for a parent to request information regarding the safest and most effective medication available. Regardless of the presence of a disorder, a parent will always look to improve the health and well-being of their child if an opportunity presents itself.

Childhood neurodevelopmental disorders are multifaceted in nature, influenced by biological, psychosocial, genetic and environmental factors, necessitating a multidimensional focus for treatment. There are a number of neurodevelopmental disorders characterised by unique cognitive and behavioural deficits, including attention-deficit/hyperactivity disorder (ADHD), autism spectrum disorder (ASD), learning disorder, dyslexia and intellectual disability. Associated symptoms can lead to problems with early learning, reduced motivation for participation in schoolwork or activities, and delays in cognitive and social development (Hinshaw 1992; Faraone et al. 1993; Greven et al. 2012; Barkley 2014). Although these disorders differ dramatically in the distinction and severity of symptoms, the benefits of treating the common symptoms between them, can have a highly valuable impact for a number of families and for the children in terms of their schooling and overall quality of life.

18.2 HISTORICAL USE OF *BACOPA MONNIERI* IN AYURVEDA

Bacopa monnieri (L) Wettst., or 'Brahmi', from the plant family *Scrophulariaceae*, is a perennial creeping herb that thrives in damp soils and marshes throughout the subcontinent and is classified as a nootropic (i.e. a cognitive enhancer; Stough et al. 2008). Figure 18.1 illustrates the white flowers that blossom on the plant throughout most of the year. Bacopa is used within the Ayurvedic medicinal system as an adaptogenic, a natural medicine that promotes an individual's ability to deal with stress and stress-related situations (Andrade et al. 2000), as well as promoting improved memory, learning ability and concentration (Pole 2013). The chief chemical constituents of the herb are saponins, or more specifically, Bacopa saponins, denoted *bacoside A* and *B* (Singh et al. 1988). Bacoside A can be further broken down into *Bacopasides* A_1, A_2, A_3, A_4 and A_5 (Deepak and Amit 2004).

The Ayurvedic medicinal system is one of the oldest healthcare systems in the world, promoting a holistic view of health (Meulenbeld 2002), utilising the synergistic properties of organic resources and prescribing individualised treatments, rather than the more accepted single target, single treatment management (Verpoorte et al. 2005). Ayurveda is derived from the ancient Sanskrit texts the *Charaka Samhita*, the *Sushruta Samhita* and the *Bhela Samhita*, which date back to sixth century BCE (Meulenbeld 2002). Bacopa is also known as *Brahmi*, a name derived from that of the Hindu god of creation, *Brahma*. Brahma is considered the equivalent of *Prajapati*, the primeval first god, and in earlier texts, Brahma is considered the supreme god in the triad of great Hindu gods that also includes *Shiva* and *Vishnu* (Cartwright 2015). The historical benefits of Bacopa consumption are memorialised by their association with Brahma's creation of the ancient Hindu texts, the four *Vedas*, with *Veda* meaning 'wisdom; knowledge', which is related to *Vid* meaning 'to know' (Lowitz and Datta 2005). The word Brahmi also derives from the term *Brahman*, the Hindu term used for *universal consciousness* and can be directly translated as *the energy* or *Shakti* (Pole 2013).

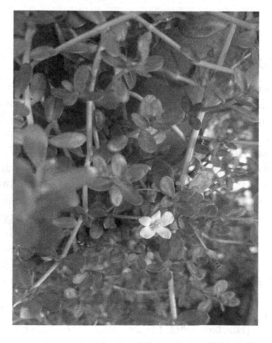

FIGURE 18.1 *Bacopa monnieri* plant with a blossoming white flower.

The use of *Bacopa monnieri* dates back to sixth century CE, with its name mentioned on ancient parchments and touted as a *medhya rasayana*, an intervention for the relief of mental deficiencies (Caldecott 2006). During this era, scholars would consume Bacopa to improve their ability to learn scripture and sacred hymns (Chatterji et al. 1965). While many reports discuss the use of Bacopa as an 'enhancer' of cognition in the healthy, it has also been touted to improve deficits experienced by those with neurological disorders, including Alzheimer's, Parkinson's and childhood disorders such as ADHD (Pole 2013). In these cases, Bacopa *treats* a disorder, bringing the deficient cognitive levels back to within a normal range. This differs from its proposed use as a *cognitive enhancer* in healthy subjects, where it boosts cognitive functioning beyond normal levels. These recent findings have led to an increase in the number of investigations into what it is exactly that Bacopa can do to improve not only cognitive functioning, but enhance mood, reduce stress and attenuate deficiencies in those experiencing age-related cognitive decline.

The holistic approach of the Ayurvedic medicinal system utilises the unique benefits of multiple extracts in polyherbal formulations. Bacopa is commonly used in these formulations to treat child and adolescent developmental disorders by encouraging a positive synergistic effect greater than that provided by any of the individual treatments alone. Polyherbal research in child and adolescent populations is an area of study requiring increased examination to ensure the benefits and risks of every vitamin, plant extract and natural compound have been adequately assessed in stringently controlled clinical trials (Kean et al. 2017). Despite the aura of safety associated with the natural medicinal world, the unrestrained use of supplements, not to mention the combination of these supplements, may pose health risks unforeseen by Ayurvedic practitioners. In a recent review investigating the effects of Bacopa-dominant polyherbal preparations, the authors reported significant improvements in various symptoms associated with clinical and non-clinical functioning (Kean et al. 2017). These studies highlight the efficacy of Ayurvedic medicinal system practices when treating this population and are listed in Table 18.1, however, the authors are keen to point out the inconsistencies with which many of these previous studies have been designed and executed.

18.3 PRECLINICAL RESEARCH INTO *BACOPA MONNIERI* (L) WETTST.

Preclinical research has been able to establish the efficacy of Bacopa in improving the learning, memory and memory retention of rats (Malhotra and Das 1959; Singh et al. 1988; Singh and Dhawan 1997). In an extension to these findings, preclinical research demonstrated various central nervous system (CNS) actions of Bacopa, including antioxidant (Bhattacharya et al. 2000), antidepressant (Sairam et al. 2002) and nootropic (Hota et al. 2009b) effects.

The active components in Bacopa, seen in Figure 18.2a and b, responsible for the increases seen in cognitive functioning are called *bacosides A* and *B* (Vishwakarma et al. 2016). Bacopa also contains alkaloids, saponins and sterols that contribute to its pharmacological effects. *In vivo* studies have examined extracts containing only these bacosides and similar significant improvements in the areas of memory and learning were found (Singh et al. 1988).

Work investigating Bacopa's neurological mechanisms demonstrate beta amyloid scavenging activities (Holcomb et al. 2006), protection against beta amyloid–induced cell death (Limpeanchob et al. 2008), modulation of fronto-cortical and hippocampal acetylcholine levels (Bhattacharya et al. 1999) and modulation of cholinergic neuron densities (Uabundit et al. 2010). The particular findings have facilitated the development of working dementia models to investigate the plausibility of Bacopa as an intervention in Alzheimer's and age-related cognitive decline (Morgan and Stevens 2010).

TABLE 18.1
Significant Effects of Polyherbal Formulations with Bacopa in Children and Adolescents

Author	Intervention	Design	Population	Results	True Cognitive Abilities
D'souza and Chavda (1991)	Mentat (BM: 144–288 mg/d)	Randomised Double-Blind Placebo Controlled	3–16 yrs Behavioural problems	Hyperactivity (ES: 6.55) Tractability (ES: 5.57) Habituation (ES: 5.20) Negative effects (ES: 4.31) Social (ES: 4.88) Academia (ES: 3.52) Impulsivity (ES: 5.10)	Language behaviour* Learning* Hyperactivity* Impulsivity* Attention* Peer relations*
Patel (1991)	Mentat (BM: 288 mg/d)	Randomised Double-Blind Placebo Controlled	2–7 yrs (approx.) Hyperkinesis	N/A	N/A
Dave et al. (1993a, 1993b)	Mentat (BM: 864 mg/d)	Randomised Double-Blind Placebo Controlled	1–18 yrs Mental retardation	Behaviour (ES: 5.77)	Reasoning* Hyperactivity* Peer relations* Aggression*
Quadri (1993)	Mentat (BM: 272–544 mg/d)	Randomised Double-Blind Placebo Controlled	4–12 yrs Mental retardation; Behavioural issues	N/A	N/A
Kalra et al. (2002)	Mentat (BM: 272 mg/d)	Randomised Double-Blind Placebo Controlled	6–12 yrs ADHD diagnosed	N/A	N/A

(Continued)

TABLE 18.1 (*Continued*)
Significant Effects of Polyherbal Formulations with Bacopa in Children and Adolescents

Author	Intervention	Design	Population	Results	True Cognitive Abilities
Upadhyay et al. (2002)	Mentat tablet or syrup (BM: Unknown)	Randomised Double-Blind Placebo Controlled	11–16 yrs Learning disability	Mentat Tablet: Coding (TES: 1.48) Sequential (TES: 1.77) Full-scale I.Q. (TES: 0.94) Arithmetic (TES: 1.41) Digit span (TES: 1.14) Mentat Syrup: Coding (TES: 1.95) Sequential (TES: 2.45) Full-scale I.Q. (TES: 1.78) Performance I.Q. (TES: 1.40) Arithmetic (TES: 2.39) Digit span (TES: 1.52)	Number facility[b] Mental speed[b]
Ojha (2007)	Manas Niyamak yoga granule (BM: 200 mg/kg/d)	Randomised Double-Blind Placebo Controlled	6–15 yrs ADHD diagnosed	Attention (TES: 1.96) Reaction time (TES: 3.73)	Visual perception[b] Hyperactivity[b] Impulsivity[a] Attention[a]
Katz et al. (2010)	Compound herbal preparation (BM: Unknown)	Randomised Double-Blind Placebo Controlled	6–12 yrs ADHD diagnosed	Response time (ES: 0.70) Variability (ES: 1.02) Overall (ES: 1.11)	Visual perception[**] Impulsivity[**] Attention[**]

(Continued)

TABLE 18.1 (*Continued*)

Significant Effects of Polyherbal Formulations with Bacopa in Children and Adolescents

Author	Intervention	Design	Population	Results	True Cognitive Abilities
Dutta et al. (2012)	Memomet (BM: 250 mg/d)	Randomised Double-Blind Placebo Controlled	6–12 yrs ADHD diagnosed	MISIC (ES: 0.90) CPRS (ES: 0.86)	Reasoning* Language behaviour* Number facility* Mental speed* Free recall* Associative memory* Auditory memory*

a   Significant treatment effect at *p* < 0.05 level.

b   Significant treatment effect at *p* < 0.01 level.

*   Significant at *p* < 0.05 level over placebo.

**   Significant at *p* < 0.01 level over placebo.

ADHD – attention-deficit/hyperactivity disorder; BM – *Bacopa monnieri*; ES – Cohen's d effect size (versus placebo); mg/d – milligrams per day; mg/kg/d – milligrams per kilogram per day; TES – treatment effect size (change from baseline); WISC – Wechsler's Intelligence Scale for Children; yrs – years.

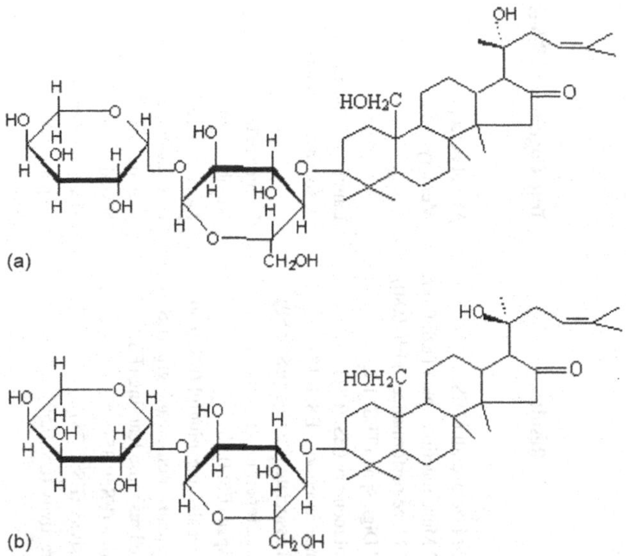

FIGURE 18.2 (a) Bacoside A (Levorotatory). (b) Bacoside B (Dextrorotatory). (From Bacopin, Chemical Constituents, Vishwakarma, Kumari and Khan 2016.)

18.4 MODERN USE OF *BACOPA MONNIERI* (L) WETTST.

Bacopa has a history of improving mental functions in clinical and non-clinical populations. Preclinical work was able to establish the efficacy of *Bacopa monnieri* in improving cognitive deficits or enhancing normal cognitive capabilities (Malhotra and Das 1959; Singh and Dhawan 1997; Hota et al. 2009a). Using randomised, double-blind, placebo-controlled chronic intervention trials, significant improvements in various cognitive functions have been reported. In a recent review, it was reported in nine of seventeen RCT studies that Bacopa significantly improved *free recall* in healthy adults consuming Bacopa (Pase et al. 2012). This supports the Ayurvedic idea that Bacopa functions as a *memory tonic*, enabling the user to improve recall characteristics of their memory.

18.5 NOOTROPIC AND ADAPTOGENIC EVIDENCE FOR *BACOPA MONNIERI* IN HEALTHY ADULT POPULATIONS

As the historical use of Bacopa has indicated improvements in memory, cognition and mood, most of the more recent research has investigated its effects upon specific components of cognition. Observations from acute studies have shown mixed results, with some indicating positive cognitive and mood outcomes at the standard adult dose (320 mg per day; Downey et al. 2013; Benson et al. 2014), whereas others reported no effects of treatment on cognitive performance (Nathan et al. 2001). Given the mixed results of acute studies, the majority of research has focused on chronic administration with an average administration period of 12 weeks (Pase et al. 2012). Stough et al. (2001) investigated the effects of an extract of the herb on cognitive outcomes in a sample of 46 healthy adults (mean age 39 years). The study reported that participants consuming 320 mg of *Bacopa monnieri* per day for 12 weeks showed significantly improved *mental speed* and *free recall* (Stough et al. 2001). In 2008, Stough and colleagues published further results reporting improvements in *visual perception* in a sample of 107 healthy adults (mean age 43 years) consuming the same extract and dose as previously (Stough et al. 2008). In an RCT, Roodenrys et al. (2002) reported significant improvements in memory retention and a reduced rate of forgetting in 76 healthy adults. Morgan and Stevens (2010) recruited a sample (*n* = 98) of healthy older adults (>55 years) reporting significant improvements in tests of *free recall* in those consuming Bacopa over those taking the placebo. Finally, Barbhaiya et al. (2008) and Calabrese et al. (2008) ran chronic

TABLE 18.2

Benefits of Bacopa in Children and Adolescents Across Cognitive, Behavioural and Intelligence

Author	Intervention	Design	Population	Results	True Cognitive Abilities
		Single Extract Studies			
Sharma et al. (1987)	Bacopa syrup (BM: 1050 mg/d)	Open-label Placebo controlled	6–8 yrs Healthy	WISC Maze overall (TES: 1.43) WISC Maze reaction time (TES: 0.66) WISC Maze performance (TES: 0.80) WISC Digit span (TES: 1.13)	Visual perception[a] Memory span[b]
Negi et al. (2000)	MemoryPlus (BM: 100mg/d)	Randomised Double-blind Placebo controlled	6–12 yrs ADHD diagnosed	Logical memory (ES: 0.81) Sentence repetition (ES: 0.13) Paired associate learning (ES: 0.50)	Language behaviour[**] Associative memory[**]
Asthana et al. (2001)	Standardized *Bacopa monnieri* extract (BM: 100 mg/d)	Randomised Double-blind Placebo controlled	6–12 yrs ADHD diagnosed	Sentence repetition (ES: 0.45) Digit span (ES: 0.28) Word recall – meaningful (ES: 0.36) Word recall – non-meaningful (ES: 0.43) Delayed response learning (ES: 0.27) Attention (ES: 0.35) Impulsivity (ES: 0.78) Hyperactivity (ES: 0.59)	Language behaviour[***] Number facility[**] Mental speed[***] Free recall memory[**] Memory span[***] Visual memory[*] Meaningful memory[**] Hyperactivity[***] Attention[***]

(Continued)

TABLE 18.2 (*Continued*)

Benefits of Bacopa in Children and Adolescents Across Cognitive, Behavioural and Intelligence

Author	Intervention	Design	Population	Results	True Cognitive Abilities
		Single Extract Studies			
Dave et al. (2008)	Bacomind (BM: 225 mg/d)	Open label	4–18 yrs I.Q. 70–90	Digit span Repeating words Visual reproduction Repeating sentences	Language behaviour[a] Mental speed[a] Visual memory[a] Auditory memory[a] Meaningful memory[a]
Dave et al. (2014)	Bacomind (BM: 225 mg/d)	Open label	6–12 yrs ADHD diagnosed	Restlessness Impulsivity Attention-Deficit Self-control Psychiatric problems Learning problems	Hyperactivity[a] Impulsivity[a] Attention[a] Learning[a]

Source: Kean, J. D. et al., *Medicines*, 4, 86, 2017.

[a] Significant treatment effect at *p* < 0.05 level.

[b] Significant treatment effect at *p* < 0.01 level.

* Significant at *p* < 0.05 level over placebo.

** Significant at *p* < 0.01 level over placebo.

***Significant at *p* < 0.001 level over placebo.

ADHD – attention-deficit/hyperactivity disorder; BM – *Bacopa monnieri*; ES – Cohen's d effect size (versus placebo); mg/d – milligrams per day; I.Q. – intelligence quotient; TES – treatment effect size (change from baseline); WISC – Wechsler's intelligence scale for children; yrs – years.

Bacopa intervention studies on older adults (65 years+). Calabrese et al. (2008) reported improvements in *visual perception* and *free recall* ($n = 54$), whereas Barbhaiya et al. (2008) reported improvements in *associative memory, memory span* and also, *free recall* ($n = 65$). The consistency in the results highlights the efficacy of Bacopa in this population upon cognitive outcomes. With outcomes demonstrating improvements in memory-related functioning in older populations, these results indicate a promising future for Alzheimer's and dementia-related research.

Bacopa is also considered an *anxiolytic*, in that it ameliorates feelings of anxiety and associated symptoms (Gohil and Patel 2010). In a preclinical trial, an extract of Bacopa demonstrated similar levels of anxiolytic activity to the benzodiazepine *lorazepam* (Bhattacharya and Ghosal 1998). However, where lorazepam induced episodes of amnesia, Bacopa demonstrated memory enhancement while also reducing symptoms of anxiety. Sairam et al. (2002) described a significant antidepressant activity of Bacoside A extract in a rat model similar to the levels seen in studies of *imipramine*, a widely used tricyclic antidepressant.

In humans, the anxiolytic effects of Bacopa have shown mixed results. Stough et al. (2001) reported significant reductions in anxious states, a finding that was replicated by Calabrese et al. (2008), who reported a decrease in depression as well as combined state-trait anxiety scores in a sample of older adults (mean age 73.5 years). A trend towards significance was reported on mood measures in a dose-range study by Benson et al. (2014) in 17 healthy adult volunteers, which also demonstrated some adaptogenic factors. An adaptogen is defined as a non-toxic herbal medicine that increases a person's resistance to anxiety and stress (EMEA 2008). A follow-up study by Stough et al. (2008) was unable to replicate their findings and a study by Roodenrys et al. (2002) reported no significant improvements in symptoms of anxiety in healthy adults. Despite these findings, the significance of the cognitive results may encourage healthy adults or adults with some memory impairment to begin treating themselves with Bacopa. In doing this, people may experience improvements in anxiety and stress. Whether this is related to the improved cognitive outcomes or is a secondary benefit of the herbal medicine has not yet been verified by the literature.

18.6 NOOTROPIC EVIDENCE FOR *BACOPA MONNIERI* IN CHILD AND ADOLESCENT POPULATIONS

It is a difficult thing to investigate the benefits of a relatively novel medication in a vulnerable population. The increased level of ethical scrutiny coupled with the complex nature of developmental psychology and neuroscience, means that many complementary and alternative medicine research investigations are restricted in their design and overall application. In clinical populations, the restrictive nature of the research can be even more stringent. In recent clinical settings, Bacopa has demonstrated improvements in attention, cognition, intelligence and behaviour in children diagnosed with attention-deficit/hyperactivity disorder (ADHD). These findings potentiate the use of Bacopa as an alternative treatment for ADHD and other developmental disorders with similar symptomology (Kalra et al. 2002; Katz et al. 2010; Dutta et al. 2012; Bhalerao et al. 2013). The research discussed here has demonstrated that chronic intervention with Bacopa has yielded consistent efficacy in terms of cognitive benefits (Stough et al. 2001, 2008; Roodenrys et al. 2002; Barbhaiya et al. 2008; Calabrese et al. 2008; Morgan and Stevens 2010; Mandal et al. 2011), as well as having anxiolytic capabilities (Bhattacharya et al. 2000; Russo et al. 2003; Dhanasekaran et al. 2007; Kapoor et al. 2009). Yet despite these encouraging results in healthy adults (Stough et al. 2001, 2008; Nathan et al. 2004; Morgan and Stevens 2010; Pase et al. 2012; Downey et al. 2013), very little research has focused on the efficacy of Bacopa within child and adolescent populations in acute or chronic settings.

A recent systematic review provided some of the first evidence for the use of Bacopa in clinical and non-clinical child and adolescent populations (Kean et al. 2016). The review outcomes support previous findings that *Bacopa monnieri* improves elements of human cognition (Stough et al. 2001, 2008; Nathan et al. 2004; Morgan and Stevens 2010; Pase et al. 2012; Downey et al. 2013).

The research corroborated the outcomes from adult studies and has been listed in Table 18.2, with multiple extracts providing similar improvements across various cognitive domains (Sharma et al. 1987; Negi et al. 2000; Asthana et al. 2001; Dave et al. 2008).

In 1987, Sharma, Chaturvedi and Tewari conducted the first clinical trial investigating a Bacopa extract in a sample population of healthy children. The team were investigating a 3-month intervention using a powdered form of Bacopa (350 mg per teaspoonful) compared to placebo in a group of school-aged children ($N = 40$; mean age 6.25 years). Significant outcomes were reported for overall score, reaction time and performance on the Wechsler's Intelligence Scale for Children (WISC) *Maze* as well as the *Digit Span Test* (Wechsler 1949). Improved scores on the Maze task highlight an increase in the child's ability to plan ahead and were associated with better visuomotor and perceptual capabilities. Better scores on the digit span test demonstrate improvements in short-term memory and increased attention and focus (Nicholson and Alcorn 1993). Further testing included the *Raven's Coloured Progressive Matrices* (RCPM; Raven 1958) and the *Bender Gestalt for Children* (BGTC; Koppitz 1960, 1964), but the researchers did not report any further significant findings. Despite these findings, the results here are derived from *change-from-baseline* analysis, which may reduce the significance of the findings in the context of the studies that followed using between-group statistical analysis.

In 2000 and 2001, two studies investigated Bacopa extracts providing the same amount of Bacopa to their respective participants per day (Negi et al. 2000; Asthana et al. 2001). Both studies investigated the efficacy of Bacopa upon the symptoms of attention-deficit/hyperactivity disorder (ADHD) using tests of memory and behavioural rating scales. Both studies reported significant sustained improvements in language behaviour, free recall memory and visual recall. These domains are associated with improvements in a child's vocabulary, spelling and auditory processing and comprehension, as well as various aspects of memory recall. The results here demonstrate the consistency in cognitive outcomes when research designs and extracts are uniform.

18.7 EVIDENCE FOR THE SAFETY AND TOLERABILITY OF *BACOPA MONNIERI* IN CHILD AND ADOLESCENT POPULATIONS

The complexity of conducting a clinical trial among children and adolescents stems from the ability of the research team to monitor and capture any adverse events that may occur to inform the scientific community of the possible dangers associated with the drug being investigated. In Table 18.3, each study to investigate a single extract of Bacopa and a polyherbal extract including Bacopa has been revisited with every side effect and adverse event outlined. In most of the included studies the authors were careful to monitor for any adverse events reported by participants. In one single-extract study, reports of abdominal pain and stomach were reported in a single participant who continued the study thereafter (Asthana et al. 2001). The same side effects were reported in another trial, in which side effects included stomach upset and vomiting in three participants, all of whom continued their participation once the symptoms ceased (Dave et al. 2008). All other trials reported no side effects of the treatment (Negi et al. 2000; Dave et al. 2014), with one study failing to declare any recorded safety measures or side effects (Sharma et al. 1987). Due to the limited number of studies, it is problematic to gauge the outright safety of *Bacopa monnieri* in the population of children and adolescents; however, each study that reported adverse events for the drug reported mild gastric upset, which is consistent with adult studies (Stough et al. 2008; Morgan and Stevens 2010). In the single-extract studies, there was an average dropout rate of 13% among the studies. This was similar in the polyherbal studies, with an average dropout rate of 9.89% among studies. Two studies from the polyherbal group failed to report any dropouts (D'souza and Chavda 1991; Patel 1991). Side effects associated with the polyherbal formulas followed similar patterns, with participants reporting stomach upset (Dave et al. 1993a,b) and some participants reporting changes in diet (Negi et al. 2000; Asthana et al. 2001). Four studies from the polyherbal group failed to report any information

TABLE 18.3

Safety and Tolerability of Bacopa in Children and Adolescents

Author	Intervention	Population	Side Effects	Safety and Tolerability
		Single-Extract Studies		
Sharma et al. (1987)	Bacopa Syrup (BM: 1050 mg/d)	6–8 yrs Healthy	Not reported	Unknown
Negi et al. (2000)	MemoryPlus (BM: 100 mg/d)	6–12 yrs ADHD diagnosed	None	Appears safe and tolerable. Reported increased appetite in active treatment group
CDRI Lucknow (2001)	Standardized *Bacopa monnieri* Extract (BM: 100 mg/d)	6–12 yrs ADHD diagnosed	None	Appears safe and tolerable. Reported increased appetite in active treatment group
Dave et al. (2008)	Bacomind (BM: 225 mg/d)	4–18 yrs I.Q. 70–90	Mild	Appears safe and mostly tolerable. Nausea and vomiting in three participants. All continued the study
Dave et al. (2014)	Bacomind (BM: 225 mg/d)	6–12 yrs ADHD diagnosed	Mild	Appears mostly safe and tolerable. Diarrhoea reported in two children. Neither continued the study
		Polyherbal Studies		
D'souza and Chavda (1991)	Mentat (BM: 144–288 mg/d)	3–16 yrs Behavioural problems	Not reported	Unknown
Patel (1991)	Mentat (BM: 288 mg/d)	Unknown	None	Appears safe and tolerable
Dave et al. (1993a, 1993b)	Mentat (BM: 864 mg/d)	1–18 yrs Mental retardation	Not reported	Unknown
Quadri (1993)	Mentat (BM: 272–544 mg/d)	4–12 yrs Mental retardation Behavioural issues	None	Appears safe and tolerable
Kalra et al. (2002)	Mentat (BM: 272 mg/d)	6–12 yrs ADHD diagnosed	Not reported	Unknown
Upadhyay et al. (2002)	Mentat tablet or syrup (BM: Unknown)	11–16 yrs Learning disability	Not reported	Unknown
Ojha (2007)	Manas Niyamak Yoga Granule (BM: 200 mg/kg/d)	6–15 yrs ADHD diagnosed	None	Appears safe and tolerable
Katz et al. (2010)	Compound Herbal Preparation (BM: Unknown)	6–12 yrs ADHD diagnosed	Mild	Appears safe and tolerable. All adverse events were considered mild. No difference between treatment groups
Dutta et al. (2012)	Memomet (BM: 250 mg/d)	6–12 yrs ADHD diagnosed	None	Appears safe and tolerable

Source: Kean, J.D. et al., *Complement. Ther. Med.*, 29, 56–62, 2016; Kean, J.D. et al., *Medicines*, 4, 86, 2017.

regarding the presence or absence of side effects (D'souza and Chavda 1991; Dave et al. 1993b; Kalra et al. 2002; Upadhyay et al. 2002). Research in this area requires complete transparency, particularly in such a vulnerable population. Without it, clinicians and other researchers cannot be confident in its safe use to treat clinical and non-clinical populations.

Overall, the extracts investigated appear to be safe and tolerable among child and adolescent populations in both clinical and non-clinical settings.

18.8 CONCLUSION

The current evidence indicates that chronic use of Bacopa may provide significant benefits to cognitive outcomes associated with memory in child and adolescent populations. Despite the significance of these outcomes, the studies discussed are not wholly homogenous. Differing doses as well as cultivation and harvesting practices make direct comparisons between the studies complicated. The key component *Bacoside A* differs in quantity between extracts, highlighting the fact that variances in cognitive outcomes may be linked to the quality of the extract being investigated. Regardless of the extract used, the key findings indicate that *Bacopa monnieri* is efficacious in terms of cognitive outcomes. In future research, the consistency with which the plant is grown, harvested and extracted will be of vital importance if the herb is to be considered a legitimate alternative for modern pharmaceutical interventions.

REFERENCES

Andrade, C., Aswath, A., Chaturvedi, S. K., Srinivasa, M. and Raguram, R. (2000). A double-blind, placebo-controlled evaluation of the anxiolytic efficacy of an ethanolic extract of withania somnifera. *Indian Journal of Psychiatry*, **42**(3), 295–301.

Asthana, O. P., Srivastava, J. S., Gupta, R. C., Negi, K. S., Jauhari, N., Singh, Y. D., et al. (2001). *Clinical Evaluation of Bacopa monniera Extract on Behavioural and Cognitive Functions in Children Suffering from Attention Deficit Hyperactivity Disorder*. Varanasi, India: Central Drug Research Institute (CDRI). Unpublished.

Bacopin. (2001). Chemical Constituents. Retrieved from http://bacopin.com/chemical.htm

Barbhaiya, H. C., Desai, R. P., Saxena, V. S., Pravina, K., Wasim, P., Geetharani, P., et al. (2008). Efficacy and tolerability of BacoMind® on memory improvement in elderly participants – A double blind placebo controlled study. *Journal of Pharmacology and Toxicology*, **3**(6), 425–434.

Barkley, R. A. (2014). *Attention-Deficit Hyperactivity Disorder: A Handbook for Diagnosis and Treatment*. New York: Guilford Publications.

Benson, S., Downey, L. A., Stough, C., Wetherell, M., Zangara, A. and Scholey, A. (2014). An acute, double-blind, placebo-controlled cross-over study of 320 mg and 640 mg doses of *Bacopa monnieri* (CDRI 08) on multitasking stress reactivity and mood. *Phytotherapy Research*, **28**(4), 551-559. doi:10.1002/ptr.5029

Bhalerao, S., Munshi, R., Nesari, T. and Shah, H. (2013). Evaluation of Brāhmī ghṛtam in children suffering from Attention Deficit Hyperactivity Disorder (Study I). *Ancient Science of Life*, **33**(2), 123–130. doi:10.4103/0257-7941.139057.

Bhattacharya, S. K., Bhattacharya, A., Kumar, A. and Ghosal, S. (2000). Antioxidant activity of *Bacopa monniera* in rat frontal cortex, striatum and hippocampus. *Phytotherapy Research*, **14**, 174–179.

Bhattacharya, S. K. and Ghosal, S. (1998). Anxiolytic activity of a standardized extract of *Bacopa monniera*: An experimental study. *Phytomedicine*, **5**(2), 77–82.

Bhattacharya, S. K., Kumar, A. and Ghosal, S. (1999). Effect of *Bacopa monniera* on animal models of Alzheimer's disease and perturbed central cholinergic markers of cognition in rats. *Research Communications in Pharmacology and Toxicology*, **4**(3&4), 1–12.

Calabrese, C., Gregory, W. L., Leo, M., Kraemer, D., Bone, K. and Oken, B. (2008). Effects of a standardized *Bacopa monnieri* extract on cognitive performance, anxiety, and depression in the elderly: A randomized, double-blind, placebo-controlled trial. *Journal of Alternative and Complementary Medicine*, **14**(6), 707–713.

Caldecott, T. (2006). "Brahmi". *Ayurveda: The Divine Science of Life*. Philadelphia, PA: Elsevier/Mosby.

Cartwright, M. (2015). Brahma. *Ancient History Encyclopedia*. Retrieved from https://www.ancient.eu/Brahma/ [Accessed 4 March 2018].

Chatterji, N., Rastogi, R. P. and Dhar, M. L. (1965). Chemical examination of *Bacopa monniera* Wettst: Part II—Isolation of chemical constituents. *Indian Journal Chemistry*, **3**, 24–29.

D'souza, B. D. and Chavda, K. B. (1991). Mentat in hyperactivity and attention deficiency disorders – A double-blind, placebo-controlled study. *Probe*, **3**, 227–232.

Dave, U., Chauvan, V. and Dalvi, J. (1993a). Evaluation of BR-16 A (Mentat) in cognitive and behavioural dysfunction of mentally retarded children a placebo-controlled study (Study I). *Indian Journal of Pediatrics*, **60**, 423–428.

Dave, U., Chauvan, V. and Dalvi, J. (1993b). Evaluation of BR-16 A (Mentat) in cognitive and behavioural dysfunction of mentally retarded children a placebo-controlled study (Study II). *Indian Journal of Pediatrics*, **60**, 423–428.

Dave, U. P., Dingankar, S. R., Saxena, V. S., Joseph, J. A., Bethapudi, B., Agarwal, A. and Kudiganti, V. (2014). An open-label study to elucidate the effects of standardized *Bacopa monnieri* extract in the management of symptoms of attention-deficit hyperactivity disorder in children. *Advances in Mind-Body Medicine*, **28**(2), 10–15.

Dave, U. P., Wasim, P., Joshua, J., Geetharani, P., Murali, B., Mayachari, A. et al. (2008). BacoMind®: A cognitive enhancer in children requiring individual education programme. *Journal of Pharmacology and Toxicology*, **3**(4), 302–310.

Deepak, M. and Amit, A. (2004). The need for establishing identities of 'bacoside A and B', the putative major bioactive saponins of Indian medicinal plant *Bacopa monnieri*. *Phytomedicine*, **11**, 264–268.

Dhanasekaran, M., Tharakan, B. and Holcomb, L. A. (2007). Neuroprotective mechanisms of Ayurvedic antidementia botanical *Bacopa monniera*. *Phytotherapy Research*, **21**, 965–969.

Downey, L. A., Kean, J., Nemeh, F., Lau, A., Poll, A., Gregory, R. et al. (2013). An acute, double-blind, placebo-controlled crossover study of 320 mg and 640 mg doses of a special extract of *Bacopa monnieri* (CDRI 08) on sustained cognitive performance. *Phytotherapy Research*, **27**(9), 1407–1413. doi:10.1002/ptr.4864.

Dutta, B., Barua, T. K., Ray, J., Adhikari, A., Biswas, S., Banerjee, S. et al. (2012). A study of evaluation of safety and efficacy of memomet, a multi herbal formulation (memomet) in the treatment of behavioural disorder in children. *International Journal of Research in Pharmaceutical Sciences*, **3**(2), 282–286.

EMEA, E. M. A. (2008). *Committee on Herbal Medicinal Products (HMPC): Reflection Paper on the Adaptogenic Concept*. Retrieved from http://www.ema.europa.eu/docs/en_GB/document_library/Scientific_guideline/2009/09/WC500003646.pdf

Faraone, S. V., Biederman, J., Lehman, B. K., Spencer, T., Norman, D., Seidman, L. J. et al. (1993). Intellectual performance and school failure in children with attention deficit hyperactivity disorder and in their siblings. *Journal of Abnormal Psychology*, **102**(4), 616–623.

Gohil, K. J. and Patel, J. J. (2010). A review on *Bacopa monniera*: Current research and future prospects. *International Journal of Green Pharmacy*, **4**(1), 1–9.

Greven, C. U., Rijsdijk, F. V., Asherson, P. and Plomin, R. (2012). A longitudinal twin study on the association between ADHD symptoms and reading. *Journal of Child Psychology and Psychiatry*, **53**(3), 234–242. doi:10.1111/j.1469-7610.2011.02445.x.

Hinshaw, S. P. (1992). Academic underachievement, attention deficits, and aggression: Comorbidity and implications for intervention. *Journal of Consulting and Clinical Psychology*, **60**(6), 893.

Holcomb, L. A., Dhanasekaran, M. and Hitt, A. R. (2006). *Bacopa monniera* extract reduces amyloid levels in PSAPP mice. *Journal of Alzheimer's Disease*, **9**, 243–251.

Hota, S. K., Barhwal, K. and Baitharu, I. (2009a). *Bacopa monniera* leaf extract ameliorates hypobaric hypoxia induced spatial memory impairment. *Neurobiology of Disease*, **34**, 23–39.

Hota, S. K., Barhwal, K., Baitharu, I., Prasad, D., Singh, S. B. and Ilavazhagan, G. (2009b). *Bacopa monniera* leaf extract ameliorates hypobaric hypoxia induced spatial memory impairment. *Neurobiology of Disease*, **34**(1), 23–39. doi:10.1016/j.nbd.2008.12.006.

Kalra, V., Zamir, H., Pandey, R. M. and Kulkarni, K. S. (2002). A randomized double blind placebo-controlled drug trial with Mentat in children with attention deficit hyperactivity disorder. *Neuroscience Today*, **6**(4), 223–227.

Kapoor, R., Srivastava, S. and Kakkar, P. (2009). *Bacopa monnieri* modulates antioxidant responses in brain and kidney of diabetic rats. *Environmental Toxicology and Pharmacology*, **27**(1), 62–69. doi:10.1016/j.etap.2008.08.007.

Katz, M., Levine, A. A., Kol-Degani, H. and Kav-Venaki, L. (2010). A compound herbal preparation (CHP) in the treatment of children with ADHD: A randomized controlled trial. *Journal of Attention Disorders*, **14**(3), 281–291.

Kean, J. D., Downey, L. and Stough, C. (2016). A systematic review of the Ayurvedic medicinal herb *Bacopa monnieri* in child and adolescent populations. *Complementary Therapies in Medicine*, **29**, 56–62. doi:10.1016/j.ctim.2016.09.002.

Kean, J. D., Downey, L. and Stough, C. (2017). Systematic overview of *Bacopa monnieri* (L.) Wettst. dominant poly-herbal formulas in children and adolescents. *Medicines*, **4**(4), 86.

Koppitz, E. M. (1960). The Bender Gestalt Test for children: A normative study. *Journal of Clinical Psychology*, **16**(4), 432–435. doi:10.1002/1097-4679(196010)16:4<432::AID-JCLP2270160431>3.0.CO;2-E.

Koppitz, E. M. (1964). *The Bender Gestalt Test for Young Children*. New York: Grune and Stratton.

Limpeanchob, N., Jaipan, S. and Rattanakaruna, S. (2008). Neuroprotective effect of *Bacopa monnieri* on beta-amyloid-induced cell death in primary cortical culture. *Journal of Ethnopharmacology*, **120**, 112–117.

Lowitz, L. and Datta, R. (2005). *Sacred Sanskrit Words*. Berkeley, CA: Stone Bridge Press.

Malhotra, C. L. and Das, P. K. (1959). Pharmacological studies of *Herpestis monniera*, Linn., (Brahmi). *Indian Journal of Medical Research*, **47**(3), 294–305.

Mandal, A. K., Hedge, S. and Patki, P. S. (2011). A clinical study to evaluate the efficacy and safety of 'Bacopa' caplets in memory and learning ability: A double blind placebo controlled study. *Australian Journal of Medical Herbalism*, **23**(3), 122–125.

Meulenbeld, G. J. (2002). *A History of Indian Medical Literature*. Leiden, the Netherlands: Koninklijke Brill NV.

Morgan, A. and Stevens, J. (2010). Does *Bacopa monnieri* improve memory performance in older persons? Results of a randomized, placebo-controlled, double-blind trial. *Journal of Alternative and Complementary Medicine*, **16**(7), 753–759.

Nathan, P. J., Clarke, J., Lloyd, J., Hutchison, C. W., Downey, L. and Stough, C. (2001). The acute effects of an extract of *Bacopa monniera* (Brahmi) on cognitive function in healthy normal subjects. *Human Psychopharmacology*, **16**(4), 345–351.

Nathan, P. J., Tanner, S., Lloyd, J., Harrison, B., Curran, L., Oliver, C. and Stough, C. (2004). Effects of a combined extract of Ginkgo biloba and *Bacopa monniera* on cognitive function in healthy humans. *Human Psychopharmacology*, **19**(2), 91–96.

Negi, K., Singh, Y., Kushwaha, K., Rastogi, C., Rathi, A., Srivastava, J. et al. (2000). Clinical evaluation of memory enhancing properties of Memory Plus in children with attention deficit hyperactivity disorder. *Indian Journal of Psychiatry*, **42**(suppl. 2), 4.

Nicholson, C. L. and Alcorn, C. L. (1993). Interpretation of the WISC-III and its subtests. *Presentation at the Annual Meeting of the National Association of School Psychologists*, Washington, DC.

Ojha, N. K., Kumar, A. and Rai, M. (2007). Clinical study on the role of an ayurvedic compound (manas niyamak yoga) and shirodhara in the management of adhd in children. *Journal of Ayurveda*, **1**, 39–47.

Pase, M., Kean, J., Sarris, J., Neale, C., Scholey, A. and Stough, C. (2012). The cognitive-enhancing effects of *Bacopa monnieri*: A systematic review of randomized, controlled human clinical trials. *Journal of Alternative and Complementary Medicine*, **18**(7), 647–652. doi:10.1089/acm.2011.0367.

Patel, R. B. (1991). Experience with Mentat in hyperkinetic children. *Probe*, **3**, 271.

Pole, S. (2013). *Ayurvedic Medicine: The Principles of Traditional Practice*. London, UK: Singing Dragon.

Quadri, A. A. (1993). Mentat (BR-16a) in mentally retarded children with behavioural problems. *Current Medical Practice*, **37**, 121.

Raven, J. C. (1958). *Coloured Progressive Matrices Set A, Ab, B*. London, UK: H.K. Lewis.

Roodenrys, S., Booth, D. and Bulzomi, S. (2002). Chronic effects of Brahmi (*Bacopa monnieri*) on human memory. *Neuropsychopharmacology*, **27**, 279–281.

Russo, A., Izzo, A. A. and Borrelli, F. (2003). Free radical scavenging capacity and protective effect of *Bacopa monniera* L. on DNA damage. *Phytotherapy Research*, **17**, 870–875.

Sairam, K., Dorababu, M., Goel, R. K. and Bhattacharya, S. K. (2002). Antidepressant activity of standardized extract of *Bacopa monniera* in experimental models of depression in rats. *Phytomedicine*, **9**(3), 207–211.

Sharma, R., Chaturvedi, C. and Tewari, P. V. (1987). Efficacy of *Bacopa Monnieri* in revitalizing intellectual functions in children. *Journal of Research Education in Indian Medicine*, **1**, 12.

Singh, H., Rastogi, R. P., Srimal, R. C. and Dhawan, B. N. (1988). Effect of bacosides A and B on avoidance responses in rats. *Phytotherapy Research*, **2**(2), 70–75.

Singh, H. K. and Dhawan, B. N. (1997). Neuropsychopharmacological effects of the Ayurvedic nootropic *Bacopa monniera* Linn. (Brahmi). *Indian Journal of Pharmacology*, **29**, 359–365.

Stough, C., Downey, L. A. and Lloyd, J. (2008). Examining the nootropic effects of a special extract of *Bacopa monniera* on human cognitive functioning: 90 day double-blind placebo-controlled randomized trial. *Phytotherapy Research*, **22**, 1629–1634.

Stough, C., Lloyd, J., Clarke, J., Downey, L. A., Hutchison, C. W., Rodgers, T. and Nathan, P. J. (2001). The chronic effects of an extract of *Bacopa monniera* (Brahmi) on cognitive function in healthy human subjects. *Psychopharmacology*, **156**(4), 481–484.

Uabundit, N., Wattanathorn, J., Mucimapura, S. and Ingkaninan, K. (2010). Cognitive enhancement and neuroprotective effects of *Bacopa monnieri* in Alzheimer's disease model. *Journal of Ethnopharmacology*, **127**(1), 26–31. doi:10.1016/j.jep.2009.09.056.

Upadhyay, S. K., Saha, A., Bhatia, B. D. and Kulkarni, K. S. (2002). Evaluation of the efficacy of mentat in children with learning disability: A placebo-controlled double-blind clinical trial. *Neurosciences Today*, **3**, 184–188.

Verpoorte, R., Choi, Y. H. and Kim, H. K. (2005). Ethnopharmacology and systems biology: A perfect holistic match. *Journal of Ethnopharmacology*, **100**(1–2), 53–56. doi:10.1016/j.jep.2005.05.033.

Vishwakarma, R. K., Kumari, U. and Khan, B. M. (2016). Memory booster plant *Bacopa monniera* (Brahmi): Biotechnology and molecular aspects of bacoside biosynthesis. In: Tsay, H. S., Shyur, L. F., Agrawal, D., Wu, Y. C. and Wang, S. Y. (Eds.), *Medicinal Plants - Recent Advances in Research and Development*. Singapore: Springer.

Wechsler, D. (1949). *Wechsler Intelligence Scale for Children; Manual*. Oxford, UK: The Psychological Corp.

19 Recent Insights on the Role of Natural Medicines in Immunostimulation

Isabella Muscari, Sabrina Adorisio, Trinh Thi Thuy, Tran Van Sung and Domenico V. Delfino

CONTENTS

19.1 INTRODUCTION: THE IMMUNE SYSTEM

The immune system is highly controlled and can distinguish self from non-self components of the body. In doing so, the immune system confers tolerance to the self and protection against non-self agents, including pathogens, transplanted cells and organs, allergens and transformed cells. The immune system can be subdivided based on the two main immune responses, namely innate and adaptive, which interact with each other reciprocally (see Figure 19.1).

Innate immunity: Innate immunity is the first line of defence against non-self antigens. It displays relatively low specificity and its main effectors are cells such as mononuclear phagocytes (macrophages/monocytes), dendritic cells, granulocytes and natural killer (NK) cells. These effector cells all produce and release defensive molecules upon stimulation by non-self molecules. *Pattern recognition receptors* (PRRs) on innate immune cells sense molecules called *pathogen-associated molecular patterns* (PAMPs), which are expressed by pathogens. Among PRR, *toll-like receptors* (TLRs) are the most common. Binding and stimulation of TLR by PAMP triggers a cascade of biochemical events that leads to activation of the NF-κB transcription factor and type I and II interferons that, in turn, modulates the transcription of pro-inflammatory genes such as those that express cytokines (Adorisio et al. 2017). The products of these target genes are responsible for mounting the innate immune response against pathogens.

Adaptive immunity: In contrast to innate immunity, adaptive immunity is characterised by a high degree of specificity and the generation of memory against a specific pathogen (Flajnik 2018). The main effectors are T lymphocytes, which mediate cellular immunity, and B lymphocytes, which mediate humoral immunity by producing soluble antibodies (also known as immunoglobulins). Immunoglobulins expressed on B-cells are receptors that recognise small regions of soluble antigens (proteins, polysaccharides or lipids)

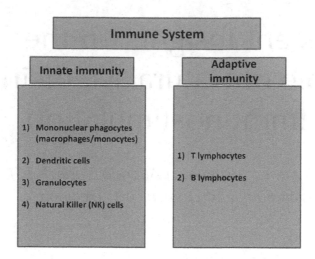

FIGURE 19.1 The organisation of immune system with its cells. Division of immune system in innate and adaptive immunity with the cells belonging to each sub-system.

called epitopes. T lymphocytes use the T cell receptor (TCR) expressed on their surface to recognise antigen expressed on the surface of antigen presenting cells (APCs), such as macrophages, dendritic cells and B-cells. APCs promote the enzymatic digestion of antigen through proteasomal degradation and expose the resulting antigenic peptides on their surface in association with major histocompatibility complex (MHC) class I or II molecules. The peptide-MHC class II complex is recognised by TCR expressed on CD4+ T helper (Th) cells, and stimulates their differentiation into different effector (Th1, Th2, Th9, Th17) or regulatory T (Treg) cell subsets. Activation of CD8+ T cytotoxic cells is triggered by recognition of the peptide-MHC class I complex by TCR expressed on the cell surface. In order to become fully activated, CD4+ and CD8+ T lymphocytes also require co-stimulatory signals mediated by APC and interaction with T cell-associated receptors that stimulate cytokine production. In fact, cytokines play an important role as T cell effector molecules (Flajnik 2018).

19.2 CONVENTIONAL IMMUNOSTIMULANTS

Strengthening the immune response is an important therapeutic goal in treating selected diseases. However, the efficacy of available drugs is generally still not completely satisfactory.

Immunostimulants could be useful in treating all conditions of immunodeficiency or viral and bacterial infections. These drugs have been used in cancer therapy as adjuvants (Cabo et al. 2017). The development of immunomodulatory drugs for cancer therapy is based on the assumption that progressive mutations of neoplastic cells are monitored by the immune system during tumour development in order to remove cancer cells through immunosurveillance functions. Cancer cells can also express MHC-associated *non-self* peptides that induce tolerance instead of the immune response. This immune anergic state is due, at least in part, to the lack of CD4+ Th cell stimulation by cancer cells and the resulting scarcity of cytokines important for activating the immune response against the malignant cells. Stimulation of cytokine production or administration of cytokines can eliminate tolerance, thereby contributing to an efficient anti-tumour immune response. The anergic state is also due to infiltration of Treg cells to the interior of the tumour mass that represents a new target of immunostimulation.

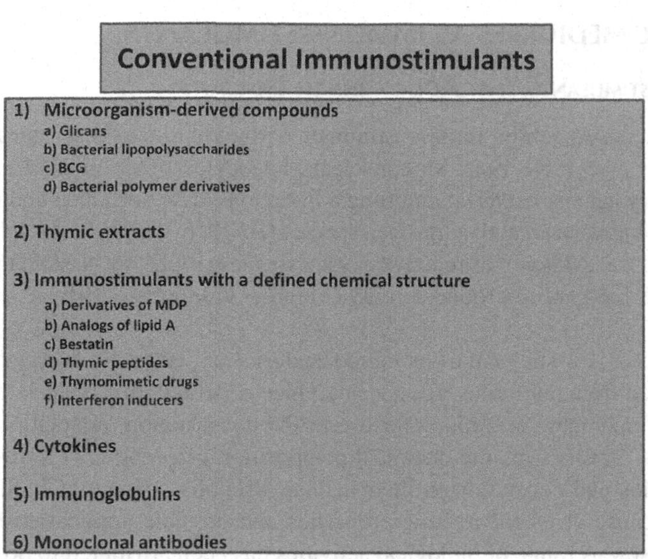

Conventional Immunostimulants

1) **Microorganism-derived compounds**
   a) Glicans
   b) Bacterial lipopolysaccharides
   c) BCG
   d) Bacterial polymer derivatives

2) **Thymic extracts**

3) **Immunostimulants with a defined chemical structure**
   a) Derivatives of MDP
   b) Analogs of lipid A
   c) Bestatin
   d) Thymic peptides
   e) Thymomimetic drugs
   f) Interferon inducers

4) **Cytokines**

5) **Immunoglobulins**

6) **Monoclonal antibodies**

FIGURE 19.2 Conventional immunostimulants. Immunostimulant drugs currently used in therapy of low immune response medical conditions.

The most commonly used immunostimulant drugs today are shown in Figure 19.2 and can be grouped as follows:

1. *Microorganism-derived compounds*
   a. *Glycans* are commonly derived from fungi and have the ability to activate macrophages, leading to an increase in their bactericidal and tumouricidal effects and increased production of pro-inflammatory cytokines, such as interleukin (IL)-1, tumour necrosis factor (TNF-α) and colony stimulating factors (CSFs)
   b. *Bacterial lipopolysaccharides*, such as *lipid A*, that stimulate B lymphocytes and macrophages
   c. *BCG* (attenuated *Mycobacterium bovis*) and extracts of mycobacterium cell wall, such as *muramyl dipeptide* (MDP), that stimulate NK cells and T lymphocytes
   d. *Bacterial polymer derivatives*
2. *Thymic extracts*, including raw thymic extracts or peptides purified from thymus (known also as thymic hormones)
3. *Immunostimulants with a defined chemical structure*
   a. *Derivatives of MDP* that activate macrophages and increase the production of IL-1, TNF-α, and CSFs
   b. *Analogues of lipid A*
   c. *Bestatin*
   d. *Thymic peptides*, such as thymosin-α
   e. *Thymomimetic drugs*, such as *levamisole, ditiocarb* or *inosine*
   f. *Interferon (IFN) inducers*, such as *PolyAU* and *Poly IC derivatives*
4. *Cytokines (IL-2, interferons, G-CSF, GM-CSF, IL-3)*
5. *Immunoglobulins*
6. *Monoclonal antibody ipilimumab* inhibits T cell activation by blocking immune checkpoints, such as CTLA-4 expressed on T lymphocytes, and by binding to B7-1 and B7-2 receptors expressed by APC. The last generation of these drugs include *nivolumab* and *pembrolizumab*, which block the interaction between PD1 expressed on the surface of T lymphocytes and PDL1, its receptor on APC (Cabo et al. 2017).

19.3 NATURAL MEDICINES AS IMMUNOSTIMULANTS

19.3.1 IMMUNOSTIMULANTS THAT ACT ON INNATE IMMUNITY

Most natural products that exhibit immunostimulant activity mainly exert their functions by acting on innate immunity (see Table 19.1). Mononuclear phagocytes function as effector cells of innate immunity, especially against bacterial and fungal infections. They produce and release nitric oxide (NO) radicals, also known as reactive nitrogen species (RNS), by the inducible NO synthase (iNOS) and superoxide (O_2^-), also known as reactive oxygen species (ROS), by NADPH phagocyte oxidase. Both ROS and RNS have antimicrobial activity (Vallejos-Vidal et al. 2016).

Propolis. Propolis is a sticky dark-coloured material collected by worker bees from leaf buds or exuded from numerous tree species. Once collected, this material is enriched with salivary and enzymatic secretions for use in the construction, adaptation and protection of their hives. In this way, the chemical composition of propolis is a direct reflection of the bee species and vegetation in their habitat. Propolis shows potential as an effective medicine because of its therapeutic properties and possible applications in the pharmaceutical industry. A range of biological activities has been attributed to propolis, including

TABLE 19.1
Influence of Natural Medicine in Immunity

Natural Medicine	Innate Immunity	Adaptive Immunity
Propolis	Mononuclear phagocytes	
Wheatgrass	Monocytes	
Juzen-taiho-to (JTT)	Macrophages	
Streptazolin	Macrophages	
Lichen polysaccharides	Macrophages	
Quercetin	?	?
Caulerpin	?	?
Beta-glucan	Macrophages, neutrophils	
AHCC	?	?
Angelica sinensis	Bone marrow	Thymus, spleen
Hippophae rhamnoides	?	?
Ocimum sanctum	Bone marrow	
Kaempferitrin	Macrophages, NK	
Hederagenin	Dendritic cells	
Curcumin		Thymus, cytotoxic T lymphocyte, Treg
Andrographolide		Cytotoxic T lymphocytes
Genistein		Th1 lymphocytes
Berberine		Treg, splenocytes
Echinacea purpurea		B lymphocytes, CD4$^+$, CD8$^+$ T cells
Nigella sativa		B lymphocytes, CD4$^+$, CD8$^+$ T cells
Squalene		Immunogenicity
Syzygium cumini		Splenic lymphocytes

(Continued)

TABLE 19.1 (*Continued*)
Influence of Natural Medicine in Immunity

Natural Medicine	Innate Immunity	Adaptive Immunity
Zingiber officinalis		Splenocytes, humoral immunity
Epigallocatechin gallate		CD8⁺ T lymphocytes, Th1 response
Lutein		Splenocytes
Withania somnifera		B and T lymphocytes
Rhodiola rosea		T- lymphocytes and Th1 response
Glycyrrhiza glabra		CD4 and CD8⁺ T cells
Asparagus racemosus		Th1/Th2 response
TMP-A	Macrophages	Lymphocytes
LDG-A	Macrophages	Lymphocytes
Abrus precatorius L.	?	?
Bee pollen	Macrophages, NK cells, Mast cells	Splenocytes, IgE
Vivartana	Bone marrow	Thymocytes, splenocytes
Panax ginseng	Bone marrow	Thymocytes, splenocytes
Resveratrol	NK cells, PBMC	T lymphocytes, B lymphocytes, Treg
Allium sativum	Macrophages	T lymphocytes
Bromelain		T lymphocytes
Tinospora cordifolia	Bone marrow dendritic cells	T lymphocytes
Agelasphins		NKT cells

immunomodulatory, antibacterial, fungicidal, anti-inflammatory, healing, anaesthetic and anticarcinogenic effects (Possamai et al. 2013). Propolis has immunostimulatory effects on mononuclear phagocytes of human blood that has been exposed to the fungus *Candida albicans* due to release of ROS. When adsorbed to polyethylene glycol (PEG), Brazilian propolis induces an increase in superoxide release by phagocytes. Therefore, propolis may potentially be an additional natural product that can be used for a variety of therapies (Possamai et al. 2013). Propolis has also been studied for its anti-tumour activity. In particular, a water-soluble derivative of propolis (WSDP) significantly increased tumour growth inhibition and the survival of tumour-bearing mice treated with cisplatin and hyperthermal intraperitoneal chemotherapy (HIPEC). This effect was accompanied by increased macrophage cytotoxicity against tumour cells. Thus, WSPD increased macrophage activity and tumour cell sensitivity to HIPEC, as well as reducing cisplatin toxicity on normal cells (Orsolic et al. 2013).

Wheatgrass. Another natural product that acts on phagocytes is wheatgrass, particularly the oligosaccharides derived from wheatgrass, including WG-PS3. Wheatgrass refers to the young grass of the common monocot wheat plant *Triticum aestivum*. Today, wheatgrass is one of the most widely used supplemental health foods and is available in many health food stores as fresh product, tablets, frozen juice and powder. Wheatgrass contains vitamins, minerals, enzymes, amino acids, polysaccharides and large amounts (70%) of chlorophyll. In traditional medicine, the health benefits of wheatgrass include improved digestion, blood pressure reduction, heavy metal detoxification from the bloodstream, immune stimulation and gout alleviation. Moreover, different papers suggest anti-tumour activities, antioxidant properties and therapeutic effects in distal ulcerative colitis. In addition, wheatgrass may help prevent diabetes and heart disease. Studies of the immunostimulatory mechanism of WG-PS3 have demonstrated that wheatgrass stimulates the expression of surface molecules and Th1 cytokines in human peripheral blood mononuclear cells, particularly CD69, CD80, CD86, IL-12, and TNF-α. The immunomodulator compound was identified as maltoheptaose, which activates monocytes by stimulating Toll-like receptor 2 (TLR-2), a receptor that can sense pathogens (Tsai et al. 2013).

Juzen-taiho-to (JTT). This oriental herbal formulation is immunostimulatory and widely used in East Asia to improve the immunological functions of cancer patients. Specifically, studies have shown that JTT stimulates macrophages to upregulate ICAM-1. The extent of this macrophage-stimulating activity depends on the chemical form of JTT. For example, JTT is much more active in lipid nanoparticle form (Hasson et al. 2014).

Streptazolin. This is a newly isolated natural product with macrophage-stimulating activity that is produced by screening a panel of microbe products. Streptazolin induces the production of immunostimulatory cytokines and stimulates the NF-κB pathway via phosphatidylinositide 3-kinase (PI3K) signalling (Perry et al. 2015).

Lichen polysaccharides. These substances enhance the production of NO by macrophages, which increases production of various cytokines, including IL-10, IL-12, IL-1β, TNF-α and IFN-α/β. Thus, lichen polysaccharides provide a source for the discovery of novel therapeutic agents (Shrestha et al. 2015).

Quercetin. A flavonol belonging to the family of polyphenols, quercetin is found in a variety of foods including tea, capers, red onions, broccoli, berries, grapevines and apples. Quercetin has a variety of pharmacological effects. In a clinical trial that evaluated inflammatory biomarkers, quercetin exerted a slight pro-inflammatory effect, depending on the apolipoprotein E genotype of healthy men (Jantan et al. 2015).

Caulerpin. This is a marine bisindole alkaloid isolated from the marine algae *Caulerpa*. A red algae *Chondria armata* was successfully tested as an immunostimulant (Lunagariya et al. 2017).

Beta-glucan. Besides their role in innate immunity, macrophages play a critical role in the immune response against tumours. Tumour-associated macrophages (TAM) consist of two phenotypes, M1 and M2, that are the result of a switch from classical activated macrophages. M1 macrophages produce IL-12, TNF-α, ROS and NO and exert tumouricidal activity. They transform into the M2 phenotype, which produce low levels of MHC class II, IL-12 and TNF-α with high levels of vascular endothelial growth factor (VEGF), arginase-1, prostaglandin E2 (PGE2) and IL-10. TAM promote tumour evasion and limit the efficacy of chemotherapy. The natural product beta-glucan is derived from yeast, fungi, bacteria or barley. Upon binding to its receptor dectin-1, beta-glucan converts immunosuppressive TAMs, M2 bone marrow-derived macrophages, to an M1 immunostimulant phenotype, resulting in reduced tumour formation and induction of macrophage reprogramming (Liu et al. 2015). Beta-glucan can also be produced by filamentous fungi, such as *Aspergillus sojae*, particularly when they are cultivated through solid-state fermentation on rapeseed meal. In this circumstance, the extract obtained has immunostimulant activity, such as activation of blood neutrophils and upregulation of IL-1β in the presence of stimulated mouse bone marrow-derived macrophages. These effects were not observed in unfermented fungi (Sutter et al. 2017). Notably, natural products can act as adjuvants during chemotherapy to increase the immune response against cancer (Lozada-Requena et al. 2015). A sulphated β(1,4)-glucan, methyl hydroxyethyl cellulose sulphate (MHCS) demonstrated a stimulatory effect on fish immune cells, as well as enhancing expression of cytokines, such as IL-1β, TNF-α1 and 2, IFN-α2, and iNOS (Kareem et al. 2018).

Active Hexose-Correlated Compound (AHCC). This is a mushroom extract derived from several species of *Basidiomycetes*, including Shiitake (*Lentinus edodes*) and Shimeji (*Lyophyllum shimeji*). AHCC is composed of a mixture of amino acids, minerals, polysaccharides and lipids enriched in α-1,4-linked glucans. AHCC is an immunostimulant that is used to improve the quality of life of patients affected by different types of cancer. AHCC increases apoptosis of acute myeloid leukaemia cells *in vitro* and reduces blast counts and increases the survival time *in vivo* (Fatehchand et al. 2017).

Angelica sinensis. Compounds isolated from *A. sinensis*, among others, have immunostimulant effects. Specifically, *A. sinensis* polysaccharide (ASP) 1 and 3, which are present in root extracts, promote haematopoiesis in bone marrow by increasing the thymus and spleen index (Kim et al. 2017).

Hippophae rhamnoides **(also called sea buckthorn).** This plant has been used in India and Tibet for its immunostimulatory properties. Studies demonstrate that *Hippophae rhamnoides* reduces corticosterone levels in plasma of whole-body irradiated rats (Kim et al. 2017).

Ocimum sanctum **(also known as Tulsi or Indian holy basil).** Used in Ayurvedic medicine, this medicinal plant has immunostimulatory properties because two flavonoids contained in it have been reported to protect against radiation-induced chromosomal aberrations and stem cell death in bone marrow (Kim et al. 2017).

Kaempferitrin. Isolated from *Justicia spicigera*, this flavonoid induces phagocytosis in human macrophages *in vitro*, increases the level of NO and H_2O_2 production and induces NK activity against tumours (Mohamed et al. 2017).

Hederagenin. Saponins are natural surface-active glycosides that are produced mainly by plants that possess many pharmacological properties, including immunostimulatory effects (Marrelli et al. 2016). One such immunostimulant is the component QS-21 (Fernandez-Tejada et al. 2016) of the complex saponin adjuvant mixture Quil A, which is isolated from *Quillaia saponaria*. In an attempt to produce a new immunostimulant based on the structure of QS-21, hederagenin, a sugar contained in *Hedera helix*, was selected for modification due to its structural similarity to QS-21. The most active saponin, 3-O-(manp(1→3) Glcp) hederagenin, demonstrated stimulatory effects at high concentration in cell culture as evaluated using the activation markers MHC class II and CD86 in murine bone marrow dendritic cells (Greatrex et al. 2015).

19.3.2 Immunostimulants That Act on Adaptive Immunity

Curcumin. This is a natural diarylheptanoid found in the rhizome of *Curcuma longa*. Among its numerous pharmacological properties, such as anticancer and anti-inflammatory effects (Jantan et al. 2015), curcumin is also considered an immunostimulant because it stimulates the production of thymocytes (Pozzesi et al. 2014), inhibits the reduction in effector cytotoxic T lymphocytes and suppresses the Treg response by downregulating anti-inflammatory cytokines, such as IL-4, IL-10 and TGF-β, in tumour-transplanted mice. Moreover, curcumin inhibits PGE2 release, which suppresses the expression of the common cytokine receptor gamma chain (Υc) and Bcl-2 in T lymphocytes, thus improving their proliferation and expansion (Mohamed et al. 2017).

Andrographolide. This is a diterpenoid lactone found in *Andrographis paniculata* that is commonly known for its extensive anti-inflammatory properties. However, administration of this compound resulted in upregulation of CD markers and increased TNF-α production, thus increasing the activity of cytotoxic T lymphocytes (Rajagopal et al. 2003; Jantan et al. 2015).

Genistein. This is a natural phytoestrogen present in soy. Genistein is known as a strong anti-inflammatory agent, and has also been reported to exhibit some immunostimulant properties.

Specifically, genistein has been shown to switch T-cell differentiation towards a Th1 phenotype by increasing IL-4 expression and inhibiting IFN-γ production in collagen-induced arthritis (Wang et al. 2008).

Berberine. This is an isoquinoline alkaloid with a broad spectrum of pharmacological effects and is the main active component in plants, such as *Berberis* spp. and goldenseal. Berberine is known for its immunosuppressive activity. However, recent studies have demonstrated that injection of berberine at high doses decreases the number of Treg cells and IL-10 production in murine splenocytes, thus providing support for its immunostimulatory activity (Karimi et al. 2017).

***Echinacea purpurea* and *Nigella sativa*.** Extracts from these two plants have immunostimulatory effects. They have been used together with Egyptian hepatitis C E1 and E2 protein-encoding constructs used to immunise mice in an effort to significantly increase CD4$^+$ and CD8$^+$ T lymphocyte responses (Shawky et al. 2015).

Squalene. This is a cholesterol precursor and its immunostimulatory properties can be used as vaccine adjuvants with advantages comparable to traditional aluminium salt adjuvant. In particular, *in vivo* studies reported that, compared to larger particle sizes, 80-nm squalene particles exhibited the strongest immunogenicity when tested in a mouse model using Respiratory Syncytial Virus Fusion protein (RSV.p) as a model antigen (Iyer et al. 2015).

***Syzygium cumini* (also known as jamun).** Used in traditional Indian medicine, *S. cumini* leaf extracts protect lymphocytes against radiation-induced DNA damage and suppress radiation-induced lipid peroxidation and DNA damage in the spleen of mice (Kim et al. 2017).

***Zingiber officinale*.** Administration of *Z. officinale* extracts to γ-irradiated mice enhanced spleen weight, splenocyte proliferation, humoral immunity and secretion of cytokines including IL-1β and IL-3 in the spleen of mice, indicating alleviation of radiation-induced immunosuppression (Kim et al. 2017).

Epigallocatechin gallate. This is a flavonoid isolated from green tea that increases the number of cytotoxic CD8$^+$ T lymphocytes infiltrating the tumour microenvironment. These cells induce a direct cytotoxic effect on the tumour cells, as well as enhance the release of IL-12 to induce a Th1 response against the tumour (Mohamed et al. 2017).

Lutein. This is a carotenoid that stimulates IFN-γ mRNA expression and suppresses the effects of IL-10 in splenocytes of mammary tumour–bearing mice (Mohamed et al. 2017).

***Withania somnifera* Dunal [also known as Ashwagandha (Salicaceae)].** The root of this plant has been shown to exert an immunostimulant effect. Extracts raise the levels of IFN- γ, IL-2, and GM-CSF while lowering TNF-α in mice treated with cyclophosphamide. The myeloprotective property of *Withania somnifera* Dunal has been attributed to its ability to increase white blood cell counts and elevate antibody titres. Moreover, reports have demonstrated that *Withania somnifera* Dunal upregulates Notch-1, which plays a role in various stages of B and T lymphocyte development (Kaur et al. 2017).

***Rhodiola rosea* (also known as golden root or arctic root).** This plant belongs to the *Crassulaceae* family and is used for treating different diseases in traditional medicine. Studies have proposed that *Rhodiola rosea* exerts immunopotentiating effects. Specifically, its ethanolic root extract inhibits T lymphocyte apoptosis, thus increasing their number and the expression of Th1 cytokines (IFN-γ, IL-2, and IL-12) (Kaur et al. 2017).

***Glycyrrhiza glabra* (Fabaceae).** Commonly known as liquorice, this plant stimulates various immune cells. Studies have demonstrated the effect of ingesting *Glycyrrhiza* herbal tincture for 7 days on the expression of CD69, which is an activation marker, on CD4$^+$ and CD8$^+$ T cells (Kaur et al. 2017).

***Asparagus racemosus*.** This member of the Linn. (Shatavari), family *Liliaceae*, augments the Th1/Th2 response (Kaur et al. 2017).

19.3.3 IMMUNOSTIMULANTS THAT ACT ON BOTH INNATE AND ADAPTIVE IMMUNITY

TMP-A. Fungi are traditionally classified as a separate kingdom from plants, animals and bacteria. These organisms contain polysaccharides in fruiting bodies, mycelium and the fermentation broth of edible and medicinal fungi. These active compounds possess different pharmacological properties, such as anti-tumour activity, immunostimulation and anti-oxidation effects. TMP-A is a novel polysaccharide isolated from the fungus *Tricholoma matsutake*, which belongs to the subgenus *Tricholoma*, is widely distributed in East Asia, consumed as food, and used in traditional medicine. This non-starch polysaccharide has been shown to inhibit bacteria such as *Micrococcus lysodeikticus*. Moreover, TMP-A has been shown to exert anti-tumour activity *in vivo*, suggesting a possible role in cell-mediated immunity. TMP-A also promotes proliferation of spleen cells *in vitro* and stimulates phagocytosis by mouse peritoneal macrophages. Thus, this study demonstrates that TMP-A stimulates the adaptive and innate immune responses through lymphocyte and macrophage activation, respectively (Hou et al. 2013a).

LDG-A. This is another non-starch polysaccharide isolated from the fungus *Lactarius deliciosus* (L. ex Fr.) Gray, and it has been reported that LDG-A exerts anti-tumour activity in mice *in vivo*. This effect was hypothesised to be the consequence of stimulating the cell-mediated immune response since it promotes significant activation of lymphocytes and macrophages by increasing the level of cytokines such as IL-6, TNF-α, and NO (Hou et al. 2013b).

Abrus precatorius L. This plant, which is commonly called *gunja* or jequirity, is used in traditional medicine in India and Ceylon to treat a variety of diseases. Studies indicate that *Abrus precatorius* L. possesses immunostimulatory and antibacterial properties and may be the source of pure compounds to discover its mechanism of immunostimulation (Garaniya and Bapodra 2014).

Bee pollen. This is a bee product of plant origin that varies in its chemical composition depending on the flora present in various climate zones. More than 250 biologically active substances have been isolated from bee pollen. The polysaccharide fraction stimulates immunological activity by increasing the macrophage number and promoting splenocyte and NK cell proliferation. Moreover, this fraction stimulates the activation of mast cells by immunoglobulin E (IgE; Rzepecka-Stojko et al. 2015).

Vivartana. This is a polyherbal formulation with immunostimulant activity that is used to counteract the side effects of cyclophosphamide (CTX) chemotherapy. Vivartana increased the number of leukocytes and the haemoglobin level. In addition, vivartana prevented the loss of organ weight by increasing the number of splenocytes, thymocytes and bone marrow cells. Furthermore, vivartana exhibited hepatoprotective activity. Taken together, these results indicate that vivartana has high potential as an immunostimulant and chemoprotectant against CTX-induced immunosuppression in mice (Gnanasekaran et al. 2015, 2017).

Panax ginseng. This is a well-known medicinal plant used extensively in China and Korea. *P. ginseng* promotes recovery from spleen and thymus damage induced by radiation exposure in mouse models. An acidic polysaccharide of ginseng was demonstrated to enhance the proliferation of bone marrow cells and splenocytes, as well as increase the production and release of cytokines, including IL-1, IL-2, IL-4, IL-6, IL-12, IFN-γ and TNF-α, in irradiated mice (Kim et al. 2017).

Resveratrol. This compound is present in foods such as grapevine and red wine. Resveratrol increases the CD4$^+$/CD8$^+$ T-cell ratio (Pozzesi et al. 2007) and enhances T cell proliferation. In addition, this immunostimulant improves the B-cell-mediated immune response and increases the level of serum antibodies. Moreover, resveratrol exhibits a strong stimulatory effect on NK cells and suppresses the release of IL-6, IL-10 and IL-1ra in human

PBMCs that were reported to possess tumour promoter activity. Resveratrol shows an inhibitory effect on the expansion and proliferation of Treg suppressor immune cells in the spleen of tumour-bearing mice (Mohamed et al. 2017).

Allium sativum (**garlic**). This plant stimulates the immune response and induces immune effector cells against tumours. Aged garlic extract induces macrophage-mediated phagocytosis and T lymphocyte-mediated cytotoxicity against sarcoma. In addition, garlic enhances the release of pro-inflammatory cytokines (IL-2, IL-12, TNF-α and IL-10) and NO production in macrophages (Mohamed et al. 2017).

Tinospora cordifolia. This plant belongs to the *Menispermaceae* family and is used in Ayurvedic medicine as an immunostimulant. Studies demonstrate that an arabinogalactan polysaccharide (G1-4A) isolated from *Tinospora cordifolia* increased the differentiation of bone marrow-derived dendritic cells (BMDCs), leading to activation of cytotoxic T lymphocytes. Furthermore, BMDCs increased their killing capacity by releasing NO (Kaur et al. 2017).

Agelasphins. These constitute a class of natural glycolipids derived from the Okinawan marine sponge *Agelas mauritianus*, which has potent anti-tumour activity as a consequence of robust immunostimulation. Even more potent immunostimulants in the form of a simple α-galactosylceramide (α-GalCer) have been developed from these glycolipids. This compound was further modified to increase the immunostimulatory effect, resulting in a potent CD1d ligand that stimulates mouse invariant natural killer T (iNKT) cells to selectively enhance Th1 cytokine production (Hossain et al. 2016).

19.4 CONCLUSIONS

Despite the development of pharmaceutical and chemical factories in the second half of the twentieth century, nature continues to be an invaluable source of medicines. The search for new natural medicines is active not only in developing countries, but also in highly developed countries with expanding interest in holistic medicine. Researching natural medicines is important because of (1) the possibility of discovering novel drugs and novel drug targets; (2) the ability to treat diseases where conventional medicines fail, due to poor efficacy and/or safety profiles; and (3) the possibility for natural drugs to serve as mimics for the chemical synthesis of novel drugs. Natural medicine may particularly benefit the field of immunostimulation, which is still poorly represented by conventional medicines. Thus, the discovery and testing of new natural products can greatly improve the prognosis of immune-depressed patients that require additional therapy beyond conventional medicine.

REFERENCES

Adorisio, S., Fierabracci, A., Muscari, I., Liberati, A. M., Ayroldi, E., Migliorati, G., et al. (2017). SUMO proteins, Guardians of immune system. *Journal of Autoimmunity*, **84**, 21–28.

Cabo, M., Offringa, R., Zitvogel, L., Kroemer, G., Muntasell, A. and Galluzzi, L. (2017). Trial watch: Immunostimulatory monoclonal antibodies for oncological indications. *Oncoimmunology*, **6**(12), e1371896.

Fatehchand, K., Santhanam, R., Shen, B., Erickson, E. L., Gautam, S., Elavazhagan, S., et al. (2017). Active hexose-correlated compound enhances extrinsic-pathway-mediated apoptosis of Acute Myeloid Leukemic cells. *PLoS One*, **12**(7), e0181729.

Fernandez-Tejada, A., Tan, D. S. and Gin, D. Y. (2016). Development of improved vaccine adjuvants based on the saponin natural product QS-21 through chemical synthesis. *Accounts of Chemical Research*, **49**(9), 1741–1756.

Flajnik M. F. (2018). A cold-blooded view of adaptive immunity. *Nature Reviews Immunology*, **18**(7), 438–453.

Garaniya, N. and Bapodra, A. (2014). Ethno botanical and phytophrmacological potential of *Abrus precatorius* L.: A review. *Asian Pacific Journal of Tropical Biomedicine*, **4**(Suppl 1), S27–S34.

Gnanasekaran, S., Sakthivel, K. M. and Chandrasekaran, G. (2015). Immunostimulant and chemoprotective effect of vivartana, a polyherbal formulation against cyclophosphamide induced toxicity in Swiss albino mice. *Journal of Experimental Therapeutics & Oncology*, **11**(1), 51–61.

Gnanasekaran, S., Sakthivel, K. M. and Chandrasekaran, G. (2017). Immunostimulant and chemoprotective effect of vivartana, a polyherbal formulation against cyclophosphamide induced toxicity in swiss albino mice. *Journal of Experimental Therapeutics & Oncology*, **11**(1), 51–61.

Greatrex, B. W., Daines, A. M., Hook, S., Lenz, D. H., McBurney, W., Rades, T., et al. (2015). Synthesis, formulation, and adjuvanticity of monodesmosidic saponins with olenanolic acid, hederagenin and gypsogenin aglycones, and some C-28 ester derivatives. *ChemistryOpen*, **4**(6), 740–755.

Hasson, T. H., Takaoka, A., de la Rica, R., Matsui, H., Smeureanu, G., Drain, C. M., et al. (2014). Immunostimulatory lipid nanoparticles from herbal medicine. *Chemical Biology & Drug Design*, **83**(4), 493–497.

Hossain, M. I., Hanashima, S., Nomura, T., Lethu, S., Tsuchikawa, H., Murata, M., et al. (2016). Synthesis and Th1-immunostimulatory activity of alpha-galactosylceramide analogues bearing a halogen-containing or selenium-containing acyl chain. *Bioorganic & Medicinal Chemistry*, **24**(16), 3687–3695.

Hou, Y., Ding, X., Hou, W., Song, B., Wang, T., Wang, F., et al. (2013b). Immunostimulant activity of a novel polysaccharide isolated from lactarius deliciosus (L. ex Fr.) Gray. *Indian Journal of Pharmaceutical Sciences*, **75**(4), 393–399.

Hou, Y., Ding, X., Hou, W., Zhong, J., Zhu, H., Ma, B., et al. (2013a). Anti-microorganism, anti-tumor, and immune activities of a novel polysaccharide isolated from Tricholoma matsutake. *Pharmacognosy Magazine*, **9**(35), 244–249.

Iyer, V., Cayatte, C., Guzman, B., Schneider-Ohrum, K., Matuszak, R., Snell, A., et al. (2015). Impact of formulation and particle size on stability and immunogenicity of oil-in-water emulsion adjuvants. *Human Vaccines & Immunotherapeutics*, **11**(7), 1853–1864.

Jantan, I., Ahmad, W. and Bukhari, S. N. (2015). Plant-derived immunomodulators: An insight on their preclinical evaluation and clinical trials. *Frontiers in Plant Science*, **6**, 655.

Kareem, N., Yates, E., Skidmore, M. and Hoole, D. (2018). In vitro investigations on the effects of semi-synthetic, sulphated carbohydrates on the immune status of cultured common carp (Cyprinus carpio) leucocytes. *Fish & Shellfish Immunology*, **74**, 213–222.

Karimi, G., Mahmoudi, M., Balali-Mood, M., Rahnama, M., Zamani Taghizadeh Rabe, S., Tabasi N., et al. (2017). Decreased levels of spleen tissue CD4$^+$CD25$^+$Foxp3$^+$ regulatory T lymphocytes in mice exposed to berberine. *Journal of Acupuncture and Meridian Studies*, **10**(2), 109–113.

Kaur, P., Robin, Makanjuola, V. O., Arora, R., Singh, B. and Arora, S. (2017). Immunopotentiating significance of conventionally used plant adaptogens as modulators in biochemical and molecular signalling pathways in cell mediated processes. *Biomedicine & Pharmacotherapy = Biomedecine & Pharmacotherapie*, **95**, 1815–1829.

Kim, W., Kan,g J., Lee, S. and Youn, B. (2017). Effects of traditional oriental medicines as anti-cytotoxic agents in radiotherapy. *Oncology Letters*, **13**(6), 4593–4601.

Liu, M., Luo, F., Ding, C., Albeituni, S., Hu, X., Ma, Y., et al. (2015). Dectin-1 Activation by a natural product beta-glucan converts immunosuppressive macrophages into an M1-like phenotype. *Journal of Immunology*, **195**(10), 5055–5065.

Lozada-Requena, I., Nunez, C. and Aguilar, J. L. (2015). Melanoma immunotherapy: Dendritic cell vaccines [*Inmunoterapia en melanoma: vacunas de celulas dendriticas*]. *Revista Peruana de Medicina Experimental y Salud Publica*, **32**(3), 555–564.

Lunagariya, J., Bhadja, P., Zhong, S., Vekariya, R. and Xu, S. (2017). Marine natural product bis-indole Alkaloid caulerpin: Chemistry and biology. *Mini Reviews in Medicinal Chemistry*, **2017**, doi: 10.2174/1 3895575176661709271542231.

Marrelli, M., Conforti, F., Araniti, F. and Statti, G. A. (2016). Effects of saponins on lipid metabolism: A review of potential health benefits in the treatment of obesity. *Molecules*, **21**(10), pii: E1404.

Mohamed, S. I. A., Jantan, I. and Haque, M. A. (2017). Naturally occurring immunomodulators with antitumor activity: An insight on their mechanisms of action. *International Immunopharmacology*, **50**, 291–304.

Orsolic, N., Car, N., Lisicic, D., Benkovic, V., Knezevic, A. H., Dikic, D., et al. (2013). Synergism between propolis and hyperthermal intraperitoneal chemotherapy with cisplatin on ehrlich ascites tumor in mice. *Journal of Pharmaceutical Sciences*, **102**(12), 4395–4405.

Perry, J. A., Koteva, K., Verschoor, C. P., Wang, W., Bowdish, D. M. and Wright, G. D. (2015). A macrophage-stimulating compound from a screen of microbial natural products. *The Journal of Antibiotics*, **68**(1), 40–46.

Possamai, M. M., Honorio-Franca, A. C., Reinaque, A. P., Franca, E. L. and Souto, P. C. (2013). Brazilian propolis: A natural product that improved the fungicidal activity by blood phagocytes. *BioMed Research International*, **2013**, 541018.

Pozzesi, N., Fierabracci, A., Thuy, T. T., Martelli, M. P., Liberati, A. M., Ayroldi E., et al. (2014). Pharmacological modulation of caspase-8 in thymus-related medical conditions. *The Journal of Pharmacology and Experimental Therapeutics*, **351**(1), 18–24.

Pozzesi, N., Gizzi, S., Gori, F., Vacca, C., Cannarile, L., Riccardi, C., et al. (2007). IL-2 induces and altered CD4/CD8 ratio of splenic T lymphocytes from transgenic mice overexpressing the glucocorticoid-induced protein GILZ. *Journal of Chemotherapy*, **19**(5), 562–569.

Rajagopal, S., Kumar, R. A., Deevi, D. S., Satyanarayana, C. and Rajagopalan, R. (2003). Andrographolide, a potential cancer therapeutic agent isolated from *Andrographis paniculata*. *Journal of Experimental Therapeutics & Oncology*, **3**(3), 147–158.

Rzepecka-Stojko, A., Stojko, J., Kurek-Gorecka, A., Gorecki, M., Kabala-Dzik, A., Kubina, R., et al. (2015). Polyphenols from bee pollen: Structure, absorption, metabolism and biological activity. *Molecules*, **20**(12), 21732–21749.

Shawky, H., Maghraby, A. S., Solliman, Mel D., El-Mokadem, M. T., Sherif, M. M., Arafa, A., et al. (2015). Expression, immunogenicity and diagnostic value of envelope proteins from an Egyptian hepatitis C virus isolate. *Archives of Virology*, **160**(4), 945–958.

Shrestha, G., St Clair, L. L. and O'Neill, K. L. (2015). The immunostimulating role of lichen polysaccharides: A review. *Phytotherapy Research*, **29**(3), 317–322.

Sutter, S., Thevenieau, F., Bourdillon, A. and De Coninck, J. (2017). Immunomodulatory properties of filamentous fungi cultivated through solid-state fermentation on rapeseed meal. *Applied Biochemistry and Biotechnology*, **182**(3), 910–924.

Tsai, C. C., Lin, C. R., Tsai, H. Y., Chen, C. J., Li, W. T., Yu, H. M., et al. (2013). The immunologically active oligosaccharides isolated from wheatgrass modulate monocytes via Toll-like receptor-2 signaling. *The Journal of Biological Chemistry*, **288**(24), 17689–17697.

Vallejos-Vidal, E., Reyes-Lopez, F., Teles M. and MacKenzie, S. (2016). The response of fish to immunostimulant diets. *Fish & Shellfish Immunology*, **56**, 5634–69.

Wang, J., Zhang, Q., Jin, S., He, D., Zhao, S. and Liu, S. (2008). Genistein modulate immune responses in collagen-induced rheumatoid arthritis model. *Maturitas*, **59**(4), 405–412.

20 Clinical Trial Protocol for Herbal Drugs
Perspectives of India

Tuhin Kanti Biswas

CONTENTS

20.1   INTRODUCTION

तदेव युक्तं भैषज्यं यद् आरोग्याय कल्पते।

स चैव भिषजां श्रेष्ठ रोगेभ्य यः प्रमोचयेत्।।

च. सं. सु. १/१३४

Tadeva Yuktam Bhaisajyam Yad Aarogaayao Kalpate /
Sa Chaiva Bhisajaam Shreshtha Rogebhya Ja Pramochayet //

(***Charaka Samhita, Sutra Sthanam, Chapter 1, Verse 134***)

According to the *Charaka Samhita*, an ancient Ayurvedic text, the Indian traditional system of medicine described that an agent that can bring about a cure is a correct drug (any varieties of medicines including natural product of herbal origin) and it is only he who can relieve patients of their ailments that is the best physician. Treatment with herbs is a long heritage of India in different traditional systems, and successful management of disease can be defined as those that satisfy the aims of the *Charaka Samhita*. The medical system of India was introduced long ago, as an outcome of the academic synthesis during its progressive transformation, since the inception of the Aryans. *Ayurveda*, a classical Indian system of medicine, is one of the outcomes among these processes of revolution. The other traditional and complementary system medicines introduced later in India are Unani, Siddha, Tibia and Naturopathy. Homeopathy, in spite of its origin in Germany, included as a part of the Indian traditional and complementary system of medicine, as it is widely practiced in certain parts of the country. India is a country with diverse varieties of natural products, especially herbal drugs, probably due to wide range of geographical and climatic variations. In all these categories of traditional system of medicine, plants are used abundantly for various medicinal formulations to combat different ailments. There are also several non-institutional traditional systems of medicine in different parts of India, which are practiced in some pockets and are limited to a specific community. India has more than 427 tribal communities that use in practice natural products, particularly herbal drugs, for primary healthcare management (Jain and Patole 2001). According to the Government of India 2011 census data, the tribal population in India is about 8.6% of the total population, almost all of whom depend upon native medicinal plants, known as folk medicine, for their healthcare management. Studies suggest that the tribal and ethnic communities in India as part of their healthcare systems use more than 8000 species of plants and approximately 25,000 folk medicine–based formulations (Sharma et al. 2016). Among these tribes, the Santal, who inhabit the Chota Nagpur area of West Bengal, Bihar and Jharkhand State of India, are reported to use several varieties of medicinal plants for the treatment of about 305 types of diseases or disease symptoms (Bodding 1986). Most of these treatments are created by the Santal expert engaged in healthcare called *Ojha* (traditional Santal practitioner). In southern India, particularly in the Thodu hills of Kerala, there is tribal group called the Kani, who are well known for the practice of herbal medicine and for rendering treatment of a number of diseases (Xavier et al. 2014). The Kani usually prepare medicines with non-timber minor forest products in various forms from 37 medicinal plants to treat 14 categories of diseases (Xavier et al. 2014).

Besides the traditional healer, there are systemic traditional practices of medicine, particularly Ayurveda, which have been practiced in India for several thousands. Ayurveda provides much information on ethnic folklore practices and traditional aspects of therapeutically important medicines. Ayurveda is gaining global acceptance primarily due to its holistic therapeutic practice, extensive profound conceptual basis and survival of its medicines since prehistoric times (Mukherjee et al. 2017). It has been reported that in Ayurveda detailed descriptions and therapeutic uses of a large number of medicinal plants are available in different classical texts. *Charaka Samhita* (1500 BCE) and *Sushruta Samhita* (1000 BCE) refer to 341 and 395 medicinal plants, respectively,

TABLE 20.1

Priority Area of Clinical Trial on Traditional System of Medicine Recommended by the Ministry of AYUSH, Government of India

Sl	Ayurveda and Siddha System		Homeopathy	
	First Priority	Second Priority	First Priority	Second Priority
1	Lifestyle-related disorders	Musculoskeletal disorders	Depressive neurosis	Alzheimer's disease
2	Metabolic disorders	Fever	Tuberculosis	Rheumatoid arthritis
3	Peptic ulcer	Diarrhoea (including dysentery)	Multidrug resistance tuberculosis	Cervical and lumber spondylosis
4	Psoriasis	Indigestion and anorexia	COPD including chronic bronchitis and emphysema	RTI and PID
5	Malnutrition	Skin diseases	Psoriasis	Filariasis
6	Reproductive Child Health (RCH) including infertility and contraceptives	Eye and ENT diseases	Polycystic ovarian disease	Kala-a-zar
7	Benign prostate enlargement	Secondary/tertiary healthcare relating issues	Menopause	Parkinson's disease
8	Preventive cardiology-hypertension, obesity		HIV infection	Gastro oesophageal reflux disorders (GERD)
9	Urolithiasis		Malignant and pre-malignant conditions	Irritable bowel syndrome
10	General health promotion (Rasyana/Medhya Rasayana)		Diabetes mellitus	Hepatitis B and C
11	Mental health/memory relating disorders		Hypothyroidism	Chronic renal disorders
12	Sports medicine		Hyperthyroidism	Oro-dental disorders
13	Liver disorders (Hepatitis B)		Systemic hypertension	Alcohol and drug abuse and de-addiction studies as protective therapy
14	Primary healthcare relating issues		Allergic disorders	Iatrogenic disease
15	Malaria		Viral infection	
16	Filaria		Reproductive and child health	
17	Rheumatoid arthritis			
18	Menstrual disorders			
19	Reproductive tract infection			
20	Cancer			
21	Bronchial asthma, upper respiratory tract infection			
22	Neurological disorders			

while 902 medicinal plants are described in the text *Ashtanga Hridaya* (600 CE). The Ayurvedic Pharmacopoeia of India (API), published by the Government of India, has described in detail about 395 medicinal plants in a scientific manner (Vassou et al. 2016). Like Ayurveda, Unani is the next traditional system of medicine practiced in India widely. It has been reported that about 90% of Unani drugs are composed with medicinal plants to treat several types of diseases (Itrat 2016). All these medicinal plants are used in different forms, like crude dried powder, ointment, oil, decoctions and liniments. Despite the large number medicinal plants that have been described in different classical texts from the Ayurveda and Unani traditions and the basic pharmacological analysis that has evaluated their biological properties, it is rare that clinical trials of these herbal products have been conducted in a scientific manner. Siddha and Sowa-Rigpa are two other systems of Indian traditional medicine that are included under the broad head AYUSH by the Government of India. The Siddha system is popular in southern India and deals with the patient, environment, age, sex, race, habits, mental framework, habitat, diet, appetite, physical condition and physiological constitution of the diseases for its treatment, which is individualistic in nature. Medicinal plants are one of the weapons in Siddha for the management of different diseases, most of which are similar to Ayurveda and Unani. Sowa-Rigpa is one of the oldest traditional systems of medicine in India and is practiced mainly in Leh and Ladakh, Himachal Pradesh, Arunachal Pradesh, Sikkim and Darjeeling. This system of Indian traditional medicine is effective for the treatment of certain limited diseases such as bronchial asthma, bronchitis and arthritis (AYUSH Systems Annual Report 2016–2017). Herbal preparations are the main source of drugs in this system, too. However, scientific clinical trials have been undertaken in the Ayurveda and Unani systems of medicine. Approaches are made in the current article to discuss the scope and present protocol for undertaking clinical trials with herbal drugs referred to in various classical traditional systems of medicine in India.

20.2   PRIORITY AREA FOR CLINICAL TRIALS WITH HERBAL DRUGS FROM INDIAN TRADITIONAL MEDICINE

There are an enormous number of medicinal plants in India used by different traditional and classical practitioners for the purpose of treatment of different diseases or symptoms of diseases. It is reported that out of total 15,000 species of higher plants in India, medicinal uses are attributed to over 1500 species (Chakrabarti et al. 2007). Although a wide range of medicinal plants are described in different indigenous system of medicine in India, but only limited numbers of them have been scientifically screened for clinical trial. The committee of the Ministry of AYUSH has categorised the priority area for clinical trials owing to their efficacy in real practice (http://www.ayush.gov.in/sites/default/files/EMR). In this clarification, there are two categories of prioritisation – primary and secondary – and these priorities differ from one system to the other (Table 20.1). Besides AYUSH, the Ayurvedic Biology division of the Department of Science and Technology, Government of India, and Indian Council of Medical Research (ICMR) also encourage clinical research with herbal drugs from traditional Indian systems of medicines in some certain priority areas.

20.3   SINGLE-HERB BASED CLINICAL TRIAL

Although most of the therapeutic modules of different traditional system of medicine in India are designed with multidrug compositions, but there are descriptions of several single herbs that were screened for clinical trial in various important areas. Some of those described have been found to be therapeutically potent on the basis of these trials, as reported in different scientific journals.

20.3.1   ANTI-STRESS EFFECT OF *WITHANIA SOMNIFERA*

Withania somnifera Dunal (Solanaceae) is a popular medicinal plant, commonly known as ashwagandha, and is mentioned in almost all traditional systems of Indian medicine for its adaptogenic, antioxidant, anticancer, anxiolytic, antidepressant, cardioprotective, thyroid modulating, immuno-modulating, antibacterial, antifungal, anti-inflammatory, neuroprotective, cognitive enhancing and haematopoietic activities. The adaptogenic activity of this plant is very popular and the aqueous extract of the root of the plant at a dose of 300 mg day^{-1} was screened on 34 patients suffering with stress of different origins assessed on the basis of the perceived stress (PSS) scale. The effect was compared with respect to an equal number of patients treated with a placebo drug. Subjects were screened on the basis of the PSS scale, DASS (Depression Anxiety Stress Scale) questionnaire and a 28-item version of the General Health questionnaire (GHQ-28) at 15-day intervals up to 60 days. Serum cortisol levels were also estimated on day '0' and '60'. A highly significant ($p < 0.001$) result was observed in the *W. somnifera* treated group with respect to the placebo control treated group as observed on the basis of the PSS, DASS and GHQ-28 parameters, as well as serum cortisol level, which indicates its potent adaptogenic activity (Chandrasekhar et al. 2012). However, adverse events like nasal congestion (rhinitis), constipation, cough and cold, drowsiness and decreased appetite were seen in the ashwagandha group. However, all these adverse effects are not serious health problem.

20.3.2 Antidiabetic Property of *Gymnema sylvestre*

Gymnema sylvestre R. Br. (Apocynaceae), commonly known as gurmar, is a mystery of the nature as it causes the loss of sensation of sweet taste upon chewing the leaves of the plant. The plant is described in *Sushruta Samhita* of Ayurveda by the name of Meshashringi for therapeutic use in *Madhumeha* (diabetes mellitus). Many pharmacological and chemical studies have been performed with this plant by different scientists and potent biological activities of low molecular weight extracts have been observed. It is reported in a study that the aqueous extract of the high molecular weight could stimulate insulin secretion both *in vivo* and *in vitro* human models (Al-Romaiyan et al. 2010). The *in vivo* study was carried out on 11 patients with type 2 diabetes mellitus (T2DM) with an aqueous extract of *G. sylvestre* at a dose of 1 g/day in two equal divided doses before meals continuously for 60 days. The mean postprandial blood glucose level was reduced from 291 $\pm$ 10 to 236 $\pm$ 30 mg/dL ($p < 0.02$) after 60 days of therapy. This result was supported with the evidence of significant increase level of serum insulin from 24 $\pm$ 09 to 32 $\pm$ 06 µU/mL ($p < 0.001$) with corresponding increase of serum C-peptide level 298 $\pm$ 42 to 447 $\pm$ 48 pmol/L ($p < 0.05$). Owing to the result of the *in vivo* study, the *in vitro* effect of *G. sylvestre* was examined for insulin secretion from human islets using a multi-channel, temperature-controlled perifusion system. Perifusion of human islets with buffer supplemented with 0.125 mg/mL *G. sylvestre* at a sub-stimulatory concentration (2 mM) of glucose evoked an approximately two fold increase in insulin secretion (217 $\pm$ 18% basal, $p < 0.001$). Subsequent exposure to 20 mM glucose following *G. sylvestre* treatment induced a further increase in insulin secretion. Increasing the glucose concentration from 2 to 20 mM (10–30 min) resulted in the expected biphasic pattern of glucose-induced insulin secretion. This study reflects that *G. sylvestre* may have a direct stimulatory effect on insulin secretion from β-cell of islets of Langerhans to combat T2DM. The clinical trial with *G. sylvestre* was undertaken after its thorough safety and efficacy study at a preclinical level on rat and mouse models.

20.3.3 *Curcuma longa* as a Drug for Peptic Ulcer and Cancer Therapy

Indian traditional system of medicine became popular in 1995 due to protests against the patenting of an Indian medicinal plant haridra (turmeric) by the US government (US Patent 5401504), which India won in 1997 after a long legal fight. The plant *Curcuma longa* Linn (family *Zingiberaceae*), commonly known as haridra, is popularly used for multiple therapeutic purposes like anti-inflam-matory, analgesics, antibacterial and antitumour activity (Araujo and Leon 2001). In addition to detailed chemical and pharmacological research carried out with this plant, extensive clinical trials have been undertaken in many different therapeutic areas. Evaluation of *C. longa* for its activity against peptic ulcer is one such example. In one study, the crude powder of *C. longa* at a dose of

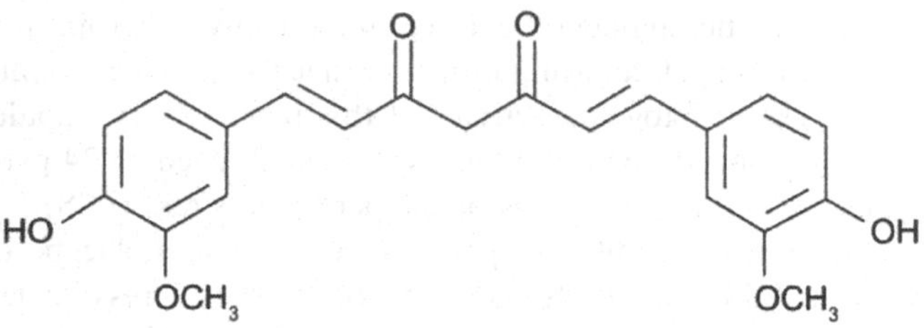

FIGURE 20.1   Curcumin, the active chemical constituent of *Curcuma longa*.

3 g in five divided doses daily for up to 12 weeks was administered to 49 patients diagnosed with peptic ulcers on the basis of clinical symptoms and endoscopic examination. The ulcer sizes varied between 0.5 to 1.5 cm in diameter. After 4 weeks of treatment, ulcers were absent in 12 cases (DU 9 and GU 3). Eighteen cases (DU 13 and GU 5) had absence of ulcer after 8 weeks of treatment. Nineteen cases (DU 14 and GU 5) did not have ulcers after 12 weeks of treatment. Detailed blood biochemistry like blood sugar, BUN, creatine, uric acid, total protein including albumin and globulin, liver function tests, lipid profiles and electrolytes like sodium, potassium, calcium, chloride, phosphorus and bicarbonate were estimated for all the patients and were found to have no adverse effect after treatment with *C. longa* (Prucksunand et al. 2001). The active chemical constituent of the plant, curcumin (diferuloylmethane; Figure 20.1) is reported for its anticancer activity in various type of carcinoma. Probably the first indication of curcumin's anticancer activities in human participants was shown in 1987 by Kuttan et al., who conducted a clinical trial involving 62 patients with external cancerous lesions. Topical curcumin was found to produce remarkable symptomatic relief, as evidenced by reductions in smell, itching, lesion size and pain. Since then, curcumin, either alone or in combination with other agents, has demonstrated potential effects in patients suffering from colorectal cancer, pancreatic cancer, breast cancer, prostate cancer, multiple myeloma, lung cancer, oral cancer, and head and neck squamous cell carcinoma (HNSCC; Gupta et al. 2013).

20.3.4   CARDIORESPIRATORY IMPROVEMENT WITH *EMBLICA OFFICINALIS*

Incidence of cardiorespiratory problems is increasing worldwide and the same scenario is also reflected in India due to various causes like smoking, environmental pollution, over exposure to stress and strain, and urbanisation. In accordance with the report of the National Commission of Macroeconomics and Health (NCMH 2005), diseases like tuberculosis, COPD (chronic obstructive pulmonary disease), bronchial asthma and heart diseases are becoming devastating the country and the rough annual cost for an individual patient with acute COPD is 32,000 INR, including hospitalisation (NCMH 2005). Development of drugs is, therefore, an urgent issue to prevent cardiorespiratory problems. *Emblica officinalis* Gaertn. (family Euphorbiaceae), commonly known as amla, is traditionally reputed for various biological activities including immunomodulation, anti-ulcer and anti-ageing. The aqueous extract of the fruit of the plant containing at least 60% w/w low molecular weight hydrolysable tannins, consisting of emblicanin-A, emblicanin-B, pedunculagin and punigluconin as screened by HPLC (Figure 20.2), was tested for clinical efficacy in 30 male subjects aged between 20 and 60 years, with excessive (>15 cigarettes/day) and long smoking history (>10 years), chronic cough, poor immune status (recurrent infection), compromised cardiovascular status (assessed based on cardiac parameters like ECG) and lipid profile, decreased appetite and digestive function, poor libido and willing to give informed consent. Patients were divided into two groups with 20 patients in group 'I' and 10 patients in group 'II', who received 500 mg of *E. officinalis* extract (coded as *Capros*) and placebo, respectively, for 60 days. The study revealed that subjects who were treated with *E. officinalis* extract experienced a significant increase in serum HDL level (25.6%), thus reducing their cardiac risk by 25%–28%. Lipoprotein (a), a putative risk

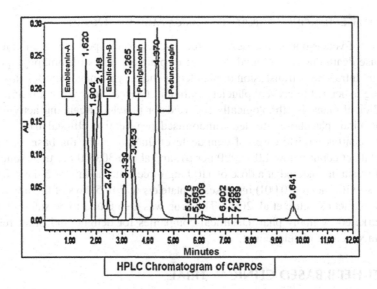

FIGURE 20.2 High-performance liquid chromatography analysis of *E. officinalis* aqueous extract. (Courtesy of Natreon Inc., India.)

factor for atherosclerotic diseases, such as coronary heart disease and stroke, was reduced by 20.5%. There was no sign of deterioration in respiratory fitness as evident from the values of forced expiratory volume (FEV1) [2.43 ± 0.16 and 2.36 ± 0.14 on 0 day and 60 day, respectively], forced vital capacity (FVC) [2.61 ± 0.15 and 2.52 ± 0.14 on 0 day and 60 days respectively] and the percentage ratio of FEV1 and FVC (FEV1: FVC) [92.03 ± 1.41 and 92.99 ± 1.61 on day 0 and day 60, respectively]. Chromosomal aberration is a common phenomenon in chronic smokers, which can be identified by study of mitotic index, and the present study showed that the mitotic index was significantly lower, indicating prevention of DNA damage (Biswas et al. 2014).

20.3.5 Wound Healing Potential of *Pterocarpus santalinus*

The healing of wounds is a natural phenomenon but it may lack quality, promptness and aesthetics, especially during occurrence of non-healing complicated wounds. Therapeutic manipulation is needed to overcome these drawbacks. In modern medicine, there is no direct wound-healing drug. Topical antibiotics are sometimes used for this purpose, but these have no direct role in the healing of wounds. In Ayurveda, 164 medicinal plants are described for their wound healing activity in the parlance of *Vranaropaka* drugs (Biswas and Mukherjee 2003). *Pterocarpus santalinus* Linn (family Fabaceae), commonly known as red sandalwood, is an important medicinal plant under this group, which was clinically screened in a pilot study for its wound healing property. An ointment of the heartwood of the plant (15%, w/w) was evaluated on six patients of lower extremity wounds on the basis of the wound contraction size (mm²), wound index, granulation, epithelialisation, neo-vascularisation and routine haematological parameters. The study revealed that the wounds were closed within 15–30 days, with improved physical and haematological parameters. Neutrophil counts were decreased promisingly with increase lymphocyte count, indicating successful collagenesis (Biswas et al. 2004a). This study was performed on the basis of the significant result obtained in initial pharmacological screening of the plant on 8 mm full thickness punch and burn wounds in rats on the basis of the physical parameters like wound contraction size (mm²), wound index, healing period (days), tensile strength (g); molecular markers like tissue DNA, RNA, protein and hydroxyproline; PAGE study and histological screening of wound tissues (Biswas et al. 2004b).

20.3.6 Platelet-Enhancing Property of *Carica papaya* in Dengue

Among varieties of vector-borne diseases, dengue fever is now appearing as an alarming disease, which may cause death due to profound decrease of platelet counts (thrombocytopenia) followed by haemorrhage. Intravenous transfusion of platelets is the only management for this condition and therefore, a drug is needed to prevent platelet inhibition. *Carica papaya* Linn (family Caricaceae), an Indian medicinal plant, is ethnologically reported for platelet enhancing activity and a multi-centric, double-blind, placebo-controlled, randomised prospective clinical trial was undertaken in five separate centres on 300 cases of dengue fever diagnosed on the basis of the serum NS_1 positive with platelet count below 1,000,000 per µL and above 30,000 per µL. Aqueous extract of *C. papaya* leaf was administered at a dose of 1100 mg three times a day for 5 days. It was observed that there were significant ($p < 0.001$) increases of platelets within 5 days of therapy on treatment of *C. papaya* leaf extract (Kasture et al. 2016). The drug was also found to be safe in human subjects and is now marketed by many pharmaceutical companies for dengue and other related diseases requiring enhancement of platelet count.

20.4 MULTI-HERB BASED CLINICAL TRIAL

20.4.1 Clinical Trial of Triphala

Ayurveda and other traditional systems of medicine are mainly based on various multi-herb formulations for the treatment of different diseases. There are many groups of drugs that are uniquely combined in a sequence since antiquity for very specific clinical application, and *triphala* is such a combination, which is composed of equal quantities (1:1:1) of three medicinal plants of Indian origin: *Terminalia chebula* Retz. (family Combretaceae) commonly known as Haritaki, *Terminalia bellirica* Linn. (family Combretaceae) commonly known as Bibhitak and *Emblica officinalis* Gaertn. (family Euphorbiaceae), commonly known as Amla. Each individual ingredient of Triphala possesses a specific biological property, but the combined form of these three drugs exhibits other activities than the individual ingredients, including antioxidant, digestive, laxative and anticancer effects (Kumar 2014). A clinical trial of this herbal combination was undertaken to qualify its well-being property in terms of bowel-regulating activity and well-being performance on 160 patients of either sex ranging from 15 to 75 years on the basis of the subjective parameters of bowel movement concerns such as constipation, undigested food materials in the stool, belching, abdominal pain, sleep, appetite and thirst. Patients were divided into two groups; the test compound-treated group consisted of 120 patients in three sub-groups, with 40 patients in each sub-group – one each for two separate market samples of *triphala*, as well as one for a standard *triphala* preparation – and one placebo control group of 40 patients. Drugs (triphala or placebo) were administered at a dose of 5 g per day for 30 days duration to all patients. The study showed that amount of stool (g) significantly improved in all three triphala-treated groups with respect to the placebo-treated group. There were also significant improvements to frequency of stool, undigested food content and colour and consistency of the stool. Associated physical symptoms like odour of stool, mucus in stool, flatulence and abdominal pain were also significantly improved. Psychological symptoms like mental concentration and sleep were also improved significantly (Mukherjee et al. 2006). The most important fact of this clinical trial is that the research was carried out purely on the basis of subjective parameters without involving any objective parameters.

20.4.2 Hepato-Protective Effect of *Picrorhiza kurroa* and *Tinospora cordifolia* Combination

There are number of drugs in modern medicine that may cause hepatotoxicity. Statin is one such drug that is used as a lipid-lowering agent in cardiovascular disease, which may cause hepatotoxicity due to elevation of serum aminotransaminase levels. In a clinical study with 50 complete cases of hyperlipidaemia treated with statin at a dose of 20 mg per day, patients were divided into two equal groups (25 in each group) and were treated with a combination of the medicinal plant Katuki (*Picrorhiza kurroa* Royle Ex benth., family Plantaginaceae) processed in Guduchi (*Tinospora cordifolia* Wild, family Menispermaceae) in a dose of 4 g per day in two divided doses for a period of 3 months and no additional supplementary drugs respectively. It was observed that after 90 days of treatment, serum bilirubin, AST (SGOT), ALT (SGPT) and serum alkaline phosphatase levels were significantly improved in the trial group compared to the control group, indicating the potentiality of this two-drug combination for it hepatoprotective effects in patients of hyperlipidaemia treated with statin (Harbans and Sharma 2011).

20.4.3 APPETITE STIMULATION ACTIVITY OF TRIKATU

Like Triphala, a combined drug with three components of medicinal plants with similar qualities is called Trikatu or Triusana, owing to the property of being pungent (*katu*) in taste. The medicinal plant rhizome of *sunthi* or ginger (*Zingiber officinalis* Roscoe, family Zingiberaceae), fruit of *pippali* or long pepper (*Piper longum* L., family Piperaceae) and the fruit of *maricha* or black pepper (*Piper nigrum* L., family Piperaceae) are family members of this group of drug which is widely popular in Ayurveda for various activities as

पिप्पली मरीच शुण्ठी त्रिभिः त्रयो उष्णं उच्यते।

दीपनं श्लेष्म मेदोघ्न कुष्ठ पीनसनाशनम।।

जयेत अरोचकम सामं मेहगुल्म गलामयान।

- शारंगधर संहिता, ६/१२-१३

Pippali Maricha Šhunthi Tribhih Trayo Uşanam Uchyate /
Dīpanam Šhleshma Medoghna Kuştha Pinasa Nāsanam //
Jayet Arochakam Sāmam Mehagulma Galāmayan //

– Shāramgadhar Samhitā, 6/12–13

That is, *pippali*, *sunthi* and *maricha* in the combination known as triusana are beneficial for stimulation of secretion for gastric juices, alleviation of cough and cold, obesity, obstinate skin diseases, rhinitis, appetite enhancer, control diabetes and have a cleansing effect on the throat (Srikanthamurthy 2003). Presence of piperine in this combination has been established by HPTLC fingerprinting, which is reported to be the most important chemical component for various therapeutic activities of this combination (Vyas et al. 2011). Taking the lead of the classical description of Ayurveda as well as modern chemical fingerprinting, an attempt at clinical evaluation of this compound's appetite-enhancing activity on the basis of the Ayurvedic methodology of examination of patients was undertaken. A total of 60 patients with dyspepsia were selected for this study, who were divided into groups 'A', who received the powder form of trikatu in a dose of 2 g twice daily, and group 'B', who received the classical Ayurvedic formulation *Agnitundi Vati*, used conventionally for the same purpose, in a dose of 250 mg twice a day. After 21 days of treatment with these two groups of drugs, it was observed that effect of trikatu was significantly better than the other group on the basis of the classical symptoms assessed on the basis of the arbitrary score (Singh 2012).

20.5 MARKETING AND PRODUCT POSITIONING

There is enormous scope for the marketing of Ayurvedic and herbal drugs of Indian origin in the near future at home and abroad. It is reported that the Indian Ayurvedic drug market is estimated to be about 80 billion INR consisting of products manufactured and marketed by thousands of small and medium-scale units and a dozen large companies (Francis 2016). Clinical trial of drugs manufactured by different herbal and Ayurvedic pharmaceutical companies are essential to achieve this target to compete with leading countries in this field. However, most of the pharmaceutical houses for herbal drugs are merely interested in conducting clinical trial of their drugs. There are some reports of clinical trials of herbal drug formulations by some of the Indian pharmaceutical houses, but most of them conducted this with limited infrastructure for clinical trial set up in the companies. Moreover, the trial results are not published in any significant journals. This situation is probably due to the fact that there is no mandatory stricture for undertaking clinical trials of herbal drug formulation by the company, once they have received the good manufacture practice (GMP) certification. Moreover, regulations state that herbal drugs formulated in accordance with classical formulation are not required to be subject to any further clinical trial. Although marketing of these herbal formulations may not be hampered within the country, positioning in the global market may be affected due to proper follow-up of clinical trials.

20.6 CLINICAL TRIAL PROTOCOL OF HERBAL DRUGS: REGULATION OF THE GOVERNMENT OF INDIA

20.6.1 GOOD CLINICAL PRACTICE

The Ministry of AYUSH, Government of India, has established specific guidelines regarding good clinical practice for Ayurveda, Siddha and Unani medicine (GCP-ASU; India 2013a). The guidelines include relevant compound protocol, ethical and safety considerations, monitoring systems, record keeping, data handling and quality assurance. The most important issues that are discussed in the guideline are phases of clinical trial for ASU drugs and/or patent or proprietary drugs. Four phases, including human pharmacology (phase I), therapeutic exploratory trials (phase II), therapeutic confirmatory trials (phase III) and pot marketing trials (phase IV), are described in detail for these traditional Indian systems of medicine. This protocol differs from conventional clinical trials on the basis of concept and design, as the preclinical trial method is not included. The drugs described in the ASU system are recommended to have a direct trial on healthy volunteers for the evaluation of safety and efficacy on human subjects as evidence of their use dates back several generations. However, the use of standard comparative drugs, specified inclusion and exclusion criteria, randomisation, blinding techniques are required. Ethical issues are emphasised in the guideline, which has been described in accordance with the guideline of the Indian Council of Medical Research (ICMR 2006).

20.6.2 ETHICAL ASPECT OF CLINICAL TRIAL ON INDIAN HERBAL DRUGS

Research on the herbal drugs of the traditional Indian system of medicine are now become very popular worldwide, and many scientists of modern medicine and other biological science desire to pursue clinical research with these agents. ICMR, Government of India, has published a general guideline regarding clinical trial protocols for Ayurveda, Unani, Siddha and medicinal plants, as well as ethical issues for human clinical trials (ICMR 2006). The guideline describes how every clinical trial should receive necessary permission for conducting clinical trials from their respective institutional ethics committee (IEC). The IEC should consist of 8–12 members, of which the Member Secretary, who will conduct the meeting, must be a representative from the host institute, and the head of the institute should not be selected for that post. A maximum of two members, including the Member Secretary from the host institute, will be selected to represent the IEC. The Chairman should always be a person outside the institute and preferably from a higher post of any organisation. Other members of the committee should be persons like clinicians, basic scientists (preferably pharmacologists), legal persons(s), layperson(s) and social scientists. There must be one ethicist in the committee with previous experience of participating in IEC meeting or trained for IEC from the outside. The main role of the IEC is to examine the safety aspect of the protocol with assessment of risks and benefit, if any. The IEC protocol varies from general clinical protocols on the basis of highlighting the aspects of safety and efficacy. The members of the IEC should also carefully examine whether the fundamental ethical perspectives, like trilingual informed consent form (ICF), are designed in accordance with WHO–Helsinki declaration (World Medical Association 2011) in which one language must be local. Besides ICF, the members of the IEC should also carefully examine the subject information sheet (SIS) for the healthy volunteers/patients to make him/her aware about the basic knowledge of the clinical trial in colloquial language.

20.6.3 DCGI CLEARANCE

The IEC of any institute is officially recognised in India by the Drug Control General of India (DCGI). The official registration of an IEC is done by the DCGI (Evangelin et al. 2017). However, the IEC of ASU drugs in different institutes does not come under the direct jurisdiction of the DCGI, so the registration of the IEC for ASU drugs is not needed. The government of India plans in the near future to implement rules for recognition of IEC by DCGI or other authorised organisations.

20.6.4 CLINICAL TRIAL REGISTRATION

Every clinical trial protocol on herbal drugs must be registered under the specific pro forma of the clinical trial registry of India (CTRI; www.ctri.nic.in). This registration is to be done through the online system to obtain a registration number after a thorough examination of the protocol, and unless it is done prior to initiation of the clinical trial and after obtaining permission from the IEC, no scientific publication can take place in any reputed national or international journal. In a study of clinical trials of Ayurvedic drugs, very few publications in this field are registered under the CTRI (Sridharan and Sivaramakrishnan 2016), indicating that more quality evidence is required for clinical research in this field.

20.6.5 NATIONAL HEALTH PORTAL

Recently, the Government of India introduced a National Health Portal for discussion of various health-related issues, including the role of medicinal plants for the prevention and control of some diseases. The portal mentions that herbs such as black pepper, cinnamon, myrrh, aloe, sandalwood, ginseng, red clover, burdock, bayberry and safflower are used to heal wounds, and that turmeric is useful to prevent and control infections due to bacteria (India 2016). However, most of this information is based on reports published in different books and scientific journals and is mainly designed to disseminate knowledge to a general audience.

20.6.6 CCRAS

The Central Council for Research on Ayurvedic Sciences (CCRAS) is the main regulatory body in India for conducting clinical trials with various Ayurvedic drugs, including medicinal plants following the standard guidelines. The CCRAS has identified 1690 clinical trials on medicinal plants from outside the India, while there are 102 studies on medicinal plants at the combined level of fundamental and clinical trials in India (India 2015).

20.6.7 CCCEM: EVIDENCE FROM CLINICAL TRIALS

Like the CCRAS, the Central Council for Research on Unani Medicine (CCRUM) is another regulatory body for clinical trials with Unani medicines. Most of the clinical studies of Unani medicine are found to be limited within the academic space of post-graduate studies and are rarely cited in larger journals. CCRUM has published a guidebook with detailed descriptions of traditional terms in an attempt to bridge the gap between modern language and traditional Unani medicine like *baras* as vitiligo, *nār fārsī* as eczema, *waja'-a-mafaṣil* or rheumatoid arthritis, *katharat-i-shahm al-dam* or hyperlipidaemia, and so forth (India 2013b).

20.6.8 Traditional Knowledge Digital Library

The Traditional Knowledge Digital Library (TKDL) program deals with the documentation of existing knowledge within Ayurvedic systems of medicine. It is imperative to safeguard the sovereignty of traditional Ayurvedic knowledge to protect it from being misused via patenting of non-patentable inventions. Although this knowledge is in the public domain, the patent office does not have a mechanism to access this information to deny patent rights. Obtaining patents for all such medicinal uses is impossible. It is also extremely costly and time-consuming to fight patents granted to others. Thus, bringing such knowledge into an easily accessible format to forestall wrongful patents is one of the goals of the TKDL (http://www.tkdl.res.in). It is an original proprietary database, which is fully protected by national and international intellectual property rights laws. The core of the project is the innovative approach in the form of Traditional Knowledge Resource Classification (TKRC), which enables conversion of 140,000 pages of information, containing 36,000 formulations described in 14 Ayurvedic texts, into patent-compatible format in various languages, including the translation of Sanskrit *shlokas* not only into Hindi, but also into other language such as English, French, German, Spanish and Japanese. The information includes names of plants, Ayurvedic description of diseases under their modern names, therapeutic formulations, and so on (Katoch et al. 2017).

20.7 NEW JOURNEY

Therapy with herbal drugs for the prevention, control and cure of several diseases is a worldwide practice. In India, it has been popular since time immemorial. Evidence-based knowledge has tremendous importance for the development of a therapeutic model with herbal drugs, but scientific evaluation is also needed to re-establish its potentiality in the modern scientific world. The World Health Organization is also looking for improvement of the clinical trial procedure for herbal drugs used in different traditional and complementary systems of medicine practiced in different parts of world, including India. Although clinical trials with various herbal formulations are now being conducted as thesis projects in postgraduate courses from different AYUSH systems in India, they are not entering the limelight due to the lack of proper documentation. Clinical trials with herbal drugs are now becoming a tough job, because they must cross several hurdles to reach their goal. The new journey for clinical trials with herbal drugs can be fulfilled by satisfying all the necessary regulations. Categorisation of trial fields is the first and foremost work. Herbal drugs have been used for a long time in India, but there are certain limitations to clinical use, such as most antidiabetic herbal drugs can lower blood glucose level up to a certain limit in T2DM, but no effect has so far been established in T1DM. Every clinical scientist should limit themselves to considering these practical implications. A survey of the literature and accumulation of knowledge from traditional folklore practitioners is also important for finding new directions for this journey. A detail field survey with a specialist team of scientists having profound knowledge in the identification of plants and their uses may be beneficial for collecting information. The knowledge of herbal drugs for therapeutic uses is described in different texts from many traditions, including Ayurveda, Siddha, Unani, and homeopathy, but the cross communication between traditional practitioners, modern medical experts and natural product chemists may bring a fruitful and practical.

The medicinal plants selected for clinical trial should be properly authenticated by a recognised organisation, and the Botanical Survey of India is the leading institute for this purpose. Voucher specimen of each individual plant should be preserved properly for future reference. There are certain diseases like stress disorders, irritable bowel syndrome or pain management, where subjective parameter using certain standardised scales (e.g. Ham 'A' and Ham 'D' scale for anxiety and depression respectively) are enough to assess the clinical efficacy of herbal drugs during clinical trial, but most diseases are now diagnosed with the help of sophisticated biochemical, haematological, genetic, radio-imaging or cytological investigations alongside clinical features, which are to be incorporated to a maximum limit to establish the actual disease, as well as to exclude differential diagnosis, so that the successful outcome of the clinical trial can be achieved in a rational way.

Randomisation of patients/subjects with more than one trial drug or doses of drugs is an essential condition to be followed strictly in the new journey. There are several procedures for the randomisation of patients, of which stratified randomisation and in-group randomisation are the two most important methods; different groups of patient are distributed in a balance manner under stratified randomisation, but in the other method patients are randomised according to specifications of group of treatment or condition of variations of clinical features (University of Chicago 2015).

Blinding is another necessary issue for this new journey for clinical trials with herbal drugs. A blind—or blinded—experiment is an experiment in which information about the test is masked (kept) from the participant, to reduce or eliminate bias, until after a trial outcome is known. It is understood that bias may be intentional or unconscious, so no dishonesty is implied by blinding. Blinding can be of different categories such as single, double, triple, masking and allocation concealment, but in clinical trial double blinding is common, which refers to keeping study participants, investigators and data assessors unaware of the allocated treatment or therapy, so that they are not influenced psychologically or physically by that knowledge (Bang et al. 2004). Use of comparator drug is also important for development of drugs from herbal origin. Comparators may be standard in relation to the selection of specified diseases or placebo control. Placebo therapy has neither an enhancing role nor a decreasing property for the disease process, but the use of a placebo is ethically contraindicated for some diseases like diabetes mellitus, bronchial asthma or cardiovascular disorders where stoppage of conventional management may cause a flare up of the disease condition. Selection of standard comparator is also to be done in a rational way in accordance with the disease condition. There may be more than one group of standard comparator drugs, attention should be given to selection based on the modus operandi. Cross-over studies may sometimes be helpful for two or more than two doses of any test drugs to reduce the chances of bias. In this condition, a period of 7–10 days is required as washout period. Meta-analysis of data revealed from the end of the study should be done critically, so that the research outcome is not challengeable and can be used for the benefit of mankind. Finally, applications of standard clinical trial phases from preclinical safety and efficacy studies (phase '0') to the post marketing survey (phase IV) are needed for the development of proper drugs from herbal origins.

20.8 FUTURE TRENDS

The trend of undertaking clinical trial with plant drugs is still lagging behind. However, due to increased awareness of regulations on herbal drug research implemented by the Government of India, the tendency to conduct clinical trials of herbal drug formulations is increasing among different manufacturers of such drugs. The import, manufacture, distribution and sale of herbal drugs described in traditional medicine are regulated by the Drug and Cosmetic Act of 1940 and the Drugs and Cosmetic Rules 1945. In 1993, an expert committee appointed by the Indian government developed guidelines for the safety and efficacy of herbal medicines that were intended to be incorporated into the Drugs and Cosmetics Act and rules. In 2001, the Central Drugs Standard Control Organisation of the Directorate General of Health Services issued GCP guidelines. These guidelines recommend approaches for clinical trials of herbal remedies and medicinal plants (Singh et al. 2004). The trend for clinical trials with herbal drugs is found to be under consideration since 2001 in a specified manner. Some of the manufacturing organisations used to claim the efficacy of a multi-ingredient herbal formulation on the basis of the accumulation of reports on clinical trials of individual drugs available in the published data, but this attitude may be a false interpretation, as the summation of reports may not exhibit the effect specified on the biological system. Separate clinical trials are required in the near future with multi-ingredient formulations of herbal drug to establish claims. Clinical trials of single or multi-ingredient herbal drug formulations and the study of herb–herb interaction is an important issue for new formulations. Attempts are also to be taken in the near future for clinical trials of herbal drugs in combinations with certain modern drugs to potentiate their therapeutic action, as well as to reduce untoward effects from either of the components.

The clinical trial of the anti-tubercular drug rifampicin boosted with piperine, derived from the Indian medicinal plant *Piper longum*, showed that it not only reduces the hepatotoxic effect of rifampicin but also increase its bioavailability (Patel et al. 2017). In addition to the programme proposed above, it may also be proposed to have a detailed multi-centric clinical trial of each herbal formulation so that unique drugs can be developed from Indian medicinal plants for the benefit of common sufferers in specific therapeutic areas.

REFERENCES

Araujo, C. A. C., and Leon, L. L. (2001). Biological activities of *Curcuma longa* L. *Memórias do Instituto Oswaldo Cruz*, **96**, 723–728.

Al-Romaiyan, A., Liu, B., Asare-Anane, H., et al. (2010). A novel *Gymnema sylvestre* extracts stimulates insulin secretion from human islets *in-vivo* and *in vitro*. *Phytotherapy Research*, **24**, 1370–1376.

Bang, H., Ni, L., and Davis, C. E. (2004). Assessment of blinding in clinical trial. *Controlled Clinical Trials*, **25**, 143–156.

Biswas, T. K., Chakrabarti, S., Pandit, S., et al. (2014). Pilot study evaluating the use of *Emblica officinalis* standardized fruit extract in cardio-respiratory improvement and anti-oxidant status of volunteers with smoking history. *Journal of Herbal Medicine*, **4**, 188–194.

Biswas, T. K., Maity, L. N. and Mukherjee, B. (2004a). The clinical evaluation of *Pterocarpus santalinus* Linn ointment on lower extremity wounds: A preliminary report. *International Journal of Lower Extremity Wounds*, **3**(4), 227–232.

Biswas, T. K., Maity, L. N. and Mukherjee, B. (2004b). Wound healing potential of *Pterocarpus santalinus* Linn: A pharmacological evaluation, *International Journal of Lower Extremity Wounds*, **3**(3), 143–150.

Biswas, T. K., and Mukherjee, B. (2003). Plant medicine of Indian origin for wound healing activity: A review. *International Journal of Lower Extremity Wounds*, **2**(1), 25–39.

Bodding, P. O. (1986). *Studies in Santal Medicine and Connected Folklore*. Calcutta, India The Asiatic Society.

Chakrabarti, S., Biswas, T. K., and Mukherjee, B. (2007). Antidiabetic plants: Scientific appraisal at a glance. In J. N. Govil, V. K. Singh and N. T. Siddique, eds., *Recent Progress in Medicinal Plants: Natural Products II*. New Delhi, India: Studium Press. pp. 275–339.

Chandrasekhar, K., Kapoor, J. and Anishetty, S. (2012). A prospective, randomized double-blind, placebo-controlled study of safety and efficacy of a high-concentration full spectrum extract of *Ashwagandha* root in reducing stress and anxiety in adults. *Indian Journal of Psychological Medicine*, **34**, 255–262.

Evangelin, L., Mounica, N. V. N., Reddy, V. S., et al. (2017). Regulatory process and ethics for clinical trials in India. *Pharma Innovation*, **6**, 165–169.

Francis, P. A. (2016). Clinical trials for AYUSH drugs. *PharmaBiz*. First published: 6 April 2016. Available from: http://www.pharmabiz.com/NewsDetails.aspx?aid=94429&sid=3

Gupta, S. C., Patchva, S., and Aggarwal, B. B., (2013). Therapeutic roles of curcumin: Lessons learned from clinical trial. *AAPS Journal*, **15**, 195–218.

Harbans, S., and Sharma, Y. K. (2011). Clinical evaluation of the hepatoprotective effect of Katuki (*Picrorhiza kurroa* Royle ex benth) and processed in Guduchi (*Tinosppora cordifolia*, Wild) Miers in patients receiving lipid lowering drugs (statin). *Indian Journal of Traditional Knowledge*, **10**, 657–660.

India. Central Council for Research in Ayurvedic Sciences (CCRAS). (2015). *Research publications in Ayurvedic sciences*. New Delhi, India: Government of India, Ministry of AYUSH.

India. Ministry of AYUSH. (2013a). *Good Clinical Practice Guidelines for Clinical Trials in Ayurveda, Siddha and Unani Medicine (GCP-ASU)*. New Delhi, India: Government of India, Ministry of AYUSH. pp. 1–61.

India. Ministry of AYUSH. (2013b). Institutional network of Central Council for Research on Unani Medicine. In: *Unani System of Medicine: The Science of Health and Healing*, New Delhi, India: Government of India, Ministry of AYUSH. pp. 76–78.

India. Ministry of AYUSH. (2017). *Annual Report 2016–2017*. New Delhi, India: Ministry of AYUSH.

India. Ministry of Health and Family Welfare. (2005). *Disease burden in India, estimation and causal analysis*. New Delhi, India: Government of India, Ministry of Health and Family Welfare. 1–6.

India. Ministry of Health and Family Welfare. (2016). Introduction and importance of medicinal plants and herbs. *National Health Portal: Unani Medicine*. Available from: http://www.nhp.gov.in/introduction-and-importance-of-medicinal-plants-and-herbs_mtl [Acessed 19 November 2017].

Indian Council of Medical Research (ICMR). (2006). Basic responsibilities of ethical review; Clinical evaluation of traditional Ayurveda, Siddha, Unani (ASU) remedies and medicinal plants. In: *Ethical Guidelines for Biomedical Research on Human Participants.* New Delhi, India: ICMR.

Itrat, M. (2016). Research in Unani medicine: Challenges and way forward. *Alternative and Integrative Medicine,* **5**, 1–4.

Jain, A. K., and Patole, S. N. (2001). Less known medicinal values of plants among some tribal and rural communities of Panchmari forest (MP). *Ethnobotany,* **13**, 96–100.

Kasture, P. N., Nagabhusan, K. H., and Kumar, A. (2016). A multi-centric, double blind, placebo controlled, randomized, prospective study to evaluate the efficacy and safety of *Carica papaya* leaf extract, as empirical therapy for thrombocytopenia associated with dengue fever. *Journal of the Association of Physicians of India,* **64**, 15–20.

Katoch, D., Sharma, J. S., Banerjee, S., et al. (2017). Government policies and initiatives for development of Ayurveda. *Journal of Ethnopharmacology,* **197**, 25–31.

Kumar, A. (2014). A review of traditional anticancer nanomedicine—triphala. *Pharma Innovation,* **3**(7), 60–66.

Mukherjee, P. K., Harwansh, R. K., Bahadur, S., et al. (2017). Development of Ayurveda: Tradition to trend. *Journal of Ethnopharmacology,* **197**, 10–24.

Mukherjee, P. K., Ray, S., Bhattacharyya, S., et al. (2006). Clinical study of triphala-a well known phytomedicine from India. *Iranian Journal of Pharmacology and Therapeutics,* **5**, 51–56.

Patel, N., Jagannath, K., Vora, A., et al. (2017). A randomized, controlled, phase III clinical trial to evaluate the efficacy and tolerability of risorine with conventional rifampicine in the treatment of newly diagnosed pulmonary tuberculosis. *Journal of the Association of Physicians of India,* **65**, 48–54.

Prucksunand, C., Indrasukhsri, B., Leethochawalit, M., et al. (2001). Phase II clinical trial on effect of long turmeric (*Curcuma longa* Linn) on healing of peptic ulcer. *Southeast Asian Journal of Tropical Medicine and Public Health,* **32**, 208–215.

Sharma, N. K., Singh, P. K., Pramanik, V., et al. (2016). Meeting report: Traditional ethnomedicinal knowledge of Indian tribes, National Workshop cum Seminar organised by Faculty of Science, Indira Gandhi National Tribal University, Amarkanta, 9–1, March 2015, *Current Science,* **110**, 486–487.

Singh, A. K. (2012). Clinical evaluation of Trikatu as appetite stimulant (agnivardhan). *Journal of Pharmaceutical and Scientific Innovation,* **1**, 50–4.

Singh, H. P., Sharma, S., Chauhan, S. B., et al. (2004). Clinical trials of traditional herbal medicine in India: Current status and challenges. *International Journal of Pharmacognosy,* **1**, 415–421.

Sridharan, K. and Sivaramakrishnan, G. (2016). Clinical trials in Ayureda: Analysis of clinical trial registry of India. *Journal of Ayurveda and Integrative Medicine,* **7**, 141–143.

Srikanthamurthy, K. R., ed. (2003). *Saramgadhar Samhita – A treatise on Ayurveda.* Varanasi, India: Chaukhambha Orientalia.

University of Chicago, Center for Research Informatics. (2015). Randomization module. *REDCap Training with CRI.* Available from: http://cri.uchicago.edu/wp-content/uploads/2015/12/REDCap-Randomization-Module.pdf.

Vassou, S. L., Nithaniyal, S., Raju, B., et al. (2016). Creation of reference DNA barcode library and authentication of medicinal plant raw drug used in Ayurvedic medicine. *BMC Complementary and Alternative Medicine,* **16**, 186–192.

Vyas, A., Jain, V., Singh, D., et al. (2011). TLC densitometric method for the estimation of piperine in Ayurvedic formulation trikatu churna. *Oriental Journal of Chemistry,* **27**, 301–304.

World Medical Association. (2011). Declaration of Helsinki: Ethical principles for medical research involving human subjects. *Bulletin of the World Health Organization,* **79**, 373–374.

Xavier, T.M., Kannan, M., Lija, L., et al. (2014). Ethnobotanical study of Kani tribes in Thoduhills of Kerala, South India. *Journal of Ethnopharmacology,* **152**, 78–90.

21 Nanotechnology and Anti-Ageing Skin Care

B. Fibrich, I.A. Lambrechts and N. Lall

CONTENTS

21.1 INTRODUCTION

21.1.1 THE SKIN

The skin can be described as a single sheet-like organ containing cells of various embryonic origin that plays a pivotal role in our daily lives by serving primarily as a crucial barrier of defence against external stress. It therefore assumes a number of important physiological functions and plays an important role in how we are perceived in society. This has put ageing treatments in the forefront of research and the cosmetic industry. The skin is distinguished by three main layers, namely the epidermis, dermis and subcutaneous fat layer (Figure 21.1). The epidermis is the outermost layer of the

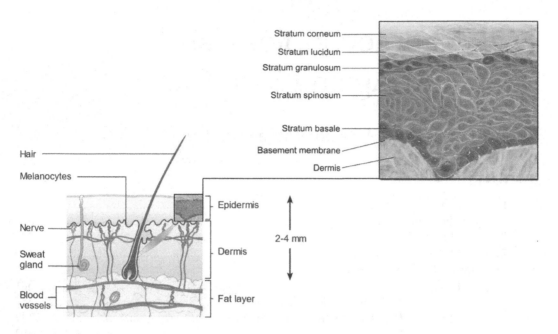

FIGURE 21.1   (See color insert.) The three main layers of skin, namely the epidermis, dermis and subcutaneous or fat layer. (Courtesy of Cancer Research UK, 2014.)

skin and is composed of two main cell types, keratinocytes and melanocytes, which strategically form 4–5 layers (depending on the locale of the body). Keratinocytes and melanocytes are formed as part of the primary ectoderm during early embryonic development. The former is responsible for the production of collagen, while the latter arise from neural crest cells and are responsible for the production of melanin. Together these cells form the stratum corneum (the outermost layer comprised of dead cells lacking a nucleus and organelles), the stratum lucidum (a translucent layer present only on thicker skin found on the palms of the hands and soles of the feet), the stratum granulosum (containing more granular cellular bodies such as keratohyalin and lamellar bodies, responsible for hydrophobicity and barrier functions), the stratum spinosum (where keratinisation begins) and the innermost layer of the epidermis, the stratum basale (the basal layer containing undifferentiated cells and oestrogen receptors).

Connective tissues such as the dermis originate from the mesoderm during embryonic development and contain cellular structures of ectodermal origin such as sweat glands. The dermis forms the bulk of the skin separating cutaneous from non-cutaneous tissue and is comprised of the reticular and papillary layers. These layers contain blood vessels and are more fibrous when compared to the cellular epidermis, however, a few of the cell types that can be found include histiocytes, mast cells and fibroblasts. In addition to housing blood vessels, lymph vessels and nerves, the dermis confers the structural integrity to the skin through the presence of structural components. These fibrous structural components include collagen (97.5%), of which 12 different types have been identified, and elastin (2.5%). Forty per cent of the body's collagen is produced in the skin by fibroblasts. It confers pliability to the skin and runs parallel to the skin, while elastin is responsible for the elasticity of the skin and occurs as a network. Glycosaminoglycans are also found within the dermis and stratum spinosum and are produced by both fibroblast cells as well as keratinocytes. Subtypes found within the skin include dermatan sulphate, chondroitin sulphate and hyaluronic acid, and these are responsible for binding water and affording the skin its soft texture. Sufficient water in the dermis also protects lower tissues from compression. Although controversial, glycosaminoglycans have been thought to remain stable with age, however, hyaluronic acid, found at elastin-collagen junctions, has been noted to decline with age and is thought to contribute to ageing of the skin. Lastly, the subcutaneous layer contains blood vessels that protrude into the dermis to supply the skin with nourishment. This layer provides definition to the contouring of the face and acts as a cushion (Calleja-Agius et al. 2013).

21.1.2 SKIN AGEING

Skin ageing can be categorised as either intrinsic (also known as chronological) or extrinsic, ageing depending on the causative agents (Pandel et al. 2013). Intrinsic ageing is the result of genetic predisposition and the passage of time. Contributing factors to this type of ageing include hormones (for example decreasing levels of oestrogen) and telomere shortening. Telomeres are short genetic sequences at the end of chromosomes that act to protect the lifespan of cells. After each cell cycle, these ends become increasingly shorter until cellular senescence ensues. In addition to this, telomeres have the propensity to diminish oxidative stress in cells.

Extrinsic ageing, on the other hand, is dependent on external factors such as lifestyle (nutrition, smoking, sleeping positions and alcohol ingestion) and environmental stress (pollution and sun exposure; Ganesan and Choi 2016). This type of ageing is also often referred to as actinic or photo-ageing as ultraviolet (UV) radiation from the sun is the largest contributor. UV rays may either be classified as UV-A, -B, or -C, depending on their wavelength. The inability of UV-C rays to penetrate the ozone layer render them the least concern, however, UV-A rays are able to penetrate the epidermis, while UV-B rays penetrate the deeper dermis (Jung et al. 2014).

The pathways for both intrinsic and extrinsic ageing are similar, with one difference being the initiating factor for each and the severity of the outcome. These factors in both instances incite the production of free radicals, which interact undesirably with biological molecules in the skin to disrupt homeostatic physiological processes. This is accompanied by chronic inflammation and abnormal degradation of the structural components of the dermis. These changes are then visualised as thinning of the epidermis, reduced surface area of the dermal-epidermal junction, reduced transfer of nutrients between the layers of the skin, and reduced synthesis of structural components and enhanced degradation of these very structural components. Photo-ageing is characterised by the progressive alteration of the extracellular matrix of the dermis that includes collagen fibres and elastin. This is because prolonged sun exposure and UV radiation induces matrix metalloproteinase (MMP) activity that results in the breakdown of type-I collagen fibres, the most abundant protein in the dermis, and elastin. During this time, dermal repair is impaired due to the inhibition of fibroblasts that prevent procollagen production that accumulates when the skin is exposed to repeated UV irradiation. Advanced stages of actinic collagenolysis result in the decrease of mechanical tension in the dermis, which results in reduced collagen production by dermal fibroblasts (Sachs et al. 2013). The resulting phenotype thus exhibits deep and fine rhytides (wrinkles), lentigines (age spots), telangiectasia (broken blood vessels), moulted pigmentation and sallowness. Intrinsic ageing, on the other hand, contributes to dermal thinning by approximately 20% with menopause in women specifically, which is compounded by extrinsic ageing. After the menopausal period, the skin is thought to thin by a further 1.13% per annum, with collagen decreasing by 2.1% per annum (Calleja-Agius et al. 2013).

Another contributing factor to ageing of the skin has been identified as glycation. This is because advanced glycation end products (AGEs) bind to, and irreversibly modify, proteins in the dermis, such as collagen. These AGEs are formed when a reducing sugar is adduced to an amino group, which is most commonly the ε-amino group of a lysine residue, resulting in the formation of a Schiff base that is rearranged to an Amadori compound, the precursor of AGEs (Yazdanparast and Ardestani 2007; Kim et al. 2012; Parengkuan et al. 2013; West et al. 2014; Kim and Park 2017).

The different types and contributing factors to skin ageing all have the following in common: they are inevitable processes that result in thinning and sagging of the skin, the formation of wrinkles, a reduction in the production of sebum, dry skin, loss of texture and the appearance of age spots (Ganesan and Choi 2016).

21.1.3 SKIN HYDRATION

Healthy skin requires immense amounts of water, which is dependent on the rate of cutaneous evaporation. As previously mentioned, glycosaminoglycans play crucial roles in the hydration of the skin as they bind water. The diminishing capacity of glycosaminoglycans thus holds consequences for the hygroscopic properties of the skin with age. In addition to these, cells associated with the stratum corneum are lipid-rich and play vital roles in preventing water loss.

Drying and flakiness of the skin is often associated with the elderly, particularly in women due to hormonal perturbations associated with menopause. This is a consequence of the diminishing function of sebaceous and sweat glands as they become less responsive to stimuli. This is associated with reduced oestrogen levels; however, oestrogen replacement therapy has been noted to rectify this (Calleja-Agius et al. 2013). The manifestation of dry skin could also be attributed to the loss of the skin barrier function and a decrease in recovery with increasing age. This shift in the skin barrier function has demonstrated to result in a greater susceptibility to dry skin and desquamation (Baumann 2007).

Desquamation can be defined as the progressive shedding of corneocytes from the surface of the skin due to the degradation of cohesive forces between corneocytes in the stratum corneum. The stratum corneum plays a crucial role in cutaneous homeostasis, regulating levels of oxidative stress, microbial levels, UV penetration, hydration and the skin barrier function (Elias 2005; Mustoe 2008). The ability of the stratum corneum to perform this wide range of critical functions is attributed to the presence of proteins such as involucrin and loricrin, lipids, ceramides, triacylglycerides, free fatty acids, stearyl esters, water, and cholesterol sulphate. The presence and concentration of cholesterol sulphate is what governs intracellular cohesion and, consequently, desquamation. In the stratum corneum the adhesive corneodesmosome is found as a specialised desmosome that is associated with lectin-like desquamin, corneodesmosin, the intracellular lipid enamel and van der Waal's forces that play a role in holding the corneocytes and lipid lamellae together. Various enzymes extruded from lamellar bodies are responsible for the degradation of these structures and include proteinases such as glycosidase, lipases, trypsin-like enzymatic activity and chymotryptic enzymes. The activity of these enzymes is influenced by the water content of the skin. When the water content of the stratum corneum is low, enzyme activity is inhibited, resulting in abnormal desquamation. Therefore, the water content of the stratum corneum is essential for both the mechanical properties of the tissue and the normal shedding of the skin. Aged skin has also been associated with an increase in trans-epidermal water loss (TEWL), leaving the stratum corneum exposed and more susceptible to environmental factors that could potentially cause the skin to become dry (Hashizume 2004; Baumann 2007; Guillou et al. 2010).

Injury to the stratum corneum holds consequences, such as loss of barrier function and derangements in the healing process such as overcompensation and dysregulation. This is seen as scar formation, where scar tissue can illustrate a disrupted barrier function for up to 1 year compared to normal skin post-injury. Disruptions in the hydration of the skin as a result of impaired barrier function result in a pro-inflammatory response within the skin that may culminate in skin disorders such as ichthyosis, dermatitis and psoriasis. Topical applications of moisturisers and emollients have been shown to improve skin hydration in the treatment of such conditions (Sharma and Sharma 2012).

The importance of skin hydration, not only for skin health, but also in the repair of perturbations to the skin, is exemplified in studies that have observed healing of mucosal wounds in a liquid environment occurs with minimal scarring and accelerated reduction in inflammatory responses when compared to skin wounds (Sharma and Sharma 2012). Studies have confirmed that attempting to mimic the liquid environment by application of silicone gels, for example, to wounded skin enhances restoration thereof, highlighting and confirming the importance of hydration in optimal wound healing, however, the mechanisms by which the epidermis is able to detect the difference in hydration remains unknown.

21.2 TRADITIONAL MEDICINE

Current skin care therapies have been shown to have harmful effects on the skin due to the presence of active ingredients such as mono-, di-, and triethanolamines, and sodium laureth sulphate that could be irritating to the skin and result in adverse reactions such as photo-allergic reactions and allergic contact dermatitis (Ganesan and Choi 2016). Recently the potential use of traditional herbal medicines in skin care products has become a subject of intense research. Traditional herbal medicine provides a largely unexplored source of useful actives for the development of modern skin care formulations. Several advantages have been linked to the use of natural skin care products because they are hypoallergenic and are readily absorbed by the skin (Wang et al. 2006; Mukherjee et al. 2011). One of the most ancient traditional medicines, dating to 5000 BCE, originates from India and is known as Ayurveda. Ayurveda uses about 200 herbs, minerals and formulations to promote healthy, younger-looking skin. The use of natural skin products has become popular in Asia and many other countries due to its significant ability to treat and prevent skin ageing (Mukherjee et al. 2011, 2012).

21.2.1 Plants for Skin Ageing

Plants are becoming increasingly popular in the field of cosmeceuticals due to their perceived safety and the plethora of activity that they offer. Anti-ageing therapies are no longer one-dimensional, but rather a three-dimensional venture that considers multiple targets in the ageing cascade. Furthermore, modern anti-ageing therapies seek not only to treat the symptom, but rather the cause. Current treatments include strategies to scavenge free radicals, enhance cellular turnover rates inhibit proteases responsible for degradation of the structural components within the dermis and anti-glycation.

Many herbs, fruits, vegetables and whole grains are known to contain antioxidants and polyphenols that are able to scavenge free radicals and metabolic by-products that delay the early onset of ageing. These antioxidants restore the skin's elasticity to slow down and reverse the effects of skin ageing. Studies have revealed antioxidants such as vitamins A and E, co-enzyme Q10, ferulic acid, idebenone, pycnogenol, silymarin and squalene ameliorate environmental damage to the skin and promote self-repair. Botanical antioxidants have also exhibited metal chelating properties and ultraviolet protection in addition to their antioxidant potential. These antioxidants can be classified into flavonoids, carotenoids and polyphenols that are divided into classes of chemicals: anthocyanins, bioflavonoids, catechins, hydroxybenzoic acids, hydroxycinnamic acids and proanthocyanidins (Mukherjee et al. 2011).

21.2.1.1 *Malus pumila* Mill.

M. pumila (Figure 21.2a), commonly referred to as the apple tree, is a deciduous tree well known for its fruit. Originating in Central Asia, it is now cultivated globally. A combination of *Malus pumila* plant stem cell extract, creatine, urea and palmitoyl tripeptide-38 was investigated for its effects on human senescent fibroblasts as well as clinical and instrumental anti-ageing effects. The study found that 71% of the treated women exhibited a visible reduction in wrinkles, specifically crow's feet, with 68% exhibiting notable changes as soon as 7 days after staring treatment. This was accompanied by a significant increase in dermal density and skin elasticity. Metabolic functions in human senescent cultured fibroblasts were also found to be more efficient once treated with the serum at 0.1% and 1%, with a significant reduction in the production of reactive oxygen species (Sanz et al. 2015). In another study, a fruit extract exhibited the highest anti-glycation propensity in a collagen model, indicating promising anti-ageing activity where glycation is the mechanism at play (Parengkuan et al. 2013). Apples may also serve as anti-ageing components based on their ability to scavenge free radicals due to the presence of phenolic compounds such as quercetin, procyanidin B2, epicatechin and hesperetin (Chondrogianni et al. 2010). In addition, other reports of pharmacological activity indicate *M. pumila* to have anticancer, neurodegenerative and cardioprotective activity (Shiseido Co. 2010).

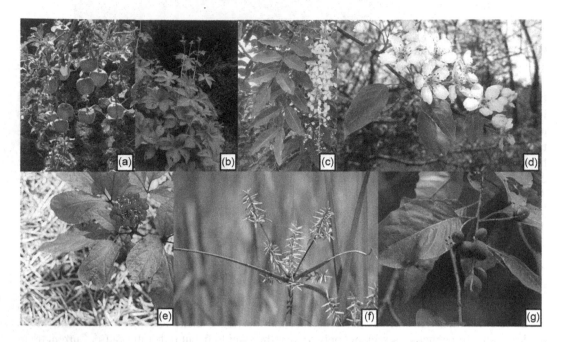

FIGURE 21.2 (See color insert.) Plants used in anti-ageing skin care therapies: (a) *Malus pumila* (Aomorikuma 2007); (b) *Humulus japonicus* (United States Department of Agriculture 2012); (c) *Cassia fistula* (Conrad 2008); (d) *Pyrus pyrifolia* (Quert 2010); (e) *Panax ginseng* (Lohrie 2006); (f) *Cyperus rotundus* (Jose 2009); and (g) *Terminalia chebula* (Zhangzhugang 2013).

21.2.1.2 *Humulus japonicus* Siebold & Zucc.

H. japonicus (Figure 21.2b), from the Cannabaceae family, is a weedy perennial herb originating in Korea and China that has spread to the Western world where it is considered invasive. Traditionally, it has been reported to treat hypertension, pneumonia, diarrhoea, tuberculosis and leprosy in Chinese medicine, and similarly, in Korea, it is also used in the treatment of pulmonary tuberculosis, hypertension and cervical lymphadenitis. Pharmacological investigations have revealed extracts of *H. japonicus* to possess antimycobacterial activity (affirming its traditional uses) as well as antioxidative, antibacterial, antimutagenic, antitumour and anti-inflammatory activity. Some investigations surrounding the bioactive components have revealed the presence of flavonoids, lupulones, phenolics and terpenes (Sung et al. 2015). The anti-ageing activity of *H. japonicus* has been patented along with members of the same genus, *H. scandens*, *H. lupulus* and *H. yunnanensis* to 'treat, prevent, control, ameliorate, inhibit, and/or reduce dermatological signs of chronologically or hormonally aged or photo-aged skin, such as fine lines, wrinkles, and sagging skin, to improve the aesthetic appearance of skin by inhibiting C-reactive protein secretion or production' (Patent US7642062 B2). A study by Sung et al. (2015) investigated the antioxidant and anti-ageing ability of ethanolic extracts of *H. japonicus* through modulation of the AMPK-SIRT 1 pathway using yeast and human fibroblast cells. The results found that the extract was capable of extending the lifespan of yeast cells and upregulating longevity associated proteins (AMP-activated protein kinase and sirtuin 1) while diminishing oxidative stress by inhibiting the generation of reactive oxygen species (Sung et al. 2015).

21.2.1.3 *Cassia fistula* L.

Commonly known as the golden shower, *C. fistula* (Figure 21.2c) is found across Asia. Ayurvedic medicine reports *C. fistula* to be useful for the treatment of skin diseases, gout, rheumatism, leprosy, diabetes, pruritus, as a laxative and for haematemesis (Manonmani et al. 2005; Bhalodia et al. 2012).

Previous studies have confirmed its antidiabetic properties and also indicated it to have anticancer and antimicrobial activity (Luximon-Ramma et al. 2002; Duraipandiyan and Ignacimuthu 2007). A study by Limtrakul et al. (2016) investigated the anti-ageing potential through considering matrix-metalloproteinase-2 (MMP-2), collagenase and tyrosinase inhibition as these are key enzymes involved in the degradation of the structural components within the extracellular matrix of the dermis. Synthesis of collagen and hyaluronic acid were also considered and the butanolic flower extract was found not only to be able to upregulate the synthesis of structural components but also inhibit the degradative enzymes investigated as well as tyrosinase (Limtrakul et al. 2016).

21.2.1.4 *Pyrus pyrifolia* var. *culta* Nakai

Pyrus pyrifolia (Figure 21.2d), commonly known as the Chinese, Japanese, Taiwanese, Korean and sand pear, is found in East Asia. The fruits of this tree are commonly eaten. Traditional reports mention *P. pyrifolia* to be used for the treatment of asthma and hypertension, while pharmacological investigations have revealed the aqueous ethanol bark extract to inhibit protein glycation and have good antioxidant activity. An aqueous ethanol callus extract has been found to reduce the signs of ageing due to its ability to scavenge the DPPH free radical, upregulate the expression of procollagen type I, reduce the transfer of melanin and enhance human fibroblast proliferation (Kim and Park 2017).

21.2.1.5 *Panax ginseng* L.

P. ginseng (Figure 21.2e) is popular in traditional medicine throughout Asia and is known to enhance physical and sexual performance, as well as to exert neuroprotective and anticancer effects. Pharmacological investigations have revealed antioxidant and anti-inflammatory effects, which may explain its benefits when topically applied to the skin. Polysaccharides, polyacetylenes and ginsenosides have previously been identified, with ginsenosides being thought to be the most important. Approximately 50 different ginsenosides have been identified from the roots alone. Often to preserve the stability and bioactivity of the compounds, the raw material is processed by drying or steaming. Depending on the processing mechanism employed, various kinds of ginseng are produced.

White ginseng is produced by drying the raw material, while red ginseng is produced by drying and steaming the raw material. Black ginseng is produced through nine repeated cycles of drying and steaming the raw material. The biological activity of these extracts may further be manipulated through fermentation, which has been done with black ginseng, for example, using *Saccharomyces cerevisiae*.

Fermented black ginseng was found to enhance the quantity of procollagen type-I proteins while reducing the expression of MMP-1, -2, and 9. The expression of TIMP-2 was also found to be enhanced. MMPs, or matrix metalloproteinases, are proteins that degrade collagen within the skin. With exposure to UV radiation, MMP gene expression can be upregulated up to five fold, making them some of the most UV-inducible genes known. TIMPs, or tissue inhibitors of matrix metalloproteinases, are endogenous inhibitors responsible for the modulation of MMP activity. With age, however, their expression has been shown to decline. Plants that have the potential to restore the crucial balance between proteases such as MMPs and anti-proteases such as TIMPs thus hold potential for anti-ageing therapies (Pham et al. 2017). Another study confirmed the use of enzyme-modified red ginseng as an anti-wrinkle agent when topical application reduced UVB-induced skin ageing in human dermal fibroblasts and hairless mice (Hwang et al. 2015). Ginsenoside Rb1 has anti-ageing activity due to its ability to increase type-I collagen production and suppression of UV-induced apoptosis. Similarly, ginsenoside F1 has been shown to protect human keratinocytes from UVB-induced apoptosis, too (Lee et al. 2003).

21.2.2 PLANTS FOR SKIN HYDRATION

Xerosis or skin dryness is normally the result of an abundant loss of water from the skin, most prevalent on the face, arms lower legs and sides of the abdomen. The dehydration of the skin can be prevented by moisturisers that support the skin and enhance the flexibility of the skin. As discussed earlier in this chapter, the stratum corneum plays a pivotal role in maintaining the skin's moisture. A balance needs to be maintained between the water content of the skin, the stratum corneum and the skin surface lipids. A disruption in the balance can result in a loss of skin moisture. In order to restore the water content of the skin, moisturising treatments need to perform the following functions: (1) reduce TEWL, (2) enhance water content, (3) reinstate the lipids' ability to attract, grasp and redistribute water and (4) refurbish the skin barrier (Ali et al. 2013). Various products are currently available to improve skin moisture and maintain the normal conditions of the skin, employing three main mechanisms, namely, occlusion, which prevents the evaporation of skin moisture by forming a greasy film on the surface of the skin that prevents water loss and delaying premature ageing; humectants, which attract and retain moisture; and deficient materials which may include phenolic compounds and antioxidants not only for protection from external factors but also to treat various other skin disorders (Dal'Belo et al. 2006; Guillou et al. 2010; Ali et al. 2013; De Azevedo Ribeiro et al. 2015; Ganesan and Choi 2016).

Organic ingredients that are often incorporated into moisturisers include hydroxy and hyaluronic acids. Hydroxy acids, also commonly referred to as fruit acids, are carboxylic acids by nature that occur in an alpha or beta conformation according to molecular structure. Examples include tartaric, lactic, citric, glycolic, salicylic, malic and lactobionic acids. They achieve restored hydration by promoting desquamation of the stratum corneum. Salicylic acid has also been incorporated into a range of anti-ageing formulations.

Hyaluronic acid is found at points where collagen and elastin meet, as previously discussed, and plays important roles in maintaining hydration, firmness and tissue repair of the skin.

21.2.2.1 *Aloe barbadensis* Miller (*Aloe vera*)

Aloe vera (Figure 21.3a) is well known for its skin healing properties and the extract is widely used in many skin care cosmeceutical products. Numerous studies have reported its medicinal potential when applied topically to burns, inflammatory skin disorders, sunburns and wounds. *In vivo* studies done by Dal'Belo et al. (2006) on 20 female volunteers found that a vehicle supplemented with

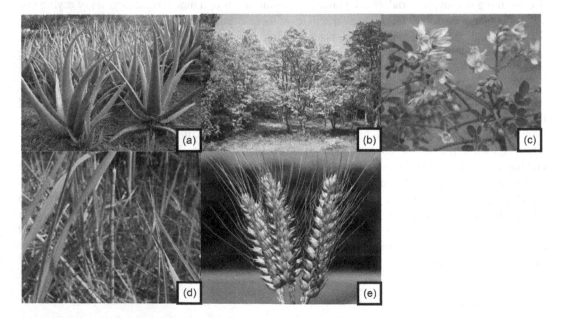

FIGURE 21.3   (See color insert.) Plants for skin moisturising therapies: (a) *Aloe barbadensis* (Maari 2012); (b) *Cedrela sinensis* (Willow 2007); (c) *Moringa oleifera* (Garg 2008); (d) *Equisetum palustre* (Peters 2006); and (e) *Triticum vulgare* (Dist 2008).

0.25% and 0.50% (w/w) freeze-dried extract of *A. barbadensis* increased the water content of the stratum corneum after a single application. After 2 weeks of application, all formulations supplemented with 0.10%, 0.25% and 0.50% (w/w) of the extract increased the water content of the stratum corneum as compared with the vehicle. The research group concluded that the aloe extract was unable to change the skin barrier function and had no effect on TEWL and therefore the extract had no occlusive properties. However, they did find that the aloe extract improved skin moisture and therefore the water content of the stratum corneum by a humectant mechanism when compared with the vehicle. They hypothesised that the activity observed could be due to the presence of alanine, arginine, glycine, histidine, serine and threonine that may increase water retention in the stratum corneum.

21.2.2.2   *Cedrela sinensis* A. Juss

Kim et al. (2010) investigated the antibacterial and skin moisturising effect of *Cedrela sinensis* shoot extract (Figure 21.3b). Clinical studies investigated the skin hydration and TEWL of a cream containing *C. sinensis* after topical application. The researchers confirmed that a cream containing *C. sinensis* extract had a 10%–15% higher skin hydrating effect compared to the placebo and an ethyl acetate fraction decreased TEWL to 6.7 g/m^2h.

21.2.2.3   *Moringa oleifera* Lam.

Moringa oleifera (Figure 21.3c) is part of the Moringaceae family and is commonly known as the drumstick tree. Traditionally the leaves are used as a purgative, for headaches, sore throat, fevers, piles, eye and ear infections, scurvy, bronchitis, catarrh and to treat sores. Bioactive compounds previously isolated from *M. oleifera* include vitamin A, vitamin B, vitamin C, β-carotene, carotenoids and phenolics (Anwar et al. 2007; Ali et al. 2013).

Studies done by Ali et al. (2013) investigated the moisturising effects of cosmetic creams containing *Moringa oleifera* aqueous methanol leaf extract. The cream with the plant extract was applied twice daily on the face for 12 weeks and measurements were carried out every 2 weeks with a tewameter and corneometer. They found that there was a continuous decrease in TEWL up until week 12 compared to the control, which had an increase in TEWL between weeks 4 and 12. A continuous increase in skin hydration was observed for the active cream compared to the control where a decrease in skin hydration was observed between weeks 8 and 12. A two-way ANOVA test confirmed that the cream with the active significantly decreased TEWL and increased skin hydration over time compared to the control with no *M. oleifera* present. They concluded that the decrease in TEWL is due to the presence of antioxidant and phenolic compounds in the extract. *M. oleifera* leaves has been reported to contain prominent levels of ascorbic acid, 106.95 mg/100 g. Ascorbic acid has been found to configure the stratum corneum barrier lipids and also has a photo-protection function that prevents inflammation, and UVB-induced immune-suppression when applied topically. In the total skin range, a concentration of 0.4–1 mg/100 g of wet-tissue weight of ascorbic acid has been found. Compounds such as kaempferol 3-O-rhamnoside, kaempferol, gallic acid, rutin, syringic acid and quercetin 3-oglucoside have been linked with protection from UV radiation and skin dryness. A large number of phenolic compounds have been identified to be present in *M. oleifera*, include ellagic, chlorogenic, ferulic and gallic acid, and the flavonoids identified were kaempferol, rutin and quercetin.

The phenolic antioxidants present in *M. oleifera* prevent impairment at a cellular level by reducing damage caused by free radicals. This results in a reduction of inflammation that protects the skin from photo-damage and an increase in collagen efficiency. The increase in skin hydration seen in the present study was hypothesised to be attributed to the rich composition of amino acids proteins such as alanine, arginine, glycine, histidine, serine and threonine present in *M. oleifera*. These amino acids improve the water retention in the stratum corneum that results in an increase in skin hydration. Vitamin A has previously been isolated from the leaves of *M. oleifera*. Vitamin A, its derivatives, and beta-carotene (provitamin A) are widely used in cosmetic products for their photo-protective properties. Vitamin B, also present in *M. oleifera* leaves, is a water-soluble nutrient that increases the attraction of water to the stratum corneum and softens the skin because it functions as a humectant. Therefore, vitamin B can effectively be used as a skin moisturiser (Lupo 2001; Ali et al. 2013).

21.2.2.4   *Equisetum palustre* L.

Equisetum palustre (Figure 21.3d), commonly known as marsh horsetail, was evaluated for its moisturising effect. A methanolic extract was incorporated into cream bases and applied to rats and mice. The maximum moisturising effect was observed for *E. palustre* compared to the control. The researchers concluded that the high moisturising activity observed could be due to the high flavonoid content of *E. palustre* (Khazaeli et al. 2011).

21.2.2.5   *Triticum vulgare* L.

Ceramides play an integral role in the normal function of the hydrolipidic barrier. Studies have investigated the topical application of ceramides on dry skin and supported the efficacy of ceramides from different plants such as in improving skin moisture. It was hypothesised that oral supplementation of ceramides could potentially improve skin hydration (Guillou et al. 2010).

In nature, a few sources of botanical ceramides include corn, konjac, rice and wheat. *Triticum vulgare*, non-genetically modified organism (GMO) wheat, is rich in ceramides that are a non-allergen (Figure 21.3e). The wheat extract has been developed in two forms, a powder and an oil. Previous studies found that the ceramide and glycosylceramides were similar in 200 mg of powder and 350 mg of oil. *In vivo* studies investigated 51 patients between the ages of 20 and 63 suffering from skin dryness. The two wheat forms were administered orally, and skin hydration was evaluated at day zero (D0) and day 84 (D84). A significant difference in skin hydration was observed at the end of the study on D84 on the arms and legs of the test subjects in the wheat oil group compared to the placebo without side effects. It was concluded that a dosage of 350 mg of wheat oil displayed a significant increase in skin hydration after a 3 month treatment in women with severely dry skin (Guillou et al. 2010).

21.3   NANOCOSMECEUTICALS

Skin care has become a priority to most individuals as the skin plays important roles in self-esteem, self-confidence and how an individual is perceived by the world. Creams are one of the most popular forms of skin care due to their convenience, ease of use and minimal invasiveness. They are also widely applicable as they can be supplemented with a wide range of active components depending on the desired effect, and therefore are versatile in the range of conditions that they are able to be applied to, for example, ageing, hydration, pigmentation disorders and acne. Combining multiple active components provides the platform for multiple targets to be addressed in any condition, thereby enhancing the therapeutic efficacy of the formulation.

These formulations are commonly supplemented with antioxidants, hyaluronic acid, hydroxy acids, ceramides, moisturisers, sunscreens, depigmenting agents, sunscreens, exfoliants, topical peptides, retinoids and one of the most popular ingredients, botanicals (Sharma and Sharma 2012). The largest concerns for the use of phyto-based skin care products are high instability and a low penetration of the active compounds, which therefore decreases compound delivery in many skin-based therapies. To overcome these challenges, nanosized compound delivery is currently being investigated to enhance the delivery of phyto-derived bioactive compounds in skin care products. By forming nanoparticles from phytocompounds, the delivery of the bioactive compounds to the target site is efficiently enhanced and the skin's protective activities are augmented. Nanocosmeceuticals that are currently undergoing investigation for their enhanced delivery of bioactive compounds in skin care products include carbon nanotubes, ethosomes, fullerenes, nanostructured lipid carriers, solid lipid nanoparticles and transfersomes to name but a few. Nanocosmeceuticals containing synthetic compounds are commercially available, although certain degrees of toxicity and skin damage have become a concern. Therefore, there is a great demand for alternative greener nano-cosmeceuticals. Nanoscale phytocompounds have become increasingly popular in products such as sunscreens, anti-ageing treatments and UV protectants (Ganesan and Choi 2016).

Vesicular systems and liposomes are examples of nanotechnology that has been introduced into skin care to enhance the therapeutic efficacy of the active components directly or facilitate site-specific delivery of the active components. Vesicular systems are delivery systems that include lipo somes, silicone vesicles and matrices and multi-walled delivery systems. Liposomes are artificial spherical submicroscopic vesicles ranging from 25 to 5000 nm in diameter. They are commonly employed delivery systems with the ability to encapsulate the active ingredients and release them deep into the dermis. Their site-specific delivery is the result of the binding of the liposome to the cell membrane where the active ingredient is directly deposited.

Niosomes, ultrasomes, photosomes and aquasomes are specialised forms of liposomes. Photosomes are of particular interest as they contain a photo-activated enzyme isolated from the marine plant *Anacystis nidulans* that, when combined with ultrasomes, yields intelligent technology that is able to combat DNA damage as a result of UV exposures. Silicone vesicles are incorporated into anti-ageing formulations to smooth out the appearance of wrinkles and give the skin a velvety texture. They are often incorporated with vitamins to nourish the skin.

Currently, solid lipid nanocarriers, nanoemulsions and nanoliposomes with active phyto-ingredients are effectively used to treat various skin disorders. Nanoemulsions have become an attractive system for many researchers in the cosmetic, pharmaceutical and food industries due to their versatility. Advantages of nanoemulsions include higher stability against coalescence, low amount of surfactant, non-toxic and non-irritancy characteristics, appearance, low viscosity and versatility of formulation. Nanoemulsions are achieved when the size of an emulsion globule reaches a size of approximately 20–500 nm. The small droplet size of nanoemulsions is useful in cosmeceuticals because the size ensures a closer contact of the product with the stratum corneum and therefore increasing the quantity of active compounds reaching the target site. Nanoemulsions are also able to improve skin layer penetration and carry active compounds into the skin, enhancing the efficacy of the active component (Bernardi et al. 2011; De Azevedo Ribeiro et al. 2015).

Particulate systems encompass micro- and nanoparticulate systems depending on the size of the components implicated. Nanoparticulate systems are submicron colloidal systems comprised of nanospheres (a matrix system) and nanocapsules (a reservoir system) with a mean particle diameter of 0.003–1 μm. The use of nanoparticulate systems allows natural products such as carotenes, vitamins, and retinol to be carried to deeper layers of the dermis where their presence is most effective. Nanospheres are particularly useful to reduce the signs of ageing as a result of UV exposures and actinic ageing (Sharma and Sharma 2012).

Solid lipid nanoparticles are novel delivery systems employed for skin hydration, protection against degradation, enhancing penetration of the active ingredients and controlled release. In addition to these, nanotopes, nanocrystals, fullerenes, and cyclodextrins are also commonly employed. Nanotopes range in size from 20 to 40 nm and are ultrasmall carriers. Vitamin E in a nanotope has illustrated deeper penetration with the propensity to diminish oxidative stress, thus reducing the onset of the ageing cascade, as well as aid in hydration of the skin (Sharma and Sharma 2012).

21.3.1 NANOMEDICINE IN AGEING

21.3.1.1 *Cyperus rotundus* L.

Gold nanoparticles are an emerging field in nanomedicine and research on this topic has attracted a lot of interest due to the reported therapeutic potential of gold nanoparticles. The benefits of gold nanoparticles include enhanced biocompatibility, high surface reactivity and diminished toxicity.

As previously discussed, glycation is a contributing factor to skin ageing, and many compounds have previously been identified as inhibitors of glycation. These compounds generally illustrate nucleophilicity. For example, aminoguanidine has been shown to be an excellent inhibitor and model for the inhibition of glycation. A study by Kim et al. (2012) aimed to investigate the ability of gold nanoparticles formed with aminoguanidine to inhibit glycation of collagen. The results found that the gold nanoparticles reduced the glycation of collaged by 56.3% compared to the control and reduced the distribution of AGEs in the lattice model (Kim et al. 2012). It has, however, been withdrawn from clinical trials due to concerns regarding the safety and efficacy of treatment. Natural inhibitors have, however, been isolated from herbal sources. In a study by Yazdanparast and Ardestani (2007) *Cyperus rotundus* (Figure 21.2f) was found to inhibit glycation in a model using fructose-mediated protein glycoxidation, an antioxidant and metal chelator. Other natural inhibitors of protein glycation include *Morinda citrifolia*, *Cornus officinalis* and *Cornus mas* (West et al. 2014).

21.3.1.2   Vitamin C and Retinoic Acid

L-Ascorbic acid, more commonly referred to as Vitamin C, and retinoic acid, more commonly known as Vitamin A, are commonly incorporated into cosmetics for their ability to scavenge free radicals, act as photoprotectants, enhance the synthesis of collagen and suppress abnormal pigmentation. Vitamin C, however, is readily oxidised and thus highly unstable, and for that reason, more stable derivatives, including ascorbyl palmitate, magnesium ascorbyl phosphate and ascorbyl tetraisopalmitate, are often used as substitutes. When ingested, they are easily converted into vitamin C, however, but this is not the same in instances of topical application. Furthermore, topically applying these derivatives also has no effect on dermal levels of antioxidants, making them ineffective for this application. Retinoic acid, on the other hand, is lipophilic, which makes it insoluble in aqueous formulations and drastically reduces the bioavailability thereof. Gold nanoparticles are becoming an increasingly popular ingredient in facial masks due to their ability to enhance skin elasticity and blood circulation. Fathi-Azarbayjani et al. (2010) developed an anti-ageing nanofibre face mask containing retinoic and ascorbic acid, collagen and gold nanoparticles. It is only wet once applied to the skin, thus preventing oxidation of unstable active ingredients that normally ensues in pre-moistened masks and enhancing the stability of the mask. The gradual dissolution of the mask once wet also exhibited slow-release and enhanced penetration of the actives (Fathi-Azarbayjani et al. 2010).

21.3.1.3   *Terminalia chebula* Retz.

T. chebula (Figure 21.2g) from the family Combretaceae is a medicinal plant reported for the promotion of longevity. Various phenolic compounds have been isolated and reported to have anti-ageing activity with the ability to inhibit tyrosinase and melanogenesis in the prevention of age spots and scavenge free radicals, including gallic acid, chebulagic and chebulinic acid, isoterchebulin, 1,3,6-tri-O-galloyl-β-glucopyranose and punicalagin (Manosroi et al. 2011). Their chemical instability during exposure to temperature, air and light limit the application and efficacy, but when combined with technology such as nanovesicles this can be averted (Boles et al. 1988; Sahin 2007). A semi-purified fraction containing gallic acid was loaded into niosomes for an anti-ageing gel. The loaded niosomes exhibited no skin irritation or cytotoxicity, a reduction in skin roughness and improvement in skin elasticity. In addition, treated cells also exhibited reduced expression levels of MMP-2, which may account for the ability of the extract to enhance skin elasticity (et al. 2011).

21.3.2   NANOMOISTURISERS

Moisturisers are one of the most prescribed products in dermatology. A number of herbal moisturisers are currently on the market claiming to be natural and safe (Kapoor and Saraf 2010). A more efficient activity has been observed for nanomoisturisers. The controlled release of active ingredients has also gained clinical relevance. It enables a more homogeneous distribution on the skin and a more efficient activity has been found in products for treating many skin disorders including xerosis (De Azevedo Ribeiro et al. 2015).

21.3.2.1 *Opuntia ficus-indica* (L.) Mill

Opuntia ficus-indica (Figure 21.4a) is a plant that grows in arid areas of Brazil. Phenolic compounds such as kaempferol and quercetin and carbohydrates such as galacturonic acid, glucose, rhamnose and arabinose have previously been identified to be present in the chemical composition of this plant. These compounds have shown potential to treat xerosis and ageing (De Azevedo Ribeiro et al. 2015). De Azevedo Ribeiro et al. (2015) explored the moisturising potential of 1% *O. ficus-indica* hydroglycolic extract characterised in an oil/water (O/W) nanoemulsion. Droplet sizes between 92.2 and 233.6 nm were obtained that presented stability for 60 days. *In vivo* studies confirmed the moisturising potential of the formulation containing the *O. ficus-indica* nanoemulsion when applied topically, compared to the placebo. Carbohydrate derivatives have formerly been linked to increasing skin hydration after topical application. Previous studies confirmed the high concentration of carbohydrates present in *O. ficus-indica* that could explain the increased moisturising effect. Compared to conventional emulsions containing *O. ficus-indica*, a nanoemulsion containing the active components allowed for an improved moisturising effect (Azevedo De Brito Damasceno 2014; De Azevedo Ribeiro et al. 2015).

21.3.2.2 *Oryza sativa* L.

Bernardi et al. (2011) investigated the moisturising effect of rice bran oil from *Oryza sativa* (Figure 21.4b) in a nanoemulsion using low energy emulsification methods. The nanoemulsion developed comprised of 10% rice bran oil, 10% surfactants sorbitan oleate/PEG-30 castor oil, 0.05% antioxidant and 0.50% preservatives formulated in distilled water. *In vivo* studies confirmed that a nanoemulsion of rice bran oil increased the moisturising variance by about 38% compared to a commercial moisturiser that only increased skin hydration with 20% after 14 days of continuous application.

21.3.2.3 *Tagetes erecta* Linn

Tagetes erecta, commonly known as the African marigold (Figure 21.4c), is traditionally used to treat wounds, ulcers and intestinal diseases. It is well known for its antiseptic, antimicrobial and antioxidant activity. The family, Compositae, is known to be rich in flavonoids such as quercetagetin with high antioxidant activity. A nanoemulsion loaded with ethyl acetate marigold flower extract (EANG) was investigated by Leelapornpisid et al. (2014) for its anti-wrinkle and skin moisturising potential. *In vivo* studies confirmed the moisturising effect of EANG compared to the placebo. The results demonstrated that the skin moisture efficiency was significantly increased after using

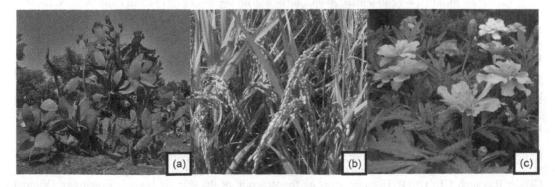

FIGURE 21.4 (See color insert.) Plants used in nanomoisturisers: (a) *Opuntia ficus-indica* (Garg 2008); (b) *Oryza sativa* (Green, 2006); and (c) *Tagetes erecta* (Starr and Starr 2007).

the EANG for 8 weeks (37.72 ± 2.07–46.42 ± 2.45) compared to the controls. The application of EANG to the lower forearm twice daily for 8 weeks produced significant improvement in the appearance of wrinkles compared to the controls. It was concluded that a nanoemulsion loaded with marigold flower extract was effective in increasing skin moisture and reducing the appearance of wrinkles. The anti-wrinkle and moisturising efficacy was attributed to the high antioxidant capacity of the marigold flower extract. Moreover, the EANG showed better stability, efficiency and wrinkle reduction and moisturising efficacy compared to the extract alone and can be used as a promising anti-ageing and moisturising cosmeceutical product.

21.4   CONCLUSION

There is an increasing need for safe and more effective skin therapies to diminish and improve the appearance of aged and dry skin. Several synthetic skin care products have been linked to a number of adverse reactions. The use of plants in skin therapies is still at its infant stage, although they have been used for centuries in traditional medicine. It is important to keep in mind that although plant extracts are considered to be a safer alternative to conventional therapies, they should still be used with caution. Not all plant extracts are safe to use on the skin and many can result in allergic contact dermatitis and other adverse effects. Therefore, the safety and efficacy of plant extracts should be investigated as with synthetic compounds.

Current skin care therapies have demonstrated a lack of efficacy due to the size of bioactive compounds which are sometimes unable enter the skin. Skin care based therapies are becoming more aware of the advantages of nanosized phyto-based bioactive compounds. Nanocosmeceuticals have led many researchers in search of novel moisturising, UV-protecting, skin brightening and anti-ageing therapies. These therapies have shown a higher efficacy than conventional therapies. Nanocosmeceuticals with phyto-based bioactive compounds are more stable, maintain higher amounts of bioactive compounds in the skin and enhance the skin for an extended time. Further research is needed for phyto-based bioactive compounds for their moisturising and wrinkle reduction efficacy as current studies have only just begun to scratch the surface of what appears to be a very promising platform for skin care.

REFERENCES

Ali, A., Akhtar, N., Khan, M. S., Rasool, F., Iqbal, F. M., Khan, M. T., Din, M. U. and Elahi, E. (2013). Moisturizing effect of cream containing *Moringa oleifera* (Sohajana) leaf extract by biophysical techniques: *In vivo* evaluation. *Journal of Medicinal Plants Research*, 7(8), 386–391. doi:10.5897/jmpr12.504.

Anwar, F., Latif, S., Ashraf, M. and Gilani, A. H. (2007). *Moringa oleifera*: A food plant with multiple medicinal uses. *Phytotherapy Research*, 21(1), 17–25. doi:10.1002/ptr.2023.

Azevedo De Brito Damasceno, G. (2014). *Obtenção de extratos da Opuntia ficus-indica (L.) Mill e suas aplicações em formulações cosméticas: Avaliação in vivo do sensorial e da eficácia hidratante.* Natal, RN, Brazil: Universidade Federal do Rio Grande do Norte.

Baumann, L. (2007). Skin ageing and its treatment. *Journal of Pathology*, 211(2), 241–251. doi:10.1002/path.2098.

Bernardi, D. S., Pereira, T. A., Maciel, N. R., Bortoloto, J., Viera, G. S., Oliveira, G. C. and Rocha-Filho, P. A. (2011). Formation and stability of oil-in-water nanoemulsions containing rice bran oil: *In vitro* and *in vivo* assessments. *Journal of Nanobiotechnology*, 9(1), 44. doi:10.1186/1477-3155-9-44.

Bhalodia, N. R., Nariya, P. B., Acharya, R. N. and Shukla, V. J. (2012). *In vitro* antibacterial and antifungal activities of *Cassia fistula* Linn. fruit pulp extracts. *AYU*, 33, 123–129.

Boles, J.S., Crerar, D.A., Grissom, G., Key, T.C. (1988). Aqueous thermal degradation of gallic acid. *Geochimica et Cosmochimica Acta*, 52, 341–344.

Calleja-Agius, J., Brincat, M. and Borg, M. (2013). Skin connective tissue and ageing. *Best Practice & Research Clinical Obstetrics and Gynaecology*, 27, 727–740. doi:10.1016/j.bpobgyn.2013.06.004.

Cancer Research UK. (2014). Diagram showing the structure of the skin. *Wikimedia Commons*. [Viewed 1 December 2017]. Available from: https://commons.wikimedia.org/wiki/File:Diagram_showing_the_structure_of_the_skin_CRUK_371.svg.

Chondrogianni, N., Kapeta, S., Chinou, I., Vassilatou, K., Papassideri, I. and Gonos, E. S. (2010). Anti-ageing and rejuvenating effects of quercetin. *Experimental Gerontology*, **45**, 763–771.

DalBelo, S. E., Rigo Gaspar, L. and Berardo Gonçalves Maia Campos, P. M. (2006). Moisturizing effect of cosmetic formulations containing *Aloe vera* extract in different concentrations assessed by skin bioengineering techniques. *Skin Research and Technology*, **12**(4), 241–246. doi:10.1111/j.0909-752X.2006.00155.x.

De Azevedo Ribeiro, R., de Andrade Gomes Barreto, S., Ostrosky, E., Rocha-Filho, P., Veríssimo, L. and Ferrari, M. (2015). Production and characterization of cosmetic nanoemulsions containing *Opuntia ficus-indica* (L.) mill extract as moisturizing agent, *Molecules*, **20**(2), 2492–2509. doi:10.3390/molecules20022492.

Duraipandiyan, V. and Ignacimuthu, S. (2007). Antibacterial and antifungal activity of *Cassia fistula* L.: An ethnomedicinal plant. *Journal of Ethnopharmacology*, **112**, 590–594.

Elias, P. M. (2005). Stratum corneum defensive functions: An integrated view. *Journal of Investigative Dermatology*, **125**(2), 183–200. doi:10.1111/j.0022-202X.2005.23668.x.

Fathi-Azarbayjani, A., Qun, L., Chan, Y. W. and Chan, S. Y. (2010). Novel vitamin and gold-loaded nanofiber facial mask for topical delivery. *AAPS PharmSciTech*, **11**(3), 1164–1170. doi:10.1208/s12249-010-9475-z.

Ganesan, P. and Choi, D.-K. (2016). Current application of phytocompound-based nanocosmeceuticals for beauty and skin therapy. *International Journal of Nanomedicine*, **11**, 1987–2007. doi:10.2147/IJN.S104701.

Guillou, S., Ghabri, S., Jannot, C., Gaillardà, E., Lamourà, I. and Boisnic, S. (2010). The moisturizing effect of a wheat extract food supplement on women's skin: A randomized, double- blind placebo-controlled trial. *International Journal of Cosmetic Science*, **3**(2), 137–143. doi:10.1111/j.1468-2494.2010.00600.x.

Hashizume, H. (2004). Skin aging and dry skin. *Journal of Dermatology*, **31**(8), 603–609. doi:10.1111/j.1346-8138.2004.tb00565.x.

Hwang, E., Park, S.-Y., Jo, H., Lee, D.-G., Kim, H.-T., Kim, Y. M., Yin, C. S. and Yi, T. H. (2015). Efficacy and safety of enzyme-modified *Panax ginseng* for anti-wrinkle therapy in healthy skin: A single-center, randomized, double-blind, placebo-controlled study. *Rejuvenation Research*, 18(5), 449–457.

Jung, H., Shin, J., Park, S., Kim, N., Kwak, W. and Choi, B. (2014). *Pinus densiflora* extract protects human skin fibroblasts against UVB-induced photoaging by inhibiting the expression of MMPs and increasing type I procollagen expression. *Toxicology Reports*, 1, 658–666. doi:10.1016/j.toxrep.2014.08.010.

Kapoor, S. and Saraf, S. (2010). Assessment of viscoelasticity and hydration effect of herbal moisturizers using bioengineering techniques. *Pharmacognosy Magazine*, **6**(24). doi:10.4103/0973-1296.71797.

Khazaeli, P., Sharififar, F., Amiri, F., Heravi, G. and Heravi, G. (2011). Evaluation of moisturizing effect of methanolic extract of five medicinal plants incorporated into cream bases using impedance and extensiometry methods. *Journal of Drugs in Dermatology*, **10**(10), 1116–1121.

Kim, H. J. and Park, J. W. (2017). Anti-aging activities of *Pyrus pyrifolia* var culta plant callus extract. *Tropical Journal of Pharmaceutical Research*, **16**(7), 1579–1588.

Kim, J., Hong, C., Koo, Y., Choi, H. and Lee, K. (2012). Anti-glycation effect of gold nanoparticles on collagen. *Biological & Pharmaceutical Bulletin*, **35**(2), 260–264.

Kim, S.-Y., Lee, M.-H., Jo, N.-R. and Park, S.-N. (2010). Antibacterial activity and skin moisturizing effect of *Cedrela sinensis* A. Juss shoots extract. *Journal of the Society of Cosmetic Scientists of Korea*, **36**(4), 315–321.

Lee, E. H., Cho, S. Y., Kim, S. J., Shin, E. S., Chang, H. K., Kim, D. H., Yeom, M. H., Woe, K. S., Lee, J., Sim, Y. C. and Lee, T. R. (2003). Ginsenoside F1 protects human HaCaT keratinocytes from ultraviolet-B-induced apoptosis by maintaining constant levels of Bcl-2. *Journal of Investigative Dermatology*, **121**, 607–613.

Leelapornpisid, P., Kiattisin, K., Jantrawut, P. and Phrutivorapongkul, A. (2014). Nanoemulsion loaded with marigold flower extract (Tagetes Erecta Linn) in gel preparation as anti-wrinkles cosmeceutical. *International Journal of Pharmacy and Pharmaceutical Sciences*, **6**(2), 231–236.

Limtrakul, P., Yodkeeree, S., Thippraphan, P., Punfa, W. and Srisomboon, J. (2016). Anti-aging and tyrosinase inhibition effects of *Cassia fistula* flower butanolic extract. *BMC Complementary and Alternative Medicine*, **16**, 497. doi:10.1186/s12906-016-1484-3.

Lupo, M. P. (2001). Antioxidants and vitamins in cosmetics. *Clinics in Dermatology*, **19**(4), 467–473. doi:10.1016/S0738-081X(01)00188-2.

Luximon-Ramma, A., Bahorun, T., Soobrattee, M. A. and Aruoma, O. I. (2002). Antioxidant activities of phenolic, proanthocyanidin, and flavonoid components in extracts of *Cassia fistula*. *Journal of Agricultural and Food Chemistry*, **50**, 5042–5047.

Manonmani, G., Bhavapriya, V., Kalpana, S., Govindasamy, S. and Apparanantham, T. (2005). Antioxidant activity of *Cassia fistula* (Linn.) flowers in alloxan induced diabetic rats. *Journal of Ethnopharmacology*, **97**, 39–42.

Manosroi, A., Jantrawut, P., Akihisa, T., Manosroi, W., Manosroi, J. (2011). *In vitro* and *in vivo* skin anti-aging evaluation of gel containing niosomes loaded with a semi-purified fraction containing gallic acid from *Terminalia chebula* galls. *Pharmaceutical Biology*, **49**(11), 1190-1203. doi: 10.3109/13880209.2011.576347.

Mukherjee, P. K., Maity, N., Nema, N. K. and Sarkar, B. K. (2011). Bioactive compounds from natural resources against skin aging. *Phytomedicine*, **19**, 64–73. doi:10.1016/j.phymed.2011.10.003.

Mukherjee, P. K., Nema, N. K., Venkatesh, P. and Debnath, P. K. (2012). Changing scenario for promotion and development of Ayurveda: Way forward. *Journal of Ethnopharmacology*, **143**, 424–434.

Mustoe, T. A. (2008). Evolution of silicone therapy and mechanism of action in scar management. *Aesthetic Plastic Surgery*, **32**, 82–92.

Pandel, R., Poljšak, B., Godic, A. and Dahmane, R. (2013). Skin photoageing and the role of antioxidants in its prevention. *ISRN Dermatology*, **2013**, 930164. doi:10.1155/2013/930164.

Parengkuan, L., Yagi, M., Matsushima, M., Ogura, M., Hamada, U. and Yonei, Y. (2013). Anti-glycation activity of various fruits. *Anti-Aging Medicine*, **10**(4), 70–76.

Pham, Q. L., Jang, H.-J. and Kim, K.-B. (2017). Anti-wrinkle effect of fermented black ginseng on human fibroblasts. *International Journal of Molecular Medicine*, **2017**, 681–686. doi:10.3892/ijmm.2017.2858.

Sachs, D. L., Ritti, L., Chubb, H. A., Orringer, J., Fisher, G. and Voorhees, J. J. (2013). Hypo-collagenesis in photoaged skin predicts response to anti-aging cosmeceuticals. *Journal of Cosmetic Dermatology*, **12**, 108–115.

Sahin N.O. (2007). Chapter 4. Niosomes as nanocarrier systems. *Nanomaterials and Nanosystems for Biomedical Applications*. Mozafari MR, Ed., Springer, Dordrecht, the Netherlands, pp. 67–81.

Sanz, M. T., Campos, C., Milani, M., Foyaca, M., Kurdian, K. and Trullas, C. (2015). Biorevitalizing effect of a novel facial serum containing apple stem cell extract, pro-collagen lipopeptide, creatine, and urea on skin aging signs. *Journal of Cosmetic Dermatology*, **15**(1), 24–30.

Sharma, B. and Sharma, A. (2012). Future prospect of nanotechnology in development of anti-ageing formulations. *International Journal of Pharmacy and Pharmaceutical Sciences*, **4**(3), 57–66.

Sung, B., Chung, J.-W., Bae, H.-R., Choi, J.-S., Kim, C.-M. and Kim, N.-D. (2015). *Humulus japonicus* extract exhibits antioxidative and anti-aging effects via modulation of the AMPK SIRT1 pathway. *Experimental and Therapeutic Medicine*, **9**(5), 1819–1826. doi:10.3892/etm.2015.2302.

Shiseido Co, Ltd. (2010). External skin preparation, whitener, antioxidant and anti-aging agent. Inventors: Rikako Suzuki, Kiyotaka Hasegawa, Kiyoshi Sato, Ken Kusakari and Tokiya Yokoi. 3 August. Appl: 20 February 2012. US Patent US20120141400A1.

Wang, K.-H., Lin, R.-D., Hsu, F.-L., Huang, Y.-H., Chang, H.-C., Huang, C.-Y. and Lee, M.-H. (2006). Cosmetic applications of selected traditional Chinese herbal medicines. *Journal of Ethnopharmacology*, **106**, 353–359. doi:10.1016/j.jep.2006.01.010.

West, B. J., Uwaya, A., Isami, F., Deng, S., Nakajima, S. and Jensen, C. J. (2014). Antiglycation activity of iridoids and their food sources. *International Journal of Food Science*, **2014**, 276950.

Wikimedia commons: Amorikuma (2007): *Malus pumila*; Conrad (2008): *Cassia fistula*; Jose (2009): *Cyperus rotundus*; Dist (2008): *Triticum vulgare;* Garg (2008): *Opuntia ficus-indica* & *Moringa oleifera*; Green (2006): *Oryza sativa*; Lohrie (2006): *Panax ginseng*; Maari (2012): *Aloe barbadensis*; Peters (2006): *Equisetum palustre*; Quert (2010): *Pyrus pyrifolia*; Starr (2007): *Tagetes erecta*; United States Department of Agriculture (2012): *Humulus japonicus*; Willow (2007): *Cedrela sinensis*; Zhangzhugang (2013): *Terminalia chebula*. [Available from: https://commons.wikimedia.org] [Last accessed: 2017-12-19].

Yazdanparast, R. and Ardestani, A., 2007. *In vitro* and *in vivo* antioxidant and free radical scavenging activity of *Cyperus rotundus*. *Journal of Medicinal Food*, **10**(4), 667–674. doi:10.1089/jmf.2006.090.

Section V

Reviews

22 *Anredera cordifolia* (Ten.) v. Steenis
A New Emerging Cure with Polypharmacological Effects

Elin Yulinah Sukandar and Dhyan Kusuma Ayuningtyas

CONTENTS

22.1 INTRODUCTION

Anredera cordifolia (Ten.) v. Steenis is known as Madeira vine, heart-leaf Madeira vine, mignonette vine, sweet mignonette (Western), lamb's tail vine (Australia), *enredadera del mosquito* or *parra de madeira* (Mexico), *enredadera papa* (Brazil), *binahong* (Indonesia), *luna luna* (Chile), *luo kui shu, de san chi* (China), *madeiraranker* (South Africa) and *madeiraranka* (Sweden). It is native to tropical and sub-tropical areas of Southern America, notably Bolivia, Paraguay, Brazil, Uruguay and Argentina. The plant spread from South America via Spanish and Portuguese traders at an early date (Wagner et al. 1999; Vivian-Smith et al. 2007). At present, *Anredera cordifolia*

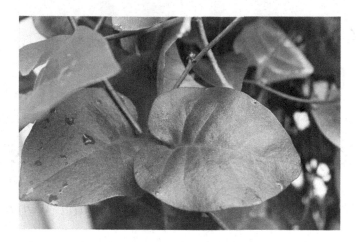

FIGURE 22.1 **(See color insert.)** The heart leaf of *Anredera cordifolia*.

is extensively distributed and cultivated around the world, either as an ornamental or medicinal plant. It has been globally distributed through China, Japan, Israel, India, some parts of Africa, the United States, Mexico, Caribbean, Australia, New Zealand and its surrounding islands, which demonstrates that this plant can grow in sub-tropical and tropical climate areas (Cagnotti et al. 2007; see Figure 22.1).

A limited number of reviews of *Anredera cordifolia* have been conducted. Currently, there is no detailed review on the phytochemical, pharmacological and toxicological properties of *Anredera cordifolia*. Predictably, this is rooted in the limited amount of research on *Anredera cordifolia* itself. Hence most of the studies in this review come from the authors' own research. This review will focus not only on the phytochemistry and pharmacological properties of *Anredera cordifolia* in more detail, but also on economic and botanical aspects of *Anredera cordifolia*, its scientific application and future prospects.

22.2   BOTANICAL DESCRIPTION

Anredera cordifolia comes from the genus *Anredera* Juss., named after Spanish word 'enredadera' which means creeping or climber plant (Wagner et al. 1999; Vivian-Smith et al. 2007). The family is Basellaceae, which includes up to 12 species of perennial, twining or scandent, succulent or muci-laginous, often tuberous vines (Sperling and Bittrich 1993). *Anredera cordifolia* has various syn-onyms, including *Boussingaultia cordifolia* Ten., *Boussingaultia gracilis* (Miers), *Boussingaultia cordata* (Sprenger), *Boussingaultia gracilis* f. *pseudobaselloides* (Hauman), and *Boussingaultia gracilis* f. *typica* (Hauman; Eriksson 2007). The taxonomic hierarchy of *Anredera cordifolia* can be seen below:

Kingdom	Plantae
Subkingdom	Viridiplantae
Superdivision	Embryophyta
Division	Tracheophyta

Subdivision	Spermatophyta
Class	Magnoliopsida
Superorder	Caryophyllanae
Order	Caryophyllales
Family	Basellaceae
Genus	*Anredera* Juss
Species	*Anredera cordifolia* (Ten.) v. Steenis

Sperling and Bittrich (1993) stated in their books that *Anredera cordifolia* was a twining or scandent succulent vine, producing annual or short-lived shoots from thickened stem bases, tuberous crowns or tubers. Inflorescence is an axillary or terminal raceme, and the bracteoles are persistent or deciduous. Its flowers are bisexual or functionally unisexual, sweetly scented with sepals sometimes more or less strongly keeled, white or yellowish to reddish. The stamens are free to the base or shortly connate. The style is single, trilobed or divided nearly at the base. Fruit a nutlet, partly or completely enclosed by the persistent dry perianth, with sepals sometimes forming a broad-winged keel (Figure 22.2).

Eriksson (2007) notes that *Anredera cordifolia* is renowned by its distinctly pedicellate flowers with a perianth that dries dark brown and spreads also in fruit, with a distinct three-part style.

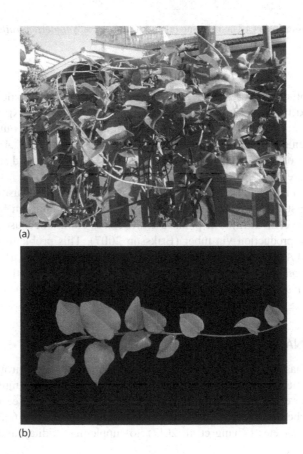

(a)

(b)

FIGURE 22.2 **(See color insert.)** The plant of *Anredera cordifolia*.

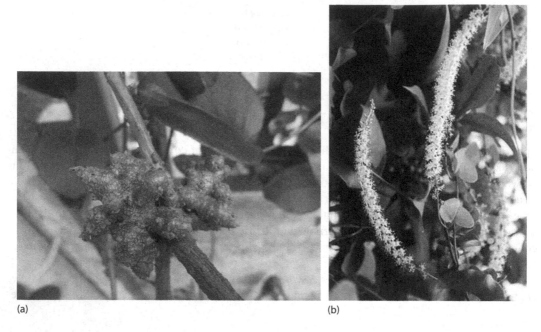

(a)   (b)

FIGURE 22.3   (See color insert.) The rhizome (a) and flower (b) of *Anredera cordifolia*.

The flowers of the other species having a three-part style tend to dry pale. The inflorescences are usually large and richly branched with numerous flowers, which explain its popularity in some countries as an ornamental plant. It usually reproduces by its tuber outside its native areas. The fruit has not been observed in some countries (Wagner et al. 1999). *Anredera cordifolia* is an evergreen climber on hedges or other plants, has flashy rhizomes and white or yellowish to reddish flowers (Figure 22.3).

Anredera cordifolia is considered a major problem in some areas. In Australia and African forests, these plants are strictly regulated because they are invasive and can harm native plants in those countries (Boyne et al. 2013). The plants are difficult to control because of their rapid growth and easy vegetative reproduction via tuber (Eriksson 2007). This problem may be a blessing in disguise for the use of *Anredera cordifolia* as an herbal medicine, particularly in developing countries. *Anredera cordifolia* may act as a cheap and easy to produce alternative medicine because it grows in various climates, is easy to cultivate, and grows rapidly, showing favourable features for an alternative medicine.

22.3   TRADITIONAL USE

Anredera cordifolia has been used traditionally to treat many diseases around the world. In its native area, South America, *Anredera cordifolia* has been used to treat injuries (wound healing) and infections (Heisler et al. 2012) as an antibacterial and antifungal (Paz et al. 1996), and to treat toothache and headache (Hilgert 2001). In other countries, *Anredera cordifolia* has also been used traditionally to treat diabetes (Zhang et al. 2017), to supplement kidney and strengthen lumbus,

Traditional Use of *Anredera cordifolia* (Ten.) Steenis

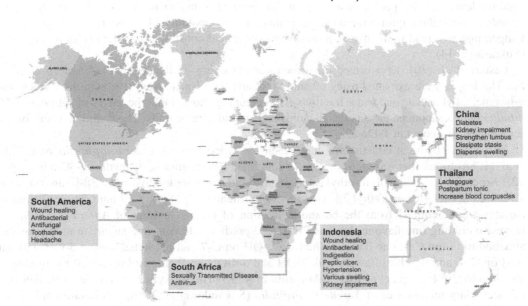

China
Diabetes
Kidney impairment
Strengthen lumbus
Dissipate stasis
Disperse swelling

Thailand
Lactagogue
Postpartum tonic
Increase blood corpuscles

South America
Wound healing
Antibacterial
Antifungal
Toothache
Headache

Indonesia
Wound healing
Antibacterial
Indigestion
Peptic ulcer,
Hypertension
Various swelling
Kidney impairment

South Africa
Sexually Transmitted Disease
Antivirus

FIGURE 22.4 **(See color insert.)** Traditional use of *Anredera cordifolia* in various countries.

dissipate stasis and disperse swelling (Zhou et al. 2011) in China; to treat sexually transmitted diseases (Tshikalange et al. 2005) and act as an antivirus (Mulaudzi et al. 2015) in South Africa; act as a galactagogue, postpartum tonic and to increase blood corpuscles in Thailand (Panyaphu et al. 2011); and to treat injury, thrush, indigestion, peptic ulcer, hypertension, various swellings (inflammation), acne, urinary tract inflammation, kidney inflammation and kidney impairment in Indonesia (Hariana 2013; Savitri 2015).

The methods of preparation in traditional use were varied, considering the multiple purposes of *Anredera cordifolia* use. To treat injury or skin infection, the leaves could be put directly on the site of injury. Some people preferred extracting the sap by crushing fresh leaves and putting the sap on the site of injury, while some preferred using the sap in compresses with pieces of clean cloth, cotton or gauze, saturated in hot water (Heisler et al. 2012). Although less traditional, a book about prescriptions for herbal healing by Balch (2012) described the use of Madeira vine for swollen eyelids caused by *Staphylococcus aureus* infection. The most common preparation was a decoction, where fresh or dried leaves of *Anredera cordifolia* were boiled with water (Hariana 2013). While less common, there have also been suggestions to make a juice of fresh *Anredera cordifolia* leaves (Hidayat and Napitupulu 2015; Figure 22.4).

22.4 PHYTOCHEMICAL

Various parts of *Anredera cordifolia*, such as the leaf, stem and tuber, have been used traditionally to treat many diseases. Phytochemical screening results for the stem, leaves and tuber of *Anredera cordifolia* showed terpenoid, steroid, glycoside and alkaloid contents, while its flower contains terpenoids, steroids and glycosides (Astuti et al. 2011; Leliqia et al. 2017). Most studies have mainly used the leaves, as this part is the most plentiful resource from *Anredera cordifolia*. The leaves of *Anredera cordifolia* require a rapid drying method, as they contain high moisture. Aeration at room temperature will lead to the degradation of some chemical constituents as the leaves retain water (Sukrasno 2014).

Lestari et al. (2015) performed phytochemical screening on the leaves of *Anredera cordifolia*. The leaves were extracted using ethanol 70%, and then fractionated to obtain three fractions: *n*-hexane, ethyl acetate and water fractions. The screening showed that the leaves of *Anredera cordifolia* contain saponins, flavonoids, alkaloids and steroid/triterpenoids. The complete result of the screening is presented in Table 22.1.

Numerous chemical constituents have been identified from *Anredera cordifolia* parts. Lin et al. (1988) found that *Anredera cordifolia* contained larreagenin A, 3β-hydroxy-30-horoleana-12,19-dien-28-oic acid with its ethyl ester, ursolic acid and 28-ethyl hydrogen 3β-hydroxyolean-12-ene-28,29-dioatea and ethyl 3β-hydroxy-30-horoleana-12, 18-dien-29-oate. Three flavonoid isolates were obtained from the butanolic fraction of ethanol extract of *Anredera cordifolia* leaves, including one flavone that has 7-OH and predicted having one sugar (monoglycoside) attached to O- on C-5, one flavone which has –OH on C-7 and predicted having 5-OH without -OH on C-4, and the third flavone with 7-OH and o-diOH on B ring and predicted having sugar attached to C-5 (Leliqia et al. 2017). Apigenin or 4′,5,7-trihydroxyflavon and oleanolic acid are the secondary metabolites of *Anredera cordifolia* (Sukandar et al. 2016). Chromatography profiles of *Anredera cordifolia* revealed the existence of apigetrin (apigenin-7-glucoside) and rutin (Leliqia et al. 2017).

Methanol extract of *Anredera cordifolia* leaves contained 8-glucopyranosyl-4′,5,7-trihydroxyflavone compound (Djamil et al. 2012), and boussingoside (A1, A2, B, C, E), momordin and larreagenin A (Espada et al. 1990, 1997). Qiong et al. (2007) successfully isolated two flavanols and four flavones from *Anredera cordifolia*, which were identified as bougracol A, 4,7-dihydroxy-5-methoxy-8-methyl-6-formyl-flavane, 7-O-methyllunonal, 5,7-dihydroxy-6,8-dimethyl-2-phenyl-4H-1-benzopyran-4-one, desmosflavone and demethoxymatteucinol. Vitexin or 8-glucopyranosyl-4′5″7-trihydroxyflavone was also found in the leaves

TABLE 22.1
Phytochemical Screening of *Anredera cordifolia*

	Crude Drug	Ethanol Extract	*n*-Hexane Fraction	Ethyl Acetate Fraction	Water Fraction
Saponin	+	+	+	+	+
Quinone	–	–	–	–	–
Flavonoid	+	+	+	+	+
Tannin	–	–	–	–	–
Alkaloid	+	+	+	+	+
Steroid/ Triterpenoid	+	+	+	+	+

Source: Lestari, D. et al., *IJPCR*, 7, 435–439, 2015.

(Mulia et al. 2017). Abou-Zeid et al. (2007) analysed the volatile constituents of the aerial parts of *Anredera cordifolia* and found that the major compounds were phytol (15.33%), alpha-pinene (9.0%) and 6,10,14-trimethyl pentadecanone (6.12%). This research also analysed the lipoidal matter which was fractionated into non-saponifiable and saponifiable matters with neophytadiene (7.72%), 5-phenyl dodecane (7.41%) and 5-phenyl undecane (6.08%) as major compounds of non-saponifiable matter. The chemical structure of several isolates from *Anredera cordifolia* can be seen in Figures 22.5–22.8.

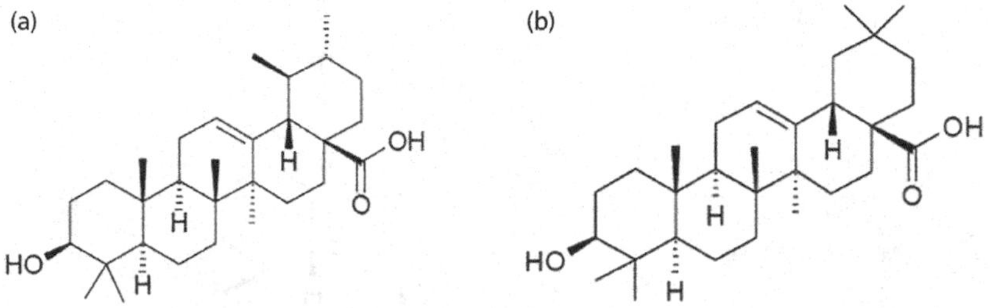

FIGURE 22.5   The chemical structure of ursolic acid (a) and its isomer oleanolic acid (b).

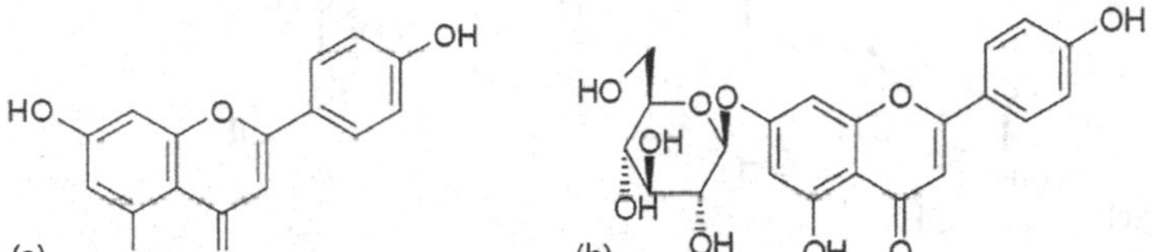

FIGURE 22.6   The chemical structure of apigenin (a) and apigetrin (b).

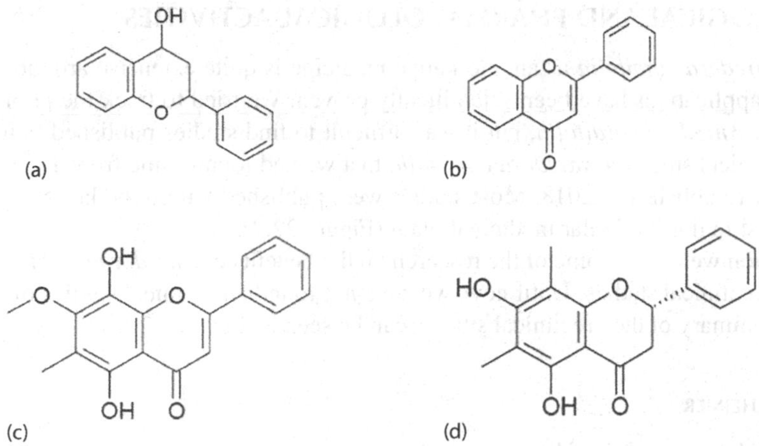

FIGURE 22.7   The chemical structure of flavanol (a), flavone (b), desmosflavone (c) and demethoxymatteucinol (d).

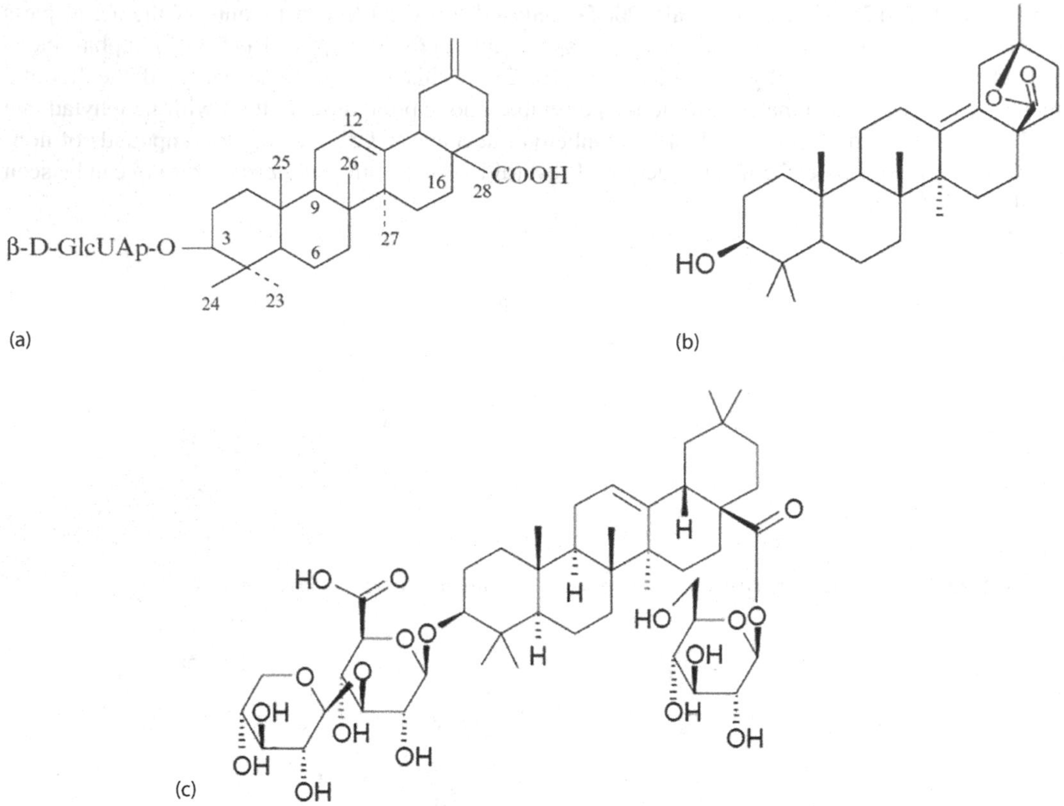

FIGURE 22.8   The chemical structure of boussingoside A1 (a), momordin IIc (b) and larreagenin A (c).

22.5   BIOLOGICAL AND PHARMACOLOGICAL ACTIVITIES

The use of *Anredera cordifolia* as an alternative medicine is quite extensive around the world, but not all of the applications have been scientifically proven. We tried to track the published journals about study of *Anredera cordifolia*, but it was difficult to find studies published before the 2000s. The first preclinical study on *Anredera cordifolia* that we had found came from 1994, while the latest one was just published in 2018. Most studies were published within the last 5 years, indicating the new interest in this particular medicinal plant (Figure 22.9).

In this section we review some of the research on the benefits of *Anredera cordifolia* as an herbal medicine in preclinical studies. Until now, we have not found any clinical studies of *Anredera cordifolia*. The summary of the preclinical studies can be seen in Table 22.2.

22.5.1   ALZHEIMER

Regulation of the expression of both amyloid precursor protein (APP) and tau proteins is vital in understanding the cause of Alzheimer's disease (AD). Tasi et al. (2015) conducted research to investigate the potential of *Anredera cordifolia* in targeted search using the internal ribosome entry site (IRES) of tau and amyloid-β precursor protein. Results indicated that memantine could reduce the activity of both the APP and tau IRES at a concentration of ~10 µM (monitored by secreted alkaline phosphatase or SEAP activity) without interfering with the cap-dependent translation as monitored by the β-galactosidase assay. Based on previous results, Tasi et al. (2015) made a preparation called NB34, which was an *Anredera cordifolia* extract fermented with *Lactobacillus* spp. In this study,

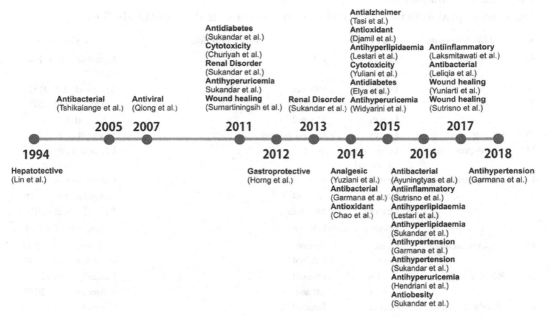

FIGURE 22.9 Timeline of preclinical studies of *Anredera cordifolia*.

TABLE 22.2
Pharmacological Activities of *Anredera cordifolia* and Its Related Metabolites

No	Effect/Activity	Part Used	Extract/Fraction	References
1	Alzheimer	Not mentioned	Extract was fermented with *Lactobacillus* spp.	Tasi et al. (2015)
2	Analgesic	Leaves	Ethanol	Yuziani et al. (2014)
3	Anti-inflammatory	Leaves	Ethanol	Laksmitawati et al. (2017)
		Leaves	Ethyl alcohol	Sutrisno et al. (2016)
4	Antibacterial	Leaves	Ethanol	Garmana et al. (2014)
		Roots	Chloroform, water	Tshikalange et al. (2005)
		Leaves	Ethanol, and then fractionated using *n*-hexane and ethyl acetate	Leliqia et al. (2017)
			Gradually extraction by reflux using *n*-hexane, ethyl acetate and ethanol 96%, respectively	
		Leaves	Ethanol	Ayuningtyas (2016)
		Leaves	Metabolite	Pitaloka and Sukandar (2017)
5	Antioxidant	Leaves	Ethanol, and then fractionated using ethyl acetate, methanol, *n*-hexane, *n*-buthanol	Djamil et al. (2017)
		Leaves	Ethanol, methanol	Chao et al. (2014)
6	Antiviral	Leaves	Ethanol	Qiong et al. (2007)
		Rhizomes	Purified protein	Chuang et al. (2007)
7	Anti-dyslipidaemia	Leaves	Ethanol, and then fractionated using *n*-hexane, ethyl acetate, and water fractions	Lestari et al. (2015)
		Leaves	Ethanol, and then fractionated using *n*-hexane, ethyl acetate, and water fractions	Lestari et al. (2016)
		Leaves	Ethanol	Sukandar et al. (2016)

(Continued)

TABLE 22.2 (*Continued*)
Pharmacological Activities of *Anredera cordifolia* and Its Related Metabolites

No	Effect/Activity	Part Used	Extract/Fraction	References
8	Cytotoxicity	Leaves	Ethanol	Churiyah and Wijaya (2011)
		Leaves	Ethanol	Yuliani et al. (2015)
9	Diabetes	Leaves	Methanol	Sukandar et al. (2011)
		Leaves	Ethanol	Elya et al. (2015)
10	Gastroprotective	Leaves	Extract powder	Horng et al. (2012)
11	Hepatoprotective	Leaves, stems, brood bud	Water	Lin et al. (1994)
12	Antihypertension	Leaves	Ethanol	Garmana et al. (2016)
		Leaves	Ethanol	Sukandar et al. (2016)
		Leaves	Metabolite	Sukandar et al. (2016)
		Leaves	Ethanol	Garmana et al. (2018)
13	Hyperuricaemia	Leaves	Ethanol	Widyarini et al. (2015)
		Herb	Ethanol	Hendriani et al. (2016)
14	Renal disorder	Leaves	Ethanol	Sukandar et al. (2011)
		Leaves	Ethanol	Sukandar et al. (2013)
15	Weight reduction (anti-obesity)	Leaves	Ethanol	Sukandar et al. (2016)
16	Wound healing	Leaves	Ethanol	Yuniarti and Lukiswanto (2017)
		Leaves	Ethanol	Sumartiningsih (2011)
		Leaves	Ethanol	Sutrisno (2017)

NB34 showed functions similarly to memantine in both IRES of APP and tau. The water Maze test also showed positive results, in which NB34 could improve the spatial memory of a high fat diet–induced neurodegeneration in apolipoprotein E-knockout (ApoE$^{-/-}$) mice.

22.5.2 ANALGESIC AND ANTI-INFLAMMATORY

In a preclinical study using Wistar rats, ethanolic extracts of *Anredera cordifolia* leaves at doses 100, 200 and 400 mg/kg body weight (bw) showed an analgesic effect. This study used the plantar test method to compare the analgesic effect of *Anredera cordifolia* with diclofenac sodium (2.25 mg/kg bw). In this study, administration of *Anredera cordifolia* resulted in significantly longer time to feel early pain compared to negative control ($P < 0.05$), even at the smallest dose. The analgesic effect was dose-dependent, so the maximum response was produced at a dose of 400 mg/kg bw. The dose of 400 mg/kg bw showed comparable results to diclofenac sodium 2.25 mg/kg on the Duncan test. The researcher proposed that *Anredera cordifolia* exerts an analgesic effect by inhibiting the synthesis of prostaglandins (Yuziani et al. 2014).

It is known that drugs like NSAIDs exert their analgesic and anti-inflammatory activity by the inhibition of cyclooxygenase (COX) activity, in which prostaglandins are synthesised by the constitutively expressed COX-1(Vane and Botting 1997). Thus, a substance that had an analgesic effect was highly probable to have an anti-inflammatory effect as well. The first study observed an anti-inflammatory effect of *Anredera cordifolia* leaves (ethanol extract) on lipopolysaccharide-induced murine macrophage cell line (RAW 264.7). Anti-inflammatory activity was determined by measuring parameters such as interleukin-1β (IL-1 β), tumour necrosis factor (TNF-α), nitric oxide (NO) and IL-6. Extracts of *Anredera cordifolia* at concentrations of 150, 250 and 500 μg/mL were toxic to cell line, which was indicated by low viability in this study. *Anredera cordifolia* showed significant decreases of TNF-α, IL-1 and IL-6 level in cell line at concentration of 50, 50, and 10 μg/mL, respectively. *Anredera cordifolia* showed the lowest decrease in NO level at a concentration of 50 μg/mL, but this was not comparable to normal cells. This study exhibited the potential of *Anredera cordifolia* as an anti-inflammatory by the inhibitory activity of inflammatory mediators including TNF-α, IL-1β, IL-6 and NO. Flavonoids are predicted to be responsible in showing the anti-inflammatory activity of *Anredera cordifolia* (Laksmitawati et al. 2017).

Another study investigated the anti-inflammatory properties of *Anredera cordifolia* extract in combination with *Centella asiatica* using human red blood cell (RBC)-membrane stabilisation assay. In this study, both *Anredera cordifolia* and *Centella asiatica* were extracted using ethyl alcohol. The extract concentrations used in this study was 100, 200, 400 and 800 μg/mL. Diclofenac sodium with the same concentration as the extracts was used as the standard drug. The results showed that *Anredera cordifolia* extract alone, *Centella asiatica* extract alone, and the extract combination could inhibit the haemolysis of RBC in hypotonic solution. The optimum concentration was 100 μg/mL for *Anredera cordifolia* extract, 400 μg/mL for *Centella asiatica* extract and 50 μg/mL of both extracts for the combination. Diclofenac sodium as a standard drug showed optimum inhibition at a concentration of 400 μg/mL. The result showed that the maximum inhibition of haemolysis activity was shown in combination of 50 μg/mL of both extracts, which was the lowest concentration of the combinations, although the rising concentration in combination did not show a significant elevation in inhibiting haemolysis. From the experiment, the extract showed an ability to inhibit haemolysis of RBC in hypotonic solution and HRBC membrane showed similarity with lysosome membrane. During inflammation, the lysosomal enzyme is released and produces several characteristics of inflammation. The ability to stabilise lysosomal membrane is predicted to prevent inflammation. *Anredera cordifolia* ultimately possessed am anti-inflammatory effect at a lower concentration than the standard drug used in this study (Sutrisno et al. 2016).

22.5.3 Antibacterial

Numerous studies have been conducted to prove the antibacterial properties of *Anredera cordifolia*. The idea came from the traditional use of *Anredera cordifolia* to treat infection and injury. People in Brazil used the leaves to 'pull out the dirt inside injury' (Heisler et al. 2012), which was believed to be pus, a sign of infection.

A study by Garmana et al. (2014) showed that ethanol extract of *Anredera cordifolia* leaves exhibited antibacterial activities towards *Bacillus cereus*, *Bacillus subtilis*, Methicillin-Susceptible *Staphylococcus aureus* (MSSA), Methicillin-Resistant Coagulase-Negative *Staphylococcus* (MRCNS), *Escherichia coli*, and *Pseudomonas aeruginosa* with minimum inhibitory concentrations (MIC) of 256, 256, 512, 512, 256 and 256 μg/mL, respectively. Tshikalange et al. (2005) focused on evaluating the antibacterial activities of aqueous and chloroform extracts of *Anredera cordifolia* on sexually transmitted diseases. In this study, aqueous and chloroform extracts did not differ in activities. *Anredera cordifolia* showed antibacterial activities towards *Bacillus pumilus*, *Bacillus subtilis*, *Staphylococcus aureus*, *Enterobacter cloacae*, *Escherichia coli*, *Klebsiella pneumoniae*, *Pseudomonas aeruginosa*, *Serratia marcescens* and *Enterobacter aerogenes* in the standard petri dish *in vitro* bioassays with MIC 50, 60, 60, 50, 60, 60, 60, 60 and 60 mg/mL respectively. The Gram-positive bacteria appeared to be more susceptible to the antibacterial properties of the extracts (water and chloroform) than the Gram-negative ones.

Leliqia et al. (2017) further investigated the antibacterial activity of *Anredera cordifolia* by testing the extract and its fractions. In this study, Leliqia et al. extracted the crude drug using two methods. The first method was extraction by reflux using ethanol 96% and then fractionated by liquid-liquid extraction using *n*-hexane and ethyl acetate. The second method was gradual extraction by reflux using *n*-hexane, ethyl acetate and then ethanol 96%. The ethanolic extract, *n*-hexane and ethyl acetate fractions of *Anredera cordifolia* from the first method had antibacterial activity against *Staphylococcus aureus*, MRSA, *Bacillus subtilis*, and *Bacillus cereus* (MIC 0.26–0.51 mg/mL).

However, the *n*-hexane and ethyl acetate extract from the second method had a broad spectrum of antibacterial activity that could inhibit the growth of *S. aureus*, MRSA, *B. subtilis*, *P. aeruginosa* and *E. coli* (MIC 0.26–0.51 mg/mL). The results of this study can be seen in Table 22.3.

Leliqia et al. also determined the bactericidal and bacteriostatic activities using minimum bactericidal concentration (MBC) to MIC ratio in this study. Bacteriostatic activity has been defined as a ratio

TABLE 22.3
Antibacterial Activities of *Anredera cordifolia* Extracts and Fractions

Bacteria	(mg/mL)	Extraction Method				Amoxicillin
		EE	HF	EAF	WF	
S. aureus						
MIC		0.51[a]	0.26[a,b]	0.51[a]	1.02	0.5[c]
MBC		>4.01	>4.01	>4.01	>4.01	0.5
MSSA						
MIC		2.05	2.05	4.01	>4.01	8
MBC		>4.01	>4.01	>4.01	>4.01	8
MRSA						
MIC		0.51[a]	1.02	1.02	>4.01	32[c]
MBC		>4.01	2.05	2.05	>4.01	32
B. subtilis						
MIC		2.05	0.51[a]	1024	>4.01	4[c]
MBC		4.01	4.01	4.01	>4.01	4
B. cereus						
MIC		4.01	0.51[a]	>4.01	>4.01	0.5[c]
MBC		>4.01	1.02	>4.01	>4.01	2
P. aeruginosa						
MIC		1.02	>4.01	>4.01	>4.01	16[c]
MBC		2.05	>4.01	>4.01	>4.01	32
E. coli						
MIC		>4.01	>4.01	>4.01	>4.01	1[c]
MBC		>4.01	>4.01	>4.01	>4.01	1
E. coli H7 (O156)						
MIC		>4.01	2.05	>4.01	>4.01	32
MBC		>4.01	4.01	>4.01	>4.01	32
ESBL *E. coli*						
MIC		4.01	1.02	2.05	>4.01	>256
MBC		>4.01	2.05	>4.01	>4.01	>256

Source: Modified from Leliqia et al. (2015). With permission.

EE: ethanolic extract of *Anredera cordifolia* leaves, HF: *n*-hexane fraction, EAF: ethyl acetate fraction, WF: water fraction, MIC: minimum inhibitory concentration, MBC: minimum bactericidal concentration.

[a] Had antibacterial potential.

[b] Significant difference compared to other extracts and fractions of *Anredera cordifolia* which had antibacterial potential against the same bacteria ($P < 0.05$).

[c] Significant difference compared to extracts and fractions of *Anredera cordifolia* which had antibacterial potential against the same bacteria ($P < 0.05$).

of MBC to MIC > 4 and bactericidal activity had ratio MBC to MIC < 4. In this study, EE had bacteriostatic activity, while HF had bactericidal activity except its activity toward *B. cereus* and *P. aeruginosa*.

Another study by Ayuningtyas (2016) showed that *Anredera cordifolia* showed antituberculosis activity toward susceptible and resistant strains of *Mycobacterium tuberculosis*. Antituberculosis activity was evaluated against susceptible H37Rv and two MDR strains (isoniazid-ethambutol resistant and rifampicin-streptomycin resistant) of *M. tuberculosis* using proportion method on Löwenstein–Jensen (LJ) medium for 8 weeks. Although *Anredera cordifolia* showed MIC > 1000 µg/mL towards *M. tuberculosis*, the extract still exhibited antituberculosis activity by showing more than 70% reduction in colony number, even at the smallest concentration. The study also showed increase in the reduction in colony number when combining *Anredera cordifolia* with the first line regimen of antituberculosis drugs.

Jiménez-Arellanes et al. (2013) suggested that the antituberculosis activity of *Anredera cordifolia* originated from the existence of ursolic acid and its isomer oleanolic acid. This claim was further supported by Pitaloka and Sukandar (2017), who used the same evaluation method as Ayuningtyas (2016). The results showed that MIC of ursolic acid was 50 µg/mL against three different strains of *Mycobacterium tuberculosis*, including the resistant strains. In addition, the combination of ursolic acid and tuberculosis drugs displayed a synergistic interaction and no antagonism resulting from the combination was observed in this study.

22.5.4 ANTIOXIDANT

In vitro test of antioxidant activity can be conducted by a few different methods, such as DPPH (1,1-diphenyl-2-picrylhydrazyl) free radical, trolox equivalent antioxidant capacity (TEAC) and oxygen radical absorbance capacity (ORAC) assays. Methanol extract of *Anredera cordifolia* leaves could scavenge DPPH radical with IC_{50} 53.11 µg/mL. Fractionation from ethanol extract were hexane, ethyl acetate and butanolic fractions gave IC_{50} DPPH 256.23, 57.96, and 132.39 µg/mL, respectively. The 8-glucopyranosyl-4′,5,7-trihydroxyflavone compound that was successfully isolated from ethyl acetate extract of *Anredera cordifolia* leaves could also scavenge DPPH radical with IC_{50} 68.07 µg/mL (Djamil et al. 2017)

Chao et al. (2014) also evaluated the antioxidant activities of *Anredera cordifolia* using different methods. Result showed that methanolic extract had IC_{50} of DPPH 1173.32 µg/mL. Using TEAC assay, methanolic and ethanolic extract showed IC_{50} 36.22 and 21.04 µg/mL, respectively. Meanwhile by using ORAC assay, the extract exhibited antioxidant activity with ORAC-hydrophilic value 202.59 µmol Trolox/g dry weight and ORAC-lipophilic value 157.75 µmol Trolox/g dry weight. The hydrophilic extract appeared to be more effective than the lipophilic extract in this study. Phytochemical screening results showed that *Anredera cordifolia* extract contained polyphenols (equal to 5.81 mg gallic acid/g dry weight), flavonoids (equal to 40 mg quercetin/g dry weight) and flavonols (equal to 6.92 mg quercetin/g dry weight, 781.28 µg myricetin/g dry weight, 455.16 µg morin/g dry weight).

Antioxidant activities mainly comes from flavonoids, which have been known for their significant antioxidant and chelating properties. Their cardioprotective effects stem from the ability to inhibit lipid peroxidation, chelate redox-active metals and attenuate other processes involving reactive oxygen species. The capability of flavonoids to inhibit free-radical mediated events is dictated by their chemical structure, which is based on the flavan nucleus, the number and positions, and substitutions influence radical scavenging and chelating activity (Heim et al. 2000).

22.5.5 ANTIVIRAL

Inhibiting the cleavage activation of a virus may prove beneficial to treat viral infection. This step plays an important part in the viral replication cycle that permits viral-endosome fusion. It can be done by targeting trypsin-like host proteases that are responsible for the cleavage (Hamilton et al. 2014). Thus, the antivirus activity can be evaluated by measuring the trypsin inhibition activity.

The first study that investigated the antiviral activity of *Anredera cordifolia* was done by Qiong et al. (2007), who successfully isolated two flavanols and four flavones from ethanol extract of *Anredera cordifolia* leaves. The author suggested that bougracol A, 4,7-dihydroxy-5-methoxy-8-methyl-6-formyl-flavane and demethoxymatteucinol presented weak anti-HIV activity with EC_{50} 45.09, 48.73, 55.47, and 82.75 μmol/L, respectively, and had TI (trypsin inhibitor) value 1.41, 1.20, 7.15 and >8.51, respectively.

The rhizome of *Anredera cordifolia* contained one major (23 kDa) protein band under non-reducing condition in the SDS-PAGE, named tentatively ancordin. Ancordin showed trypsin inhibitory activity in the SDS-PAGE gel, which was found not only in rhizomes but also in aerial tubers, although there were few in the fresh leaves of *Anredera cordifolia*. The results showed that purified ancordin exhibited 0.0428 μg trypsin inhibition/μg ancordin. Ancordin also stimulated NO production in RAW264.7 cell without showing any cytotoxic effect (Chuang et al. 2007).

22.5.6 ANTIDYSLIPIDAEMIA

Anredera cordifolia has down a highly beneficial effect as an anti-hyperlipidaemic. Lestari et al. (2015) evaluated the anti-hyperlipidaemic effects on male Wistar rats given high fat food and pure cholesterol. In this study, simvastatin 3.6 mg/kg bw was used as a standard drug. The result showed that administration of *Anredera cordifolia* leaf extract at 50, 100 and 200 mg/kg bw decreased blood cholesterol level by 55.29%, 63.45% and 67.70%, respectively, compared to the statin and negative control group 78.58% and 46.52%, respectively. Triglycerides were decreased 61.64% in statin group; 41.08%, 47.59% and 50.66% in *Anredera cordifolia* leaf extract at doses 50, 100 and 200 mg/kg bw, respectively; and 20.17% in the negative control group. Meanwhile LDL level decreased 97.14% in statin group; 81.31%, 89.01% and 95.33% in the 50, 100 and 200 mg/kg bw *Anredera cordifolia* leaf extract, respectively; and 69.69% in the negative control group. There did not appear to be any significant increase in HDL level for all of extracts. It was concluded that *Anredera cordifolia* leaf extract at doses 50, 100 and 200 mg/kg bw significantly reduced total cholesterol level, triglycerides and LDL level compared to negative control group ($P < 0.05$) and had no influence in HDL level. Lestari et al. also evaluated the ability of *Anredera cordifolia* to reduce endothelial fat content and showed that extract at doses 50, 100 and 200 mg /kg bw could reduce fat deposits in the endothelial cells of blood vessels.

Lestari et al. (2016) further investigated the same activity using various fractions of *Anredera cordifolia*. The crude drug was extracted by reflux using ethanol 96%, and then fractionated by liquid-liquid extraction to obtain three fractions: *n*-hexane, ethyl acetate and water fractions. Results showed all fractions could reduce the total cholesterol significantly ($P < 0.05$) compared to the negative control group. The result demonstrated that ethyl acetate fraction from ethanol leaf extract of *Anredera cordifolia* was very efficient in reducing total cholesterol level. In the negative control group, the total cholesterol level also decreased 57.1%, which might be due to the replacement of high cholesterol feed by normal feed. Based on this data, it can be concluded that by diet only the total cholesterol level would decrease slowly by itself, but administration of *Anredera cordifolia* provided a faster way to reduce total cholesterol level.

Another study by Sukandar et al. (2016) evaluated the anti-hyperlipidaemic activity of *Anredera cordifolia* leaves alone and in combination with *Morus nigra* (mulberry) leaf extract. Simvastatin 3.6 mg/kg bw was used as the standard drug. The rats were divided into seven groups: normal, control, simvastatin 3.6 mg/kg bw, *Anredera cordifolia* leaf extract 100 mg/kg bw (A100), *Morus nigra* leaf extract 200 mg/kg bw (M200), combination of *Anredera cordifolia* extract 50 mg/kg and *Morus nigra* 100 mg/kg (A50+M100), and combination of *Anredera cordifolia* extract 100 mg/kg bw and *Morus nigra* 200 mg/kg bw (A100+M200). There were significant differences ($P < 0.05$) between groups M200, A50+M100, and A100+M200 compared to the control group at day 14, with the reduction of total cholesterol level 33.68%, 34.39% and 44.81%, respectively and reduction of triglyceride level 36.86%, 37.16% and 49.99%, respectively. It was concluded that the combination of both extracts (A100+M200) showed considerably better activity than either *Anredera cordifolia* extract or *Morus nigra* extract alone.

The anti-obesity effect of *Anredera cordifolia*, particularly the secondary metabolites api-genin and apigetrin, was studied further *in silico*. This study was conducted to investigate *in silico* interaction between apigenin and apigetrin with 3-hydroxy-3-methyl-glutayl-co-enzyme A (HMG Co-A) reductase, to find the most favourable binding site as well as to predict the binding mode. HMG Co-A reductase is the rate-controlling enzyme of the mevalonate pathway, which produces cholesterol and other isoprenoids. Results showed binding affinity and inhibition constants of R-mevalonate were Ei = −4.2 kcal/mol, Ki = 836.78 µM; apigenin Ei = −7.0 kcal/mol, Ki = 7.43 µM; apigetrin Ei = −5.9 kcal/mol, Ki = 47.53 µM; simvastatin Ei = −8.2 kcal/mol; Ki = 0.98 µM; atorvastatin Ei = −8.4 kcal/mol; Ki = 0.7 µM. Apigenin had a better binding interaction than api-getrin. This research indicated the potential of apigenin to be developed as an anticholesterol drug (Lestari et al. 2017).

22.5.7 Cytotoxicity

Churiyah and Wijaya (2011) conducted a preliminary study to investigate the cytotoxicity of *Anredera cordifolia* against MCF-7 and T47D breast cancer cell lines after being extracted with several concentrations of ethanol of 90%, 70%, 50% and 30%. Cytotoxic analysis indicated that increasing ethanol concentration as the solvent resulted in decreasing IC_{50} value, hence the 90% ethanol showed the highest toxicity. *Anredera cordifolia* extracted with ethanol 90% showed IC^{50} 60.35 and 68.75 µg/mL on T-47D cells and MCF-7 cells, respectively.

Another study was conducted by Yuliani et al. (2015) to evaluate the cytotoxicity effect of *Anredera cordifolia* on different cell lines using HeLa cells, a model of stress inducing-p53 cervi-cal cancer cells. Cytotoxic study on HeLa cells was designed by a 3-[4,5-dimethylthiazol-2-yl]-2,5 diphenyltetrazolium bromide (MTT) test and further apoptotic induction assay was determined by the annexin V-FITC method. Extract of *Anredera cordifolia* leaves showed cytotoxic activity and promoted apoptosis in HeLa cells with IC_{50} value 75 µg/mL. The extract did not increase level expression of p53 in cells, hence it was predicted the cytotoxic activity of *A. cordifolia* leaf extract on HeLa cells was through a p53-independent pathway.

22.5.8 Diabetes

Anredera cordifolia also has effect in lowering blood glucose level and in repairing damage of β-pancreas cells. The extract was tested on diabetic Swiss Webster mice induced by alloxan. *Anredera cordifolia* was administrated for 14 days and blood glucose levels were measured after 7 and 14 days. The pancreas cells of treated mice were observed histologically on day 14. The research showed that the methanol extract of *Anredera cordifolia* leaves at a dose of 50, 100 and 200 mg/kg bw could lower blood glucose levels significantly compared to the control group ($P < 0.05$) on both day 7 or day 14 and increased the number and repaired the damage of β-pancreas cells (Sukandar et al. 2011). Another researcher conducted an *in vitro* study that reported that the ethanol extract of *Anredera cordifolia* leaves could inhibit α-glycosidase with IC_{50} 54.24 µg/mL, while extract 62.5 µg/mL also gave 74.03% inhibition to α-amylase and 10.70% inhibition to DPP IV (Elya et al. 2015).

22.5.9 Gastroprotective

Horng et al. (2015) investigated the effect of *Anredera cordifolia* on gastric mucosal protection. A lesion on gastric mucosa was induced using ethanol. *Anredera cordifolia* extract powder at doses of 250, 500 and 1250 mg mg/kg bw significantly reduced ulcer index (16.0%, 12.6% and 16.2%, respectively) compared to the negative control (31.1%). In histopathological evaluation, ethanol caused moderate to severe/high acute degeneration/necrosis with deep ulceration and haemorrhage on the mucosal layer and submucosal oedema of the stomach. The amelioration of gastric mucosal lesions in histopathological observation was also found in pretreatment of Madeira vine extract powders. The author proposed that *Anredera cordifolia* possessed significant free radical scavenging activity, which could be involved in biological function of gastric mucosa protective activity.

22.5.10 HEPATOPROTECTIVE

Hepatoprotective effect of *Anredera cordifolia* was studied against CCl_4 and D-galactosamine (D-GalN) induced hepatotoxicity in rats. The administration of the brood bud extract (300 mg/kg) was more potent than indomethacin (10 mg/kg). The aqueous extracts were proven to significantly lower the acute increase in serum SGOT and SGPT levels caused by CCl_4 and D-GalN. Histological changes such as necrosis, fatty change, ballooning degeneration, inflammatory infiltration of lymphocytes and Kupffer cells around the central vein (CCl_4-induced hepatotoxicity) and portal vein (D-GalN induced hepatotoxicity) were simultaneously improved by the treatment with aqueous extracts (leaf, stem, brood bud) of *Anredera cordifolia* (Lin et al. 1994).

22.5.11 HYPERTENSION

Garmana et al. (2016) conducted preliminary research to verify the antihypertensive effect of *Anredera cordifolia* leaves. The antihypertensive effect was examined in adrenaline-induced rats to increase the heart rate. Heart rate was measured by non-invasive tail cuff. The diuretic effect was also examined by modified Lipschitz method. Extract was tested at doses of 50, 100 and 200 mg/kg body weight. *Anredera cordifolia* leaf extract of 50 mg/kg bw reduced the heart rate that was induced by adrenaline ($P < 0.05$). It showed a weak diuretic effect compared to furosemide.

Sukandar et al. (2016) performed another study to investigate the vasodilation effect and mechanism of an ethanolic extract of *Anredera cordifolia*, *Sonchus arvensis* L and ursolic acid. Isolated rabbit aortic and frog heart aortic rings were placed in an organ bath and precontracted with norepinephrine (2.9×10^{-3} mM) and potassium chloride (40 μM) before the addition of ethanolic extract of *Anredera cordifolia*, *Sonchus arvensis* L and ursolic acid. The heart of anesthetised frog was exposed and placed in an organ bath to be precontracted by norepinephrine (2.9×10^{-3} mM). The vasodilation response was evaluated in the duration of aortic contraction and the decrease of frequency and amplitude pattern of the frog heart. Ethanolic extract of *Anredera cordifolia* (0.9 mg/mL) produced significant vasodilation of the norepinephrine precontracted rabbit aortic rings ($P < 0.05$), but did not produce vasodilation of potassium chloride precontracted rabbit aortic rings. The vasodilation response to an ethanolic extract of *Anredera cordifolia* may have resulted through NO, because the pretreatment of the isolated rabbit aortic rings with methylene blue inhibited the NO-mediated vasodilation. Moreover, the extract exhibited vasodilation of the frog heart, which appeared to be mediated by inhibition of β1-adrenoreceptor. In addition, the pattern of vasodilation appeared to be similar with vasodilation induced by bisoprolol (2.5). In addition, the ursolic acid compound did not produce any vasodilation effect on the norepinephrine and potassium chloride pre-contracted rabbit aortic rings, but exhibited vasodilation of the frog heart, which have been mediated by β1-adrenoreceptor inhibition.

The previous study was continued by Sukandar et al. (2016) who investigated the vasodilation and the mechanism of action of oleanolic acid and apigenin, secondary metabolites of *Anredera cordifolia*. This study used the same method as the previous study. Oleanolic acid (0.5 μg/mL) produced significant vasodilation of the norepinephrine precontracted rabbit aortic rings ($P < 0.05$) but not with methylene blue followed with norepinephrine. In addition, oleanolic acid did not produce vasodilation in rings precontracted with potassium chloride. Moreover, oleanolic acid exhibited vasodilation in the frog heart. Apigenin (0.05 μg/mL) produced a vasodilation effect on the norepinephrine, methylene blue followed by norepinephrine and potassium chloride precontracted rabbit aortic rings ($P < 0.05$). Moreover, apigenin exhibited vasodilation of the frog heart. The authors concluded that oleanolic acid exhibited vasodilation by facilitating the release of NO and inhibition of $\beta 1$-adrenoreceptors, whereas, the apigenin exhibited a vasodilation effect by facilitating the inhibition of calcium channel and $\beta 1$-adrenoreceptors.

Garmana et al. (2018) published a continuation of their previous research to further prove the antihypertensive effect of *Anredera cordifolia* in dexamethasone-induced hypertensive rat and to determine the release of NO. In this study, ethanol extract of Madeira vine (EEMV), ethyl acetate fraction (EF), and water fraction (WF) could reduce systolic blood pressure at day 14 with a diastolic blood pressure (DBP) reduction of 26.8, 34.1 and 40.5 mmHg, respectively. DBP began to decrease from day 8 in the EEMV group, with a DBP reduction of 24.1 mmHg. In the HF, EF and WF groups, decreases in DBP occurred on day 14, which were 22.0, 24.5 and 35.4 mmHg, respectively. NO level in rat serum was increased significantly at 90 min after administration of EEMV 100 mg/kg bw and WF 40.73 mg/kg bw. Increase in NO levels due to EF administration with a dose of 1.66 mg/kg bw was not significantly different compared to the control group. The mechanism of ethanol extract of Madeira vine leaves and its WF was most likely due to vasodilation effect through the NO-pathway, whereas EF could have other mechanism(s) of action.

22.5.12 HYPERURICAEMIA

A research to investigate the xanthine oxidase (XO) inhibitory activity and the ability to reduce serum uric acid levels of 70% ethanol extracts of *Anredera cordifolia* (ACE) and *Sonchus arvensis* (SAE) leaves, and its combinations was conducted. The anti-hyperuricaemic activity was evaluated *in vivo* on male Wistar rats, which were induced by a high-purine diet and potassium oxonate (PO). The reduction of serum uric acid levels after extract administration was observed and compared to allopurinol. The inhibitory activity of XO was determined by measuring uric acid formation by UV spectrophotometry. The IC_{50} results obtained for ACE, SAE and the combination of both with a ratio of 1:1 were 635.25, 1345.93 and 846.32 µg/mL, respectively. The IC_{50} of allopurinol as reference was 0.88 µg/mL. Results of the anti-hyperuricaemic assay showed that uric acid levels of the group administered with allopurinol, ACE, SAE and the combination of both extracts were significantly lower compared to the positive control group at 120 and 150 minutes after PO induction ($P < 0.05$), but the combination extracts exhibited additive effect in lowering serum uric acid levels (Widyarini et al. 2016). Hendriani et al. (2016) reported the percentages of XO inhibitory activity *in vitro* at the concentration 50, 100 and 200 µg/mL of *Anredera cordifolia* extract were 49.71 ± 12.01, 53.24 ± 8.24, and $66.20 \pm 9.69\%$ respectively, while the IC_{50} value was 66.20 µg/mL.

22.5.13 KIDNEY DISORDER

Another study was conducted to determine the activity of *Anredera cordifolia* leaf extract on renal function improvement in renal failure conditions. A rat model of renal failure was developed by administrating gentamicin 100 mg/kg bw and piroxicam 3.6 mg/kg for 8 days. *Anredera cordifolia* extract at doses 50, 100 and 150 mg/kg bw were given from day 8 for 4 weeks. After four weeks of therapy, *Anredera cordifolia* extract at doses of 50, 100 and 150 mg/kg bw decreased creatinine levels (0.02 ± 0.17, 0.07 ± 0.13 and 0.05 ± 0.12 mg/dL) significantly compared to the positive control group. Urea level also decreased significantly at a dose of 150 mg/kg bw. The same dose also significantly influenced renal index. Histological results in the three test groups also showed improvement in renal cells after administration of the extract. All doses of *Anredera cordifolia* provided improvements to the kidney function (Sukandar et al. 2011).

The previous study was continued by combining *Anredera cordifolia* with *Zea mays* L. hair (corn silk). Rats were divided into the positive control group, the group treated with 75 mg/kg bw of corn silk, the group treated with 100 mg/kg bw of *Anredera cordifolia*, two groups treated with graded doses of a combination of corn silk and *Anredera cordifolia*, and the negative control group. Administration of the extract combination at half dose resulted in marked depletion of serum creatinine and urea, which was comparable to the results in the corn silk and *Anredera cordifolia* treated groups. In addition, the extract combination was shown to reduce the kidney index compared to positive control group. The combination was further revealed to reduce renal damage histologically. Administration of the extract combination was demonstrated to attenuate kidney oxidative stress, as shown by the reduction in lipid peroxidation and the increased activity of antioxidant enzymes, such as catalase and superoxide dismutase (SOD). Taken together, results of this study suggest that corn silk in combination with *Anredera cordifolia* possesses renal function improving activity that is slightly better compared to the activity of each extract alone. The results further indicate that reduction of oxidative stress by each extract as well as their combination might be beneficial for the repair of renal damage (Sukandar et al. 2013).

22.5.14 WEIGHT REDUCTION (ANTI-OBESITY)

Weight reduction may help many conditions because overweight or obesity is one of the health problems that can promote cardiovascular risk diseases such as hypertension, hyperlipidaemia, atherosclerosis and diabetes mellitus. The anti-obesity effect was evaluated on obese rats induced with a high-carbohydrate diet. A high-carbohydrate diet was given *ad libitum* for 30 days to rats in all groups, except to the negative control group. The results showed that ethanol extract of *Anredera cordifolia* leaves at a dose of 100 mg/kg bw had the lowest increment of body weight (59.97 ± 5.63%) among other groups, and it was significantly lower ($P < 0.05$) compared to positive control group (76.11 ± 8.50%). The percentage of the food index and faeces index did not differ significantly among all test groups. The author concluded that ethanol extract of *Anredera cordifolia* leaves at a dose of 100 mg/kg bw showed potential as an anti-obesity agent by inhibiting the increment of the body weight of obese rats induced by a high-carbohydrate diet, without affecting their appetite and bowel movement (Sukandar et al. 2016).

22.5.15 WOUND HEALING

Wound healing was one of the most widespread traditional uses of *Anredera cordifolia*, so numerous studies had investigated this claim. Yuniarti and Lukiswanto (2017) conducted a study to evaluate the ability of *Anredera cordifolia* to heal burn injuries with an animal model. In this research, there were four treatment groups: G0 (sulfadiazine), G1 (2.5% extract of *Anredera cordifolia*), G2 (5% extract of *Anredera cordifolia*), and G3 (10% extract of *Anredera cordifolia*), which were given skin burns using hot metal plates. Each treatment was given topically 3 times a day for 14 days. Microscopic observation of the wound healing process on the collagen deposition, polymorphonuclear infiltration, angiogenesis and fibrosis showed that G2 had a significantly better healing result compared to the rest of the groups ($P < 0.05$), while group G0 was significantly better than G1 and G3 ($P < 0.05$). A study by Sumartiningsih (2011) also showed a similar result, but for a blunt trauma injury (haematoma). Nevertheless, the administration of *Anredera cordifolia* for 3 days resulted in a significant drop of 5% in cell inflammation and a 2% increase of fibroblast (cell membrane) count. Ethanol extract of *Anredera cordifolia* alone and in combination with *Centella asiatica* extract induced the proliferation of fibroblast cell line 3T3/NIH. The combination consisted of 100 µg/mL of *Anredera cordifolia* extract and 100 µg/mL *Centella asiatica* extract showed a better result in inducing cell proliferation compared to the reference drug SanoSkin® Melladerm® with the same concentration (Sutrisno 2017).

Various components may be responsible for the wound healing ability of *Anredera cordifolia*. Saponin is thought to influence the activity and synthesis of TGF-β1 and modifications of the receptors TGF-β1 and TGF-β2 in fibroblasts. Saponins play a role as agents for angiogenesis by regulating VEGF that increases the mitogenic activity of endothelial cells in the formation of blood vessels during the proliferative phase. Tannins and alkaloids have shown antioxidants and antimicrobial activities that help the wound healing process by keeping the wound area from free radicals and pathogenic bacteria. Lastly, flavonoids have potential for their antioxidant, antibacterial, anti-ageing, antileukemic and vasodilator activity (Hanafiah et al. 2017).

22.6 SAFETY

Anredera cordifolia extract was very well tolerated. No mortality was observed at the single administration in acute toxicity study even at the highest dose of 15 g/kg bw. In sub chronic toxicity study, *Anredera cordifolia* ethanol extract up to dose of 1 g/kg bw did not cause mortality and behavioural changes. There were no significantly differences in body weight development, relative organ weight, haematology or blood biochemistry in rats treated by *Anredera cordifolia* extract compared with control group ($P > 0.05$). Histology observations also showed that heart, lung, liver, kidney and spleen had no difference with the control group (Salasanti et al. 2014). Ethanolic extract of *Anredera cordifolia* at doses of 100, 400 and 1000 mg/kg bw in rat did not show any teratogenic effect (Sukandar et al. 2014). To date, a chronic toxicity study of *Anredera cordifolia* has not yet been conducted.

22.7 ECONOMIC ASPECT

Anredera cordifolia is not an expensive medicine. As mentioned, the plant is considered problematic in some countries because of its invasiveness. Personally, we believe this characteristic is a blessing in disguise for the development of *Anredera cordifolia* as an herbal medicine. This plant is very easy to cultivate and grows rapidly in various climates, showing a prospect to be mass produced with low cost.

The dried leaves can be bought for 50,000–150,000 IDR (US$3.50–$10.50) per kg in Indonesia. The yield of ethanol extract varied between 15%–20% of dried leaves. *Anredera cordifolia* was commonly marketed in dried extract form, which was formulated into a capsule in Indonesia. The capsule was mostly packed into a bottle contained 30–120 capsules for a certain duration of treatment, usually from 2 weeks to 2 months, depends on the posology. The price varied considerably, because Indonesia has divided the herbal medicine into three categories. The first is *jamu*, an herbal medicine with its efficacy claimed empirically; the second is a *standardised herbal medicine* with its efficacy claim proven in preclinical study and its raw material standardised; and the third is *fitofarmaka*, the efficacy of which is proven by clinical study. *Jamu* is considered cheapest because it does not need to fund any scientific research, but it still lacks the backing of efficacy and safety data to convince the populace.

Policies about herbal medicines differ in each country, but some aspects remain the same. *Anredera cordifolia* has clearly shown multiple pharmacological activities in preclinical study. The road to develop this herbal medicine may be taxing, but it is worth being developed commercially.

22.8 FUTURE PROSPECT

Anredera cordifolia has many pharmacological activities which had been proven in preclinical trials as mentioned earlier in this paper. Although limited in number, some studies have also evaluated the pharmacological properties in combination with another medicinal plant. Future research may progress on the combination of *Anredera cordifolia* with other plants. Future research should also consider *Anredera cordifolia* not only as an alternative medicine, but how it may work as a complementary medicine with conventional drugs. Research may progress by combining *Anredera cordifolia* with conventional drugs to enhance the existent pharmacological activities, and this may help in cases such as drug resistance.

Anredera cordifolia has shown polypharmacological activities in preclinical study. This aspect gives a new possibility to advance research by using *Anredera cordifolia* alone to treat several diseases simultaneously. Furthermore, *Anredera cordifolia* contains several active compounds, and preclinical trials have shown that some of these can be isolated and then developed into new medicine. Ultimately, future research should be extended to clinical studies of *Anredera cordifolia*.

REFERENCES

Abou-Zeid, A. H. S., Soliman, F. M., Sleem, A. A. and Mitry, M. N. R. (2007). Phytochemical and bio-activity investigations of the aerial parts of *Anredera cordifolia* (Ten.) v. Steenis. *Bulletin of the National Research Centre (Cairo)*, **32**(1), 1–33.

Astuti, S. M., Sakinah, M., Andayani, R. and Awalluddin, R. (2011). Determination of saponin compound from *Anredera cordifolia* (Ten) v. Steenis plant (binahong) to potential treatment for several diseases. *Journal of Agricultural Science*, **3**(4), 224–232. doi:10.5539/jas.v3n4p224

Ayuningtyas, D. K. (2016). In vitro *antituberculosis activity of selected medicinal plants as a complementary therapy in inhibiting susceptible and multi-drug resistant* Mycobacterium tuberculosis. Bandung, Indonesia: Bandung Institute of Technology.

Balch, P. A. (2012). *Prescription for Herbal Healing*. Penguin: New York.

Boyne, R.L., Osunkoya, O.O. and Scharaschkin, T. (2013). Variation in leaf structure of the invasive Madeira vine (*Anredera cordifolia*, *Basellaceae*) at different light levels. *Australian Journal of Botany*, **61**(5), 412–417.

Cagnotti, C., Mc Kay, F. and Gandolfo, D. (2007). Biology and host specificity of *Plectonycha correntina lacordaire* (Chrysomelidae), a candidate for the biological control of *Anredera cordifolia* (tenore) v. Steenis (Basellaceae). *African Entomology*, **15**(2), 300–309. doi:10.4001/1021-3589-15.2.300

Chao, P.Y., Lin, S., Lin, K., Liu, Y., Hsu, J., Yang, C. M. and Lai, J. (2014). Antioxidant activity in extracts of 27 indigenous Taiwanese vegetables. *Nutrients*, **6**(5), 2115–2130. doi:10.3390/nu6052115

Chuang, M. T., Lin, Y. S. and Hou, W. C. (2007). Ancordin, the major rhizome protein of Madeira-vine, with trypsin inhibitory and stimulatory activities in nitric oxide productions. *Peptides*, **28**(6), 1311–1316. doi:10.1016/j.peptides.2007.04.011

Churiyah, T. and Wijaya, F. A. (2011). Preliminary cytotoxic activity of ethanolic *Anredera cordifolia* (Ten.) v. Steenis leaf extracts with different concentrations of ethanol. In *Proceedings of the 2nd International Symposium on Temulawak and the 40th Meeting of National Working Group on Indonesia Medicinal Plant*. Bogor, Indonesia: Institute of Research and Community Services, Bogor Agricultural University. pp. 375–378.

Djamil, R., Wahyudi, P. S., Wahono, S. and Hanafi, M. (2012). Antioxidant activity of flavonoid from *Anredera cordifolia* (Ten) v. Steenis leaves. *International Research Journal of Pharmacy*, **3**(9), 241–243.

Djamil, R., Winarti, W., Zaidan, S. and Syamsudin, A. (2017). Antidiabetic activity of flavonoid from binahong leaves (*Anredera cordifolia*) extract in alloxan induced mice. *Journal of Pharmacognosy & Natural Products*, **3**(2), 2–5. doi:10.4172/2472-0992.1000139

Elya, B., Handayani, R., Sauriasari, R., Azizahwati, Hasyyati, U. S., Permana, I. T. and Permatasari, Y. I. (2015). Antidiabetic activity and phytochemical screening of extracts from Indonesian plants by inhibition of alpha amylase, alpha glucosidase and dipeptidyl peptidase IV. *Pakistan Journal of Biological Sciences*, **18**(6), 273–278. doi:10.3923/pjbs.2015.279.284

Eriksson, R. (2007). A synopsis of Basellaceae. *Kew Bulletin*, **62**(2), 297–320.

Espada, A., Riguera, R. and Jiménez, C. (1997). Boussingoside E: a new triterpenoid saponin from the tubers of *Boussingaultia baselloides*. *Journal of Natural Products*, **60**(1), 17–19. doi:10.1021/np960392g

Espada, A., Rodriguez, J., Villaverde, M. C. and Riguera, R. (1990). Hypoglucaemic triterpenoid saponins from *Boussingaultia baselloides*. *Canadian Journal of Chemistry*, **68**(11), 2039–2044. doi:10.1139/v90-312.

Garmana, A. N., Sukandar, E. Y. and Fidrianny, I. (2014). Activity of several plant extracts against drug-sensitive and drug-resistant microbes. *Procedia Chemistry*, **13**, 164–169. doi:10.1016/j.proche.2014.12.021

Garmana, A. N., Sukandar, E. Y. and Fidrianny, I. (2016). Preliminary study of blood pressure lowering effect of *Anredera cordifolia* (Ten.) v. Steenis on Wistar rats. *International Journal of Pharmacognosy and Phytochemical Research*, **8**(2), 300–304.

Garmana, A. N., Sukandar, E. Y. and Fidrianny, I. (2018). Antihypertension study of *Anredera cordifolia* (Ten). v. Steenis extract and its fractions in rats through dexamethasone induction and nitric oxide release. *Asian Journal of Pharmaceutical and Clinical Research*, **11**(1), 278–282.

Hanafiah, O. A., Hanafiah, D. S., Bayu, E. S., Abidin, T., Ilyas, S., Nainggolan, M. and Syamsudin, E. (2017). Quantity differences of secondary metabolites (saponins, tannins, and flavonoids) from binahong plant extract (*Anredera cordifolia* (Ten.) v. Steenis) treated and untreated with colchicines that play a role in wound healing. *World Journal of Dentistry*, **8**(4), 296–299.

Hariana, A. (2013). *262 Tumbuhan Obat Dan Khasiatnya*. Penebar Swadaya Grup.

Heisler, E. V., Badke, M. R., Andrade, A. and Rodrigues, M. G. S. (2012). Popular knowledge about the use of plant *Anredera cordifolia* (fat leaf) [Saber popular sobre a utilização da planta *Anredera cordifolia* (folha gorda)]. *Florianopolis*, **21** (4), 937–944.

Hendriani, R., Sukandar, E. Y., Anggadiredja, K. and Sukrasno. (2016). In vitro evaluation of xanthine oxidase inhibitory activity of selected medicinal plants. *International Journal of Pharmaceutical and Clinical Research*, **8**(4), 235–238.

Hidayat, S.R. and Napitupulu, R.M. (2015). *Kitab Tumbuhan Obat*. Cibubur, Jakarta, Indonesia: AgriFlo.

Hilgert, N. I. (2001). Plants used in home medicine in the Zenta River Basin, Northwest Argentina. *Journal of Ethnopharmacology*, **76**(1), 11–34. doi:10.1016/S0378-8741(01)00190-8

Horng, C. T., Chao, H., Lee, C., Hsueh, C. and Chen, F. (2012). Gastro protective effect of Madeira vine against ethanol-induced gastric mucosal lesion in rat. *Asian Journal of Chemistry*, **24**, 765–768.

Jiménez-Arellanes, A., Luna-Herrera, J., Cornejo-Garrido, J., López-García, S., Castro-Mussot, M., Meckes-Fischer, M., Mata-Espinosa, D., Marquina, B., Torres, J. and Hernández Pando, R. (2013). Ursolic and oleanolic acids as antimicrobial and immunomodulatory compounds for tuberculosis treatment. *BMC Complementary and Alternative Medicine*, **13**, 258.

Laksmitawati, D. R., Widyastuti, A., Karami, N., Afifah, E., Rihibiha, D. D., Nufus, H. and Widowati, W. (2017). Anti-inflammatory effects of *Anredera cordifolia* and *Piper crocatum* extracts on lipopolysaccharide-stimulated macrophage cell line. *Bangladesh Journal of Pharmacology*, **12**(1), 35–40. doi:10.3329/bjp.v12i1.28714

Leliqia, N. P. E., Sukandar, E. Y. and Fidrianny, I. (2017a). Antibacterial activities of *Anredera cordifolia* (Ten.) v. Steenis leaves extracts and fractions. *Asian Journal of Pharmaceutical and Clinical Research*, **10**(12), 10–13.

Leliqia, N. P. E., Sukandar, E. Y. and Fidrianny, I. (2017b). Overview of efficacy, safety and phytochemical study of *Anredera cordifolia* (Ten.) v. Steenis. *Pharmacology Online*, **1**, 124–131.

Lestari, D., Sukandar, E. Y. and Fidrianny, I. (2015). *Anredera cordifolia* leaves extract as antihyperlipidemia and endothelial fat content reducer in male Wistar rat. *International Journal of Pharmaceutical and Clinical Research*, **7**(6), 435–439. doi:10.22159/ajpcr.2016.v9i6.13628

Lestari, D., Sukandar, E. Y. and Fidrianny, I. (2016). *Anredera cordifolia* leaves fraction as an antihyperlipidemia. *Asian Journal of Pharmaceutical and Clinical Research*, **9**(6), 6–8. doi:10.22159/ajpcr.2016.v9i6.13628

Lestari, D., Sukandar, E. Y. and Fidrianny, I. (2017). In silico study of apigenin and apigetrin as inhibitor of 3-hydroxy-3-methyl-glutayl-coenzyme a reductase. *Asian Journal of Pharmaceutical and Clinical Research*, **10**(11), 11–14.

Lin, C. C., Sung, T. C. and Yen, M. H. (1994). The antiinflammatory and liver protective effects of *Boussingaultia gracilis* var. pseudobaselloides extract in rats. *Phytotherapy Research*, **8**(4), 201–207. doi:10.1002/ptr.2650080403

Lin, H. Y., Kuo, S. C., Chao, P. D. L. and Lin, T. D. (1988). A new sapogenin from *Boussingaultia gracilis*. *Journal of Natural Products*, **51**(4), 797–798. doi:10.1021/np50058a028

Mulaudzi, R. B., Ndhlala, A. R. and Van Staden, J. (2015). Ethnopharmacological evaluation of a traditional herbal remedy used to treat gonorrhoea in Limpopo Province, South Africa. *South African Journal of Botany*, **97**, 117–122. doi:10.1016/j.sajb.2014.12.007

Mulia, K., Muhammad, F. and Krisanti, E. (2017). Extraction of vitexin from binahong (*Anredera cordifolia* (Ten.) v. Steenis) leaves using betaine: 1,4 Butanediol Natural Deep Eutectic Solvent (NADES). *AIP Conference Proceedings*, 1823. doi:10.1063/1.4978091.

Panyaphu, K., Van On, T., Sirisa-Ard, P., Srisa-Nga, P., Chansakaow, S. and Nathakarnkitkul, S.(2011). Medicinal plants of the Mien (Yao) in Northern Thailand and their potential value in the primary healthcare of postpartum women. *Journal of Ethnopharmacology*, **135**(2), 226–237. doi:10.1016/j.jep.2011.03.050

Paz, E. A., Cerdeíras, M. P., Fernández, J., Ferreira, F., Moyna, P., Soubes, M., Vázquez, A., Vero, S. and Bassagoda, M. J. (1996). Screening of Uruguayan medicinal plants for antimicrobial activity. Part II. *Journal of Ethnopharmacology*, **53**(2), 111–115. doi:10.1016/0378-8741(96)01428-6

Pitaloka, D. A. E., and Sukandar, E. Y. (2017). In vitro study of ursolic acid combination first-line antituberculosis drugs against drug-sensitive and drug-resistant strains of Mycobacterium tuberculosis. *Asian Journal of Pharmaceutical and Clinical Research*, **10**(4), 8–10. doi:10.22159/ajpcr.2017.v10i4.16582

Qiong, G., Ma, Y., Zhang, X., Wang, R., Zhou, J., Zheng, Y. T. and Chen, J. (2007). One new flavanoid and anti-HIV active constituents from *Boussingaultia gracilis* Miers var. Pseudobaselloides Bailey. *Chemical Journal of Chinese Universities (Chinese)*, **28**, 1508–1511.

Salasanti, C. D., Sukandar, E. Y. and Fidrianny, I. (2014). Acute and sub chronic toxicity study of ethanol extract of *Anredera cordifolia* (Ten.) v. Steenis leaves. *International Journal of Pharmacy and Pharmaceutical Sciences*, **6**(5), 348–352.

Savitri, A. (2015). *Tanaman Ajaib! Basmi Penyakit Dengan TOGA (Tanaman Obat Keluarga)*. Bibit Publisher.

Sperling, C.R. and Bittrich, V. (1993). Basellaceae. In K. Kubitzki, J. G. Rower and V. Bittrich, eds., *Flowering Plants: Dicotyledons*. New York: Springer. pp. 143–146.

Sukandar, E. Y., Fidrianny, I. and Adiwibowo, L. F. (2011a). Efficacy of ethanol extract of *Anredera cordifolia* (Ten.) v. Steenis leaves on improving kidney failure in rats. *International Journal of Pharmacology*, **7**(8), 850–855. doi:10.3923/ijp.2011.850-855

Sukandar, E. Y., Fidrianny, I., Nofianti, T. and Safitri, D. (2016a). Subchronic toxicity study of corn silk (*Zea mays* L.) in combination with binahong (*Anredera cordifolia* (Ten.) v. Steenis) leaves on Wistar rats. *Asian Journal of Pharmaceutical and Clinical Research*, **9**(1), 274–278.

Sukandar, E. Y., Kurniati, N. F. and Nurdianti, A.F. (2016b). Antiobesity effect of ethanol extract of *Anredera cordifolia* (Ten) v. Steenis leaves on obese male Wistar rats induced by high-carbohydrate diet. *International Journal of Pharmacy and Pharmaceutical Sciences*, **8**(4), 171–173.

Sukandar, E. Y., Qowiyyah, A. and Larasari, L. (2011b). Efek ekstrak metanol daun binahong (*Anredera cordifoolia* (Ten.) v. Steenis) terhadap gula darah pada mencit model diabetes melitus. *Jurnal Medika Planta*, **1**(4), 1–10.

Sukandar, E. Y., Ridwan, A. and Sukmawan, Y. P. (2016c). Vasodilation effect of oleanolic acid and apigenin as a metabolite compound of *Anredera cordifolia* (Ten.) v. Steenis on isolated rabbit aortic and frog heart. *International Journal of Research in Ayurveda & Pharmacy*, **7**(5), 82–84. doi:10.7897/2277-4343.075200

Sukandar, E. Y., Sigit, J. I. and Adiwibowo, L. F. (2013). Study of kidney repair mechanisms of corn silk (*Zea mays* L. hair)-binahong (*Anredera cordifolia* (Ten.) v. Steenis) leaves combination in rat model of kidney failure. *International Journal of Pharmacology*, **9**(1), 12–23. doi:10.3923/ijp.2013.12.23

Sukandar, E.Y., Safitri, D. and Aini, N. N. (2016d). The study of ethanolic extract of binahong leaves (*Anredera cordifolia* (Ten.) v. Steenis) and mulberry leaves (*Morus nigra* L.) in combination on hyperlipidemic induced rats. *Asian Journal of Pharmaceutical and Clinical Research*, **9**(6), 288. doi:10.22159/ajpcr.2016.v9i6.14412

Sukrasno. (2014). Changes in secondary metabolite contents following crude drug preparation. *Procedia Chemistry*, **13**, 57–62. doi:10.1016/j.proche.2014.12.006

Sulistiyani, D. A. and Ariyani, R. (2011). Extract of lempuyang gajah (*Zingiber zerumbet* L.) tea infusion reduced blood cholesterol. In *Proceedings of the 2nd International Symposium on Temulawak and the 40th Meeting of National Working Group on Indonesia Medicinal Plant*. Bogor, Indonesia: Institute of Research and Community Services, Bogor Agricultural University. pp. 267–270.

Sumartiningsih, S. (2011). The effect of binahong to hematoma. *World Academia of Science, Engineering and Technology*, **78**(6), 743–745.

Sutrisno, E. (2017). *Wound healing in vivo and in vitro study of binahong (Anredera cordifolia (Ten.) v. Steenis) leaves and pegagan (Centella Asiatica (L.) Urban) herbs ethanolic extract*. Bandung, Indonesia: Bandung Institute of Technology.

Sutrisno, E., Adnyana, I. K., Sukandar, E. Y. Fidrianny, I. and Aligita, W. (2016). Anti-inflammatory study of *Anredera cordifolia* leaves and *Centella asiatica* herbs and its combinations using human red blood cell-membrane stabilization method. *Asian Journal of Pharmaceutical and Clinical Research*, **9**(5), 78. doi:10.22159/ajpcr.2016.v9i5.11973

Tasi, Y., Chin, T., Chen, Y., Huang, C. and Lee, S. (2015). Potential natural products for Alzheimer's disease: Targeted search using the internal ribosome entry site of tau and amyloid-β precursor protein. *International Journal of Molecular Sciences*, **16**, 8789–8810. doi:10.3390/ijms16048789

Tshikalange, T. E., Meyer, J. J. M. and Hussein, A. A. (2005). Antimicrobial activity, toxicity and the isolation of a bioactive compound from plants used to treat sexually transmitted diseases. *Journal of Ethnopharmacology*, **96**(3), 515–519. doi:10.1016/j.jep.2004.09.057

Vane, J. R. and Botting, R. M. (1997. Mechanism of action of aspirin-like drugs. *Seminars in Arthritis and Rheumatism*, **26**(6 Suppl 1), 2–10. doi:10.1016/S0049-0172(97)80046-7

Vivian-Smith, G., Lawson, B. E., Turnbull, I. and Paul, O. D. (2007). The biology of Australian weeds 46. *Plant Protection Quarterly*, **22**(1), 2–10.

Wagner, W. L., Herbst, D. R. and Sohmer, S. H. (1999). *Manual of the flowering plants of Hawai'i, Vol 1 and 2*. Honolulu, HI: University of Hawai'i and Bishop Museum Press.

Wijayanti, D., Setiatin, E. T. and Kurnianto, E. (2017). Study on postpartum estrus of guinea pigs (*Cavia cobaya*) using *Anredera cordifolia* leaf extract. *Veterinary World*, **10**(4), 375–379. doi:10.14202/vetworld.2017.375-379.

Yuliani, S. H., Anggraeni, C. D., Sekarjati, W., Panjalu, A., Istyastono, E. P. and Setiawati, A. (2015). Cytotoxic activity of *Anredera cordifolia* leaf extract on HeLa cervical cancer cells through p53-independent pathway. *Asian Journal of Pharmaceutical and Clinical Research*, **8**(2), 328–331.

Yuniarti, W. M. and Lukiswanto, B. S. (2017). Effects of herbal ointment containing the leaf extracts of Madeira vine (*Anredera cordifolia* (Ten.) v. Steenis) for burn wound healing process on albino rats. *Veterinary World*, **10**(7), 808–813. doi:10.14202/vetworld.2017.808-813.

Yuziani, Harahap, U. and Karsono. (2014). Evaluation of analgesic activities of ethanolic extract of *Anredera cordifolia* (Ten.) v. Steenis leaf. *International Journal of PharmTech Research*, **6**(5), 1608–1610.

Zhang, Z., Shen, C., Gao, F., Wei, H., Ren, D. and Lu, J. (2017). Isolation, purification and structural characterization of two novel water-soluble polysaccharides from *Anredera cordifolia*. *Molecules*, **22**(8), 1276.

Zhou, J., Xie, G. and Xiajian, Y. (2011). *Encyclopedia of traditional Chinese medicines: Volume 5 Isolated compounds (T-Z) references TCM plants and congeners*. New York: Springer.

23 Medicinal Properties of Ginger (*Zingiber officinale* Roscoe)

Jamuna Prakash

CONTENTS

23.1 INTRODUCTION

Health and nutrition are inherently linked with longevity and diseases. While good eating habits can take care of the nutritional needs of the body, the phytochemical constituents of foods can delay the process of ageing and prevent diseases. The role of diet is now being considered beyond providing basic nutrients to protect the body from diseases. The dietary patterns of human beings have gradually evolved over the years from what was grown and available locally to a much more diverse form where ingredients or prepared foods could be outsourced from any corner of the world. New ingredients or new foods have been introduced into diets. Trade and transport between nations have made many ingredients available on the market shelf all around. Traditionally, the use of spices was more or less restricted to the places where they were grown, mostly tropical and Asian countries, but spices are now used worldwide on account of their easy availability.

The science of nutrition progressed from the discovery of nutrients and the study of their functions, metabolism, requirements and recommendations. However, there were far more functions of foods observed than could be accounted for by the presence of known nutrients. These were mainly related to disease prevention or healing properties of foods and the components responsible for these. These properties were also being used traditionally in many ethnic populations. Considerable data has been collected regarding the composition and health benefits of all classes of foods, starting from whole grains, fruits and vegetables, to herbs, spices and condiments. Among these, ginger is a widely grown and used spice both in fresh and dry form for cooking as well as for medicinal purposes. This chapter deals briefly with the nutritional and medicinal properties of ginger.

23.2 HISTORY OF USE

Spices and condiments are wonder ingredients used for imparting a specific desirable flavour to dishes. A characteristic feature of spices is the small amount used for generating a delectable aroma. Spices are also used for their medicinal quality and cosmetic purposes, and many of them find mention in traditional documents. The use of ginger is documented in the ancient civilisations of India and China. Many travellers from European countries have mentioned abundant cultivation and use of ginger and other spices in India and Sri Lanka (Achaya 1994). It is possible that its use was prevalent much earlier than documented history. Through travel and trade, as the opportunity arose, ginger spread to other regions of world and today its cultivation is widespread in tropical countries.

The ginger plant has a long history of cultivation known to originate in China and then spread to India, South East Asia, West Africa and the Caribbean (Weiss 1997; McGee 2004). The use of ginger in traditional medicine has been recorded in many documents. Ginger figures in ancient Indian scripts as *ardraka*, and in *Atharvaveda* it is referred to as *adara* (Prakash 1961). In Ayurvedic texts, dry ginger is considered as pungent and hot in potency and bitter in taste. Ginger treats vitiations of *kapha* and oedema, *vata*, colicky pain, constipation, abdominal disorders, flatulence, dyspnoea and *slipada* (Raghunathasuri 2012); *kapha* and *vata* are humoral imbalance of the body, whereas *slipada* can be associated with elephantiasis. In traditional Chinese medicine, ginger is used as a supportive remedy for spleen, stomach, and kidney disorders. In Arabic medicine, it is said to be warm and has a softening effect on the belly, it is beneficial to the body against digestive ailments such as flatulence, food toxins and constipation (Perez 2005). Ginger also has antiemetic activity and is used to prevent motion sickness, as a digestive aid and also a food preservative (Vishwakarma et al. 2002; Sontakke et al. 2003; Manusirivithaya et al. 2004). The use of ginger has also been mentioned in Western medicine. It has been used as such or as an ingredient in a specific herbal formula and also consumed as a corrective remedy against the unwanted effects of other plants (Perez 2005). In Nigeria, ginger is used to flavour a local drink called *Kunnu*. It is also an important ingredient of many herbal formulations. Its properties are listed as carminative, pungent and stimulant, and it is consumed widely for indigestion, stomach upset, malaria and fevers. Its traditional medicinal uses are also listed for abdominal pain, chest congestion, chronic bronchitis, colic and vomiting (Jatoi et al. 2007).

During the last 5 decades, many scientific studies on ginger have emerged examining its physiological effects using either animal models or human subjects. Medically, ginger is used as a stimulant and carminative and is used frequently for dyspepsia and colic. It has a sialagogue action, stimulating the production of saliva. It is also used to disguise the taste of medicines. Ginger promotes the release of bile from the gallbladder. Ginger may also decrease joint pain from arthritis, may have blood thinning and cholesterol lowering properties and may be useful for the treatment of heart diseases and lungs diseases (Kato et al. 1993; O'Hara et al. 1998; Kuschener and Stark 2003). Ginger has been found effective by multiple studies for treating nausea caused by seasickness, morning sickness and chemotherapy (Ernst and Pittler 2000). Ginger has been reported to be effective for the treatment of inflammation, rheumatism, cold, heat cramps and diabetes (Al-Amin et al. 2006; Afshari et al. 2007).

The culinary uses of ginger vary according to geographical region. It is primarily used as a spice both for its pungent strong taste and for its powerful sweet aroma. It is used in curry powders, in fresh gravies, and as an ingredient in many dishes – beverages, soups, chutneys, pickles and preserves. It is used for baked products too. When the plant matures, the taste and pungency of ginger increases; young rhizomes are juicy and fleshy with a mild taste, while juice from old rhizomes are extremely potent and sharp and is often used as a spice in oriental cuisines (Burdock 1996). Ginger can also be made into a candy, which is a very popular preserve.

Mature ginger roots are fibrous and nearly dry. They can be cooked as an ingredient in many dishes. They can be stewed in boiling water to make ginger tea, to which honey is often added as a sweetener; sliced orange or lemon fruit may also be added. The juice of ginger roots is extremely potent and is often used as a spice to flavour dishes such as seafood, mutton, snacks or stew. Powdered dry ginger root (ginger powder) is typically used to add spiciness to ginger bread and other recipes. Ginger is also made into candy and used as flavouring for cookies, crackers and cakes as well as flavour in ginger ale (a sweet, carbonated, non-alcoholic beverage), gingerbread, ginger snaps, ginger cake and ginger biscuits (McGee 2004).

23.3 PRODUCTION OF GINGER

Ginger (*Zingiber officinale* Roscoe), belonging to the family Zingiberaceae, is used as a spice the world over in fresh and dry form. The world production of ginger was 3,270,762 tonnes in the year 2016; the major producing countries are listed in Table 23.1.

Ginger is a perennial herb with thick tuberous rhizomes. Only the rhizome or the root part of the plant is used for cooking. Ginger is described as a herbaceous rhizomatous perennial, which can reach up to 90 cm in height and has purple flowers. Rhizomes of ginger plant vary from pale yellowish to brown in colour, they are thick lobed, with a strong aromatic sweet and warm odour. Leaves are long, narrow, oblong and lanceolate, 2–3 cm in width with sheathing bases, the blade gradually tapering to a point. They are arranged in simple alternate distichous manner along the stem. During the growing process, the herb develops several lateral shoots in clumps, which start drying when the plant matures. Inflorescence is solitary, lateral radical pedunculate with oblong cylindrical points. Flowers are rare, smaller in size, calyx superior, gamosepalous, three toothed open splitting on one side, corolla on the subequal to lanceolate connate greenish segments (Kawai et al. 1994; Burdock 1996).

TABLE 23.1

Major Ginger-Producing Countries of the World

Sl. No.	Country	Production (tonnes)
1	India	1,109,000
2	Nigeria	522,964
3	China, mainland	492,905
4	Indonesia	340,341
5	Nepal	271,863
6	Thailand	164,266
7	Cameroon	79,273
8	Bangladesh	77,290
9	Japan	62,244
10	Mali	38,589
11	Philippines	26,787
12	Sri Lanka	15,588
13	Malaysia	13,362
14	Ethiopia	10,892
15	Bhutan	10,182

Source: FAO, Ginger production, Food and Agriculture Data, Downloaded from www.Fao.org/Faostat/en, 2017.

23.4 NUTRITIONAL AND CHEMICAL COMPOSITION

Being a spice with a pungent flavour, ginger is used in small amounts for cooking and does not contribute immensely to the nutritional content of diets as such. Nevertheless, its regular use cannot be ignored for smaller nutrient contribution, as it does add important minerals, protein, fat and dietary fibre to diet. The nutritional composition of raw and dry ginger has been reported by many authors and some values are presented in the tables below.

The proximate composition of fresh ginger reported by different workers is compiled in Table 23.2. Fresh ginger is mostly used as an ingredient in many dishes. It has a fair amount of protein and fat. Comparatively, it also has high fibre content, though that will depend on the stage of maturity, as the tender rhizomes have lower amounts of fibre. Longvah et al. (2017) reported the content of insoluble and soluble dietary fibre in fresh ginger as 4.28 and 1.08 g/100 g, respectively. Dry ginger has a higher content of all relative constituents as it becomes concentrated upon drying (Table 23.3). Traditionally, ginger is dried in the shade, although technologies for mechanical drying are also available. Dry rhizomes have a considerable amount of protein, ranging from 5.28 to12.05 g/100 g, and fat, ranging from 1.4 to 17.11 g/100 g. The ash content is also higher, indicating it can be a rich source of minerals. Similarly, the dry rhizome is also rich in fibre on account of its cellulosic components.

TABLE 23.2
Proximate Composition of Raw Ginger

Constituent (g/100g)	References[a]				
	(1)	(2)	(3)	(4)	(5)
Moisture	73.8	70.1	88.5	76.86	81.27
Protein	4.3	3.06	1.2	8.75	2.22
Fat	2.1	7.85	0.2	5.62	0.85
Ash	1.3	1.81	1.5	2.54	1.33
Crude/Dietary fibre	1.6	9.0	1.1	2.93	5.36
Carbohydrate	16.7	8.18	7.6	–	8.97

[a] (1) Ajayi et al. (2017); (2) Agu et al. (2016); (3) El-Ghorab et al. (2010); (4) Odebunmi et al. (2010); (5) Longvah et al. (2017).

TABLE 23.3
Proximate Composition of Dry Ginger

Constituent (g/100g)	References[a]							
	(1)	(2)	(3)	(4)		(5)	(6)	(7)
Moisture	6.32	7.29	6.37	3.95	4.63	6.67	10.0	15.2
Protein	5.45	5.28	8.58	12.05	11.65	8.58	7.20	5.09
Fat	6.48	5.54	5.35	17.11	9.89	5.53	1.40	3.72
Ash	6.57	5.97	6.30	4.95	7.45	6.40	6.10	3.85
Crude/Dietary fibre	10.36	9.74	3.25	21.9	8.30	–	8.20	49.0[b]
Carbohydrate	64.82	66.26	68.15	39.70	58.21	72.84	67.0	38.35

[a] (1) Ogbuewu et al. (2014); (2) Adanlawo and Dairo (2007); (3) Otunola et al. (2010); (4) Ajayi et al. (2013); (5) Nwinuka et al. (2005); (6) El-Ghorab et al. (2010); (7) Pilerood and Prakash (2010).
[b] Insoluble fibre, 23.50 and soluble fibre 25.50 g/100 g.

TABLE 23.4
Mineral Composition of Dry Ginger

Mineral (µg/g)	References[a]					
	(1)	**(2)**	**(3)**	**(4)**		**(5)**
Zinc	4.19	4.06	0.4	4.0	3.0	9.2
Manganese	18.90	19.60	0.02	3.0	7.0	91.3
Copper	0.86	0.76	0.01	1.0	1.0	5.45
Calcium	34.55	35.66	250.8	68.0	41.0	884.0
Phosphorus	26.70	25.70	125.6	42.0	47.0	1740.0
Iron	1.59	1.44	34.6	29.0	14.0	80.0
Sodium	38.96	40.96	50.0	26.0	39.0	–
Potassium	36.34	37.34	215.0	98.0	138.0	–

[a] (1) Ogbuewu et al. (2014); (2) Adanlawo and Dairo (2007); (3) Otunola et al. (2010); (4) Ajayi et al. (2013); (5) Pilerood and Prakash (2010).

The wide range of difference seen in values reported by different workers are mostly due to different cultivars used for analysis, as well as the stage of maturity of the rhizome. The tender rhizomes have more moisture and less of other constituents, and as it matures, the moisture decreases, while the other nutrients and fibre increase.

The mineral content of dry ginger compiled in Table 23.4 shows a very large variation between different studies. This could be attributed to the growing area, as soil conditions are specifically known to affect the mineral concentrations of crop. However, further studies would be required to confirm the concentrations of minerals in ginger due to large variations observed. Apart from these, the presence of carotenoids (79 mg/100 g) and phenolic substances (840 mg/100 g) – which have antioxidant function – has also been reported in ginger (Pilerood and Prakash 2010).

The characteristic pungent flavour of ginger is attributed to certain non-volatile phenylpropanoid derived compounds, gingerols and shogaols. Zingerone is formed from gingerols, has a less pungent flavour and can be detected when ginger is cooked. Ginger contains up to 3% of an essential oil that is responsible for the fragrance of the spice. The main constituents are sesquiterpenoids with (-)-zingiberene as the main component. Other components include β-sesquiphellandrene bisabolene and farnesene, which are also sesquiterpenoids, β-sesquiphellandrene, cineol and citral (O'Hara et al. 1998). The major pungent principle of ginger – identified as 6-gingerol (1-[4′-hydroxy-3′-methoxyphenyl]-5-hydroxy-3-decanone) – has been shown to have antioxidant, anti-inflammatory and anti-tumour promoting function (Surh et al. 1998; Bode et al. 2001; Jagtap et al. 2009). Ginger oil has been associated with the prevention of skin cancer in mice and gingerols with the destruction of ovarian cancer cells (Singh et al. 2011).

23.5　ANTIOXIDANT PROPERTIES

In foods, antioxidants have been defined as 'substances in small quantities that are able to prevent or greatly retard the oxidation of easily oxidisable materials such as fats'. In biological systems it refers to 'any substance that when present at low concentrations compared to an oxidisable substrate, significantly delays or prevents oxidation of that substrate'. This includes all oxidisable substrates such as lipids, proteins, DNA and carbohydrates (Halliwell and Gutteridge 1999). Oxidative stress is the state of imbalance between the reactive oxygen species in the body and total antioxidant defences. Increased production of free radicals can overwhelm the antioxidant defences and contribute to the development of many diseases. The literature suggests that this may lead to a wide variety of conditions such as ageing, cancer, cataracts, cardiovascular diseases, rheumatoid arthritis and neurological disorders. The theory of oxidative stress on ageing and age-related degenerative diseases shows the importance of daily use of natural phytochemicals and compounds (Harman 1992).

During the various normal cellular activities in our body, different biochemical reactions take place, which continuously produce various free radicals. A free radical is any species capable of independent existence (hence the term 'free') that contains one or more unpaired electrons, an unpaired electron being one that is alone in an atomic or molecular orbital. It is this electron imbalance that gives rise in most cases to the high reactivity of the free radical, because it tends to react with other molecules to pair the electron(s) and generate a more stable species. Free radicals are also generated by exposure to sunlight, ozone and environmental pollutants.

The efficiency of endogenous antioxidant systems in different organisms may not be adequate to combat all oxidative damage, therefore the interest in the natural exogenous antioxidants like flavonoids and polyphenols in the human diet is greater. Natural antioxidants influence the safety and acceptability of the food system. They can keep food stable against oxidation and also be effective in controlling microbial growth. The traditional practice of adding antioxidants during processing can still play a very important role, because the added compounds have the potential to enhance the activity of the inherent antioxidant systems (Stoilova et al. 2007).

Spices are traditionally recognised for their medicinal properties, some of which can be attributed to the presence of phytochemicals. In a variety of spice extracts, the systematic evaluation of total antioxidant concentration has been conducted using *in vitro* assays, including common Indian spices, have been shown to inhibit lipid peroxidation. In one study, relative antioxidant activities from highest to lowest were found in cloves, cinnamon, pepper, ginger and garlic (Shobana and Naidu 2000). *In vitro* studies also show that ginger extract has antioxidative properties and scavenges superoxide anion and hydroxyl radicals (Cao et al. 1993; Krishnakantha and Lokesh 1993), and several studies have identified ginger with high antioxidant content (Shobana and Naidu 2000; Halvorsen et al. 2002). Several *in vivo* studies have also have determined the antioxidative capacity of spices and their constituents.

Ginger roots and their extracts have polyphenol compounds (6-gingerol, gingerol, gingerdiol, gingerdione) and other compounds that could be responsible for the antioxidant activities of ginger (Chen et al. 1986; Kikuzaki and Nakatani 1996). Ginger contains 11% gingerols, including 5% of 6-gingerol (Nazemieh et al. 2002). Although various extracts are obtained from ginger, the CO_2 extracts are richest in phenolic compounds and have a composition that is closest to the roots (Chen et al. 1986; Bartley and Jacobs 2000). At high concentration, the active component of ginger, gingerol, inhibits the ferrous ascorbate complex, which in turn induces lipid peroxidation (Reddy and Lokesh 1992). Several studies have shown that consumption of foods rich in polyphenolic antioxidants such as tea, garlic, olive oil, ginger and tomato reduce diabetic complications and protect the antioxidant system of the body (Aviram and Eias 1993; Serafini et al. 1994; Fuhrman et al. 2000, George et al. 2004).

The antioxidant potential of ginger has been studied by many workers, using both *in vitro* and *in vivo* models. It has been said that the increasing antioxidant activity of plant extracts in proportion to their concentration is related to the presence of antioxidant compounds, especially phenols (Matsufuji et al. 1998; Chu et al. 2002), and in particular, flavonoids, catechin and isocatechin (Materska and Perucka 2005; Gramza et al. 2006, Dubost et al. 2007). Some examples of the studies demonstrating antioxidant properties of ginger are compiled below.

- The total phenolic content and antioxidant activities of ginger were investigated by Kaur and Kapoor (2002). The total phenolic compound of 80% ethanolic extract was reported as 221.3 mg/100 g and the antioxidant activity was found to be 71.8 (ethanolic extract) and 65.0% (water extract).
- The total phenols of alcoholic ginger extract were reported as 870.1 mg/g dry extract (Stoilova et al. 2007). The free radical scavenging activity (FRSA) was higher than

butylated hydroxyanisole (90.1%), with IC_{50} concentration for inhibition being 0.64 µg/mL. The antioxidant activity measured by different methods at two temperatures, 37°–80°C was 73.32% and 68.2% by linoleic acid/water emulsion system evaluated by means of thiobarbituric acid reactive substances assay (TBARS); 71.6% and 65.7% inhibition of conjugated diene formation; and 79.6% and 74.8% inhibition of hydroxyl radical, respectively.

- Ahmed and Rocha (2009) analysed the total phenol content of ginger plant originating from Iraq and reported the content as 266.3 mg gallic acid equivalent (GAE)/100 g. A good correlation between antioxidant activity and phenolic content was found. *In vivo* antioxidant activity of ginger determined against lipid oxidation in brain homogenate TBARS in rat showed an activity of 32.9%–64.8% at concentration of 3.5–16.9 mg/mL. They also determined the Fe+2 chelating ability of the water extractable phytochemicals of ginger and reported an activity of 54.7%–64.1% at the concentration tested (3.5–16.9 mg/mL). The use of iron chelation is a popular therapy for management of Fe+2 associated oxidative stress in brain. The iron chelating ability of ginger is an indicator of the neuroprotective property, because iron is involved in the pathogenesis of Alzheimer's and other diseases by multiple mechanisms (Malecki and Connor 2002).

- Ghasemzadeh et al. (2010) evaluated the antioxidant activity of methanol extracts from the leaves, stems and rhizomes of two varieties of ginger (*Halia Bentong* and *Halia Bara*) to explore the potential medicinal properties of different parts of the plant. The FRSA was higher in the plant leaves, which had higher phenolic and flavonoids content than rhizomes. In contrast, the ferric reducing antioxidant potential (FRAP) activity was greater in the rhizomes than in the leaves. At low concentration, the inhibition activity in the leaves of both varieties was significantly higher than or comparable to those of young rhizomes. Between the two varieties, *Halia Bara* had higher antioxidant activity as well as total phenolic and flavonoid content than *Halia Bentong*. A positive relationship between total phenolic content and antioxidant activity was found.

- Pilerood and Prakash (2010) reported that methanolic and ethanolic extracts of ginger exhibited high total antioxidant activity of 98,825 and 91,176 µmol/g of sample. The FRSA of methanolic extract was 84.4% per 1.0 mg concentration of ginger.

- Maizura et al. (2011) reported a similar antioxidant activity of 79.0% measured by FRSA assay with a total phenolic content of 101.6 mg GAE/100 g of fresh ginger.

- El-Ghorab et al. (2010) investigated the composition of the volatile oil and antioxidant activity of ginger. The analysis of volatile oils of fresh and dried ginger showed camphene, p-cineole, R-terpineol, zingiberene and pentadecanoic acid as major components. Maximum total phenolic contents were observed in the methanol extract of fresh ginger (95.2 mg/g dry extract) followed by the hexane extract (87.5 mg/g dry extract). The FRSA of fresh and dried ginger essential oils were 83.87 and 83.03%, respectively. The FRAP of essential oils was similar to FRSA. Ginger can therefore be used as potential source of natural antioxidants in foods.

- Ginger has been shown to protect against chemical induced – in particular, organophosphate-induced – toxicity in biological systems where free radicals are involved. Exposure to pesticide chemicals leads to generation of free radicals and alterations in antioxidants or oxygen free radical scavenging enzymes. Hence, in a research study, the effect of sub-chronic malathion exposure was determined on lipid peroxidation, glutathione and related enzymes and oxygen free radical scavenging enzymes in albino rats. The malondialdehyde levels in serum, activities of superoxide dismutase, catalase and glutathione peroxidase in erythrocyte and glutathione reductase and glutathione S-transferase in serum increased on malathion administration. However, the glutathione level in whole blood was reduced. Concomitant dietary feeding of ginger (1%, w/w) significantly reduced malathion-induced lipid peroxidation and oxidative stress in the experimental animals (Ahmed et al. 2000).

- Manju and Nalini (2005) studied the chemo-preventive efficacy of ginger in an animal model against a procarcinogen-induced colon cancer by monitoring lipid peroxidation and antioxidant status. They observed that in the presence of a colon carcinogen, plasma lipid peroxidation and cancer incidence increased significantly in experimental animals, whereas enzymatic and non-enzymatic antioxidant concentrations diminished in comparison to control rats. The number of tumours, as well as the incidence of cancer, was significantly reduced on treatment with ginger. In addition, ginger supplementation at the initiation stage and also at the post-initiation stages of carcinogenesis significantly decreased circulating lipid peroxidation and increased the enzymatic and non-enzymatic antioxidants compared to unsupplemented control rats. The authors concluded that ginger supplementation can suppress colon carcinogenesis in the presence of procarcinogen.

23.6 NUTRITIONAL AND MEDICINAL PROPERTIES

As mentioned earlier, ginger has traditionally been associated with many nutritional and medicinal properties and its use has been documented. Many scientists have studied the traditional health claims attributed to ginger, and the literature is replete with reports dealing with multiple aspects of ginger for functional effect and elucidation of mechanism. These include investigations on nutritional and chemical structure and composition, antioxidant properties, hypolipidaemic, hypoglycaemic, hypocholesterolaemic, antibacterial, anti-nausea and vomiting, anticancer, anti-obesity and antidiarrheal properties.

23.6.1 HYPOLIPIDAEMIC AND HYPOGLYCAEMIC EFFECT

The root of ginger, commonly used as a spice in various foods and beverages, has also been shown to be effective in controlling diabetes and dyslipidaemia. Metabolic syndrome including obesity, dyslipidaemia, hyperglycaemia and insulin resistance that predisposes type 2 diabetes are major disease problems all around the world, and traditionally herbal medicines have been used for controlling these disorders.

Ginger extract is also known as a functional food because it possesses both nutritional and medicinal benefits. Consumption of ginger extract is said to be beneficial in attenuation of atherosclerosis development. It is associated with downregulation of macrophage-mediated oxidation of low-density lipoproteins (LDL), as well as reduction in (i) uptake of oxidised LDL by macrophages, (ii) oxidative state of LDL and (III) LDL aggregation (Fuhrman et al. 2000). All these effects lead to a reduction in the accumulation of cellular cholesterol and foam cell formation associated with early atherosclerosis.

Ginger was shown to have hypolipidaemic effect in rabbits and rats fed food containing cholesterol (Bhandari et al. 1998; Bhandari 2005). Incorporating ginger in a rat's diet significantly increases the activity of hepatic cholesterol 7-a-hydroxylase. This is a rate-limiting enzyme in the biosynthesis of bile acids and stimulates the conversion of bile acids leading to the excretion of cholesterol from the body (Srinivasan and Sambaiah 1991).

Bhandari (2005) evaluated the lipid lowering and antioxidant potential of ethanolic extract of ginger in streptozotocin induced rats and observed a significant anti-hyperglycaemic effect. The total cholesterol and triglycerides were decreased and high-density lipoprotein (HDL) cholesterol level was increased in the treatment group in comparison to the control group. As compared to normal healthy control rats, streptozotocin treatment also exhibited a significant increase in liver and pancreas lipid peroxide levels, which could be lowered in the treatment group. The results indicated that ginger can protect the tissues from lipid peroxidation and showed a significant lipid lowering activity in diabetic rats.

The hypoglycaemic and hypolipidaemic potential of ginger was demonstrated by Al-Amin et al. (2006) in rats. An aqueous extract of raw ginger was administered daily (500 mg/kg, intraperitoneally) for 7 weeks to streptozotocin (STZ)-induced diabetic rats. Raw ginger was significantly effective in lowering serum glucose, cholesterol and triacylglycerol levels in the ginger-treated diabetic rats compared with the control diabetic rats. The ginger treatment also resulted in a significant reduction in urine protein levels, maintenance of body weights and decreased water intake and urine output in diabetic rats. Thus, ginger may be of great value in managing the effects of diabetic complications in human subjects.

Nammi et al. (2009) observed a significant reduction in hepatic triglycerides and decreased heparin cholesterol levels in rats fed ethanol extract of ginger (400 mg/kg) along with a high fat diet. In parallel, the extract increased both LDL receptor mRNA and protein level and decreased HMG-CoA reductase protein expression in the liver. The metabolic control of body lipid homeostasis was attributed to enhanced cholesterol biosynthesis and reduced expression of LDL receptor sites following long-term consumption of high fat diets. The results showed restoration of transcriptional and post-transcriptional changes in LDL and HMG-CoA reductase by ginger administration with a high fat diet and provide a rational explanation for the effect of ginger in the treatment of hyperlipidaemia.

Lam et al. (2007) studied the antioxidant actions of phenolic compounds of ginger on LDL and erythrocytes using several *in vitro* oxidative systems. Results revealed that 6-gingerol showed strong inhibition against lipid peroxidation in LDL and erythrocyte membranes, providing scientific evidence to substantiate the traditional use of ginger in preventing metabolic disorder.

The effect of feeding ginger (5% of food consumed) on diabetic retinopathy, plasma AO capacity and lipid peroxidation was examined by Afshari et al. (2007) in rats. Blood samples from heart and kidneys were evaluated for plasma antioxidant capacity by FRAP assay and malondialdehyde (MDA) as indicator of lipid peroxidation. Renal samples were analysed for focal cell proliferation and glomerular and tubular structural changes. In ginger-treated diabetic rats, the MDA levels were significantly lower and plasma antioxidant capacity was higher than the other group. Diabetes induced nephropathies were also lower in the ginger-treated group. This study demonstrated that ginger caused a reduction in lipid peroxidation, a rise in plasma antioxidant capacity and a decrease in renal nephropathy.

Alizadeh-Navaei et al. (2008) studied the effect of ginger on lipid levels of hyperlipidaemic patients. Subjects were divided the into two groups, the treatment group (ginger capsules 3 g/day in 3 divided doses) and the placebo group (lactose capsule 3 g/day in 3 divided doses) given for 45 days. Lipid concentrations profiles before and after treatment was measured by enzymatic assay. Results showed a significant reduction in triglyceride, cholesterol, LDL, and very low-density lipoproteins (VLDL) levels after the study. Mean changes in triglyceride and cholesterol levels of the ginger group were significantly higher than in the placebo group ($p < 0.05$). Mean reduction in LDL level and increase in high-density lipoprotein level of the ginger group was higher than the placebo group, but the VLDL level of placebo was higher than ginger ($p > 0.05$). The results show that ginger has a significant lipid-lowering effect compared to placebo.

A recent meta-analysis of nine clinical studies by Jafarnejad et al. (2017) on ginger supplementation given as either tablets, capsules, powder or rhizome, concluded that ginger could significantly reduce fasting blood glucose, total cholesterol and triglycerides, though specific results were influenced by the clinical conditions.

23.6.2 ANTIBACTERIAL ACTIVITY

In vitro studies support that apart from antiradical activity, ginger extract also possesses antibacterial activity (Jirovetz et al. 2005). Chen et al. (2008) studied the antimicrobial activity of 18 species of Zingiberaceae plants from five genus in Taiwan. Most of the plant extracts exhibited antimicrobial activity against all tested food microorganisms, namely, *Escherichia coli*, *Salmonella enterica*, *Staphylococcus aureus* and *Vibrio parahaemolyticus*.

Malu et al. (2009) studied the antibacterial and medicinal properties of ginger. Dry ginger was extracted in different media, namely, ethanol, *n*-hexane, ethyl acetate and water, and the extract obtained was concentrated and evaporated to dryness. The dried extracts were tested for antibacterial activity against coliform bacillus, *Staphylococcus epidermidis* and Viridans Streptococcus organisms. Results showed that the solvent extracts of ginger exhibited antibacterial activity, however the water extract showed no effect. The inhibition of pathogenic organism was dose-dependent. The authors suggest that solvent extracts of ginger may be used for treating bacterial infections. The antibacterial effect of ginger may also be dose dependent, as in some studies both solvent and water extract did not show any antibacterial activity (Pilerood et al. 2013).

Azu and Onyeagba (2007) studied the antimicrobial properties of various extracts of ginger against *E. coli*, *Salmonella typhi* and *Bacillus subtilis*. The ethanolic extracts of ginger gave the widest zone of inhibition against two out of three test organisms at the concentration of 0.8 g/L. The extraction solvent and its different concentrations affected the sensitivity of two of the test organisms to the plant material. The minimum inhibitory concentration of ginger extracts on the test organisms ranged from 0.1 g/mL and they were effective against gram negative test organisms but not against gram positive test organisms.

Gao and Zhang (2010) tested the antibacterial activity of raw and processed ginger extract against gram-positive bacteria (two strains) and gram-negative bacteria (four strains) and showed its effectiveness against all organisms tested. Many studies also report that the active constituents of ginger – gingerols – are effective against *Helicobacter pylori*, which causes peptic ulcer, dyspepsia and gastric and colon cancer (Mahady et al. 2003, 2005; O'Mahony et al. 2005; Nostro et al. 2006; Siddaraju and Dharmesh 2007).

The antimicrobial activity of fresh and dry ginger oil against *Bacillus subtilis*, *Pseudomonas aeruginosa*, *Candida albicans*, *Trichoderma* spp., *Aspergillus niger*, *Penicillium* spp. and *Saccharomyces cerevisiae* was investigated by Sasidharan and Menon (2010), and the MIC values of the oils were found to range from 10 µg/mL to 1.0 µg/mL. Zingiberene was the major compound in both ginger oils. Fresh ginger oil contained geranial (8.5%) as the second main compound and had more oxygenated compounds (29.2%) compared to dry ginger oil (14.4%). The dry ginger oil also contained ar-curcumene (11%), β-bisabolene (7.2%), sesquiphellandrene (6.6%) and δ-cadinene (3.5%).

The antimicrobial activity of ginger is not only beneficial for preventing bacterial infections but also for protecting food from spoilage. Addition of ginger can protect the food from fungal and mould attack. Singh et al. (2008) investigated the antimicrobial efficacy of ginger essential oil and oleoresin against food borne pathogenic fungal and bacterial species and showed good to moderate effects with many of the species. The inhibition was found to be 100% for *Fusarium moniliforme* and essential oil was more effective than oleoresin.

23.6.3 Weight Management

Although the digestion-stimulating effect of this spice have long been known, the stimulating effect on peptic juices, such as gastric juice, bile, pancreatic and intestinal juices was a later discovery. Bile acids play a major role in the uptake of fat and any upset in fat metabolism will slow down food digestion as a whole because fatty particles cover the food elements and make them inaccessible for the action of digestive enzymes. Lipase also plays important role in fat digestion. Ginger has long been associated with reduction in body weight. The effect may be mediated by enzymatic action. When ginger was included in animal diet, there was a considerable increase in the pancreatic and intestinal lipase, indicating a better breakdown of fat particles (Platel and Srinivasan 2000).

Pilerood et al. (2016) investigated the influence of ginger and valerian on food intake, weight gain and blood parameters of adult Wistar rats. Forty rats maintained on a normal diet were divided into five groups: the control group (1) was given placebo and the others (2–5) were fed with dry ginger and valerian root powder via gavage at 3 and 6 mg levels respectively for 30 days. At the end of the study all animals were sacrificed and organs weights and biochemical indices were recorded. Results revealed that there were no significant differences between control and study group in any of blood parameters and organ weights. There was significant weight loss in both groups fed ginger in comparison to the control, although the food intake of all groups was similar. In both valerian-fed groups, there was an increase in food intake with higher weight gain. Valerian increased appetite of animals and induced lethargy in comparison to control group. Authors state that ginger possibly increased the metabolic rate, thereby decreasing body weight despite normal food intake.

23.6.4 ANTI-INFLAMMATORY ACTION

It is hypothesised that prostaglandins and other eicosanoids influence carcinogenesis through action on nuclear transcription sites and downstream gene products important in the control of cell proliferation. Non-steroidal anti-inflammatory drugs – potent inhibitors of cyclooxygenase (COX), the enzyme responsible for prostaglandins synthesis – are associated with reduced risk of several cancers (Wargovich et al. 2001). Natural products, including spices, have therefore been examined for their capacity to inhibit COX or other parts of the inflammation pathway. Ginger has been reported to interfere with inflammatory processes (Ozaki et al. 1991).

Thomson et al. (2002) studied the use of ginger as a potential anti-inflammatory and antithrombotic agent. The effect of an aqueous extract of ginger on serum cholesterol and triglyceride levels as well as platelet thromboxane-B2 and prostaglandins E-2 production was studied. An aqueous extract of raw ginger was administered daily either orally or intraperitoneally (IP) to rats for 4 weeks. A low dose of ginger (50 mg/kg) administered either orally or intraperitoneally (IP) did not cause any significant reduction in serum thromboxane-B2 levels when compared to control animals, although an oral administration caused significant changes in the serum PGE-2 at this dose. High doses of ginger (500 mg/kg) were significantly effective in lowering serum PGE-2 when given either orally or IP. However XB-2 levels were significantly lower in rats given 500 mg/kg ginger orally, but not IP. A significant reduction in serum cholesterol was observed with a high dose, and at low dose, IP treatment also showed this. There were no changes in triglyceride levels. These results suggest that ginger can be used as cholesterol lowering, antithrombotic, anti-inflammatory agent.

23.6.5 ANTIDIARRHOEAL PROPERTIES

Enterotoxigenic *Escherichia coli* heat labile enterotoxin (LT)-induced diarrhoea is the leading cause of infant death in developing countries. Chen et al. (2007) showed that ginger significantly blocks the binding of LT to cell-surface receptor GM1, resulting in the inhibition of fluid accumulation in the closed ileal loops of mice. Biological activity guided search for active components indicated zingerone to be the most likely active constituent responsible for the antidiarrhoeal efficacy of ginger. Further analysis of chemically synthesised zingerone derivatives revealed that compound 31 (2-[(4-methoxybenzyl)oxy]benzoic acid) significantly suppressed LT-induced diarrhoea in mice via an excellent surface complementarity with the B subunits of LT. Hence, ginger could be an effective herbal supplement for the clinical treatment of enterotoxigenic *Escherichia coli* diarrhoea.

23.6.6 NAUSEA AND VOMITING

Ginger has been linked with reduction of nausea and vomiting related to early pregnancy, motion sickness, chemotherapy induced nausea and post-operative nausea. Studies reporting the efficacy of ginger against nausea and vomiting suggest that in each case ginger was more effective than the placebo and was preferred for reducing nausea caused by various reasons (Ernst and Pittler 2000; Bryer 2005). Smith et al. (2004) examined the efficacy of ginger to reduce nausea or vomiting in pregnancy in comparison to vitamin B_6. A randomised controlled trial was conducted with 291 women in early pregnancy who were given either 1.05 g of ginger or 75 mg of vitamin B_6 everyday and results recorded on days 7, 14 and 21. Ginger was found to be equivalent to vitamin B_6 in reducing symptoms of nausea, dry retching and vomiting. Adib-Hajbaghery and Hosseini

(2015) examined the inhalation of ginger essence to reduce post-operative nausea and vomiting in 120 nephrectomy patients divided equally as control and experimental groups. The experimental group reported significantly lower feelings of nausea and vomiting episodes during the 6 hours post-surgery. These observations support the traditional use of ginger for preventing nausea of any kind.

23.7 TOXICITY AND ADVERSE REACTIONS

Because ginger has been used as a natural ingredient in food, it is generally considered safe. In traditional use, no toxicity has ever been reported. Systematic studies on the effect of consumption of ginger or its extracts have been reported. In a study by Rong et al. (2009), a 35-day toxicity of ginger powder in rats at the dosages of 500, 1000 and 2000 mg/kg body weight by a gavage method given daily was evaluated. Results showed that chronic administration of ginger was not associated with any mortality and abnormalities in general conditions, behaviour, growth and food and water consumption. Except for dose-related decrease in serum lactate dehydrogenase activity in males, there was no significant difference in hepatological and blood biochemical parameters between the ginger treatment group and controlled animals. No organ abnormality was seen in the ginger-fed group. Only at the highest dose, ginger led to slightly reduced absolute and relative weights of tests (by 14.4% and 11.5% respectively). A study by Pilerood et al. (2016) showed no effect of feeding a smaller quantity of ginger (3–6 mg/kg body weight) on any clinical blood parameters of rats. When ginger extract was fed to pregnant rats, the preparation was well tolerated up to 1000 mg/kg body weight. There was no effect seen on weight gain, food consumption or reproductive performance of pregnant rats. No embryotoxicity or teratogenicity was observed in fetuses, indicating that ginger was safe during pregnancy (Weidner and Sigwart 2001).

There have been few adverse reactions reported, which may include allergic reactions to ginger such as heartburn, bloating, gas, belching and nausea (particularly if taken in powdered form). Unchewed fresh ginger may result in intestinal blockage, and individuals who have had ulcers, inflammatory bowel diseases or blocked intestines may react badly to large quantities of fresh ginger. Ginger can also adversely affect individuals with gallstones, and may affect blood pressure, clotting and heart rhythms (O'Hara et al. 1998). Ginger can cause heartburn or act as a gastric irritant in higher doses (Chrubasik et al. 2005). There have also been some converse reports of ginger in pregnant rats. In a study by Wilkinson (2000), ginger tea fed to pregnant rats did not result in any maternal toxicity, however, a higher embryonic loss was observed, although surviving fetuses were reported to be heavier.

It is very unlikely that the amount of ginger generally consumed in the diet may pose any risk of interference with drugs. It may either have no reaction or sometimes can support the action of drug. There are very few specific reports on interaction of ginger with drugs. The action of the anti-coagulant drug warfarin was not influenced by intake of 1.2 g of ginger (divided in three doses taken for a week) in healthy volunteers (Jiang et al. 2005). Earlier reports have also supported this observation (Vaes and Chyka 2000; Weidner and Sigwart 2000). Ginger demonstrated a synergistic effect with nifedipine on anti-platelet aggregation in normal and hypertensive subjects. Hence, it was suggested that ginger may be effective in preventing cardiovascular and cerebrovascular complications due to platelet aggregation (Young et al. 2006).

23.8 CONCLUSION

Both traditional use and scientific evidence bring out the various physiological benefits of ginger. In particular, the medicinal properties observed are related to the gastrointestinal tract, including treatment for indigestion, constipation, nausea and vomiting, helminthiasis, peptic ulcer, dyspepsia, diabetes and hyperlipidaemia, vascular health, platelet aggregation, anti-inflammatory, anticancer, antibacterial, management of healthy weight and for muscular aches and pains.

No specific toxicity has been reported, although a few studies report a mild gastro-intestinal disturbance of heart burn and discomfort, which can be attributed to its 'hot' nature as mentioned in traditional uses. In conclusion, ginger can be used for its therapeutic properties as a safe medicine with no demonstrable adverse effects.

REFERENCES

Achaya, K. T. (1994). *Indian Foods – A Historical Companion*. Oxford University Press. New Delhi. India.

Adanlawo, I. G. and Dairo, F. A. S. (2007). Nutrient and anti-nutrient constituents of ginger (*Zingiber officinale* Roscoe) and the influence of its ethanolic extract on some serum enzymes in albino rats. *International Journal of Biological Chemistry*, **1**, 38–46.

Adib-Hajbaghery, M. and Hosseini, F. S. (2015). Investigating the effects of inhaling ginger essence on post-nephrectomy nausea and vomiting. *Complementary Therapies in Medicine*, **23**(6), 827–831. doi:10.1016/j.ctim.2015.10.002.

Afshari, A. T., Shirpoor, A., Farshid, A., Saadatian, R., Rasmi, Y., Saboory, E., Ilkhanizadeh, B. Allameh, A. (2007). The effect of ginger on diabetic nephropathy, plasma antioxidant capacity and lipid peroxidation in rats. *Food Chemistry*, **101**(1), 148–153.

Agu, C. S., Igwe, J. E., Amanze, N. N. and Oduma, O. (2016). Effect of oven drying on proximate composition of ginger. *American Journal of Engineering Research*, **5**(8), 58–61.

Ahmed, S. H. and Rocha, J. B. (2009). Antioxidant properties of water extracts for the Iraqi plants *Phoenix dactylifera, Loranthus europeas, Zingiber officinalis* and *Citrus aurantifolia*. *Modern Applied Science*, **3**(3), 161.

Ahmed, R., Seth, V., Pasha, S. and Banerjee, B. (2000). Influence of dietary ginger (*Zingiberofficinale* Rosc) on oxidative stress induced by malathion in rats. *Food and ChemicalToxicology*, **38**(5), 443–450.

Ajayi, O. A., Ola, O. O. and Akinwunmi, O. O. (2017). Effect of drying method on nutritional composition, sensory and antimicrobial properties of ginger (*Zinginber officinale*). *International Food Research Journal*, **24**(2), 614–620.

Ajayi, O. B., Akomolafe, S. F. and Akinyemi, F. T. (2013). Food value of two varieties of ginger (*Zingiber officinale*) commonly consumed in Nigeria. *ISRN Nutrition*, **2013**, 359727. doi:10.5402/2013/359727.

Al-Amin, Z. M., Thomson, M., Al-Qattan, K. K., Peltonen-Shalaby, R. and Ali, M. (2006). Anti-diabetic and hypolipidaemic properties of ginger (*Zingiber officinale*) in streptozotocin-induced diabetic rats. *British Journal of Nutrition*, **96**, 660–666.

Alizadeh-Navaei, R., Roozbeh, F., Saravi, M., Pouramir, M., Jalali, F. and Moghadamnia, A. A. (2008). Investigation of the effect of ginger on the lipid levels, a double blind controlled clinical trial. *Saudi Medical Journal*, **29**(9), 179–183.

Aviram, M. and Eias, K. (1993). Dietary olive oil reduces low density lipoproteins uptake by macrophages and decreases the susceptibility of the lipoprotein to undergo lipid peroxidation. *Annals of Nutrition and Metabolism*, **37**(2), 75–84.

Azu, N. and Onyeagba, R. (2007). Antimicrobial properties of extracts of *Allium cepa* (onions) and *Zingiber officinale* (ginger) on *Escherichia coli, Salmonella typhi* and *Bacillus subtilis*. *The Internet Journal of Tropical Medicine*, **3**(2), 1–10.

Bartley, J. P. and Jacobs, A. L. (2000). Effects of drying on flavour components in Australian grown ginger (*Zingiber officinale*). *Journal of Science of Food and Agriculture*, **80**(2), 209–215.

Bhandari, U. (2005). Effect of ethanolic extract of *Zingiber officinale* on dyslipidaemia in diabetic rats. *Journal of Ethnopharmacology*, **97**, 227–230.

Bhandari, U., Sharma, J. and Zafar, R. (1998). The protective action of ethanolic ginger (*Zingiber officinale*) extract in cholesterol fed rabbits. *Journal of Ethnopharmacology*, **61**, 167–171.

Bode, A. M., Ma, W. Y., Surh, Y. J. and Dong, Z. (2001). Inhibition of epidermal growth factor induced cell transformation and activator protein 1 activation by [6]-gingerol. *Cancer Research*, **61**(3), 850.

Bryer, E. (2005). A literature review of the effectiveness of ginger in alleviating mild -to moderate nausea and vomiting of pregnancy. *Journal of Midwifery Women's Health*, **50**, e1–e 3.

Burdock, G. A. (1996). Fenaroli's handbook of flavor ingredients. *Gordian Hamburg*, **96**, 547–549.

Cao, Z., Chen, Z., Guo, P., Zhang, S., Lian, L., Luo, L. and Hu, W. (1993). Scavenging effects of ginger on superoxide anion and hydroxyl radical. *China Journal of Chinese Materia Medica*, **18**(12), 750.

Chen, I. N., Chang, C. C., Ng, C. C., Wang, C. Y. Shyu, Y. T. and Chang, T. L. (2008). Antioxidant and anti-microbial activity of *Zingiberaceae* plants in Taiwan. *Plant Foods for Human Nutrition*, **63**(1), 15–20.

Chen, J. C., Huang, L. J., Wu, S. L., Kuo, S. C., Ho, T. Y. and Hsiang, C. Y. (2007). Ginger and its bioactive component inhibit enterotoxigenic *Escherichia coli* heat-labile enterotoxin-induced diarrhea in mice. *Journal of Agricultural and Food Chemistry*, **55**, 8390–8397.

Chen, C. C., Kuo, M. C., Wu, C. M. and Ho, C. T. (1986). Pungent compounds of ginger (*Zingiber officinale* Roscoe) extracted by liquid carbon dioxide. *Journal of Agricultural and Food Chemistry*, **34**(3), 477–480.

Chrubasik, S., Pittler, M. H. and Roufogalis, B. D. (2005). Zingiberis rhizoma: A comprehensive review on the ginger effect and efficacy profiles. *Phytomedicine*, **12**, 684–701.

Chu, Y.F., Sun, J., Wu, X. and Liu, R. H. (2002). Antioxidant and antiproliferative activities of common vegetables. *Journal of Agricultural and Food Chemistry*, **50**(23), 6910–6916.

Dubost, N. J., Ou, B. and Beelman, R. B. (2007). Quantification of polyphenols and ergothioneine in cultivated mushrooms and correlation to total antioxidant capacity. *Food Chemistry*, **105**(2),727–735.

El-Ghorab, A. H., Nauman, M., Anjum, F. M., Hussain, S. and Nadeem, M. (2010). A comparative study on chemical composition and antioxidant activity of ginger (*Zingiber officinale*) and cumin (*Cuminum cyminum*). *Journal of Agricultural and Food Chemistry*, **58**, 8231–8237.

Ernst, E. and Pittler, M. H. (2000). Efficacy of ginger for nausea and vomiting systematic review of randomized clinical trials. *British Journal of Anaesthesia*, **84**(3), 367–371.

FAO (United Nations Food and Agriculture Organization). (2017). Ginger production, Food and Agriculture Data. Downloaded from http://www.fao.org/faostat/en/#data.

Fuhrman, B., Rosenblat, M., Hayek, T., Coleman, R. and Aviram, M. (2000). Ginger extract consumption reduces plasma cholesterol, inhibits LDl oxidation and attenuates development of atherosclerosis in atherosclerotic apolipoprotein E deficient mice. *Journal of Nutrition*, **130**(5), 1124.

Gao, D. and Zhang, Y. (2010). Comparative antibacterial activities of extracts of dried ginger and processed ginger. *Pharmacognosy Journal*, **2**(15), 41–44.

George, B., Kaur, C., Kurdiya, D. and Kapoor, H. (2004). Antioxidants in tomato (*Lycopersium esculentum*) as a function of genotype. *Food Chemistry*, **84**(1), 45–51.

Ghasemzadeh, A., Jaafar, H. Z. E. and Rahmat, A. (2010). Antioxidant activities, total phenolics and flavonoids content in two varieties of Malaysia young ginger (*Zingiber officinale* Roscoe). *Molecules*, **15**(6), 4324–4333.

Gramza, A., Khokar, S., Yoko, S., Swiglo, G. A. and Korczak, J. (2006). Antioxidant activity of tea extracts in lipids and correlation with polyphenol content. *European Journal of Lipid Science and Technology*, **108**(4), 351–362.

Halliwell, B. and Gutteridge, J. M. (1999). *Free Radicals in Biology and Medicine*. Oxford, UK: Oxford University Press.

Halvorsen, B. L., Holte, K., Myhrstad, M. C. W., Barikmo, I., Hvattum, E., Remberg, S. F., Wold, A. B., et al. (2002). A systematic screening of total antioxidants in dietary plans. *Journal of Nutrition*, **132**(3), 461–471.

Harman, D. (1992). Free radical theory of ageing. *Mutation Research*, **275**(3–6), 257–266.

Jafarnejad, S., Kashavarz, S. A., Mehbubi, S., Saremi, S., Arab, A., Abbasi, S. and Djafarian, K. (2017). Effect of ginger (*Zingiber officinale*) on blood glucose and lipid concentrations in diabetic and hyperlipidemic subjects: A meta analysis of randomized controlled trials. *Journal of Functional Foods*, **29**, 127–134.

Jagtap S., Meganathan, K., Wagh, V., Winkler, J., Hescheler, J. and Sachinidis, A. (2009). Chemoprotective mechanisms of the natural compounds, epigallocatechin-3-O-galate, quercetin and curcumin against cancer and cardiovascular diseases. *Current Medicinal Chemistry*, **16**(12), 1451–1462.

Jatoi, S. A., Kikuchi, A., Gilani, S. A. and Watanabe, K. N. (2007). Phytochemical, pharmacological, and ethnobotanical studies in mango ginger (*Curcuma amada Roxb.: Zingiberaceae*). *Phytotherapy Research*, **21**(6), 507–516.

Jiang, X., Blair, E. Y. and McLachlan, A. J. (2005). Investigation of the effects of herbal medicines on warfarin response in healthy subjects: A population pharmacokinetic-pharmacodynamic modelling approach. *Journal of Clinical Pharmacology*, **46**, 1370–1378.

Jirovetz, L., Buchbauer, G., Denkova, Z., Stoyanova, A., Murgov, I. and Lien, H. (2005). Antimicrobial testing and gas chromatograph analysis of black pepper (*Piper nigrum* K.) and ginger (*Zingiber officinale* (L.) Rosc) oleoresin from Vietnam. *Euro Cosmetics*, **13**, 22–28.

Kato, M., Rocha, M. L., Carvallo, A. B., Chaves, M. E., Rana, M. C. and Olverra, F. C. (1993). Occupational exposure to neurotoxicants. Preliminary survey in five industries of caricari petrochemical complex. *Brazil Environmental Research*, **61**, 133–139.

Kaur, C. and Kapoor, H. C. (2002). Antioxidant activity and total phenolic content of some Asian vegetables. *International Journal of Food Science and Technology*, **37**(2), 153–161.

Kawai, T., Kinoshita, K., Koyama, K. and Takahashi, K. (1994). Anti-emetic principles of *Magnolia obavata* bark and *Zingiber officinale* rhizome. *Planta Medica*, **60**, 17–20.

Kikuzaki, H. and Nakatani, N. (1996). Cyclic diarylheptanoids from rhizomes of *Zingiber officinale*. *Phytochemistry*, **43**(1), 273–277.

Krishnakantha, T. and Lokesh, B. (1993). Scavenging of superoxide anions by spice principles. *Indian Journal of Biochemistry and Biophysics*, **30**(2), 133.

Kuschener, W. G. and Stark, P. (2003). Occupational toxicants exposure have an important roles in many cases of lung diseases seen in workers. Occupational lungs diseases. Part 1. Identifying work related asthma and other disorders. *Postgraduate Medicine*, **113**(4), 70–78.

Lam, R. Y. Y., Woo, A. Y. H., Leung, P. S. and Cheng, C. H. K. (2007). Antioxidant actions of phenolic compounds found in dietary plants on low density lipoprotein and erythrocytes in vitro. *Journal of American College of Nutrition*, **26**(3), 233.

Longvah, T., Ananthan, R., Bhaskarachary, K. and Venkaiah, K. (2017). *Indian Food Composition Tables*. National Institute of Nutrition, Hyderabad. India.

Mahady, G. B., Pendland, S. L., Yun, G. S., Lu, Z. Z. and Stoia, A. (2003). Ginger (*Zingiber officinale* Roscoe) and the gingerols inhibit the growth of Cag A+ strains of *Helicobacter pylori*. *Anticancer Research*, **23**, 3699–3702.

Mahady, G. B., Pendland, S. L., Stoia, A., Hamill, F. A., Fabricant, D., Dietz, B. M. and Chadwick, L. R. (2005). *In vitro* susceptibility of *Helicobacter pylori* to botanical extracts used traditionally for the treatment of gastrointestinal disorders. *Phytotherapy Research*, **19**, 988–991.

Maizura, M., Aminah, A. and Wan Aida, W. M. (2011). Total phenolic content and antioxidant activity of kesum (*Polygonum minus*), ginger (*Zingiber officinale*) and turmeric (*Curcuma longa*) extract. *International Food Research Journal*, **18**, 526–531.

Malecki, E. A. and Connor, J. R. (2002). The case for iron chelation and/or antioxidant therapy in Alzheimer's disease. *Drug Development Research*, **56**(3), 526–530.

Malu, S. P., Obochi, G. O., Tawo, E. N. and Nyong, B. E. (2009). Antibacterial activity and medicinal properties of ginger (*Zingiber officinale*). *Global Journal of Pure and Applied Sciences*, **15**(3), 365–368.

Manju, V. and Nalini, N. (2005). Chemopreventive efficacy of ginger, a naturally occurring anti-carcinogen during the initiation, post-initiation stages of 1,2 dimethyl hydrazine-induced colon cancer. *Clinica Chimica Acta*, **358**(1–2), 60–67.

Manusirivithaya, S., Sripramote, M., Tangjitgamol, S., Sheanakul, C., Leelahakorn, S., Thavaramara, T. and Tangcharoenpanich, K. (2004). Antiemetic effect of ginger in gynecologic oncology patients receiving cisplatin. *International Journal of Gynecological Cancer*, **14**(6), 1063–1069.

Materska, M. and Perucka, I. (2005). Antioxidant activity of the main phenolic compounds isolated from hot pepper fruit (*Capsicum annuum* L.). *Journal of Agricultural and Food Chemistry*, **53**(5), 1750–1756.

Matsufuji, H., Nakamura, H., Chino, M. and Takeda, M. (1998). Antioxidant activity of capsanthin and the fatty acid esters in paprika (*Capsicum annuum*). *Journal of Agricultural and Food Chemistry*, **46**(9), 3468–3472.

McGee, H. (2004). *On Food and Cooking: The Science and Lore of the Kitchen*. 2nd Edition. New York: CAB International. 425–426.

Nammi, S., Sreemantula, S. and Roufogalis, B. D. (2009). Protective effects of ethanolic extract of *Zingiber officinale* rhizome on the development of metabolic syndrome in high fat diet fed rats. *Basic and Clinical Pharmacology and Toxicology*, **104**, 366–373.

Nazemieh, H., Delazar, A., Afshar, J. and Eskandari, B. (2002). Isolation, identification and quantitative determination of gingerols in ginger roots. *Pharmaceutical Sciences*, **2**(61), 6.

Nostro, A., Cellini, L., Di Bartomolomeo, S., Cannatelli, M. A., Di Campli, E., Procopio, F., Grande, R., Marzio, L. and Alonzo, V. (2006). Effects of combining extracts (from propolis or *Zingiber officinale*) with clarithromycin on *Helicobacer pylori*. *Phytotherapy Research*, **20**, 187–190.

Nwinuka, N. M., Ibeh, G. O. and Ekeke, G. I. (2005). Proximate composition and levels of some toxicants in four commonly consumed spices. *Journal of Applied Science, Environment and Management*, **9**, 150–155.

Odebunmi, E. O., Oluwaniyi, O. O. and Bashiru, M. O. (2010). Comparative proximate analysis of some food condiments. *Journal of Applied Sciences Research*, **6**(3), 272–274.

Ogbuewu, I. P., Jiwuba, P. D., Ezeokeke, C. T., Uchegbu, M. C., Okoli, I. C. and Iloeje, M. U. (2014). Evaluation of phytochemical and nutritional composition of ginger rhizome powder. *International Journal of Agriculture and Rural Development*, **17**(1), 1663–1670.

O'Hara, M. A., Kiefer, D., Farrell, K. and Kemper, K. (1998). A review of 12 commonly used medicinal herbs. *Archives of Family Medicine*, **7**(6), 523–529.

O'Mahony, R., Al-Khtheeri, H., Weerasekera, D., Fernando, N., Vaira, D., Holton, J. and Basset, C. C. (2005). Bactericidal and anti-adhesive properties of culinary and medicinal plants against *Helicobacter pylori*. *World Journal of Gastroenterology*, **11**, 7499–7507.

Otunola, G. A., Oloyede, O. B., Oladiji, A. T. and Afolayan, A. J. (2010). Comparative analysis of the chemical composition of three spices – *Allium sativum* L. *Zingiber officinale* Rosc. and *Capsicum frutescens* L. commonly consumed in Nigeria. *African Journal of Biotechnology*, **9**(41), 6927–6931.

Ozaki Y., Kawahara, N. and Harada, M. (1991). Anti-inflammatory effect of *Zingiber cassumunar* Roxb. and its active principles. *Chemical and Pharmaceutical Bulletin*, **39**(9), 2353–2256.

Perez, N. (2005). *Zingiber officinale* Roscoe essential oil of ginger roots. *Journal of the International Federation of Aroma Therapists*, **1**, 63.

Pilerood, S. A., Oghbaei, M. and Prakash, J. (2016). Effect of *Zingiber officianale* and *Valeriana officianalis* on biochemical profile and body weights in adult Wistar rats. *European Journal of Pharmaceutical and Medical Research*, **3**(1), 239–247.

Pilerood, S. A. and Prakash, J. (2010). Nutritional composition and antioxidant properties of ginger root (*Zingiber officinale*). *Journal of Medicinal Plants Research*, **4**(24), 2674–2679.

Pilerood, S. A., Prakash, J., Shrisha, D. L. and Raveesha, K. A. (2013). Antibacterial potential of selected herbs and spices against human pathogenic bacteria. *International Journal of Pharmaceutical and Biological Archives*, **4**(4), 647–652.

Platel, K. and Srinivasan, K. (2000). Influence of dietary spices and their active principles on pancreatic digestive enzymes in albino rats. *Food/Nahrung*, **44**, 42–46.

Prakash, O. (1961). *Food and Drinks in Ancient India*. New Delhi, India: Munshi Ram Manohar Lal.

Raghunathasuri. (2012). Properties of spices. In the book, Bhojanakutulaham. Edited by P. Venkat, G. G. Gangadharan, M. A. Lakshmithathachar and M. A. Alwar. Bangalore, India: Institute of Ayurveda and integrative Medicine.

Reddy, P. A. C. and Lokesh, B. (1992). Studies on spice principles as antioxidants in the inhibition of lipid peroxidation of fat liver microsomes. *Molecular and Cellular Biochemistry*, **111**(1), 117–124.

Rong, X., Peng, G., Suzuki, T., Yang, Q., Yamahara, J. and Li, Y. (2009). A 35 day gavage safety assessment of ginger in rats. *Regulatory Toxicology and Pharmacology*, **54**(2), 118–123.

Sasidharan, I. and Menon, A. N. (2010). Comparative chemical composition and antimicrobial activity of fresh and dry ginger oils (*Zingiber officinale* Roscoe). *International Journal of Current Pharmaceutical Research*, **2**(4), 40–43.

Serafini, M., Ghiselli, A., Ferro-Luzzi, A. and Melville, C. (1994). Red wine, tea and antioxidants. *The Lancet*, **344**(8922), 626.

Shobana, S. and Naidu, A. K. (2000). Antioxidant activity of selected Indian Spices. *Prostaglandins, Leukotrienes and Essential Fatty Acids*, **62**(2), 107–110.

Siddaraju, M. N. and Dharmesh, S. M. (2007). Inhibition of gastric H(+), K(+)-ATPase and *Helicobacter pylori* growth by phenolic antioxidants of *Zingiber officinale*. *Molecular Nutrition and Food Research*, **51**, 324–332.

Singh, G., Kapoor, I. P. S., Singh, P., de Heluani, C. S., de Lampasona, M. P. and Catalan, C. A. N. (2008). Chemistry, antioxidant and anti-microbial investigation on essential oil and oleoresin of *Zingiber officinale*. *Food and Chemical Toxicology*, **46**, 3295–3302.

Singh, R., Mehta, A., Mehta, P. and Shukla, K. (2011). Antihelminthic activity of rhizome extracts of *Curcuma longa* and *Zingiber officinale* (*Zingiberaceae*). *International Journal of Pharmacy and Pharmaceutical Sciences*, **3**(Suppl. 2), 236–237.

Smith, C., Crowther, C., Wilson, K., Hotham, N. and McMillian, V. (2004). A randomized controlled trial of ginger to treat nausea and vomiting in pregnancy. *Obstetrics and Gynecology*, **103**(4), 639–645.

Sontakke, S., Thawan, V. and Naik, M. (2003). Ginger as an antiemetic in nausea and vomiting induced by chemotherapy: A randomized cross over double blind study. *Indian Journal of Pharmacology*, **35**(1), 32–36.

Srinivasan, K. and Sambaiah, G. (1991). The effect of spices on cholesterol-7a-hydroxylase activity and on serum and hepatic cholesterol levels in the rat. *International Journal for Vitamin and Nutrition Research*, **61**, 364–369.

Stoilova I., Krastanov, A., Stoyanova, A., Denev, P. and Gargova, S. (2007). Antioxidant activity of ginger extract (*Zingiber officinale*). *Food Chemistry*, **102**(3), 764–770.

Surh, Y. J., Lee, E. and Lee, J. M. (1998). Chemoprotective properties of some pungent ingredients present in red pepper and ginger. *Mutation Research/Fundamental and Molecular Mechanisms of Mutagenesis*, **402**, 259–267.

Thomson, M., Al-Qattan, K., Al-Sawan, S., Al-Naqeed, M., Khan, I. and Ali, M. (2002). The use of ginger (*Zingiber officinale*) as a potential anti-inflammatory and antithrombotic agent. *Prostaglandins, Leukotrienes, and Essential Fatty Acids*, **67**, 475–478.

Vaes, L. P. and Chyka, P. A. (2000). Interactions of warfarin with garlic, ginger, gingko or ginseng: Nature of evidence. *Annals of Pharmacotherapy*, **34**, 1478–1482.

Vishwakarma, S., Pal, S., Kasture, V. S. and Kasture, S. (2002). Anxiolytic and antiemetic activity of *Zingiber officinale*. *Phytotherapy Research*, **16**(7), 621–626.

Wargovich, M. J., Woods, C., Hollis, D. M. and Zander, M. E. (2001). Herbals, cancer prevention and health. *Journal of Nutrition*, **131**(11), 3034S.

Weidner, M. S. and Sigwart, K. (2000). The safety of ginger extract in the rat. *Journal of Ethnopharmacology*, **73**, 513–520.

Weidner, M. S. and Sigwart, K. (2001). Investigation on the teratogenic potential of a *Zingiber officinale* extract in the rat. *Reproductive Toxicology*, **15**, 1575–1580.

Weiss, E. A. (1997). *Essential Oil Crops*. Oxford, UK: CAB International, 76.

Wilkinson, J. M. (2000). Effect of ginger tea on the foetal development of Sprague-Dawley rats. *Reproductive Toxicology*, **14**, 507–512.

Young, H. Y., Liao, J. C. Chang, Y. S., Luo, Y. L., Lu, M. C. and Peng, W. H. (2006). Synergistic effect of ginger and nifedipine on human platelet aggregation: A study in hypertensive patients and normal volunteers. *American Journal of Chinese Medicine*, **34**, 545–551.

24 Single Herb to Single Phytochemical–Based Therapy for Diabetes Mellitus

Bhoomika M. Patel, Hemangi Rawal and Ramesh K. Goyal

CONTENTS

Diabetes mellitus is a group of metabolic disorders shown by increases in blood glucose levels. Over the decades, the prevalence of diabetes has continuously increased. In 1964, about 30 million people were reported to suffer from diabetes worldwide (Entmacher and Marks 1965). According to the International Diabetes Federation, there were 425 million adults with diabetes and this is expected to increase to 629 million by 2045 (International Diabetes Federation 2017). Diabetes can cause both microvascular and macrovascular complications that are the major causes of the mortality and morbidity among the people suffering from diabetes. Microvascular complications include retinopathy, nephropathy and neuropathy (Harris et al. 1992), while macrovascular complications include mainly coronary heart disease, cerebrovascular disease (stroke) and peripheral vascular disease (Tuomilehto and Rastenyte 1997). In addition to long-term complications, diabetes mellitus is also an important constituent of metabolic syndrome made up of a cluster of obesity and cardiovascular diseases. This syndrome is a major health concern, as it causes a five-fold increase in the risk of developing diabetes. Type 2 diabetes develops mainly through insulin resistance, which occurs due to the inability of the target tissue to respond to insulin, and it also contributes to morbid obesity.

The liver plays a major role in insulin resistance and is the physiological mechanism involved in handling carbohydrates, and fats to regulate energy supply and demands within the body. When there is increase in glucose levels in the system, the liver stores the excess in the form of glycogen, and when it gets lower, it converts some of the glycogen to glucose and makes it available for the body to use. Recently, there is a growing interest in the liver as one of the major organs involved in the development of insulin resistance. Moreover, leptin is a key player in the regulation of lipids in the body, and leptin itself is regulated by the liver (Martí et al. 1999). Thus, an antidiabetic agent that acts through liver could be strategically beneficial in cluster of metabolic syndrome.

There are several antidiabetic drugs available that work by targeting different organs. Sulphonylurea and meglitinides act by increasing the secretion of insulin in the pancreas (Dornhorst 2001; Gribble and Reimann 2002). GLP-1 receptor (GLP-1R) agonists (GLP-1RA) mediate their antidiabetic action by acting on the pancreas and increasing the secretion of insulin and reducing the production of glucagon while dipeptidyl peptidase 4 (DPP-4) inhibitors (DPP-4i) increase the endogenous levels of incretin by blocking the action of DPP-4 (Verspohl 2009). Sodium–glucose cotransporter 2 (SGLT-2) inhibitors (SGLT-2i) work to reduce the renal reabsorption of glucose (Bailey 2011). Thiazolidinediones and metformin are two agents acting on the liver. Thiazolidinediones (TZDs) increase the sensitivity of insulin in the skeletal muscle, adipose tissue and liver (Yki-Jarvinen 2004). Metformin decreases the concentration of glucose by increasing the insulin sensitivity peripherally and enhancing insulin-mediated glucose uptake in skeletal muscle of type 2 diabetic subjects. It is now clear that metformin causes inhibition of gluconeogenesis, causes reduction in hepatic glucose output, and lowers fasting blood glucose concentration in the liver, in addition to its other effects on peripheral use of glucose inhibiting gluconeogenesis, reducing hepatic output of glucose and reducing the fasting glucose concentration in the liver (Delibegovic et al. 2009).

With the advancements in technology and molecular biology, there has been a better understanding of diabetes and its novel targets. Despite this, diabetes mellitus has been on the rise for years (Figure 24.1). Herbal drugs have therefore been important sources for novel agents, acting by varied mechanisms and that are also considered to be safe. The World Health Organization (WHO) has also recommended standards to promote traditional/herbal drugs in national healthcare programmes because such drugs are easily available, comparatively cheap and safe, and people also

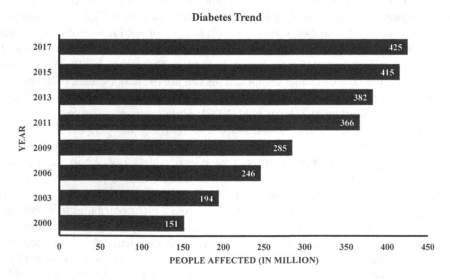

FIGURE 24.1 Trend of diabetes from 2000 to 2017.

have faith in such remedies. Scientific investigation of medicinal plants to identify novel bioactive phytochemicals with therapeutic potential has come to be the core area of research in the pharmaceutical industry today.

24.1 *ENICOSTEMA LITTORALE*: A POTENTIAL ANTIDIABETIC HERB WITH CARDIOPROTECTIVE EFFECTS

Enicostema littorale Blume is a glabrous perennial herb belonging to the *Gentianaceae* family (Kirtikar and Basu 1935). It grows all over India, although more frequently near the sea, and reaches the height of 1.5. It is called *Chota-kirayata* or *Chotachirayata* in Hindi, *Mamejavo* in Gujarati, *Nagajivha* in Bengal and *Vellarugu* or *Vallari* in Tamil. Chemically, *E. littorale* contains catechins, sterols, saponins, steroids, triterpenoids, alkaloids and volatile oil (Natarajan and Prasad 1972; Retnam and DeBritto 1988). Some of the important chemical constituents identified in the plant are glycosides like betulin, swertiamarin (Desai et al. 1966; Rai and Thakar 1966; Vishwakarma et al. 2004) and monoterpene; alkaloids like enicoflavine and gentiocrucine (Ghosal et al. 1974; Chaudhuri et al. 1975); phenolic acids such as vanillic acid, syringic acid, p-hydroxy benzoic acid, protocatechuic acid, p-coumaric acid and ferulic acid (Daniel and Sabnis 1978); and flavonoids such as apigenin, genkwanin, isovitexin, swertisin, saponarin, 5-O-glucosylswerisin and 5-O-glucosylisoswertisin (Ghoswal and Jaiswal 1980).

E. *littorale* has been used as a folk medicine for the treatment of diabetes mellitus in Western and Southern India (Gupta et al. 1962). For more than a decade, this plant has been widely studied for its antidiabetic efficacy using crude extracts and in recent years, even the active constituents have been isolated and detailed mechanistic studies have also been carried out. Surprisingly, there is a stark coincidence between *E. littorale* and metformin. Metformin was isolated from a French plant *Galega officinale*, which was reported to have anti-malarial effects and has become a first-line choice of drug in diabetes. *E. littorale* was also reported in 1947 in the Indian Medical Gazette for its anti-malarial action (Rai 1946).

24.1.1 CLINICAL STUDIES PERTAINING TO *E. LITTORALE*

E. littorale has been evaluated clinically for its antidiabetic action. In one such study, pills prepared from *E. littorale* were given to 84 patients suffering from type 2 diabetes for 9 months. The treatment caused a significant reduction in blood glucose and insulin levels and also led to an improvement in kidney function, lipid profile and blood pressure, suggesting that this herbal extract has a potent antidiabetic effects. (Upadhyay and Goyal 2004). The long-term effect of the extract was then evaluated over 5 years in selected patients of the previous study, who took *E. littorale* regularly for 5 years or more and compared with selected diabetic patients who were not taking *E. littorale* regularly for the last 5 years or more. The results suggested that the patients treated with the extract showed better glycaemic control by maintaining normal blood glucose levels and insulin sensitivity, triglycerides (as measured by lipid tolerance test) and preserved cardiac and renal functions. Additionally, the patients taking *E. littorale* regularly exhibited prevention of DNA damage as evaluated by comet assay. It was therefore concluded that the extract can be used as a safe and effective supplementary therapy for long-term management of patients with type 2 diabetes mellitus (Mansuri et al. 2009). Table 24.1 contains the summary of the studies that are described earlier.

TABLE 24.1

Summary of the Clinical Studies Pertaining to *E. littorale*

Constituent/Extract Used	Subjects Used	Key Results	References
Pills of *Enicostemma littorale*	Patients with type 2 diabetes mellitus	It caused a significant reduction in blood glucose levels and insulin levels and also lead to an improvement in kidney function, lipid profile and blood pressure	Upadhyay et al. (2004)
Pills of *Enicostemma littorale*	Patients with type 2 diabetes mellitus	The extract showed better glycaemic control by maintaining normal blood glucose levels and insulin sensitivity, lipid profile, cardiac function and does not cause DNA damage as compared to those who dint take the extract regularly but took the conventional antidiabetic medications regularly	Mansuri et al. (2009)

24.2 *IN VIVO* ANTIDIABETIC STUDIES

Moving with the concept of reverse pharmacology, various *in vivo* pharmacological studies were carried out after confirming the efficacy of *E. littorale* in diabetic patients. Different extracts of *E. littorale* have been studied in animal models of both type 1 and type 2 diabetes mellitus.

24.2.1 TYPE 1 DIABETES MELLITUS

The effect of *E. littorale* has been studied with various types of extracts in type 1 diabetes models. One of the studies by Maroo et al. (2003b) showed dose-dependent hypoglycaemic effects of an aqueous extract of *E. littorale* in alloxan-induced type 1 diabetes in male Charles Foster rats. The results suggested that when the rats were treated at different doses (0.5, 1.0, 1.5, 2.5, 3.5 g dry plant equivalent extract/100 g body wt., p.o.), the effective dose was found to be 1.5 g, which led to a significant reduction in glycosylated haemoglobin levels, glucose-6-phosphatase activity in the liver and significant increase in serum insulin levels in diabetic rats as compared to the control group. However, at the doses of 2.5 and 3.5 g, toxicity was observed, which lead to mortality among the treatment group compared to the control group. There were mild gastrointestinal tract (GIT) disturbances when the extract was given to the rats at lower doses, while at higher doses these GIT disturbances were quite profound, which could be one of the contributing factors that led to the mortality among rats treated at a higher dose. A similar study was conducted (Rajamani et al. 2013) to determine the hypoglycaemic effect of aqueous extract *E. littorale* in alloxan-induced type 1 diabetes in female albino Wistar rats, which suggested that when the plant aqueous extract was given orally for 45 days, it caused a significant reduction in blood glucose, concentration of TBARS (Thiobarbituric Acid) and HP and increased the concentration of GSH and the activities of GPx (glutathione peroxidase) and SOD (superoxide dismutase and catalase in the liver, kidney, and pancreas). It was also suggested that *E. littorale* showed greater efficacy at a dose of 2 gm/kg compared to 1 gm/kg. It was concluded that the antioxidant potential of this extract was due to the various alkaloids, sterols, catechins and flavonoids, and this was responsible for the therapeutic effect of the aqueous extract of the drug (Mishra et al. 2017). Vijayvargia et al. (2000) also conducted a study to test the hypoglycemic effects of the aqueous extract of the plant on both normoglycaemic and hyperglycaemic Charles Foster male albino rats. Alloxan was used to induced hyperglycaemia in the rats. No significant changes were observed in normoglycaemic rats, while in the hyperglycaemic rats there was a significant drop that was observed in the blood glucose levels within 30 days of treatment with the aqueous extract of the drug. Apart from the decrease in the plasma glucose levels, there was a decrease in the glycosylated haemoglobin levels and also the activity of glucose-6-phosphatase in the liver.

Although various studies concluded that the aqueous extract of this drug can be used as a potent antidiabetic agent in cases of moderate diabetes, Vishwakarma et al. (2010) showed some different observations. They reported that dose-dependent effects of aqueous extract (hot and cold) of *E. littorale* (0.5, 1 and 2 g/kg, p.o.) on streptozotocin (STZ)-induced type 1 diabetic male Sprague Dawley rats significantly reduced the elevated glucose, $AUC_{glucose}$ levels, serum cholesterol and triglyceride in the rats, but at a lower dose (0.5 g/kg) treatment with the hot aqueous extract produced a significant decrease in serum glucose and triglycerides, but the serum cholesterol and $AUC_{glucose}$ levels were not significantly altered. The study also showed that the cold extract of *E. littorale* failed to produce any changes even at the concentration of 1 or 2 g/kg. The results were related to swertiamarin content. When TLC was done with both hot and cold extracts, the active phytoconstituent swertiamarin was found to be one of the major components present only in the hot extract and not in cold the extract. Another interesting observation was the weight gain seen in the animals that were treated with a dose of 2 g/kg, which was not seen at lower doses. The results suggested that swertiamarin, a major constituent of the hot extract of *E. littorale*, might be responsible for the potent antidiabetic activity and anti-dyslipidaemic effect.

24.2.2 ACTIVITY-GUIDED STUDIES IN TYPE 1 DIABETIC ANIMAL MODEL AND TARGET IDENTIFICATION

The studies triggered detailed activity guided phytochemical studies of *E. littorale*. Having studied the aqueous extract of *E. littorale*, various alcoholic and hydro-alcoholic extract were studied by various authors in type 1 diabetes. The methanolic extract was reported to exhibit a hypoglycaemic and antioxidant effect in alloxan-induced type 1 diabetic male Charles Foster rats (Maroo et al. 2003a). The extract caused an increase in the levels of serum insulin and also improved the antioxidant status of these rats. The antioxidant effect of the extract was monitored by measuring blood GSH levels, erythrocyte CAT activity, GSH and LPO. These results also suggest that *E. littorale* has a potent antidiabetic activity, as well as a potent antioxidant activity, which could be very useful for the treatment of diabetes and has great potential for being developed as an antidiabetic agent. In another study, the methanolic extract was studied for its efficacy in diabetic neuropathy using alloxan-induced diabetes in male Charles Foster rats (Bhatt et al. 2009). The result suggested that the therapy significantly improved nociception in diabetic rats and the changes in lipid peroxidation status and antioxidant enzymes, such as superoxide dismutase, glutathione peroxidase and catalase levels observed in diabetic rats, were also significantly restored with the above treatment. The decrease in Na-K$^+$ ATPase activity was also significantly restored by *E. littorale*, which could possibly be due to the inhibition of oxidative stress and also by the amelioration of vascular function. It was therefore concluded that the plant extract has a great efficacy in treating diabetes, and it is also found to have an effect on nerve function and oxidative stress in rats suffering from diabetic neuropathy. Studies were also conducted to determine the mechanism of action of *E. littorale*. Maroo et al. (2002) conducted a study where a single dose of aqueous extract of *E. littorale* was given to alloxan-induced diabetic male Charles Foster rats. The extract caused a glucose-dependent insulin release. The insulinotropic action of aqueous extract of *E. littorale* was further investigated using pancreatic islets from the rats. When it was incubated with a Ca^{2+} chelator (EGTA) and Ca^{2+} channel blocker (nimodipine), the glucose-induced insulin release was not affected. These results suggested that the glucose-lowering effect of aqueous extract of *E. littorale* was associated with potentiation of glucose-mediated insulin release through K$^+$ATP channel-dependent pathway and which does not require Ca^{2+} influx.

Srivastava et al. (2016) carried out a study to demonstrate the potent anti-apoptotic and cytopro-tective activity of the methanolic extract of *E. littorale* in isolated islets of adult virgin male rats of Charles-Foster strain. The reactive oxygen species (ROS) of the islets was quantified by 2′,7′-dichloro-fluorescein diacetate dye staining and cell death using PS (Annexin V-FITC)/PI (propidium iodide) and FDA (fluorescein diacetate)/PI staining. Comet assay, biochemical assessment of caspase-3 and antioxidant enzyme activities along with immunoblotting of PARP-1, caspase-3, TNF-α activation and p-P38 MapK (stress kinase) induction were also performed in this study. The study suggested that the methanolic extract of *E. littorale* caused a decrease in the intracellular ROS, as well as cell death. Also, the levels of caspase-3 activity, PARP-1 cleavage, p-P38 MapK (stress kinase) activation and TNF-α levels, which had been significantly elevated earlier, were normalised. Antioxidant enzymes along with Comet assay demonstrated that pretreatment with this extract can augment antioxidant enzyme activities and can protect against DNA damage. From the above study, it was concluded that *E. littorale* protects the islets or the beta cells from oxidative stress-induced apoptosis by blocking the ROS-mediated damage of the DNA, increasing the activity of the antioxidants and suppressing the expression of the intra-islet stress kinase and pro-inflammatory cytokines. Thus it can be considered as a novel therapeutic agent that protects the islets of Langerhans at various levels against oxidative stress. Table 24.2 summarises the *in vivo* studies carried out on type 1 diabetes model rats.

TABLE 24.2

Summary of the *In Vivo* Studies Carried Out on Type 1 Diabetes Model Rats

Extract Used	Animal Model	Key Result	References
Aqueous extract	Alloxan-induced diabetes in male Charles Foster rats	At the effective dose, the extract caused a significant decrease in glycosylated haemoglobin, liver glucose-6-phosphatase activity and significant increase in serum insulin levels where as no significant differences were found between the toxicity parameters of the extract diabetic rats as compared to the control group.	Maroo et al. (2003b)
Aqueous extract	Alloxan-induced diabetes in diabetes female albino Wistar rats	It showed a decrease in the blood glucose, concentration of TBARS (thiobarbituric acid) and HP and increased the concentration of GSH and the activities of GPx (glutathione peroxidase), SOD (superoxide dismutase and catalase in liver, kidney and pancreas. It was also suggested that *Enicostema littoral* showed greater efficacy at a dose of 2 gm/kg as compared to 1 gm/kg.	Rajamani et al. (2013)
Aqueous extract	Normoglycaemic and hyperglycaemic using alloxan induced in Charles Foster male albino rats	Apart from the decrease in the plasma glucose levels, there was a decrease in the glycosylated haemoglobin levels and also the activity of glucose-6-phosphatase in the liver.	Vijayvargia et al. (2000)

(Continued)

TABLE 24.2 *(Continued)*

Summary of the *In Vivo* Studies Carried Out on Type 1 Diabetes Model Rats

Extract Used	Animal Model	Key Result	References
Aqueous extracts (hot and cold)	Streptozotocin (STZ)-induced type 1 diabetic male Sprague Dawley rats	Treatment with 1 and 2 g/kg of the hot extract significantly reduced the elevated glucose, $AUC_{glucose}$ levels, serum cholesterol and triglyceride in the rats whereas the treatment with the hot aqueous extract at 0.5 g/kg produced a significant decrease in serum glucose and triglycerides but the serum cholesterol and $AUC_{glucose}$ levels were not significantly altered. The cold extract failed to produce any changes even at the concentration of 1 or 2 gm/kg. Weight gain was seen in the subjects that were treated with a dose of 2 gm/kg that was not seen at lower doses. It suggests that the extract also causes a significant improvement in the lipid profile apart from its antidiabetic activity.	Vishwakarma et al. (2010)
Methanol extract	Alloxan-induced diabetic male Charles Foster rats	The extract caused an increase in the serum insulin levels and also improved the antioxidant status of these rats. Another interesting factor that was observed was the increase in the GSH levels and also significant decrease erythrocyte catalase activity (CAT) and lipid peroxidation (LPO). Apart from potent antidiabetic activity it also has a potent antioxidant activity.	Maroo et al. (2003a)
Methanolic extract	Alloxan-induced diabetes in male Charles Foster rats	The extract was found to have an effect on the nerve function and oxidative stress in the rats suffering from diabetic neuropathy.	Bhatt et al. (2009)
Aqueous extract	Alloxan-induced diabetic male Charles Foster rats	The results suggested that the glucose lowering effect of aqueous extract of *E. littorale* was associated with potentiation of glucose-induced insulin release through K^+ATP channel dependent pathway and does not require Ca^{2+} influx.	Maroo et al. (2002)
Methanolic extract	Islets of adult virgin male rats of Charles Foster strain	It was suggested that *Enicostema littorale* protects the islets or the beta cells from the oxidative stress induced apoptosis by blocking the ROS mediated damage of the DNA, increasing the activity of the antioxidants, suppressing the expression of the intra-islet stress kinase and pro-inflammatory cytokines.	Srivastava et al. (2016)

24.2.3   Type 2 Diabetes Mellitus

Similar to the reports of type 1 diabetes, extensive studies have also been reported with respect to effect of *E. littorale* in type 2 diabetes. A study was conducted to show the hypoglycaemic effects of the aqueous extract of *E. littorale* daily for 6 weeks in STZ-induced neonatal NIDDM (non-insulin dependent diabetes mellitus) albino Wistar rats (Murali et al. 2002). The results of the oral glucose tolerance test (OGTT) and insulin sensitivity test suggested that the extract caused a decrease in both glucose and insulin levels and also caused an increase in insulin sensitivity. Apart from these hypoglycaemic effects, the extract also produced anti-dyslipidaemic and nephroprotective effects. Thus, it was concluded that this herbal extract can be used safely in diabetics to prevent long-term complications of diabetes mellitus.

Encouraged with the results of the crude aqueous extracts, Vishwakarma et al. (2003) conducted a comparative evaluation using different fractions of aqueous extracts of the plant, including toluene, ethyl acetate, *n*-butanol and chloroform, to test its antidiabetic activity on STZ-induced neonatal NIDDM type 2 albino Sprague Dawley rats. The results suggested that there was a significant decrease in the fasting glucose and insulin levels in the rats treated with the ethyl acetate, *n*-butanol and aqueous extract of the plants compared to the control group, while the toluene and the chloroform fractions did not produce any effects on the glucose and insulin levels. The phytochemical investigations that were done suggested that the *n*-butanol and ethyl acetate fractions contain triterpenoids, coumarins, alkaloids and flavonoids. It was further suggested that the triterpenoids were responsible for the lipid-lowering activities, while the flavonoids were responsible for the antioxidant activity, which might be responsible for the observed beneficial effects that were seen with the use of *E. littorale*. Thus, it was concluded that the aqueous extract of *E. littorale* and its *n*-butanol and ethyl acetate fractions were responsible for its potent antidiabetic activity. In addition to this, these extracts were also responsible for lowering the serum lipid levels and protecting against liver and kidney dysfunction.

Hydroalcoholic fractions were also used to evaluate efficacy in a study conducted by Deepa et al. (2012). Nanocapsules of ethanolic extract of *E. littorale* were prepared and its antidiabetic efficacy was compared to the crude extract of *E. littorale* in STZ-induced diabetic male albino Wistar rats. An oral dose of 20 mg/kg nanocapsule and 2000 mg/kg of crude extract was used. Both had a similar antidiabetic effect, reducing the blood glucose, triglycerides, cholesterol, creatinine, ALT, AST and ATP levels. The nanocapsule was used in a dose 100 times lower than the crude extract and still exhibited better results within 10 days of treatment. Both nanocapsules and extract showed low expansion of the islets and reduced the number of injuries to the pancreas, and did not cause an increase in the number of islets, suggesting that the glucose-lowering effect of the plant extract is not due to the increase in the number of islets but is possibly due to the K_{ATP} mediated glucose-dependent insulin release. Thus, the authors further suggested that the nanoemulsification method can be applied for poor water-soluble ethanolic herbal extracts to reduce the dosage and time of treatment. Table 24.3 summarises the *in vivo* studies carried out on type 2 diabetes model rats.

TABLE 24.3

Summary of the *In Vivo* Studies Carried Out on Type 2 Diabetes Model Rats

Constituent/Extract Used	Animal Model	Key Result	References
Aqueous extract	Streptozotocin-induced diabetes in neonatal non-insulin dependent diabetes mellitus (NIDDM) albino rats of Wistar strain	The extract caused a decrease in both glucose and insulin levels and also caused an increase in the insulin sensitivity. Apart from these hypoglycaemic effects the extract also produced anti-dyslipidaemic and nephroprotective effects.	Murali et al. (2002)
Toluene, ethyl acetate, *n*-butanol and chloroform fraction of aqueous extracts	Streptozotocin-induced diabetes in albino Sprague Dawley rats	The aqueous extract of *Enicostema littorale* and its *n*-butanol and ethyl acetate fractions were responsible for its potent antidiabetic activity. In addition to this, these extracts are also responsible for lowering the serum lipid levels and protecting against the liver and kidney dysfunction.	Vishwakarma et al. (2003)
Ethanolic extract and nanocapsules of ethanolic extract	Streptozotocin-induced diabetic male albino Wistar rats	Both of them had a similar antidiabetic effect, reducing the blood glucose, triglycerides, cholesterol, creatinine, ALT, AST, and ALP levels. The NEL was used in a 100 times less dose than EL and still exhibited better results within 10 days of treatment. Both NEL and EL showed low expansion of the islets and reduced the number of injuries to the pancreas. Both NEL and EL did not cause an increase in the number of islets suggesting that, the glucose lowering effect of the plant extract is not due to the increase in the number of islets but it is possibly due to the K_{ATP} mediated, glucose-dependant insulin release.	Deepa et al. (2012)

24.3   ACTIVE CONSTITUENTS OF *E. LITTORALE,*
SWERTIAMARIN: CELLULAR STUDIES

Swertiamarin is a seco-iridoid glycoside and has a number of reported pharmacological effects such as hepatoprotective, anti-oedematogenic/anti-inflammatory, free radical scavenging activity and antispastic activity (Vaijanathappa and Badami 2009). Taking the leads from different fractions and extracts, different scientists have carried out several studies using active constituents of *E. littorale.* Vaidya et al. (2012a) conducted a study using swertiamarin, which is a chief constituent of *E. littorale.* Swertiamarin was given once a day for a period of 6 weeks to STZ-induced type 2 diabetes in 2-day-old pups and neonates. It caused a significant reduction in the fasting blood glucose levels, along with an increase in the insulin sensitivity index. It also demonstrated a significant reduction in serum triglycerides, cholesterol and low-density lipoprotein (LDL) levels in diabetic animals compared with diabetic control animals. Because insulin plays an important role in lipid metabolism by regulating a number of enzymes like HMG-CoA reductase and lipoprotein lipase, swertiamarin – by increasing the insulin sensitivity index or increasing insulin use – helped in the reduction of serum triglycerides, cholesterol and low-density lipoprotein levels in diabetic animals. Vaidya et al. (2012b) also conducted a similar study to determine whether gentianine, an active metabolite of swertiamarin, is responsible for its antidiabetic effect. Swertiamarin treatment had no significant effect on adipogenesis or PPAR-g and GLUT-4 mRNA expression, but it caused a significant increase in adiponectin mRNA expression. On the other hand, when treatment was done with gentianine, it caused a significant increase in adipogenesis, which was associated with a significant increase in the mRNA expression of PPAR-g, GLUT-4 and adiponectin. It was therefore suggested that the antidiabetic effect of swertiamarin is due to gentianine, an active metabolite of swertiamarin. Another study was conducted by Patel et al. (2013) to understand the molecular mechanism of swertiamarin, obtained from *E. littorale,* by comparing its molecular effects with the aqueous extract on insulin resistance in type 2 diabetes. The hypolipidaemic and insulin-sensitising effects of swertiamarin were also investigated in experimentally induced NIDDM in male Charles Foster rats. It was seen that they work by restoring G6Pase and HMG-CoA reductase activities to normal levels and restoring normal transcriptional levels of PEPCK, GK, Glut 2, PPAR-γ, leptin, adiponectin, LPL, SREBP-1c and Glut 4 genes, suggesting that the extract corrects dyslipidaemia by increasing insulin sensitivity (Qin et al. 2003). When the diabetic animals were treated with the aqueous extract and swertiamarin, it caused an increase in the insulin receptor protein synthesis and its autophosphorylation in the liver and adipose tissue, which may be responsible for the increase in the insulin sensitivity in TIIDM (Kadowaki et al. 2003). The current study proves that swertiamarin activates PPAR-γ and its regulatory genes, which causes an improvement in the fat metabolism in adipose tissues. By controlling PPAR-γ, swertiamarin maintains the status of small adipocytes that reduce the expression of leptin and TNF-α and increase the expression of adiponectin. This adiponectin improves the expression of the insulin receptors, its autophosphorylation and the downstream insulin signalling in the liver, as well as the adipose tissue, by reducing the HMG-CoA reductase activities, so swertiamarin further contributes in the treatment of dyslipidaemia. It can be considered as a drug that can regulate the different players that are involved in carbohydrate and fat metabolism in the peripheral tissues. It was therefore suggested that both treatments increased insulin sensitivity and regulated carbohydrate and fat metabolism.

Studies with swertiamarin combined with *E. littorale* clearly indicated that, in addition to its potent antidiabetic actions, *E. littorale* could also be considered as an effective alternative for dyslipidaemia and thereby plays an important role in metabolic syndrome. Dadheech et al. (2013) also conducted a study to identify new agents that stimulated differentiation of islets for which various compounds were isolated from *E. littorale,* and several *in vitro* experiments were carried out using NIH3T3 cells, as well as *in vivo* studies. Reversal of hyperglycaemia was monitored after transplanting ILCC in STZ-induced diabetic BALB/c mice using methanolic extract.

During this study, swertisin was isolated, which was found to be the most effective in differentiating NIH3T3 into endocrine cells. The glucose-mediated release of insulin (*in vitro*) and decreased FBG (fasting blood glucose; *in vivo*) in transplanted diabetic BALB/c mice suggested that there was a functional maturity of ILCC. Insulin and glucagon expression in excised islet grafts suggested that there is survival and functional integrity. This suggested that swertisin, which is a readily available differentiating agent, can be made into a therapeutic tool for the effective treatment of diabetes.

A new arena for the treatment of diabetes is created through the multipotent differentiation property of stem cells. It is known that many chemical and biochemical compounds cause stem cells to differentiate into insulin-producing cells. In view of this, Gupta et al. (2010) conducted a study to determine the islet neogenic property of the plant *E. littorale*. An active compound, SGL-1, was isolated from the methanolic extract of the plant, which was used to differentiate between two stem cell lines, PANC-1 and NIH3T3. The study suggested that SGL-1 had great islet neogenic potential and has significant islet yield compared to the serum-free medium. When the morphological, molecular and immunological characterisation was carried out of newly generated ICAs (islet-like cellular aggregates) they were found to be differentiated and positive for islet hormone. When the functional characterisation of the ICAs was done, it was seen that there was a glucose-dependent insulin release. Thus, from the data mentioned above, it can be concluded that SGL-1 isolated from the plant has great potential to increase islet cell mass to treat diabetic patients (Mishra et al. 2017). Table 24.4 summarises the studies done using the active constituents of the plant.

TABLE 24.4

Summary of the Studies Carried Out Using the Active Constituents of the Plant

Constituent	Animal Model/Cell Line	Key Result	References
Swertiamarin	Streptozotocin-induced type 2 diabetes in 2-day-old pups and neonates	It caused a significant decrease in the fasting blood glucose levels along with an increase in the insulin sensitivity index. It also a significant reduction in serum triglycerides, cholesterol and low-density lipoprotein levels in diabetic animals as compared with diabetic control animals.	Vaidya et al. (2012a)
Gentianine, active metabolite of swertiamarin	3T3-L1	Swertiamarin treatment had no significant effect on adipogenesis, or the mRNA expression of PPAR-g and GLUT-4; but it caused a significant increase in the mRNA expression of adiponectin. On the other hand, when treatment was done with gentianine it caused a significant increase in adipogenesis, which was associated with a significant increase in the mRNA expression of PPAR-g, GLUT-4 and adiponectin suggesting that the antidiabetic effect of swertiamarin is due to gentianine, an active metabolite of swertiamarin.	Vaidya et al. (2012b)

(Continued)

TABLE 24.4 (*Continued*)

Summary of the Studies Carried Out Using the Active Constituents of the Plant

Constituent	Animal Model/Cell Line	Key Result	References
Swertiamarin	Non-insulin-dependent diabetes mellitus (NIDDM) in male Charles Foster rats	The current study proves that swertiamarin, activates PPAR-γ and its regulatory genes which causes and improvement in the fat metabolism in the adipose tissues. By controlling PPAR-γ, swertiamarin maintains the status of the small adipocytes that reduce the expression of leptin and TNF-α and increase the expression of adiponectin. This adiponectin secretion improves the expression of the insulin receptors, its autophosphorylation and the downstream insulin signalling in the liver as well as the adipose tissue. By reducing the HMG-CoA reductase activities swertiamarin further contributes in the treatment of dyslipidemia.	Patel et al. (2013)
Swertisin	STZ-induced diabetic BALB/c mice	The glucose induced insulin release (*in vitro*) and decreased fasting blood glucose (FBG) (*in vivo*) in transplanted diabetic BALB/c mice suggested that there was a functional maturity of ILCC. Insulin and glucagon expression in excised islet grafts suggested survival and functional integrity.	Dadheech et al. (2013)
Compound SGL-1	Stem cell lines PANC-1 and NIH3T3	SGL-1 had great islet neogenic potential and has significant islet yield as compared to the serum free medium. When the morphological, molecular and immunological characterisation was done of newly generated islet-like cellular aggregates (ICA's) they were found to be differentiated and positive for islet hormone. When the functional characterisation of the ICAs was done, it was seen that there was a glucose dependant insulin release.	Gupta et al. (2010)

24.4 FUTURE PERSPECTIVES

Diabetes has emerged as a syndrome that not only is associated with poor quality of life but also increased rate of mortality due to several complications. Our rich source of herbal heritage has provided many lead candidate drugs including taxanes, artemisin, digoxin, vincristine and vinblastine. Such success stories serve as a boost for various researchers to carry out systematic pharmacological studies using standardised extracts and isolated active constituents. Additionally, expansions in the field of molecular biology have paved the way for precise studies focussing on the exact mechanisms of action and thereby providing key lead drug candidates. *E. littorale* is a classic example that has provided positive lead drug candidates. Currently, swertiamarin and swertisin are two lead drugs that have shown promising results, and novel compounds using computer-aided drug design can be designed, synthesised and screened in future to provide a lead antidiabetic agent. Further clinical studies of such developed compounds will bring hope not only for diabetes, but also its associated complications so as to have an improved quality of life and better survival for the society.

REFERENCES

Bailey, C. J. (2011). Renal glucose reabsorption inhibitors to treat diabetes. *Trends in Pharmacological Sciences*, **32**, 63–71.

Bhatt, N. M., Barua, S. and Gupta, S. (2009). Protective effect of *Enicostemma littorale* Blume on rat model of diabetic neuropathy. *American Journal of Infectious Diseases*, **5**(2), 106–112.

Chaudhuri, R. K., Singh, A. K. and Ghosal S. (1975). Chemical constituents of gentianaceae. XVIII. Structure of Enicoflavine. Monoterpene alkaloids from *Enicostemma hyssopifolium*. *Chemistry and Industry*, **3**,127–128.

Dadheech, N., Soni, S. and Srivastava, A. (2013). A small molecule Swertisin from *Enicostemma littorale* differentiates NIH3T3 cells into islet-like clusters and restores normoglycemia upon transplantation in diabetic balb/c mice. *Evidence-Based Complementary and Alternative Medicine*, **2013**, 280392. doi:10.1155/2013/280392.

Daniel, M. and Sabnis, S. D. (1978). Chemical systematic of family Gentianaceae. *Current Science*, **47**, 109–111.

Deepa, V., Sridhar, R., Neelakanta, R. P. and Balakrishna, M. P. (2012). Development, characterization, efficacy and repeated dose toxicity of nanoemulsified ethanolic extract of *Enicostemma littorale* in streptozotocin-induced diabetes rats. *International Journal of Phytomedicine*, **4**(1), 70–89.

Delibegovic, M., Zimmer, D., Kauffman, C., et al. (2009). Liver-specific deletion of protein-tyrosine phosphatase 1B (PTP1B) improves metabolic syndrome and attenuates diet-induced endoplasmic reticulum stress. *Diabetes*, **58**, 590–599.

Desai, P. D., Ganguly, A. K., Govindachari, T. R., Joshi, B. S., Kamat, V. N., Manmade, A. H., et al. (1966). Chemical investigation of some Indian medicinal plants: Part II. *Indian Journal of Chemistry*, **4**, 457–459.

Dornhorst, A. (2001). Insulinotropic meglitinide analogues. *Lancet*, **358**, 1709–1716.

Entmacher, P. S., and Marks, H. H. (1965). Diabetes in 1964; a world survey. *Diabetes*, **14**, 212–223.

Ghosal, S., Singh, A. K., Sharma, P. V. and Chaudhuri, R. K. (1974). Chemical constituents of Gentianaceae IX: Natural occurrence of erythrocentaurin in *Enicostemma hyssopifolium* and *Swertia lawii*. *Journal of Pharmaceutical Sciences*, **63**(6), 944–945.

Ghoswal, S. and Jaiswal, D. K. (1980). Chemical constituents of Gentianaceae XXVIII: Flavonoids of *Enicostemma hyssopifolium* (Wild.) *Verd*. *Journal of Pharmaceutical Sciences*, **61**, 53–56.

Gribble, F. M. and Reimann, F. (2002). Pharmacological modulation of KATP channels. *Biochemical Society Transactions*, **30**, 333–339.

Gupta, S., Dadheech, N., Singh, A., Soni, S. and Bhonde, R. R. (2010). *Enicostemma littorale*: A new therapeutic target for islet of neogenesis. *International Journal of Integrative Biology*, **9**(1), 50.

Gupta, S. S., Seth, C. B. and Variyar, M. C. (1962). Experimental studies on pituitary diabetes. Part I. Inhibitory effect of a few ayurvedic antidiabetic remedies on anterior pituitary extract induced hyperglycemia in albino rats. *Indian Journal of Medical Research*, **50**, 73–81.

Harris, M. I., Klein, R., Welborn, T. A., et al. (1992). Onset of NIDDM occurs at least 4–7 yr before clinical diagnosis. *Diabetes Care*, **15**(7), 815–819.

International Diabetes Federation. (2017). *IDF Diabetes Atlas*, 8th edition. Brussels, Belgium: International Diabetes Federation.

Kadowaki, T., Hara, K. and Yamauchi, T. (2003). Molecular mechanism of insulin resistance and obesity. *Experimental Biology and Medicine*, **228**(10), 1111–1117.

Kirtikar, K. R. and Basu, B. D. (1935). *Indian Medicinal Plants*. 2nd edition. Dehradun, India: Bishen Singh Mahendra Pal Singh. pp. 1655–1656.

Mansuri, M. M., Goyal, B. R., Upadhyay, U. M., Sheth, J. and Goyal, R. K. (2009). Effect of long term treatment of aqueous extract of *Enicostemma littorale* in type 2 diabetic patients. *Oriental Pharmacy and Experimental Medicine*, **9**(1), 39–48.

Maroo, J., Ghosh, A., Mathur, R., Vasu, V. T. and Gupta, S. (2003a). Antidiabetic efficacy of *Enicostemma littorale* methanol extract in alloxan-induced diabetic rats. *Pharmaceutical Biology*, **41**(5), 388–391.

Maroo, J., Vasu, V. T., Aalinkeel, R. and Gupta, S. (2002). Glucose lowering effect of aqueous extract of *Enicostemma littorale* Blume in diabetes: A possible mechanism of action. *Journal of Ethnopharmacology*, **81**(3), 317–320.

Maroo, J., Vasu, V. T. and Gupta, S. (2003b). Dose dependent hypoglycemic effect of aqueous extract of *Enicostemma littorale* Blume in alloxan induced diabetic rats. *Phytomedicine*, **10**(2–3), 196–199.

Martí, A., Berraondo, B. and Martínez, J. A. (1999). Leptin: Physiological actions. *Journal of Physiology and Biochemistry*, **55**(1), 43–49.

Mishra, N., Kaushal, K., Mishra, R. and Sharma, A. K. (2017). An Ayurvedic herb: *Enicostemma littorale* Blume: A review article. *Journal of Medicinal Plants Studies*, **5**(1), 78–82.

Murali, B., Upadhyaya, U. M. and Goyal, R. K. (2002). Effect of chronic treatment with *Enicostemma littorale* in non-insulin-dependent diabetic (NIDDM) rats. *Journal of Ethnopharmacology*, **81**(2), 199–204.

Natarajan, P. N. and Prasad, S. (1972). Chemical investigation of *Enicotemma littorale*. *Planta Medica*, **22**, 42–46.

Patel, T. P., Soni, S. and Parikh, P. (2013). Swertiamarin: An active lead from *Enicostemma littorale* regulates hepatic and adipose tissue gene expression by targeting PPAR-Γ and improves insulin sensitivity in experimental NIDDM rat model. *Evidence-Based Complementary and Alternative Medicine*, **2013**, 358673. doi:10.1155/2013/358673.

Qin, M. B., Nagasaki, M. R. and Bajotto, G. (2003). Cinnamon extract (traditional herb) potentiates *in vivo* insulin-regulated glucose utilization via enhancing insulin signalling in rats. *Diabetes Research and Clinical Practice*, **62**(3), 139–148.

Rai, B. B. (1946). *Enicostema littorale* Blume in malaria. *Indian Medical Gazette*, **81**(12), 506–508.

Rai, J. and Thakar, K. A. (1966). Chemical investigation of *Enicotemma littorale* Blume. *Current Science*, **35**, 148–149.

Rajamani, S., Thirumalai, T., Hemalatha, M., Balaji, R. and David, E. (2013). Pharmacognosy of *Enicostemma littorale*: A review. *Asian Pacific Journal of Tropical Biomedicine*, **3**(1), 79–84.

Retnam, K. R. and DeBritto, A. J. (1988). Preliminary phytochemical screening of three medicinal plants of Tirunelveli hills. *Journal of Economic and Taxonomic Botany*, **22**, 677–681.

Srivastava, A., Bhatt, N. M. and Patel, T. P. (2016). Anti-apoptotic and cytoprotective effect of *Enicostemma littorale* against oxidative stress in islets of langerhans. *Pharmaceutical Biology*, **54**(10), 2061–2072.

Tuomilehto, J. and Rastenyte, D. (1997). Epidemiology of macrovascular disease and hypertension in diabetes mellitus. In K. Alberti, P. Zimmet, R. DeFronzo, et al., eds., *International Textbook of Diabetes Mellitus*. Chichester, UK: Wiley. pp. 1559–1583.

Upadhyay, U. M. and Goyal, R. K. (2004). Efficacy of *Enicostemma littorale* in type 2 diabetic patients. *Phytotherapy Research*, **18**(3), 233–235.

Vaidya, H., Goyal, R. K. and Cheema, S. K. (2012b). Anti-diabetic activity of swertiamarin is due to an active metabolite, gentianine, that upregulates PPAR-Γ gene expression in 3T3-L1 cells. *Phytotherapy Research*, **27**(4), 624–627.

Vaidya, H., Prajapati, A., Rajani, M., Sudarsanam, V., Padh, H. and Goyal, R. K. (2012a). Beneficial effects of swertiamarin on dyslipidaemia in streptozotocin-induced type 2 diabetic rats. *Phytotherapy Research*, **26**(8), 1259–1261.

Vaijanathappa, J. and Badami, S. (2009). Antiedematogenic and free radical scavenging activity of swertiamarin isolated form *Enicostemma axillare*. *Planta Medica*, **75**, 12–17.

Verspohl, E. J. (2009). Novel therapeutics for type 2 diabetes: Incretin hormone mimetics (glucagon-like peptide-1 receptor agonists) and dipeptidyl peptidase-4 inhibitors. *Pharmacology & Therapeutics*, **124**, 113–138.

Vijayvargia, R., Kumar, M. and Gupta, S. (2000). Hypoglycemic effect of aqueous extract of Enicostemma littorale Blume (chhota chirayata) on alloxan induced diabetes mellitus in rats. *Indian Journal of Experimental Biology*, **38**(8), 781–784.

Vishwakarma, S. L., Rajani, M., Bagul, M. S. and Goyal, RK. (2004). A rapid method for the isolation of swertiamarin from *Enicostemma littorale*. *Pharmaceutical Biology*, **42**, 400–403.

Vishwakarma, S. L., Rajani, M. and Goyal, R. K. (2003). Comparative antidiabetic activity of different fractions of *Enicostemma littorale* Blume in streptozotocin induced NIDDM rats. *Oriental Pharmacy and Experimental Medicine*, **3**(4), 196–204.

Vishwakarma, S. L., Sonawane, R. D., Rajani, M., Goyal, R. K., et al. (2010). Evaluation of effect of aqueous extract of *Enicostemma littorale* Blume in streptozotocin-induced type 1 diabetic rats. *Indian Journal of Experimental Biology*, **48**(1), 26–30.

Yki-Jarvinen, H. (2004). Thiazolidinediones. *New England Journal of Medicine*, **351**, 1106–1118.

25 Phytochemical, Pharmacological and Therapeutic Profile of *Bacopa monnieri*
A Prospective Complementary Medicine

Muhammad Shahid, Fazal Subhan, Nazar Ul Islam, Ihsan Ullah, Javaid Alam, Nisar Ahmad and Gowhar Ali

CONTENTS

25.1 INTRODUCTION

About 80% of the world population continues to use indigenous or traditional medicines for their primary healthcare needs. Traditional medicine is at present being revalued through extensive research activity on different plant species and their therapeutic constituents (Mahady 2001; Ayaz et al. 2017; Shahid et al. 2017a). *Bacopa monnieri* (Linn.) Pennell, [Syn. *Bacopa monnieri* (Linn.) Wettst., *Bacopa monniera, Monniera cuneifolia, Lysimachia monnieri, Gratiola monnieri, Herpestis monniera, Herpestis fauriei*] is commonly known as Jal Neem Buti, Brambhi, Brahmi, the thinking person's herb, water hyssop, baby tears or moneywort. It is a small creeping perennial herb from the Scrophulariaceae family that grows throughout the subcontinent in damp, wet and marshy places (Figure 25.1) (Russo and Borrelli 2005).

Bacopa monnieri occupies a predominant position in Ayurvedic medicine (Adams et al. 2007) and is traditionally used for memory enhancement, rejuvenation, increasing longevity and promoting progeny (Singh 2013), as a nervine tonic in India (Chunekar 1960), as an aphrodisiac (Loonoowella) in Sri Lanka, as a diuretic in Philippines (Russo and Borrelli 2005), as a blood purifier in the Nara desert of Pakistan (Qureshi and Raza Bhatti 2008) and recently for cognitive enhancement, antianxiety, antidepressant and for gastrointestinal disturbances (Gohil and Patel 2010).

This review summarises the available scientific information related to the botanical features and chemical studies including the identification and determination of active components and other chemical compounds contained therein. Information regarding the pharmacological studies in different organs systems and human studies available in the recent scientific literature is presented.

25.2 BOTANICAL FEATURES

Bacopa monnieri has succulent or sub-succulent, non hairy, hollow or solid, erect, quadrangular or procumbent stem; the leaves are simple, less than 2 cm long/wide, sessile, narrow or broad, opposite, evenly distributed on the stem, succulent, entire margin, rounded or obtuse apex, base obtuse or rounded or clasping, cuneate, pinnately veined without close parallel secondary venation, non-prominent midrib with non-waxy surface; flowers are single, stalked, less than 2 cm, purple or yellow, bisexual, axillary, solitary, with five or more petals or sepals and 2–5 stamens with non-hairy bracts; seeds are pitted or spiny, oblong/ellipsoid; fruit is a capsule (Russo and Borrelli 2005).

The majority of the commercial supply of *Bacopa monnieri* comes from the wild natural population (Rahman et al. 2002). In the summer and monsoon months (May to September), *Bacopa monnieri* branches proliferate and cover the entire soil surface with a network of foliage several centimetres thick, but at the onset of winter (November) the herb enters into senescence until spring (March). The crop renews its growth in summer and subsequently enters into a new season of higher rate of growth during the monsoon (Mathur et al. 2002).

The extensive use of *Bacopa monnieri* has led to its gradual reduction from natural sources (Karthikeyan et al. 2011), so techniques such as multiple shoot induction (Tiwari et al. 2006; Tiwari and Singh 2010), polyploidization (Salvio Escandón et al. 2006), cell

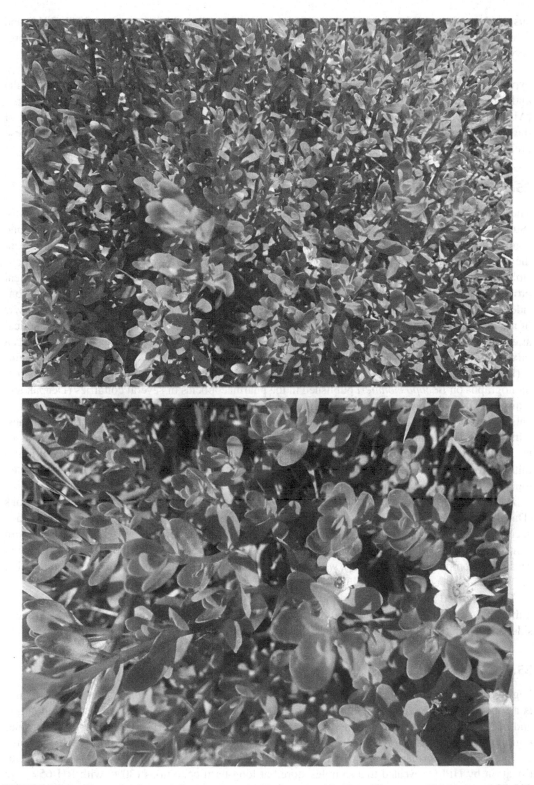

FIGURE 25.1   (See color insert.) *Bacopa monnieri* in its natural habitat. (Courtesy of Muhammad Shahid, Margalla Hills near Quaid-i-Azam University, Islamabad, Pakistan.)

suspension culture (Rahman et al. 2002), genetic transformation (Majumdar et al. 2011, 2012) and *in vitro* micropropagation (Sharma et al. 2010; Tanveer et al. 2010) have become imperative to preserve the biodiversity of the herb and provide a constant supply for pharmaceutical industries.

Bacopa monnieri is a fast-proliferating wetland species, which also grows in water and is often exposed to a large variety of pollutants, especially heavy metals like lead, manganese (Sinha and Saxena 2006), cadmium, mercury (Hussain et al. 2011), arsenic (Mishra et al. 2013), copper (Ali et al. 1998) and chromium (Shukla et al. 2007). *Bacopa monnieri* is also used as a model of the eco-genotoxicity assessment of wetland plants for the effects of pollutants contaminating these areas (Vajpayee et al. 2006).

25.3   CHEMICAL CONSTITUENTS

The major chemical constituents present in *Bacopa monnieri* are flavonoids, saponins, tannins, (Subhan et al. 2010), carotenoids (Singh et al. 2011), carbohydrates, steroids, terpenes, phenolic compounds (Shahare and D'Mello 2010) and alkaloids (Russo and Borrelli 2005). It is evident from the literature that saponins including bacosides A and B, as the primary complex mixture are responsible for the well-known nootropic effect of *Bacopa monnieri*, as well as other pharmacological properties (Calabrese et al. 2008; Shikha et al. 2009; Morgan and Stevens 2010). Bacoside A is considered as part of the major saponins, along with bacopaside I and constitutes more than 96% w/w of the total saponins of *Bacopa monnieri* (Deepak and Amit 2013). Bacoside B is in fact an optical artefact of bacoside A produced during isolation (Russo and Borrelli 2005). Bacoside A occurs as a mixture of bacoside-A_3, bacopaside-II, bacopasaponin-C, and jujubogenin isomer of bacopasaponin-C (Deepak et al. 2005). These saponins are now required to be measured for compliance to analytical monographs on *Bacopa monnieri* published in the pharmacopoeias of several countries (Deepak and Amit 2013). It is noteworthy that the dammarane-type triterpenoid saponins are the major constituents of several herbal drugs, including ginseng (Zhu et al. 2004), that have been used for centuries. Although jujubogenin glycosides have been isolated from a number of reputed medicinal plants of the Rhamnaceae and Scrophulariaceae families, *Bacopa monnieri* is unique in that – in addition to jujubogenin glycosides – pseudojujubogenin glycosides are also present and these have been reported together so far only from this medicinal plant (Garai et al. 1996; Russo and Borrelli 2005).

Bacopa monnieri possesses low levels of genetic diversity in geographically distinct accessions (Darokar et al. 2001); however, a significant variation exists in the bacoside A content of the various accessions collected from different locations (Deepak et al. 2005; Bansal et al. 2014). The saponin content of *Bacopa monnieri* is present in the highest concentration in the shoots during the rainy season (Phrompittayarat et al. 2011), with highest content of bacoside-A occurring at the completion of the growth phase (Mathur et al. 2002).

The reported chemical compounds isolated from *Bacopa monnieri* are summarised in Table 25.1. The structures of the major components of bacoside A are shown in Figure 25.2a (bacoside-A_3), 25.2b (bacopaside-II) and 25.2c (bacopasaponin-C).

25.4   ANALYSIS

High-performance liquid chromatography (HPLC) fingerprint analysis of bacoside-A shows that it is a saponin mixture with bacoside-A_3, bacopasaponin-C, jujubogenin isomer of bacopasaponin-C and bacopaside-II as major components (Deepak et al. 2005). High-performance thin-layer chromatography (HPTLC) shows an Rf value of 0.68, having a sensitivity of 46 ng and linearity in the range of 200–1200 ng (Shahare and D'Mello 2010). For stability assessment of *Bacopa monnieri*, quantification by HPLC revealed that samples stored at long-term conditions (30°C with RH 65%) are rich in bacoside A and bacopaside I components compared to storage of samples under accelerated conditions (40°C with RH 75%) (Srivastava et al. 2012). The HPLC system coupled with an evaporative light scattering detector (ELSD) for simultaneous determination of bacoside-A, bacoside-A_3,

TABLE 25.1
Reported Chemical Compounds Isolated from *Bacopa monnieri*

Chemical Compound	References
Bacopaside IX (3-*O*-{β-D-glucopyranosyl (1→4) [α-L-arabinofuranosyl-(1→2)]-β-D-glucop-yranosyl}- 20-*O*-α-L-arabinopyranosyljujubogenin)	Zhou et al. (2009)

Bacopasaponin-A
(3-*O*-α-Larabinopyranosyl-20-*O*-α-L-arabinopyranosyl-jujubogenin)
    Bacopasaponin-B
    (3-*O*-[α-L-arabinofuranosyl (1→2) α-L-arabinopyranosyl] pseudojujubogenin)
    Bacopasaponin-C
    (3-*O*-[β-D)-glucopyranosyl (1→3) {α-L-arabinofuranosyl (1→2)}α-L-arabinopyranosyl]
    pseudojujubogenin)
	Garai et al.
	(1996b)

Bacopasaponin-D (3-*O*-[α-L-arabinofuranosyl (I→2) β-D-glucopyranosyl] pseudojujubogenin)	Garai et al. (1996a)

Bacopasaponin-E
    (3-*O*-[β-D-glucopyranosyl (1→3) {α-L-arabinofuranosyl (1→2)} α-L-arabinopyranosyl]-20-
    O-(α-L-arabinopyranosyl) jujubogenin)
    Bacopasaponin-F
    (3-*O*-[β-D-glucopyranosyl (1→3) {α-L-arabinofuranosyl (1→2)} β-D-glucopyranosyl]-20-*O*-α-L-
    arabinopyranosyl) jujubogenin)
	Mahato et al.
	(2000)

Bacopaside-I
(3-*O*-α-arabinofuranosyl-(1→2)-[6-*O*-sulphonyl-β-D-glucopyranosyl-(1→3)]-α-L-arabinopyranosyl
pseudojujubogenin)
    Bacopaside-II
    (3-*O*-α-L-arabinofuranosyl-(1→2)-[β-D-glucopyranosyl (1→3)]-β-D-glucopyranosyl
    pseudojujubogenin)
	Chakravarty et al.
	(2001)

Bacopaside-III
    (3-*O*-[6-*O*-sulfonyl-*β*-D-glucopyranosyl-(1→3)]-α-L-arabinopyranosyl pseudojujubogenin)
    Bacopasaponin-G
    (3-*O*-[α-L-arabinofuranosyl-(1→2)]-α-L-arabinopyranosyl jujubogenin)
    Bacopaside-A
    ((3*R*)-1-octan-3-yl-(6-*O*-sulfonyl)-*β*-D-glucopyranoside)
    Bacopaside-B
    (3,4-dihydroxyphenylethyl alcohol (2-*O*-feruloyl)-*β*-D-glucopyranoside)
    Bacopaside-C
    ([5-*O*-*p*-hydroxybenzoyl-*β*-D-apiofuranosyl-(1f2)]-*β*-D-glucopyranoside)
	Hou et al. (2002)

Bacopaside-III
    (3-*O*-α-L-arabinofuranosyl (1→2)-β-D-glucopyranosyl jujubogenin)
    Bacopaside-IV
    (3-*O*-β-D-glucopyranosyl (1→3)-α-L-arabinopyranosyl jujubogenin)
    Bacopaside-V
    (3-*O*-β-D-glucopyranosyl (1→3)-α-L-arabinopyranosyl pseudojujubogenin)
	Chakravarty et al.
	(2003)

Bacosterol-3-*O*-β-D-glucopyranoside, Bacosine, Luteolin-7-*O*-β-glucopyranoside and Bacosterol	Bhandari et al. (2006)
Betulinic acid, Oroxindin (5,7-dihydroxy-8-methoxy-2-phenyl-4H-1-benzopyran-4-one-7-glucuronide), Wogonin (5,7-dihydroxy-8-methoxy-2-phenyl-4H-1-benzopyran-4-one)	Chaudhuri et al. (2004)

(Continued)

TABLE 25.1 (*Continued*)

Reported Chemical Compounds Isolated from *Bacopa monnieri*

Chemical Compound	References
p-Hydroxyl benzenemethanol, Ursolic acid, *p*-Hydroxyl benzoic acid, Lupeol, Loliolide, $\Delta^{5,24(28)}$-Ergostadien-3β-ol, β-Daucosterin, 28-Hydroxyllupeol, Stigmasterol-3-*O*-β-D-glucopyranoside, 3,4-Dimethoxycinnamic acid, Feruloyl glucoside, Rosavin, Ampelozigenin, Quercetin, Luteolin, Zizyotin and Apigenin	Zhou et al. (2007)
Bacobitacin-A (2,7β,16α,20R-tetrahydroxy-25-acetoxy-cucurbita-1,5,23E-triene-3,11,22-trione, Bacobitacin-B (2,20R-dihydroxy-16α,25-diacetoxy-cucurbita-1,5,23E-triene-3,11,22-trione, Bacobitacin-C (2-*O*-[{α-L-rhamnopyranosyl-(1→2)-α-L-arabifuranosyl-(1→4)}-{α-L-rhamnopyranosyl-(1→2)-α-L-arabinopyranosyl}] cucurbitacin E, Bacobitacin-D (2-*O*-[{α-L-rhamnopyranosyl-(1→2)-α-L-arabifuranosyl-(1→4)}-{α-L-rhamnopyranosyl-(1→2)-α-L-arabinopyranosyl}]-7β,16α,20R-trihydroxy-25-acetoxy-cucurbita 1,15,23E-triene-3,11,22-trione	Bhandari et al. (2007)
Monnieraside-I (α-*O*-[2-*O*-(4-hydroxybenzoyl)-β-D-glucopyranosyl]-4-hydroxyphenylethanol, Monnieraside-II (α-*O*-[2-*O*-(3-methoxy-4-hydroxycinnamoyl)-β-D-glucopyranosyl]-3,4-dihydroxyphenylethanol, Monnieraside-III (α-*O*-[2-*O*-(4-hydroxybenzoyl)-β-D-glucopyranosyl]-3,4-dihydroxyphenylethanol)	Chakravarty et al. (2002)
Bacopaside-N1 (3-*O*-[β-D-glucopyranosyl (1→3)-β-D-glucopyranosyl] jujubogenin, Bacopaside-N2 (3-*O*-[β-D-glucopyranosy l(1→3)-β-D-glucopyranosyl] pseudojujubogenin)	Sivaramakrishna et al. (2005)
Bacoside-A$_1$ (3-*O* [α-L-arabinofuranosyl (1→3) α-L-arabinopyranosyl] jujubogenin)	Jain and Kulshreshtha (1993)
Bacoside-A$_3$ (3-*O*-α-L-arabinofuranosyl-(1→2)-[β-D-glucopyranosyl-(1→3)]-β-D-glucopyranoside)	Rastogi et al. (1994)

bacopaside-I, bacopaside-II, bacopaside-X and bacopasaponin-C gives a recovery of 95.8%–99.0%, with detection limit of 0.54–6.06 µg/mL and quantification limit of 1.61–18.78 µg/mL (Bhandari et al. 2009). An HPLC system of Luna C-8 column of 3 µm material, methanol as mobile phase, flow rate of 0.5 mL/min and temperature of 40°C would enable the baseline separation of bacoside-A$_3$, bacopaside-II, bacopasaponin-C, bacopaside-IV and bacopaside-V in less than 30 min (Ganzera et al. 2004). Similarly, an HPLC system having a reversed phase C-18 column of 5 µm packing material and a mobile phase consisting of 0.05 M sodium sulphate buffer and acetonitrile in a ratio of 68.5:31.5 v/v at a flow rate of 1.0 mL/min and temperature of 30°C gives a highly specific, accurate and precise simultaneous determination of 12 major *Bacopa monnieri* saponins (Murthy et al. 2006). For rapid quantification of bacoside-A$_3$ and bacopaside-II in herbal extracts or formulation, reversed phase HPTLC and packed column supercritical fluid chromatography with photodiode array detection techniques offers good resolution and high-quality information on the major components (Agrawal et al. 2006). An HPLC system coupled to NMR and MS provides an

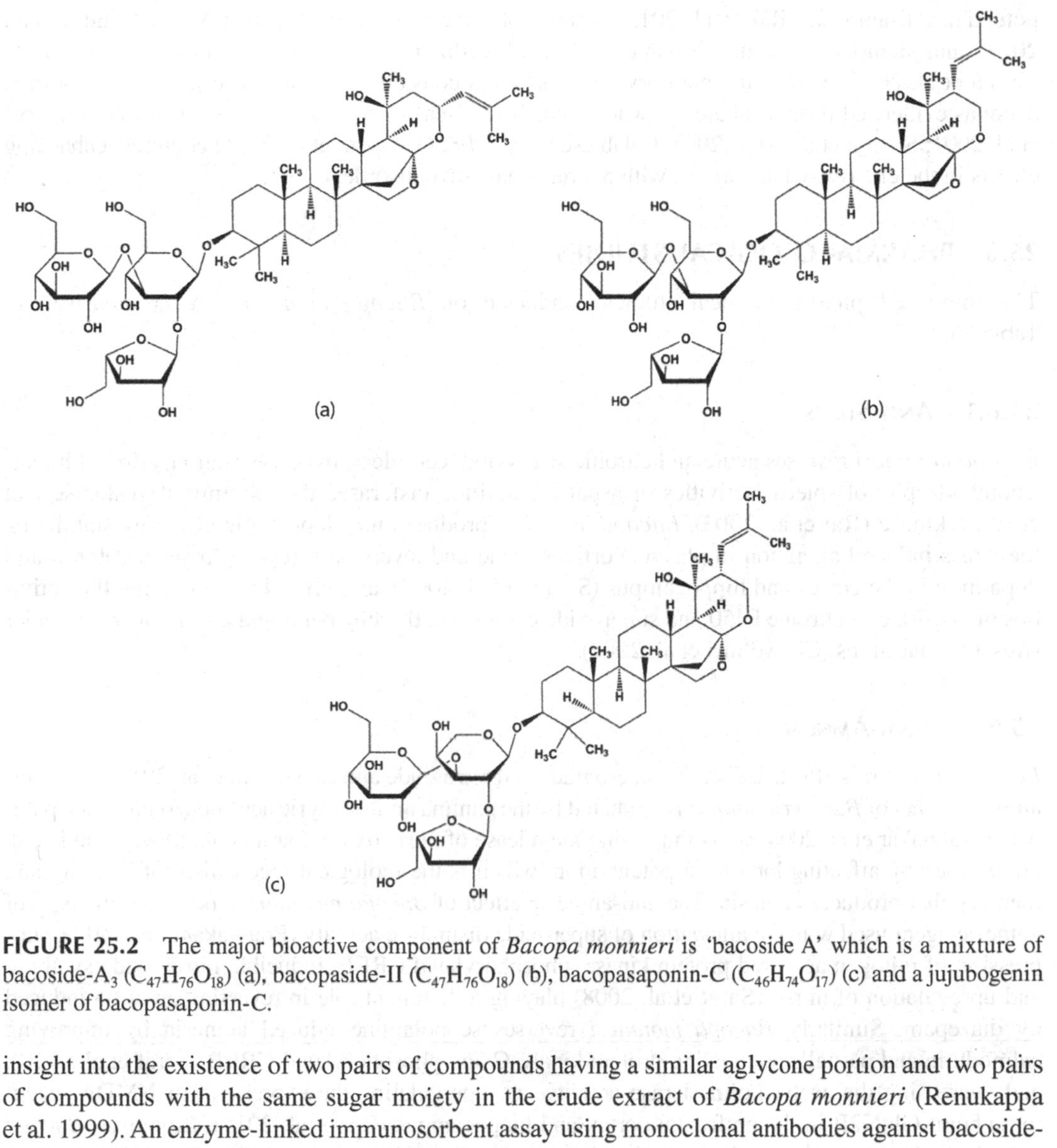

FIGURE 25.2 The major bioactive component of *Bacopa monnieri* is 'bacoside A' which is a mixture of bacoside-A$_3$ (C$_{47}$H$_{76}$O$_{18}$) (a), bacopaside-II (C$_{47}$H$_{76}$O$_{18}$) (b), bacopasaponin-C (C$_{46}$H$_{74}$O$_{17}$) (c) and a jujubogenin isomer of bacopasaponin-C.

insight into the existence of two pairs of compounds having a similar aglycone portion and two pairs of compounds with the same sugar moiety in the crude extract of *Bacopa monnieri* (Renukappa et al. 1999). An enzyme-linked immunosorbent assay using monoclonal antibodies against bacoside-A$_3$ for detection of small quantities of jujubogenin glycosides in *Bacopa monnieri* provides a precise, accurate and sensitive method, with a detection limit of 0.48 ng/mL (Tothiam et al. 2011).

25.5 STANDARDISED EXTRACTS

Recently, specific standardise extracts of *Bacopa monnieri* have emerged and are subjected to rigorous *in vitro*, animal and human clinical trials. The important standardised extracts include BacoMind (Natural Remedies; India) (Kasture et al. 2007; Pravina et al. 2007; Barbhaiya et al. 2008; Deb et al. 2008), KeenMind (Flordis; Australia) (Nathan et al. 2001; Stough et al. 2001, 2008, 2013), Bacognize capsules (Pharmanza Herbal; India) (Goswami et al. 2011), Memory Plus (Nivaran Herbal, Chennai, India) (Vohora et al. 2000), Brahmi capsule (Natural Remedies Pvt. Ltd., Bengaluru, India) (Hosamani 2009) and MediHerb Pty Ltd (Calabrese et al. 2008). Of these, the CDRI 08 extract marketed as KeenMind is a high-quality extract of *Bacopa monnieri* containing 55% bacosides (based on spectrophotometry), and it has been thoroughly studied in the Central Drug Research Institute (CDRI) in India. Research on CDRI 08 suggests that this extract of *Bacopa monnieri* has potential anti-amnesic (Rai et al. 2015), neuroprotective (Dulcy et al. 2012; Mondal and Trigun 2015), and memory-enhancing (Rajan et al. 2011; Preethi et al. 2012, 2014; Rani and Prasad 2015; Verma et al. 2015) effects in laboratory animals and is considered a safe and efficacious nootropic agent as evidenced from its acute (Downey et al. 2013; Benson et al. 2014) and chronic (Roodenrys et al. 2001; Stough et al. 2001, 2008; Calabrese et al. 2008; Goswami et al. 2011) cognitive-enhancing effects in the elderly and in patients with neurodegenerative disorders.

25.6 PHARMACOLOGICAL STUDIES

The important pharmacological studies conducted on *Bacopa monnieri* are summarised in Table 25.2.

25.6.1 ANTI-STRESS

Bacopa monnieri reverses acute and chronic stress–induced ulcer, hyperglycaemia, adrenal hypertrophy, atrophy of spleen, activities of aspartate aminotransferase, alanine aminotransferase and creatine kinase (Rai et al. 2003). *Bacopa monnieri* produces its adaptogenic effect by stabilising the stress induced alteration in plasma corticosterone and levels of norepinephrine, serotonin and dopamine in the cortex and hippocampus (Sheikh et al. 2007), as well as by modulating the activities of Hsp70, cytochrome P450 and superoxide dismutase, thereby helping the brain to work under stressful conditions (Chowdhuri et al. 2002).

25.6.2 ANTI-AMNESIC

Bacopa monnieri is effective for both anterograde and retrograde amnesia (Saraf et al. 2011). The anti-amnesic effect of *Bacopa monnieri* is mediated by the gamma aminobutyric acid-benzodiazepine pathway (Prabhakar et al. 2008) or by improving the release of nitric oxide (Saraf et al. 2009; Anand et al. 2010), thereby affecting long-term potentiation, which is the biological mechanism of learning and memory that produces amnesia. The anti-amnesic effect of *Bacopa monnieri* depends on the type of amnesic agent used with the alleviation of superoxide dismutase activity (Prabhakar et al. 2011), suppression of mitogen activated protein kinase, phosphorylated CREB, inducible nitric oxide synthase and upregulation of nitrite (Saraf et al. 2008) playing a dominant role in reversing amnesia induced by diazepam. Similarly, *Bacopa monnieri* reverses scopolamine-induced amnesia by improving calmodulin and partially attenuating protein kinase-C and phosphorylated-CREB (Saraf et al. 2010), and decreasing the acetylcholinesterase activity and upregulating the expression of NMDA receptor subunit GluN2B in the prefrontal cortex and hippocampus (Rai et al. 2015). Moreover, *Bacopa monnieri* – besides reducing the cognitive deficit side effect of phenytoin (Vohora et al. 2000) – also reduces D-galactose–induced contextual associative learning deficit by enhancing antioxidant enzyme activities and stabilising neurotransmitter release and synaptic proteins levels (Dulcy and Rajan 2009).

25.6.3 COGNITIVE ENHANCING

Bacopa monnieri is a well-known nootropic drug (Kasture et al. 2007) that has the potential to improve cognition – particularly the speed of attention (Kongkeaw et al. 2014). It produces enhanced memory retention and spatial learning performance (Vollala et al. 2010; Promsuban et al. 2017). The cognitive-enhancing effect of *Bacopa monnieri* is mediated through increased cerebral blood flow (Kamkaew et al. 2012); inhibition of acetylcholinesterase (Das et al. 2002); increased expression of serotonin reuptake transporter with increased synthesis (Charles et al. 2011) and level of serotonin (Dulcy and Rajan 2009); upregulation of the 5-HT$_{3A}$ receptor that facilitates the release of acetylcholine in the hippocampus and may activate GABAergic neurons – which enhances GABA release (Rajan et al. 2011); decreased neuronal degeneration, plasma corticosterone, oxidative stress and

TABLE 25.2

Summary of Important Pharmacological Studies on *Bacopa monnieri*

Pharmacological Effect	Treatment	Results	References
Adaptogenic	*Bacopa monnieri* 40 and 80 mg/kg po for 3 days in acute stress or 7 days in chronic stress	↓Ulcer index, adrenal gland weight ↑Spleen weight ↓Glucose level in acute stress ↑Glucose in chronic stress ↑ALT, AST and creatine kinase levels ↓Plasma corticosterone, 5HT, DA in acute stress ↑Level of NA, DA and 5-HT in chronic stress	Rai et al. (2003), Sheikh et al. (2007)
	Bacopa monnieri 20 and 40 mg/kg for 7 days	↓Expression of Hsp70 in hippocampus ↓SOD level in hippocampus ↓Cytochrome P450 enzymes activity	Chowdhuri et al. (2002)
Anticancer	Bacoside-A 15 mg/kg po for 16 weeks	↓Expression and activities of MMP-2 and MMP-9 ↓Levels of AFP, CEA and 5-nucleotidase ↓Level of lipopolysaccharide ↑Levels of vitamin C and E	(Janani et al. 2010a, 2010b)
	Cell viability was assessed at various concentrations (50–550 μg/mL) at different time intervals (12, 24 and 48 h)	↓GSH levels with induction of apoptotic cell death in S-180 cells at 550 μg/mL at 48 h	Rohini and Devi (2008)
Antiepileptic	*Bacopa monnieri* 50 mg/kg po in rats and 55 mg/kg in mice	↓Locomotor activity ↓strychnine and pentylenetetrazol-induced convulsions ↓hind limb extention ↑In the onset of hypoxia stree induced convulsions and lithium-pilocarpine induced status epilepticus	Kaushik et al. (2009)
	Bacopa monnieri and bacoside-A 300 mg/kg po for 15 days	Reverse the downregulation of GABA$_A$ receptor subunits in the cerebellum, hippocampus, striatum, cerebral cortex and enhances motor learning, memory and behavioural deficit	Mathew et al. (2010a, 2010b, 2011, 2012)
Anti-inflammatory	*Bacopa monnieri* 100 mg/kg i.p. in mice, 5, 10, 25, 50 and 100 mg/kg i.p. in rats	Inhibits prostaglandin E$_2$-induced inflammation Inhibits the activities of COX and LOX and downregulates TNF-α LPS-activated TNF-α, IL-6 and nitrite production in mononuclear cells ↑Hydroxyproline, hexosamine and hexuronic acid ↑Wound breaking strength	Channa et al. (2006), Viji and Helen (2008, 2011), Murthy et al. (2013)

(Continued)

TABLE 25.2 (Continued)

Summary of Important Pharmacological Studies on *Bacopa monnieri*

Pharmacological Effect	Treatment	Results	References
Neuroprotective	*Bacopa monnieri* 20 and 40 mg/kg for 3 weeks in rats	Restored deficit in behavioural activity ↓Lipid peroxidation ↑Reduced GSH in substantia nigra ↑Catalase, superoxide dismutase in striatum	Shobana et al. (2012)
	Bacopa monnieri 5 mg/kg ip in mice	↓Lipid peroxidation, ↓protein carbonyl contents and ↑GSH in hippocampus, striatum, cortex, cerebellum ↓Acetylcholinesterase and butyrylcholinesterase ↑Dopamine level in striatum	Shinomol et al. (2011)
	Bacopa monnieri (different doses) *in vitro* (SK-N-SH cells, a human neuroblastoma cell line and PC12, rat pheochromocytoma cells)	↑Cytoprotection Restored complex-1 and proteasomal activity ↑GSH levels ↓ROS and superoxide anions ↑γ-GCS, GST, GR, GPx ↑Nrf2, ↓Keap1, ↑pAkt Induce mitochondrial depolarization Prevent Trx1 downregulation ↓HSP90 levels ↑Tyrosine hydroxylase	Singh et al (2012, 2013)
	Bacopa monnieri 300 mg/kg po in male pups	Improve behavioural alterations ↓5-HT, ↓Nitrite levels, ↑GSH, catalase in hippocampus Preserve cerebellum histopathology	Sandhya et al. (2012)
	Bacopa monnieri 40 mg/kg po for 21 days or 5 weeks in rats	↓Accumulation of 4-HNE, TBA-RS, carbonyl content and lipofuscin granules in the cerebral cortex ↓Lipid peroxidation, protein carbonyl contents, ↑SOD levels, ↓accumulation of lipofuscin granules and nectroc alteration in hippocampal CA1 neurons Restored behavioural alterations, ↓TBARS, protein carbonyl contents, ↑GSH, GPx, SOD and CAT, ↓GR activity in the cerebellum ↓Nitrite and nitrate levels in serum	Jyoti et al. (2007), Jyoti and Sharma (2006), Sumathi et al. (2012)

(Continued)

TABLE 25.2 (*Continued*)
Summary of Important Pharmacological Studies on *Bacopa monnieri*

Pharmacological Effect	Treatment	Results	References
	Bacopa monnieri leaf powder mixed with diet	↓MDA, ROS, hydroperoxide, protein carbonyl contents, ↑GSH, catalase, glutathione peroxidase and superoxide dismutase, ↓Acetylcholinesteraase in striatum, cortex, cerebellum and hippocampus	Shinomol (2011)
	Bacopa monnieri (20, 40 and 80 mg/kg) for 2, 4 and 6 weeks in rats	↑Dendritic, processes, length and branching of amygdaloid and hippocampal CA3 neurons	Vollala et al. (2011a, 2011b)
	Bacopa monnieri in vitro (different concentrations) *in vivo* 5 mg/kg po in mice	↓MDA, ROS and hydroperoxide and protein carbonyl contents, ↑GSH, thiols, ↑activities of catalase, glutathione peroxidase and superoxide dismutase, acetylcholinesterase, butarylcholinesterase, ↓free iron, in striatum, hippocampus, cortex and cerebellum	Shinomol and Bharath (2012)
	Bacopa monnieri (25–100 μg/mL) *in vitro* (PC12, rat pheochromocytoma cells)	↓LDH release Upregulation of BDNF and MUS-1 receptor regulation Downregulation of acetylcholinesterase gene expression	Pandareesh and Anand (2013)
	Bacopa monnieri (120, 160 and 240 mg/kg) po for 8 days in rats	↑SOD, CAT, GPx, GR and GSH ↓Lipid peroxidation Attenuates ischemia-induced memory deficit Improve neurobehavioural activity ↓Infarct size ↓Nitric oxide, lipid peroxidation ↑Catalase, glutathione peroxidase	Saraf et al. (2010)
	Bacopa monnieri (20, 40 and 80 mg/kg) po for a total of 3 weeks in rats	Improves spatial memory Ameliorate cholinergic neurons densities in hippocampus	Uabundit et al. (2010)
	Bacopa monnieri (100 μg/mL) *in vitro* (primary cortical cell culture)	↓ROS levels Promotes cells survival ↓Acetylcholinesterase activity	Limpeanchob et al. (2008)
	Bacopa monnieri 50 mg/kg po for 15 days	Improve cognitive performance ↓Lipid peroxidation and protein carbonyl contents, ↑GSH, SOD, CAT, GSH-Px, GR, GST, ↓acetylcholinesterase activity in cortex and hippocampus	Saini et al. (2012)
	Bacopa monnieri 50 mg/kg po for a total of 72 days	Improves non-spatial short-term memory, spatial working memory and long term fair memory ↑pSer896-NMDAR, pThr286-CaMKII, ↑BDNF mRNA in the hippocampus Reverse ChAT downregulation Attenuates ChAT positive cells in the medial septum ↓Acetylcholinesterase activity in the cortex	Le et al (2013)

increased cytochrome-c activity, with concomitant increase in the ATP levels (Hota et al. 2009); increased protein kinase activity with increased protein content; decreased norepinephrine level; downregulation of Hif-1α and upregulation of *Fmr-1* expression; increased levels of antioxidant enzymes and differential regulation of the activity of histone acetylation and protein phosphatases (PP1a, PP2A) in the hippocampus (Dhawan and Singh 1996; Khan et al. 2014; Preethi et al. 2014; Rani and Prasad 2015); increased synaptic plasticity (Preethi et al. 2012); stimulation of thyroid function (Kar et al. 2002); restoration of NR1 expression and binding of REST/NRSF to NR1 promoter (Verma et al. 2015); and increased vesicular glutamate transporter type 2 (VGLUT2) in the prefrontal cortex (Piyabhan and Wetchateng 2014). Moreover, *Bacopa monnieri* restores the cognitive deficits related to cerebral ischemia, and this protective effect has been attributed in part to the presence of bacopaside-I via PKC and PI3K/Akt mechanisms (Le et al. 2015).

25.6.4 NEUROPROTECTIVE

Bacopa monnieri has a potential neuroprotective effect (Zandar and Zain 2010; Nannepaga et al. 2014). *Bacopa monnieri*, by virtue of its antioxidant effect, inhibits neuronal oxidative stress injury (Shinomol 2011; Hosamani et al. 2014) and protects against autism by normalising locomotor activity, anxiety, increasing social behaviour, enhancing serotonin level in the hippocampus and improving histopathological changes in the cerebellum (Sandhya et al. 2012). It also protects the cerebral cortex (Jyoti et al. 2007) and hippocampus by inhibiting lipid accumulation and protein damage (Jyoti and Sharma 2006), prevents cerebral ischemia reperfusion injury (Rehni et al. 2007), enhances dendritic length and arborisation of amygdala (Vollala et al. 2011a) and hippocampal CA$_3$ neurons (Vollala et al. 2011b) and modulates cholinergic and dopaminergic functions by enhancing muscarinic receptor binding in hippocampus and dopamine D$_2$ receptor binding in corpus striatum (Yadav et al. 2011). *Bacopa monnieri* also protects the striatum and other brain regions by inhibiting lipid peroxidation and protein oxidative damage (Shinomol and Bharath 2012), protects against brain ischemic injury by decreasing nitrite and lipid peroxidation and enhancing the activities of catalases (Saraf et al. 2010), protects astrocytes by inhibiting DNA damage (Russo et al. 2003), protects the cerebellum by increasing catalase and superoxide dismutase activities and enhances motor performance (Sumathi et al. 2012), ameliorates the alteration in the expression of two glutamate binding subunits, NR2A and NR2B (Mondal and Trigun 2015), and decreases the immunodensity of glutamate/*N*-methyl-D-aspartate receptor subtype 1 (NMDAR1) in the CA2/3 regions of hippocampus and dentate gyrus (Piyabhan and Wetchateng 2014). *Bacopa monnieri* ameliorates cognitive dysfunction by protecting cholinergic system and enhancing synaptic plasticity–related signalling and BDNF transcription (Le et al. 2013). Bacoside A is effective against cigarette smoke–induced neuropathological changes and restores the changes at the neurotransmitter level, lipid peroxidation states, mitochondrial functions, membrane alterations and apoptotic damage in the brain (Vani et al. 2015). Moreover, *Bacopa monnieri* mitigates sodium fluoride induced behavioural, biochemical and neuropathological alterations by improving memory, cholinesterase levels and antioxidant enzymes and prevents the degeneration of nerve fibres in the brain (Balaji et al. 2015). *Bacopa monnieri* possesses a neuroprotective role in type 2 diabetes mellitus–induced brain ageing and cognitive impairments by reversing the accumulation of lipofuscin, recovering memory loss, decreasing AChE activity and enhancing dendritic spine density (Pandey and Prasad 2017). *Bacopa monnieri* exerts its effects on biological endpoints, neuroprotection and processes underlying learning and memory and Alzheimer's disease (AD) by modulating the function of the identified transcription factors involving the activation of ATF4 and NRF2, while inhibiting the function of FOXO3 (Leung et al. 2017).

25.6.5 ANTI-ALZHEIMER'S

Bacopa monnieri is effective for reducing the memory loss and neurodegeneration associated with AD, due to its strong antioxidant property, which prevents the decrease of cholinergic neurons in the

CA_1 and CA_2 areas of hippocampus (Uabundit et al. 2010), reduces the intracellular acetylcholinesterase activity, beta amyloid cortical neurotoxicity (Limpeanchob et al. 2008), beta amyloid deposition (Holcomb et al. 2004; Dhanasekaran et al. 2007) and beta amyloid conformation (Holcomb et al. 2004) and restoring the activities of Na^+K^+ ATPase and cholinesterase (Saini et al. 2012). *Bacopa monnieri* is considered a promising therapeutic agent in AD and other forms of cognitive impairment (Chaudhari et al. 2017).

25.6.6   Anti-Parkinson's

The anti-Parkinson's effect of *Bacopa monnieri* is mediated by enhancing antioxidant defences in the striatum (Shinomol et al. 2011; Hosamani 2010), which prevents the degeneration of dopaminergic neurons (Jadiya et al. 2011) and increases the level of dopamine (Nellore 2013) or inhibits its depletion (Hosamani 2009), therefore relieving depression and increasing motor coordination and learning ability (Shobana et al. 2012). Besides preserving the mitochondrial membrane potential, *Bacopa monnieri* maintains mitochondrial complex-I activity with activation of nuclear factor erythroid-2 related factor-2 pathway by modulating Keap1 expression and phosphorylation of Akt, promoting its role in cell survival (Singh et al. 2012). Furthermore, *Bacopa monnieri* improves behavioural abnormalities, reduces oxidative stress and apoptosis in the brains of transgenic *Drosophila* Parkinson's disease model flies (Siddique et al. 2014). In an *in vitro* model of Parkinson's disease, *Bacopa monnieri* ameliorated morphological damage, cell viability, and apoptosis of PC12 cells exposed to rotenone (Ramaiah and Rajendra 2017). *Bacopa monnieri*, by creating an anti-apoptotic environment [reducing apoptotic (Bax and caspase-3) and increasing the levels of anti-apoptotic (Bcl2) protein expression], facilitates nigrostriatal dopaminergic neuroprotection against MPTP-induced Parkinsonism (Singh et al. 2017).

25.6.7   Anti-Epileptic

Bacopa monnieri possessed potent antiepileptic activity (Kaushik et al. 2009; Mishra et al. 2015) and is effective against status epilepticus (Semphuet et al. 2017). The anti-epileptic effect may be due to the presence of bacoside A, which reduces impairment of the peripheral nervous system by normalising the activities of acetylcholine esterase and malate dehydrogenase in the muscle and heart while stabilising the serum levels of epinephrine, norepinephrine, T_3 and insulin (Mathew et al. 2010). Moreover, *Bacopa monnieri* increases GABA, $GABA_A$ receptor subunit, $GABA_A$ receptor binding and upregulation of GAD gene in the hippocampus (Mathew et al. 2011), cerebellum (Mathew et al. 2010a), cerebral cortex (Mathew et al. 2012), striatum (Mathew et al. 2010b), increases 5-HT, 5-HT receptor binding in the cerebellum (Krishnakumar et al. 2009a), decreases the binding and expression of $5-HT_2$ receptors (Krishnakumar et al. 2009b) while increasing the binding and expression of NMDA receptors in the hippocampus (Khan et al. 2008), reverses the alterations in 5-HT2C, NMDA receptor functions and IP3 content in the cerebral cortex (Krishnakumar et al. 2014), and interacts with T-type calcium channels (Pandey et al. 2010), thereby producing anti-epileptic activity.

25.6.8   Antidepressant

Bacopa monnieri possesses antidepressant activity (Sairam et al. 2002; Chatterjee et al. 2010) mediated through serotonergic and adrenergic system activation (Ramanathan et al. 2011). *Bacopa monnieri*, by modulating the expression of HSP-70 as well as preventing the depletion of superoxide dismutase and catalase, prevents the disabilities associated with physical fatigue (Anand et al. 2012). Moreover, *Bacopa monnieri* alleviates chronic unpredictable stress-induced depression by decreasing BDNF protein and mRNA levels in the hippocampus and frontal cortex (Banerjee et al. 2014).

25.6.9 Anti-Ageing

Bacopa monnieri has potential as a therapeutic antioxidant to reduce oxidative stress and improve age-related decline in cognitive performance (Simpson et al. 2015). *Bacopa monnieri* relieves depression and provides improvement of overall health and nutritional status in geriatrics (Mehta and Malik 2006). *Bacopa monnieri* prevents ageing-associated cognitive disorders (Kapoor et al. 2009) by preventing the formation of lipofuscin pigments and malondialdehyde (Kalamade et al. 2008). *Bacopa monnieri* exerted distinct age-related effects comparable to that of donepezil on cell-mediated immune responses through selective modulation of antioxidant enzyme activities and intracellular targets, including the modulation of ERK pathway with specific effects on CREB and Akt (Priyanka et al. 2013b). *Bacopa monnieri* has the ability to protect against ageing-related neuroendocrine and immune system abnormalities by enhancing the antioxidant enzyme activities in the brain areas, heart, thymus, spleen and mesenteric lymph nodes and increasing tyrosine hydroxylase and nerve growth factor protein levels via ERK 1/2 and NF-κB pathways in the spleen (Priyanka et al. 2013a). Moreover, *Bacopa monnieri* enhances the survival of *Caenorhabditis elegans* in different stress conditions due to its anti-stress and potent reactive oxygen species scavenging properties (Phulara et al. 2015).

25.6.10 Anti-Arthritis

Bacopa monnieri decreases foot oedema and symptoms of arthritis by inhibiting the activities of 5-lipoxygenase and cyclooxygenase-2, decreases the infiltration of neutrophils and serum IgG and IgM antibodies (Viji et al. 2010), increases the activities of β-glucuronidase, β-hexosaminidase, hyaluronidase, collagenase and cathepsin-D and protein-bound carbohydrates in the articular cartilage, decreases the activities of glycosaminoglycans and prostaglandins-E_2, downregulates interleukin-6 expression (Vijayan et al. 2011) and inhibits protein degeneration with stabilisation of the membrane (Volluri et al. 2011).

25.6.11 Anti-Asthmatic

Bacopa monnieri has a strong potential as an herbal anti-asthmatic drug (Taur and Patil 2011). *Bacopa monnieri* produces bronchodilation mediated by β-adrenoceptors (Dar and Channa 1997a), inhibition of calcium ions (Dar and Channa 1997b), and mast cell stabilisation (Samiulla et al. 2001).

25.6.12 Antimicrobial

Bacopa monnieri possesses antibacterial activity against both gram positive and gram negative bacteria (Khan et al. 2011). *Bacopa monnieri* has potent antibacterial effect against *Streptococcus pneumonia, Enterococcus faecalis, Proteus mirabilis, Klebsiella pneumonia* (Kalaivani et al. 2012), *Proteus vulgaris* (Sampathkumar et al. 2008), *Salmonella enterica* (Mandal et al. 2007), *Staphylococcus aureus, Pseudomonas aeruginosa* and *Bacillus subtilis* (Alam et al. 2011). *Bacopa monnieri* has potential antifungal activity against *Candida albicans, Aspergillus niger* (Sampathkumar et al. 2008), *Curvularia lunata, Rhizoctonia solani, Acremonium kiliense* and *Alternaria brassicicola* (Sengupta et al. 2008).

25.6.13 Anticancer

Bacopa monnieri has potential antitumour and cytotoxic properties (Sengupta et al. 1998). *Bacopa monnieri* – due to its strong chemopreventive action (Janani et al. 2010a) – causes apoptosis of sarcoma cells (Rohini and Devi 2008). The antitumour property of *Bacopa monnieri* has been attributed to the presence of stigmasterol, which causes apoptosis of cancer cells through ceramide-induced activation of protein phosphatase-2A (Ghosh et al. 2011), while the anti-metastatic property of *Bacopa monnieri* has been attributed to the presence of bacoside A that – by inhibiting the activities and expression of matrix metalloproteinases 2 and 9 – prevents cancer metastasis (Janani et al. 2010b). The presence of bacoside A in *Bacopa monnieri* enhances $CaMK_2A$ and activates $CaMK_2A$ phosphorylation ($pCaMK_2A$), which triggers high calcium release from the endoplasmic reticulum, thus causing macropinocytosis and membrane hydrostatic stress induced tumour cell death (John et al. 2017).

25.6.14 ANTIDIABETIC

By virtue of its antioxidant and anti-peroxidase properties, *Bacopa monnieri* inhibits oxidative stress and produces a significant decrease in blood glucose (Ghosh et al. 2010), as well as preventing the renal and neurological complications of diabetes mellitus by restoring various metabolic activities (Kapoor et al. 2009). Stimulation of adenosine-A_1 receptors by *Bacopa monnieri* provides protection against diabetic neuropathic pain (Sahoo et al. 2010).

25.6.15 REPRODUCTIVE FUNCTION

Bacopa monnieri causes a reversible decrease in the weight of the epididymis and reduces the number of spermatozoa. It also produces degenerative changes in the seminiferous tubules in the form of loosening of germinal epithelium with exfoliation of germ cells, intraepithelial vacuolisation and formation of giant cells (Singh and Singh 2009). Conversely, *Bacopa monnieri* has been shown to improve sperm quality, and spermatogenic cell density and steroidogenic indices in the testis (Patel et al. 2017a). Additionally, *Bacopa monnieri* is useful in improving reproductive health in males by potentiating germ cell dynamics and improving sperm quality by enhancing antioxidant enzyme activities. These beneficial effect of *Bacopa monnieri* involves phosphorylated protein kinase B (*p*-Akt)-mediated activation of nuclear factor-erythroid-2-related factor-2 (Nrf2), thereby enhancing antioxidant enzyme activities, upregulation of mitogen-activated protein kinase, MAP2K1 and MAP2K2 and suppression of MKK4 in the testis (Patel et al. 2017b).

25.6.16 ANTIHYPERTENSIVE

Bacopa monnieri, by virtue of its bacoside-A_3 and bacopaside-II content, reduces blood pressure in the aorta, mesenteric, basilar, tail and femoral arteries that is mediated through nitric oxide release from the endothelium (Kamkaew et al. 2011) and inhibition of calcium influx via both voltage and receptor operated calcium channels of the cell membrane (Dar and Channa 1999).

25.6.17 ANTI-INFLAMMATORY

Bacopa monnieri has strong anti-inflammatory activity (Vidya et al. 2011) that is mediated through decreased release of tumour necrosis factor-α and interleukin-6 from mononuclear cells (Viji and Helen 2011), inhibition of activities of cyclooxygenase-2, lipooxygenase-5 and lipooxygenase-15 (Viji and Helen 2008), inhibition of prostaglandin-E_2 production (Channa et al. 2006), and stabilisation of lysosomal membranes (Jain et al. 1994) and mast cells (Samiulla et al. 2001). The presence of bacoside A in *Bacopa monnieri* inhibits bacteria-derived proteases and is responsible for its wound-healing effect (Sharath et al. 2010). *Bacopa monnieri* reduces airway inflammation and inhibits the activities of leukotriene-C4-synthase, leukotriene-A4-hydrolase and/or cyclooxygenase-2. Moreover, it also downregulates the expression of mRNA of leukotriene-C4-synthase (Soni et al. 2014)]. Additionally, *Bacopa monnieri* and its active constituent, bacoside A, inhibit the release of inflammatory cytokines (TNF-α and IL-6) from microglial cells and inhibit enzymes (caspase 1 and 3, and matrix metalloproteinase-3) associated with inflammation in the brain (Nemetchek et al. 2017).

25.6.18 ANTIMALARIAL

Bacopa monnieri was used traditionally to treat malaria and malaria-like symptoms. The antiplasmodial effect of cyclohexane extract alone has a percent inhibition of 70% and an IC_{50} of 6.55 µg/mL, while in combination with chloroquine it has percent inhibition and IC_{50} of 89% and 4.88 µg/mL, respectively (Chenniappan and Kadarkarai 2010).

25.6.19 ANTIOXIDANT

Bacopa monnieri is a strong natural antioxidant (Anand et al. 2011) and an efficient scavenger of DPPH free radicals (Srivastava et al. 2012), peroxynitrites (Alam et al. 2010), hydrogen peroxide (Shinde et al. 2011), nitric oxide (Alam et al. 2012) and superoxide radicals (Ghosh et al. 2007). Bacoside A is responsible for the different pharmacological effects of *Bacopa monnieri* (Sudharani, 2011) due to its potential free radical–scavenging property (Anbarasi et al. 2005). *Bacopa monnieri* shows a concentration-dependent increase in free radical scavenging activity (Anand et al. 2011). The free radical scavenging action of *Bacopa monnieri* may explain its cognitive-enhancing action (Bhattacharya et al. 2000). At a concentration of 1000 µg/mL, *Bacopa monnieri* shows significant lipid peroxidation (63.34%), free radical scavenging (63.87%) and hydrogen peroxide scavenging (58.03%) properties (Sathiyanarayanan et al. 2010). Moreover, *Bacopa monnieri* possesses a cyto-protective propensity, as it ameliorates the mitochondrial and plasma membrane damage induced by hydrogen peroxide (Pandareesh et al. 2014). Additionally, *Bacopa monnieri* exhibits promising protection against hydrogen peroxide–induced oxidative stress by boosting the endogenous defence machinery, increasing glutathione levels and maintaining membrane integrity, supported by a reduction in the levels of NF200, HSP70 and mortalin (Bhatia et al. 2017).

25.6.20 GASTROPROTECTIVE

Due to the presence of flavonoids, saponins, triterpenoids and tannins, *Bacopa monnieri* inhibits gastrointestinal motility mediated by either GABA and alpha-2 receptors (Subhan et al. 2010) or by inhibition of calcium influx via receptor and voltage operated calcium channels (Dar and Channa 1999). The anti-ulcerogenic effect of *Bacopa monnieri* is mediated through increased production of prostaglandins-E, prostaglandins-I_2, inhibition of *Helicobacter pylori* (Goel et al. 2003), reduction in the secretion of acid and pepsin, increase in mucin secretion and a decrease in mucosal cell exfoliation (Sairam et al. 2001). Moreover, *Bacopa monnieri* exhibits a potent anti-emetic action by attenuating not only the dopamine upsurge in the area postrema and brain stem, but also the intestinal serotonin concentration (Ullah et al. 2014). *Bacopa monnieri* may have potential as an anti-emetic or adjunct for the prophylaxis and treatment of chemotherapy-induced (delayed) vomiting, and this beneficial effect may stem from a combination of the antioxidant, calcium channel–blocking activity, and/or anti-dopaminergic and anti-serotonergic properties of *Bacopa monnieri* (Ullah et al. 2017; Alam et al. 2017).

25.6.21 CARDIOPROTECTIVE

Bacopa monnieri by ameliorating oxidative stress thereby prevents necrosis, infiltration of inflammatory cells, oedema and vacuolar changes in the myocardium (Mohanty et al. 2009). *Bacopa monnieri* has an atheroprotective effect by virtue of its ability to lower the plasma levels of total cholesterol, triglycerides, phospholipids, low-density lipoproteins and very low-density lipoprotein, and it increases the levels of high-density lipoproteins (Kamesh and Sumathi 2012). *Bacopa monnieri* improves myocardial function following ischemia/reperfusion injury through recovery of coronary blood flow, contractile force and a decrease in infarct size (Srimachai et al. 2017).

25.6.22 HEPATOPROTECTIVE AND NEPHROPROTECTIVE

Bacopa monnieri possesses hepatoprotective activity (Ghosh et al. 2007; Menon et al. 2010). *Bacopa monnieri* protects the liver by increasing the activities of catalases that prevent the accumulation of free radicals (Ghosh et al. 2007). Bacoside A is the compound responsible for the hepatoprotective effect of *Bacopa monnieri* (Sumathi and Nongbri 2008), which reduces oxidative stress and enhances the activities of antioxidants (Janani et al. 2009). *Bacopa monnieri* prevents morphine-induced hepatotoxicity by inhibiting the enhanced synthesis of lipid peroxide (Sumathy et al. 2001). Similarly, *Bacopa monnieri*, by enhancing endogenous antioxidants, protects the kidneys from the toxicological influence of morphine (Sumathi and Devaraj 2009). Moreover, *Bacopa monnieri* has been shown to ameliorate carbon tetrachloride–induced hepatotoxicity and nephrotoxicity by preserving the histoarchitecture of the liver and kidneys and restoring the various biochemical parameters (Shahid and Subhan 2014). *Bacopa monnieri* may provide a beneficial herbal remedy for the management of opioid related hepatotoxicity and nephrotoxicity, as it restores the elevation of serum ALT, AST and creatinine and protects the liver and kidneys from the toxicological influence of morphine or street heroin (Shahid et al. 2016).

25.6.23 ANTINOCICEPTIVE

Bacopa monnieri is effective in a variety of pain conditions. *Bacopa monnieri* has shown its utility against tonic visceral chemically induced nociceptive pain and acute phasic thermal nociception in animal studies (Rauf et al. 2011). Additionally, *Bacopa monnieri* attenuates opioid tolerance, enhances opiate-induced analgesia and has a morphine-like analgesic effect without producing any tolerance to its own analgesic effect (Rauf et al. 2011, 2013). *Bacopa monnieri* is an effective analgesic in a model of diabetic neuropathy, as it allays streptozotocin-induced hyperalgesia and the protection has been afforded via stimulation of adenosine A_1-receptors (Sahoo et al. 2010). *Bacopa monnieri* and its isolated constituent bacosine attenuated diabetic neuropathic pain through modulation of oxidative-nitrosative stress and reduction in advanced glycation end product formation (Kishore et al. 2017). *Bacopa monnieri* presents marked antinociceptive properties by alleviating allodynia and hyperalgesia associated with neuropathic pain, and it may constitute a beneficial herbal remedy for the efficient management of neuropathic pain syndromes (Shahid et al. 2017b).

25.6.24 IMMUNE FUNCTION

Bacopa monnieri affects both cell and humoral mediated immunity with different actions on various immune cells (Saraphanchotiwitthaya et al. 2008). *Bacopa monnieri* activates macrophages and neutrophils to produce increase amount of immune mediators (Hule and Juvekar 2009), spleen lymphocytes to produce IgG, IgA, IgM, interferon-γ and interleukin-2 as well as decrease production of tumour necrosis factor-α (Yamada et al. 2011). *Bacopa monnieri* exerts an anti-inflammatory effect by the regulation of Th1-polarised immune responses involving suppression of NO (and TNF-α) by macrophages and IFN-g by innate lymphocytes, with sustained production of IL-10 indicates the neutralisation of Th1 activation in favour of activation of regulatory T cells (Williams et al. 2014).

25.6.25 OPIOIDS AND *BACOPA MONNIERI*

Bacopa monnieri possess antinociceptive activity (Bhaskar and Jagtap 2011) that may be mediated through opioidergic (Abbas et al. 2011) or non-opioidergic mechanisms (Abbas et al. 2013) and inhibits pharmacological effects induced by morphine (Sumathi and Veluchamy 2007). Acute and chronic administration of *Bacopa monnieri*, besides enhancing morphine's antinociceptive effects, also reduces the development and expression of morphine tolerance (Rauf et al. 2011) and is beneficial in morphine-induced hyperactivity by decreasing morphine-induced dopamine, dihydroxyphenylacetic acid, homovanillic acid and 5-hydroxyindole acetic acid upsurges in the striatum (Rauf et al. 2011). The antioxidant effect of bacoside A in *Bacopa monnieri* inhibits morphine-induced brain oxidative stress by improving the activity of ATPases, maintaining sodium, potassium, calcium and magnesium ionic equilibrium (Sumathi et al. 2011) and normalising the activities of isocitrate dehydrogenase, α-ketoglutarate dehydrogenase, succinate dehydrogenase, malate dehydrogenase, NADPH dehydrogenase and cytochrome-c oxidase (Sumathy et al. 2001). *Bacopa monnieri* is effective for the reduction of morphine-induced withdrawal symptoms (Sumathi et al. 2002). Moreover, *Bacopa monnieri*, due to its strong antioxidant potential, attenuates morphine-associated cerebellar toxicity by reverting the pathological changes in the Purkinje, basket, stellate and granule cells (Shahid et al. 2017).

25.7 CLINICAL TRIALS

The major focus of *Bacopa monnieri* clinical trials has been on its cognitive-enhancing and neuroprotective effects in healthy humans and in patients with various neurodegenerative diseases (Neale et al. 2013). In healthy humans, *Bacopa monnieri* showed significant acute cognitive effects at 1 and 2 h post treatment with a clinically standard dose of 320 mg and possessed memory enhancement qualities with faster information processing and decision-making time, along with improvement in attention or freedom of distractibility (Downey et al. 2013; Benson et al. 2014). When administered chronically for 12 weeks, *Bacopa monnieri* enhances verbal learning rate, speed of early information processing and memory consolidation, while in patients with age-associated memory impairment, *Bacopa monnieri* improves paired associated learning, mental control and logical memory (Nathan et al. 2001; Stough et al. 2001; Downey et al. 2013; Benson et al. 2014; Raghav et al. 2006). In patients with AD, *Bacopa monnieri* improves quality of life, reading, writing and comprehension, orientation of person, time and place and decreases insomnia and irritability (Goswami et al. 2011). In humans aged 40–65, *Bacopa monnieri* reduces the amount of information loss from the memory and decreases the rate of forgetfulness of newly acquired information (Roodenrys et al. 2001). In healthy older persons over 55 years of age, *Bacopa monnieri* safely improves memory retention and acquisition (Calabrese et al. 2008; Morgan and Stevens 2010). *Bacopa monnieri*, in combination with *Ginkgo biloba*, does not show any significant effect on cognitive performance (Nathan et al. 2004). *Bacopa monnieri* in polyherbal preparations improves cognitive and behavioural outcomes in children and adolescents (Kean et al. 2017).

25.8 CLINICAL USES

Bacopa monnieri is currently recognised for the treatment of mental illness and epilepsy (Russo and Borrelli 2005). The cognitive-enhancing dose of *Bacopa monnieri* standardised extract in AD patients is 300 mg twice daily for 6 months (Goswami et al. 2011), while in healthy adults it is 300 mg once a day for 12 weeks (Stough et al. 2001; Calabrese et al. 2008). *Bacopa monnieri* is available in powder, tablet, capsule and syrup dosage forms.

25.9 TOXICOLOGY

Bacopa monnieri is generally well tolerated. The hydroethanolic extract of *Bacopa monnieri* has an LD_{50} of 232 mg/kg in mice after intraperitoneal administration and toxicity is due to the presence of saponins that cause haemolysis of red blood cells (Subhan et al. 2010). The formulated *Bacopa monnieri*, BacoMind™ has an LD_{50} of 2400 mg/kg with no observed effect level of 500 mg/kg after subchronic oral toxicity testing for 90 days in rats (Joshua Allan et al. 2007). In humans, oral administration of BacoMind™ capsules at a dose of 300 mg for 15 days and 450 mg for the next 15 days showed minor side effects in the form of fullness and bloating sensations, nausea, epigastric burning, minor elevation of pulse rate and ALT and decrease levels of fasting blood glucose, AST and serum creatinine that are within normal ranges (Pravina et al. 2007). Chronic administration of an extract of *Bacopa monnieri* (KeenMind) in humans at a dose of 300 mg for 12 weeks causes a decrease in felt stress, nausea, excessive thirst, increase appetite, palpitations and headache (Stough et al. 2001). In humans combined administration of an extract containing *Bacopa monnieri* (300 mg) with Ginkgo biloba (120 mg) for 4 weeks causes nausea, palpitations, sleep disturbances, visual abnormalities, headache, dry mouth and gastrointestinal complaints (Nathan et al. 2004). *Bacopa monnieri* can contribute to herbal–drug interactions, as *Bacopa monnieri* – as well as its five individual constituents – inhibits the function of P-glycoprotein (Singh et al. 2015) and also reduces the catalytic activities of CYP3A4, CYP2C9 and CYP2C19 drug-metabolising enzymes (Ramasamy et al. 2014).

25.10 CONCLUSIONS

The scientific research on *Bacopa monnieri* suggests the huge biological potential of this plant. Many pharmacological studies using standardised extracts have been conducted and demonstrated significant anti-stress, anti-amnesic, neuroprotective, antiepileptic, anti-inflammatory, anticancer, hepatoprotective, analgesic, gastroprotective, cardioprotective and cognitive enhancing properties. *Bacopa monnieri* has multiple modes of action on the brain that may impact human cognition in an acute manner and also serve to ameliorate cognitive decline when consumed over longer periods. A battery of well-validated and sensitive neuropsychological tests have shown that the CDRI 08 extract of *Bacopa monnieri* shows promise as a cognitive enhancer across a range of ages, as evidenced from its robust acute and chronic nootropic effects exemplified as improvement in information processing and decision-making time, reduction in anxiety and a significant decrease in the rate of forgetting newly acquired information. There is mounting evidence for the utility of *Bacopa monnieri* in improving cognitive functioning in healthy humans, as well as in patients with different memory disorders. Standardised *Bacopa monnieri* preparations are well tolerated and becoming more widely used throughout the world by practitioners of complementary medicine for the treatment of mental ailments.

REFERENCES

Abbas, M., F. Subhan, N. Mohani, K. Rauf, G. Ali, M. Khan, The involvement of opioidergic mechanisms in the activity of *Bacopa monnieri* extract and its toxicological studies, *Afr. J. Pharm. Pharmacol.* 5(8) (2011) 1120–1124.

Abbas, M., F. Subhan, K. Rauf, S.N.-U.-H. Mohani, The involvement of non opioidergic mechanism in the antinociceptive and antilocomotive activity of *Bacopa monnieri, Iran. J. Pharmacol. Ther.* 11(1) (2013) 15–19.

Adams, M., F. Gmünder, M. Hamburger, Plants traditionally used in age related brain disorders – A survey of ethnobotanical literature, *J Ethnopharmacol.*, 113(3) (2007) 363–381.

Agrawal, H., N. Kaul, A. Paradkar, K. Mahadik, Separation of bacoside A3 and bacopaside II, major triterpenoid saponins in *Bacopa monnieri*, by HPTLC and SFC. Application of SFC in implementation of uniform design for herbal drug standardization, with thermodynamic study, *Acta Chromatogr.*, 17 (2006) 125–150.

Alam, J., F. Subhan, I. Ullah, M. Shahid, G. Ali, R. D. Sewell, Synthetic and natural antioxidants attenuate cisplatin-induced vomiting, *BMC Pharmacol. Toxicol.* 18(1) (2017) 4.

Alam, K., N. Parvez, S. Yadav, K. Molvi, N. Hwisa, S. Sharif, D. Pathak et al., Antimicrobial activity of leaf callus of *Bacopa Monnieri* L, *Der Pharmacia Lettre*, 3(1) (2011) 287–291.

Alam, M., M. Hossain, M. Asadujjaman, M. Islam, M. Mazumder, M. Haque, Peroxynitrite scavenging and toxicity potentail of different fractions of the ariel parts of *Bacopa monniera* Linn, *Int. J. Pharm. Sci. Res.*, 1(10) (2010) 78–83.

Alam, M.N., T.B. Wahed, F. Sultana, J. Ahmed, M. Hasan, In vitro antioxidant potential of the methanolic extract of *Bacopa monnieri* L., *Turk. J. Pharm. Sci.*, 9(3) (2012) 285–292.

Ali, G., P. Srivastava, M. Iqbal, Morphogenic response and proline content in *Bacopa monniera* cultures grown under copper stress, *Plant Sci.*, 138(2) (1998) 191–195.

Anand, A., M.K. Saraf, S. Prabhakar, Antiamnesic effect of *B. monniera* on L-NNA induced amnesia involves calmodulin, *Neurochem. Res.*, 35(8) (2010) 1172–1181.

Anand, T., M. Naika, M. Swamy, F. Khanum, Antioxidant and DNA damage preventive properties of *Bacopa Monniera* (L) Wettst, *Free Radic. Antioxidants*, 1(1) (2011) 84–90.

Anand, T., G. Phani Kumar, M. Pandareesh, M. Swamy, F. Khanum, A. Bawa, Effect of bacoside extract from *Bacopa monniera* on physical fatigue induced by forced swimming, *Phytother. Res.*, 26(4) (2012) 587–593.

Anbarasi, K., K.E. Sabitha, C.S.S. Devi, Lactate dehydrogenase isoenzyme patterns upon chronic exposure to cigarette smoke: Protective effect of bacoside A, *Environ. Toxicol. Pharmacol.*, 20(2) (2005) 345–350.

Ayaz, M., M. Junaid, F. Ullah, F. Subhan, A. Sadiq, G. Ali, M. Ovais et al., Anti-Alzheimer's studies on β-sitosterol isolated from *Polygonum hydropiper* L, *Front. Pharmacol.*, 8 (2017) 697.

Balaji, B., E.P. Kumar, A. Kumar, Evaluation of standardized *Bacopa monniera* extract in sodium fluoride-induced behavioural, biochemical, and histopathological alterations in mice, *Toxicol. Ind. Health*, 31(1) (2015) 18–30.

Banerjee, R., S. Hazra, A.K. Ghosh, A.C. Mondal, Chronic administration of *Bacopa monniera* increases BDNF protein and mRNA expressions: A study in chronic unpredictable stress induced animal model of depression, *Psychiatry Investig.*, 11(3) (2014) 297–306.

Bansal, M., A. Kumar, M.S. Reddy, Diversity among wild accessions of *Bacopa monnieri* (L.) Wettst. and their morphogenetic potential, *Acta Physiol. Plant.*, 36(5) (2014) 1177–1186.

Barbhaiya, H.C., R.P. Desai, V.S. Saxena, K. Pravina, P. Wasim, P. Geetharani, J.J. Allan et al., Efficacy and tolerability of BacoMind® on memory improvement in elderly participants – A double blind placebo controlled study, *J. Pharmacol. Toxicol.*, 3(6) (2008) 425–434.

Benson, S., L.A. Downey, C. Stough, M. Wetherell, A. Zangara, A. Scholey, An acute, double-blind, placebo-controlled cross-over study of 320 mg and 640 mg doses of *Bacopa monnieri* (CDRI 08) on multitasking stress reactivity and mood, *Phytother. Res.*, 28(4) (2014) 551–559.

Bhandari, P., N. Kumar, B. Singh, V.K. Kaul, Bacosterol glycoside, a new 13, 14-seco-steroid glycoside from *Bacopa monnieri*, *Chem. Pharm. Bull. (Tokyo)*, 54(2) (2006) 240–241.

Bhandari, P., N. Kumar, B. Singh, V.K. Kaul, Cucurbitacins from *Bacopa monnieri*, *Phytochemistry*, 68(9) (2007) 1248–1254.

Bhandari, P., N. Kumar, B. Singh, V. Singh, I. Kaur, Silica-based monolithic column with evaporative light scattering detector for HPLC analysis of bacosides and apigenin in *Bacopa monnieri*, *J. Sep. Sci.*, 32(15–16) (2009) 2812–2818.

Bhaskar, M., A. Jagtap, Exploring the possible mechanisms of action behind the antinociceptive activity of *Bacopa monniera*, *Int. J. Ayurveda Res.*, 2(1) (2011) 2.

Bhatia, G., V. Dhuna, K. Dhuna, M. Kaur, J. Singh, *Bacopa monnieri* extracts prevent hydrogen peroxide-induced oxidative damage in a cellular model of neuroblastoma IMR32 cells, *Chin. Nat. Med.* (中国天然药物), 15(11) (2017) 834–846.

Bhattacharya, S., A. Bhattacharya, A. Kumar, S. Ghosal, Antioxidant activity of *Bacopa monniera* in rat frontal cortex, striatum and hippocampus, *Phytother. Res.*, 14(3) (2000) 174–179.

Calabrese, C., W.L. Gregory, M. Leo, D. Kraemer, K. Bone, B. Oken, Effects of a standardized *Bacopa monnieri* extract on cognitive performance, anxiety, and depression in the elderly: a randomized, double-blind, placebo-controlled trial, *J. Altern. Complement. Med.*, 14(6) (2008) 707–713.

Chakravarty, A.K., S. Garai, K. Masuda, T. Nakane, N. Kawahara, Bacopasides III-V: Three new triterpenoid glycosides from *Bacopa monniera*, *Chem. Pharm. Bull. (Tokyo)*, 51(2) (2003) 215–217.

Chakravarty, A.K., T. Sarkar, K. Masuda, K. Shiojima, T. Nakane, N. Kawahara, Bacopaside I and II: Two pseudojujubogenin glycosides from *Bacopa monniera*, *Phytochemistry*, 58(4) (2001) 553–556.

Chakravarty, A.K., T. Sarkar, T. Nakane, N. Kawahara, K. Masuda, New phenylethanoid glycosides from *Bacopa monniera*, *Chem. Pharm. Bull. (Tokyo)*, 50(12) (2002) 1616–1618.

Channa, S., A. Dar, S. Anjum, M. Yaqoob, Anti-inflammatory activity of *Bacopa monniera* in rodents, *J. Ethnopharmacol.*, 104(1) (2006) 286–289.

Charles, P.D., G. Ambigapathy, P. Geraldine, M.A. Akbarsha, K.E. Rajan, *Bacopa monniera* leaf extract up-regulates tryptophan hydroxylase (TPH2) and serotonin transporter (SERT) expression: Implications in memory formation, *J Ethnopharmacol.*, 134(1) (2011) 55–61.

Chatterjee, M., P. Verma, G. Palit, Comparative evaluation of *Bacopa monniera* and *Panax quniquefolium* in experimental anxiety and depressive models in mice, *Indian J. Exp. Biol.*, 48(3) (2010) 306–313.

Chaudhari, K.S., N.R. Tiwari, R.R. Tiwari, R.S. Sharma, Neurocognitive Effect of Nootropic Drug Brahmi (*Bacopa monnieri*) in Alzheimer's Disease, *Ann. Neurosci.*, 24(2) (2017) 111–122.

Chaudhuri, P., R. Srivastava, S. Kumar, Phytotoxic and antimicrobial constituents of *Bacopa monnieri* and *Holmskioldia sanguinea*, *Phytother. Res.*, 18(2) (2004) 114–117.

Chenniappan, K., M. Kadarkarai, In vitro antimalarial activity of traditionally used Western Ghats plants from India and their interactions with chloroquine against chloroquine-resistant *Plasmodium falciparum*, *Parasitol. Res.*, 107(6) (2010) 1351–1364.

Chowdhuri, D.K., D. Parmar, P. Kakkar, R. Shukla, P. Seth, R. Srimal, Antistress effects of bacosides of *Bacopa monnieri*: Modulation of Hsp70 expression, superoxide dismutase and cytochrome P450 activity in rat brain, *Phytother. Res.*, 16(7) (2002) 639–645.

Chunekar, K., Varanasi (Hindi translation), Bhav Prakasa Nighantu Chaukhamba Bharati Publications (1960) p. 372.

Dar, A., S. Channa, Bronchodilatory and cardiovascular effects of an ethanol extract of *Bacopa monniera* in anaesthetized rats, *Phytomedicine*, 4(4) (1997a) 319–323.

Dar, A., S. Channa, Relaxant effect of ethanol extract of *Bacopa monniera* on trachea, pulmonary artery and aorta from rabbit and guinea pig, *Phytother. Res.*, 11(4) (1997b) 323–325.

Dar, A., S. Channa, Calcium antagonistic activity of *Bacopa monniera* on vascular and intestinal smooth muscles of rabbit and guinea-pig, *J. Ethnopharmacol.*, 66(2) (1999) 167–174.

Darokar, M.P., S.P. Khanuja, A. Kumar Shasany, S. Kumar, Low levels of genetic diversity detected by RAPD analysis in geographically distinct accessions of *Bacopa monnieri*, *Genet. Resour. Crop Evol.*, 48(6) (2001) 555–558.

Das, A., G. Shanker, C. Nath, R. Pal, S. Singh, H.K. Singh, A comparative study in rodents of standardized extracts of *Bacopa monniera* and Ginkgo biloba: Anticholinesterase and cognitive enhancing activities, *Pharmacol. Biochem. Behav.*, 73(4) (2002) 893–900.

Deb, D.D., P. Kapoor, R. Dighe, R. Padmaja, M. Anand, P. D'SOUZA, M. Deepak et al., In vitro safety evaluation and anticlastogenic effect of BacoMind™ on human lymphocytes, *Biomed. Environ. Sci.*, 21(1) (2008) 7–23.

Deepak, M., A. Amit, 'Bacoside B' – The need remains for establishing identity, *Fitoterapia*, 87(2013) (2013) 7–10.

Deepak, M., G. Sangli, P. Arun, A. Amit, Quantitative determination of the major saponin mixture bacoside A in *Bacopa monnieri* by HPLC, *Phytochem. Anal.*, 16(1) (2005) 24–29.

Dhanasekaran, M., B. Tharakan, L.A. Holcomb, A.R. Hitt, K.A. Young, B.V. Manyam, Neuroprotective mechanisms of ayurvedic antidementia botanical *Bacopa monniera*, *Phytother. Res.*, 21(10) (2007) 965–969.

Dhawan, B., H. Singh, Pharmacological studies on *Bacopa monniera*, an ayurvedic nootropic agent, *Eur. Neuropsychopharmacol.*, 6(1003) (1996) 144–144.

Downey, L.A., J. Kean, F. Nemeh, A. Lau, A. Poll, R. Gregory, M. Murray et al., An acute, double-blind, placebo-controlled crossover study of 320 mg and 640 mg doses of a special extract of *Bacopa monnieri* (CDRI 08) on sustained cognitive performance, *Phytother. Res.*, 27(9) (2013) 1407–1413.

Dulcy, C.P., E. Rajan, *Bacopa monniera* extract enhance the cognitive ability of rats by increasing serotonin level, *Neurosci. Res.*, 65 (2009) S110.

Dulcy, C.P., H.K. Singh, J. Preethi, K.E. Rajan, Standardized extract of *Bacopa monniera* (BESEB CDRI-08) attenuates contextual associative learning deficits in the aging rat's brain induced by D-galactose, *J. Neurosci. Res.*, 90 (2012) 2053–2064.

Ganzera, M., J. Gampenrieder, R.S. Pawar, I.A. Khan, H. Stuppner, Separation of the major triterpenoid saponins in *Bacopa monnieri* by high-performance liquid chromatography, *Anal. Chim. Acta*, 516(1) (2004) 149–154.

Garai, S., S.B. Mahato, K. Ohtani, K. Yamasaki, Bacopasaponin D-A pseudojujubogenin glycoside from *Bacopa monniera*, *Phytochemistry*, 43(2) (1996a) 447–449.

Garai, S., S.B. Mahato, K. Ohtani, K. Yamasaki, Dammarane-type triterpenoid saponins from *Bacopa monniera*, *Phytochemistry*, 42(3) (1996b) 815–820.

Ghosh, T., G.K. Dash, S.S. Nayak, Hepatoprotective activity of ethanolic extract of *Bacopa monnieri* Linn. aerial parts against CCl4-induced hepatotoxicity in rats, *Nat. Prod. Sci.*, 13(1) (2007) 61–67.

Ghosh, T., T. Kumar Maity, M. Das, A. Bose, D. Kumar Dash, In vitro antioxidant and hepatoprotective activity of ethanolic extract of *Bacopa monnieri* Linn. aerial parts, *Iran. J. Pharmacol. Ther.*, 6(1) (2007) 77–85.

Ghosh, T., T.K. Maity, P. Sengupta, D.K. Dash, A. Bose, Antidiabetic and in vivo antioxidant activity of ethanolic extract of *Bacopa monnieri* Linn. aerial parts: A possible mechanism of action, *Iran. J. Pharm. Res.*, 7(1) (2010) 61–68.

Ghosh, T., T.K. Maity, J. Singh, Evaluation of antitumor activity of stigmasterol, a constituent isolated from *Bacopa monnieri* Linn aerial parts against Ehrlich Ascites Carcinoma in mice, *Orient. Pharm. Exp. Med.*, 11(1) (2011) 41–49.

Goel, R., K. Sairam, M. Dora Babu, I. Tavares, A. Raman, In vitro evaluation of *Bacopa monniera* on anti-*Helicobacter pylori* activity and accumulation of prostaglandins, *Phytomedicine*, 10(6) (2003) 523–527.

Gohil, K.J., J.A. Patel, A review on *Bacopa monniera*: Current research and future prospects, *Int. J. Green Pharm.*, 4(1) (2010) 1–9.

Goswami, S., A. Saoji, N. Kumar, V. Thawani, M. Tiwari, M. Thawani, Effect of *Bacopa monnieri* on cognitive functions in Alzheimer's disease patients, *Int. J. Collaborat. Res. Int. Med. Public Health*, 3 (2011) 285–293.

Holcomb, L.A., M. Dhanasekaran, K.A. Young, B.V. Manyam, The effect of *Bacopa monniera* extract on neuropathology in the doubly transgenic PSAPP Alzheimer's disease mouse model, *Neurobiol. Aging*, 25 (2004) S244–S244.

Hosamani, R., Neuroprotective efficacy of *Bacopa monnieri* against rotenone induced oxidative stress and neurotoxicity in *Drosophila melanogaster*, *Neurotoxicology*, 30(6) (2009) 977–985.

Hosamani, R., Prophylactic treatment with *Bacopa monnieri* leaf powder mitigates paraquat-induced oxidative perturbations and lethality in *Drosophila melanogaster*, *Indian J. Biochem. Biophys.*, 47(2) (2010) 75–82.

Hosamani, R., G. Krishna, Muralidhara, Standardized *Bacopa monnieri* extract ameliorates acute paraquat-induced oxidative stress, and neurotoxicity in prepubertal mice brain, *Nutr. Neurosci.*, (2014) doi:10.11 79/1476830514Y.0000000149.

Hota, S.K., K. Barhwal, I. Baitharu, D. Prasad, S.B. Singh, G. Ilavazhagan, *Bacopa monniera* leaf extract ameliorates hypobaric hypoxia induced spatial memory impairment, *Neurobiol. Dis.*, 34(1) (2009) 23–39.

Hou, C.-C., S.-J. Lin, J.-T. Cheng, F.-L. Hsu, Bacopaside III, bacopasaponin G, and bacopasides A, B, and C from *Bacopa monniera*, *J. Nat. Prod.*, 65(12) (2002) 1759–1763.

Hule, A., A. Juvekar, In vitro immune response of saponin rich fraction of *Bacopa monnieri*, Linn, *Int. J. PharmTech Res.*, 1(4) (2009) 1032–1038.

Hussain, K., A. Abdussalam, P. Ratheesh Chandra, Heavy metal accumulation potential and medicinal property of *Bacopa monnieri*-a paradox, *J. Stress Physiol. Biochem.*, 7(4) (2011) 40–50.

Jadiya, P., A. Khan, S.R. Sammi, S. Kaur, S.S. Mir, A. Nazir, Anti-Parkinsonian effects of *Bacopa monnieri*: Insights from transgenic and pharmacological Caenorhabditis elegans models of Parkinson's disease, *Biochem. Biophys. Res. Commun.*, 413(4) (2011) 605–610.

Jain, P., N. Khanna, N. Trehan, V. Pendse, J. Godhwani, Antiinflammatory effects of an Ayurvedic preparation, Brahmi Rasayan, in rodents, *Indian J. Exp. Biol.*, 32(9) (1994) 633–636.

Jain, P., D.K. Kulshreshtha, Bacoside A, a minor saponin from *Bacopa monniera*, *Phytochemistry*, 33(2) (1993) 449–451.

Janani, P., K. Sivakumari, A. Geetha, B. Ravisankar, C. Parthasarathy, Chemopreventive effect of bacoside A on N-nitrosodiethylamine-induced hepatocarcinogenesis in rats, *J. Cancer Res. Clin. Oncol.*, 136(5) (2010a) 759–770.

Janani, P., K. Sivakumari, A. Geetha, S. Yuvaraj, C. Parthasarathy, Bacoside A downregulates matrix metalloproteinases 2 and 9 in DEN-induced hepatocellular carcinoma, *Cell Biochem. Funct.*, 28(2) (2010b) 164–169.

Janani, P., K. Sivakumari, C. Parthasarathy, Hepatoprotective activity of bacoside A against N-nitrosodiethylamine-induced liver toxicity in adult rats, *Cell Biol. Toxicol.*, 25(5) (2009) 425–434.

John, S., K. Sivakumar, R. Mishra, Bacoside A induces tumor cell death in human glioblastoma cell lines through catastrophic macropinocytosis, *Front. Mol. Neurosci.*, 10 (2017) 171.

Joshua Allan, J., A. Damodaran, N. Deshmukh, K. Goudar, A. Amit, Safety evaluation of a standardized phytochemical composition extracted from *Bacopa monnieri* in Sprague–Dawley rats, Food Chem. Toxicol., 45(10) (2007) 1928–1937.

Jyoti, A., P. Sethi, D. Sharma, *Bacopa monniera* prevents from aluminium neurotoxicity in the cerebral cortex of rat brain, *J. Ethnopharmacol.*, 111(1) (2007) 56–62.

Jyoti, A., D. Sharma, Neuroprotective role of *Bacopa monniera* extract against aluminium-induced oxidative stress in the hippocampus of rat brain, *Neurotoxicology*, 27(4) (2006) 451–457.

Kalaivani, T., M. Sasirekha, D. Arunraj, V. Palanichamy, C. Rajasekaran, *In vitro* evaluation of antibacterial activity of phytochemical extracts from aerial parts of *Bacopa monnieri* (L.) Wettest (Scorphulariaceae), *J. Pharm. Res.*, 5(3) (2012) 1636–1639.

Kalamade, V., M. Pillai, I. Kalamade, Effect of *Bacopa monniera* (Linn.) on lipid peroxidation and lipofuscinogenesis in prostate gland of D-galactose induced aging mice, Mus musculus, *Indian J. Exp. Biol.*, 46(7) (2008) 547–549.

Kamesh, V., T. Sumathi, Antihypercholesterolemic effect of *Bacopa monniera* Linn. on high cholesterol diet induced hypercholesterolemia in rats, *Asian Pac. J. Trop. Biomed.*, 5(12) (2012) 949–955.

Kamkaew, N., C. Norman Scholfield, K. Ingkaninan, N. Taepavarapruk, K. Chootip, *Bacopa monnieri* increases cerebral blood flow in rat independent of blood pressure, *Phytother. Res.*, 27(1) (2012) 135–138.

Kamkaew, N., C.N. Scholfield, K. Ingkaninan, P. Maneesai, H.C. Parkington, M. Tare, K. Chootip, *Bacopa monnieri* and its constituents is hypotensive in anaesthetised rats and vasodilator in various artery types, *J. Ethnopharmacol.*, 137 (2011) 790–795.

Kapoor, R., S. Srivastava, P. Kakkar, *Bacopa monnieri* modulates antioxidant responses in brain and kidney of diabetic rats, *Environ. Toxicol. Pharmacol.*, 27(1) (2009) 62–69.

Kar, A., S. Panda, S. Bharti, Relative efficacy of three medicinal plant extracts in the alteration of thyroid hormone concentrations in male mice, *J. Ethnopharmacol.*, 81(2) (2002) 281–285.

Karthikeyan, A., A. Madhanraj, S.K. Pandian, M. Ramesh, Genetic variation among highly endangered *Bacopa monnieri* (L.) Pennell from Southern India as detected using RAPD analysis, *Genet. Resour. Crop Evol.*, 58(5) (2011) 769–782.

Kasture, S., V. Kasture, A. Joshua, A. Damodaran, A. Amit, Nootropic activity of Bacomind™, an enriched phytochemical composition from *Bacopa monnieri*, *J. Nat. Remedies*, 7(1) (2007) 166–173.

Kaushik, D., A. Tripathi, R. Tripathi, M. Ganachari, S.A. Khan, Anticonvulsant activity of *Bacopa monniera* in rodents, *Braz. J. Pharm. Sci.*, 45(4) (2009) 643–649.

Kean, J.D., L.A. Downey, C. Stough, Systematic overview of *Bacopa monnieri* (L.) Wettst. Dominant Poly-Herbal formulas in children and adolescents. *Medicines*, 4(4) (2017) 86.

Khan, A.V., Q.U. Ahmed, I. Shukla, A.A. Khan, Antibacterial efficacy of *Bacopa monnieri* leaf extracts against pathogenic bacteria, *Asian Biomed.*, 4(4) (2011) 651.

Khan, M.B., M. Ahmad, S. Ahmad, T. Ishrat, K. Vaibhav, G. Khuwaja, F. Islam, *Bacopa monniera* ameliorates cognitive impairment and neurodegeneration induced by intracerebroventricular-streptozotocin in rat: behavioral, biochemical, immunohistochemical and histopathological evidences, *Metab. Brain Dis.*, 30(1) (2014) 115–127.

Khan, R., A. Krishnakumar, C. Paulose, Decreased glutamate receptor binding and NMDA R1 gene expression in hippocampus of pilocarpine-induced epileptic rats: Neuroprotective role of *Bacopa monnieri* extract, *Epilepsy Behav.*, 12(1) (2008) 54–60.

Kishore, L., N. Kaur, R. Singh, Bacosine isolated from aerial parts of *Bacopa monnieri* improves the neuronal dysfunction in streptozotocin-induced diabetic neuropathy, *J. Funct. Foods*, 34 (2017) 237–247.

Kongkeaw, C., P. Dilokthornsakul, P. Thanarangsarit, N. Limpeanchob, C.N. Scholfielde, Meta-analysis of randomized controlled trials on cognitive effects of *Bacopa monnieri* extract, *J. Ethnopharmacol.*, 151(1) (2014) 528–535.

Krishnakumar, A., P.M. Abraham, J. Paul, C. Paulose, Down-regulation of cerebellar 5-HT2C receptors in pilocarpine-induced epilepsy in rats: Therapeutic role of *Bacopa monnieri* extract, *J. Neurol. Sci.*, 284(1) (2009a) 124–128.

Krishnakumar, A., T. Anju, P.M. Abraham, C. Paulose, Alteration in 5-HT2C, NMDA receptor and IP3 in cerebral cortex of epileptic rats: Restorative role of *Bacopa monnieri*, *Neurochem. Res.*, 40(1) (2014) 216–225.

Krishnakumar, A., M. Nandhu, C. Paulose, Upregulation of 5-HT2C receptors in hippocampus of pilocarpine-induced epileptic rats: Antagonism by *Bacopa monnieri*, *Epilepsy Behav.*, 16(2) (2009b) 225–230.

Kumar, E., A.A. Elshurafa, K. Elango, T. Subburaju, B. Suresh, Cytotoxic and anti-tumor properties of ethanolic extract of *Bacopa monneri* (L) Penn, *Anc. Sci. Life*, 17(3) (1998) 228–234.

Le, X.T., H.T.N. Pham, P.T. Do, H. Fujiwara, K. Tanaka, F. Li, T. Van Nguyen et al., *Bacopa monnieri* ameliorates memory deficits in olfactory bulbectomized mice: Possible involvement of glutamatergic and cholinergic systems, *Neurochem. Res.*, 38(10) (2013) 2201–2215.

Le, X.T., H.T.N. Pham, T. Van Nguyen, K.M. Nguyen, K. Tanaka, H. Fujiwara, K. Matsumoto, Protective effects of *Bacopa monnieri* on ischemia-induced cognitive deficits in mice: The possible contribution of bacopaside I and underlying mechanism, *J. Ethnopharmacol.*, 164 (2015) 37–45.

Leung, H.-W., G. Foo, G. Banumurthy, X. Chai, S. Ghosh, T. Mitra-Ganguli, A.M. VanDongen, The effect of *Bacopa monnieri* on gene expression levels in SH-SY5Y human neuroblastoma cells, *PLoS One*, 12(8) (2017) e0182984.

Limpeanchob, N., S. Jaipan, S. Rattanakaruna, W. Phrompittayarat, K. Ingkaninan, Neuroprotective effect of *Bacopa monnieri* on beta-amyloid-induced cell death in primary cortical culture, *J. Ethnopharmacol.*, 120(1) (2008) 112–117.

Mahady, G.B. (2001). Global harmonization of herbal health claims. *J. Nutr.* 131(3), 1120S–1123S.

Mahato, S.B., S. Garai, A.K. Chakravarty, Bacopasaponins E and F: Two jujubogenin bisdesmosides from *Bacopa monniera*, *Phytochemistry*, 53(6) (2000) 711–714.

Majumdar, S., S. Garai, S. Jha, Genetic transformation of *Bacopa monnieri* by wild type strains of *Agrobacterium rhizogenes* stimulates production of bacopa saponins in transformed calli and plants, *Plant Cell Rep.*, 30(5) (2011) 941–954.

Majumdar, S., S. Garai, S. Jha, Use of the cryptogein gene to stimulate the accumulation of bacopa saponins in transgenic *Bacopa monnieri* plants, *Plant Cell Rep.*, 31(10) (2012) 1899–1909.

Mandal, S., M.D. Mandal, N.K. Pal, Antibacterial potential of *Azadirachta indica* seed and *Bacopa monniera* leaf extracts against multidrug resistant Salmonella enterica serovar Typhi isolates, *Arch. Med. Sci.*, 3(1) (2007) 14–18.

Mathew, J., S. Balakrishnan, S. Antony, P.M. Abraham, C. Paulose, Decreased GABA receptor in the cerebral cortex of epileptic rats: Effect of *Bacopa monnieri* and Bacoside-A, *J. Biomed. Sci.*, 19(1) (2012) 25.

Mathew, J., G. Gangadharan, K.P. Kuruvilla, C. Paulose, Behavioral deficit and decreased GABA receptor functional regulation in the hippocampus of epileptic rats: Effect of *Bacopa monnieri*, *Neurochem. Res.*, 36(1) (2011) 7–16.

Mathew, J., J. Paul, M. Nandhu, C. Paulose, Increased excitability and metabolism in pilocarpine induced epileptic rats: Effect of *Bacopa monnieri*, *Fitoterapia*, 81(6) (2010) 546–551.

Mathew, J., T. Peeyush Kumar, R.S. Khan, C. Paulose, Behavioral deficit and decreased GABA receptor functional regulation in the cerebellum of epileptic rats: Effect of *Bacopa monnieri* and bacoside A, *Epilepsy Behav.*, 17(4) (2010a) 441–447.

Mathew, J., S. Soman, J. Sadanandan, C.S. Paulose, Decreased GABA receptor in the striatum and spatial recognition memory deficit in epileptic rats: Effect of *Bacopa monnieri* and bacoside-A, *J. Ethnopharmacol.*, 130(2) (2010b) 255–261.

Mathur, S., M. Gupta, M. Ram, S. Sharma, S. Kumar, Herb yield and bacoside-A content of field-grown *Bacopa monnieri* accessions, *J. Herbs Spices Med. Plants*, 9(1) (2002) 11–18.

Mehta, D., A.B. Malik, Signaling mechanisms regulating endothelial permeability, *Physiol. Rev.*, 86(1) (2006) 279–367.

Menon, B.R., M. Rathi, L. Thirumoorthi, V. Gopalakrishnan, Potential effect of *Bacopa monnieri* on nitrobenzene induced liver damage in rats, *Indian J. Clin. Biochem.*, 25(4) (2010) 401–404.

Mishra, A., A.K. Mishra, O. PrakashTiwari, S. Jha, Pharmacognostic, physicochemical and phytochemical investigation of *Bacopa monnieri* L. stem and its anticonvulsant potential in laboratory animals, *Int. J. Epilepsy* (2015). doi:10.1016/j.ijep.2015.02.004.

Mishra, S., S. Srivastava, S. Dwivedi, R.D. Tripathi, Investigation of biochemical responses of *Bacopa monnieri* L. upon exposure to arsenate, *Environ. Toxicol.*, 28(8) (2013) 419–430.

Mohanty, I.R., U. Maheswari, D. Joseph, V. Moghe, *Bacopa monniera* augments endogenous antioxidants and attenuates myocardial injury, *Int. J. Integr. Biol.*, 7(2) (2009) 73–79.

Mondal, P., S.K. Trigun, *Bacopa monnieri* extract (CDRI-08) modulates the NMDA receptor subunits and nNOS-apoptosis axis in cerebellum of hepatic encephalopathy rats, *Evid. Based Complement. Alternat. Med.*, 535013 (2015).

Morgan, A., J. Stevens, Does *Bacopa monnieri* improve memory performance in older persons? Results of a randomized, placebo-controlled, double-blind trial, *J. Altern. Complement. Med.*, 16(7) (2010) 753–759.

Murthy, P.B.S., V.R. Raju, T. Ramakrisana, M.S. Chakravarthy, K.V. Kumar, S. Kannababu, G.V. Subbaraju, Estimation of twelve bacopa saponins in *Bacopa monnieri* extracts and formulations by high-performance liquid chromatography, *Chem. Pharm. Bull. (Tokyo)*, 54(6) (2006) 907–911.

Murthy, S., M. Gautam, S. Goel, V. Purohit, H. Sharma, R. Goel, Evaluation of In vivo wound healing activity of *Bacopa monniera* on different wound model in rats, *BioMed Res. Int.*, 2013(2013) (2013) 972028.

Nannepaga, J.S., M. Korivi, M. Tirumanyam, M. Bommavaram, C.-H. Kuo, Neuroprotective effects of *Bacopa monniera* whole-plant extract against aluminum-induced hippocampus damage in rats: Evidence from electron microscopic images, *Chin. J. Physiol.*, 57(5) (2014) 279–285.

Nathan, P.J., J. Clarke, J. Lloyd, C. Hutchison, L. Downey, C. Stough, The acute effects of an extract of *Bacopa monniera* (Brahmi) on cognitive function in healthy normal subjects, *Hum. Psychopharmacol.*, 16(4) (2001) 345–351.

Nathan, P.J., S. Tanner, J. Lloyd, B. Harrison, L. Curran, C. Oliver, C. Stough, Effects of a combined extract of Ginkgo biloba and *Bacopa monniera* on cognitive function in healthy humans, *Hum. Psychopharmacol.*, 19(2) (2004) 91–96.

Neale, C., D. Camfield, J. Reay, C. Stough, A. Scholey, Cognitive effects of two nutraceuticals Ginseng and Bacopa benchmarked against modafinil: A review and comparison of effect sizes, *Br. J. Clin. Pharmacol.*, 75(3) (2013) 728–737.

Nellore, J., *Bacopa monnieri* phytochemicals mediated synthesis of platinum nanoparticles and its neurores-
cue effect on 1–methyl 4–phenyl 1, 2, 3, 6 tetrahydropyridine-induced experimental Parkinsonism in
Zebrafish, *J. Neurodegener. Dis.*, 2013 (2013) 1–8.

Nemetchek, M.D., A.A. Stierle, D.B. Stierle, D.I. Lurie, The Ayurvedic plant *Bacopa monnieri* inhibits inflammatory pathways in the brain, *J. Ethnopharmacol.*, 197 (2017) 92–100.

Pandareesh, M., T. Anand, Neuromodulatory propensity of *Bacopa monniera* against scopolamine-induced
cytotoxicity in PC12 cells via down-regulation of AChE and up-regulation of BDNF and muscarnic-1
receptor Expression, *Cell. Mol. Neurobiol.*, 33(7) (2013) 875–884.

Pandareesh, M., T. Anand, P.V. Bhat, Cytoprotective propensity of *Bacopa monniera* against hydrogen peroxide induced oxidative damage in neuronal and lung epithelial cells, *Cytotechnology* (2014). doi:10.1007/
s10616-014-9767-3.

Pandey, R., S. Gupta, S. Tandon, O. Wolkenhauer, J. Vera, S.K. Gupta, Bacoside A suppresses epileptic-like
seizure/convulsion in Caenorhabditis elegans, *Seizure*, 19(7) (2010) 439–442.

Pandey, S.P., S. Prasad, Diabetes Mellitus Type 2 Induces Brain Aging and Memory Impairment in Mice:
Neuroprotective Effects of *Bacopa monnieri* Extract, *Top. Biomed. Gerontol.*, Springer, Singapore,
2017, pp. 335–355.

Patel, S.K., S. Singh, H.K. Singh, S.K. Singh, Effect of standardized extract of *Bacopa monnieri* (CDRI-08)
on testicular functions in adult male mice, *J. Ethnopharmacol.*, 197 (2017a) 101–109.

Patel, S.K., S. Singh, S.K. Singh, Standardized extract of *Bacopa monnieri* (CDRI-08): Effect on germ cell
dynamics and possible mechanisms of its beneficial action on spermatogenesis and sperm quality in
male mice, *Biochem. Biophys. Res. Commun.*, 494(1) (2017b) 34–41.

Phrompittayarat, W., K. Jetiyanon, S. Wittaya-areekul, W. Putalun, H. Tanaka, I. Khan, K. Ingkaninan,
Influence of seasons, different plant parts, and plant growth stages on saponin quantity and distribution
in *Bacopa monnieri*, *Songklanakarin J. Sci. Technol.*, 33(2) (2011) 193–199.

Phulara, S.C., V. Shukla, S. Tiwari, R. Pandey, *Bacopa monnieri* promotes longevity in Caenorhabditis elegans under stress conditions, *Pharmacogn. Mag.*, 11(42) (2015) 410–416.

Piyabhan, P., T. Wetchateng, EPA-0094–Cognitive enhancement effect of *Bacopa monnieri* on vesicular glutamate transporter 2, vglut2, in the prefrontal cortex, striatum and hippocampus of schizophrenia rat
model, *Eur. Psychiatry*, 29(1) (2014) 1.

Piyabhan, P., T. Wetchateng, Neuroprotective effects of *Bacopa monnieri* (Brahmi) on novel object recognition and NMDAR1 immunodensity in the prefrontal cortex, striatum and hippocampus of sub-chronic
phencyclidine rat model of schizophrenia, *J. Med. Assoc. Thai.*, 97(8) (2014) S50–S55.

Prabhakar, S., M.K. Saraf, A. Banik, A. Anand, *Bacopa monniera* selectively attenuates suppressed Superoxide
dismutase activity in diazepam induced amnesic mice, *Ann. Neurosci.*, 18(1) (2011) 8–13.

Prabhakar, S., M.K. Saraf, P. Pandhi, A. Anand, *Bacopa monniera* exerts antiamnesic effect on diazepam-
induced anterograde amnesia in mice, *Psychopharmacology*, 200(1) (2008) 27–37.

Pravina, K., K. Ravindra, K. Goudar, D. Vinod, A. Joshua, P. Wasim, K. Venkateshwarlu et al., Safety evaluation of BacoMind™ in healthy volunteers: A phase I study, *Phytomedicine*, 14(5) (2007) 301–308.

Preethi, J., H.K. Singh, P.D. Charles, K.E. Rajan, Participation of microRNA 124-CREB pathway: A parallel memory enhancing mechanism of standardised extract of *Bacopa monniera* (BESEB CDRI-08),
Neurochem. Res., 37(10) (2012) 2167–2177.

Preethi, J., H.K. Singh, J.S. Venkataraman, K.E. Rajan, Standardised extract of *Bacopa monniera* (CDRI-08)
improves contextual fear memory by differentially regulating the activity of histone acetylation and
protein phosphatases (PP1α, PP2A) in hippocampus, *Cell. Mol. Neurobiol.*, 34(4) (2014) 577–589.

Priyanka, H.P., P. Bala, S. Ankisettipalle, S. ThyagaRajan, *Bacopa monnieri* and 1-Deprenyl differentially
enhance the activities of antioxidant enzymes and the expression of tyrosine hydroxylase and nerve
growth factor via ERK 1/2 and NF-κB pathways in the spleen of female Wistar rats, *Neurochem. Res.*,
38(1) (2013a) 141–152.

Priyanka, H.P., R.V. Singh, M. Mishra, S. ThyagaRajan, Diverse age-related effects of *Bacopa monnieri* and
donepezil in vitro on cytokine production, antioxidant enzyme activities, and intracellular targets in
splenocytes of F344 male rats, *Int. Immunopharmacol.*, 15(2) (2013b) 260–274.

Promsuban, C., S. Limsuvan, P. Akarasereenont, K. Tilokskulchai, S. Tapechum, N. Pakaprot, *Bacopa monnieri* extract enhances learning-dependent hippocampal long-term synaptic potentiation, *Neuroreport*,
28(16) (2017) 1031–1035.

Qureshi, R., G. Raza Bhatti, Ethnobotany of plants used by the Thari people of Nara Desert, Pakistan,
Fitoterapia, 79(6) (2008) 468–473.

Raghav, S., H. Singh, P. Dalal, J. Srivastava, O. Asthana, Randomized controlled trial of standardized *Bacopa
monniera* extract in age-associated memory impairment, *Indian J. Psychiatry*, 48(4) (2006) 238–242.

Rahman, L.U., P.C. Verma, D. Singh, M.M. Gupta, S. Banerjee, Bacoside production by suspension cultures of *Bacopa monnieri* (L.) Pennell, *Biotechnol. Lett.*, 24(17) (2002) 1427–1429.

Rai, D., G. Bhatia, G. Palit, R. Pal, S. Singh, H.K. Singh, Adaptogenic effect of *Bacopa monniera* (Brahmi), *Pharmacol. Biochem. Behav.*, 75(4) (2003) 823–830.

Rai, R., H.K. Singh, S. Prasad, A special extract of *Bacopa monnieri* (CDRI-08) restores learning and memory by upregulating expression of the NMDA receptor subunit GluN2B in the brain of scopolamine-induced amnesic mice, *Evid. Based Complement. Alternat. Med.*, Article ID 254303 (2015).

Rajan, K.E., H.K. Singh, A. Parkavi, P.D. Charles, Attenuation of 1-(m-Chlorophenyl)-biguanide induced hippocampus-dependent memory impairment by a standardised extract of *Bacopa monniera* (BESEB CDRI-08), *Neurochem. Res.*, 36(11) (2011) 2136–2144.

Ramaiah, C.V., W. Rajendra, Protective role of *Bacopa monnieri* against Rotenone-induced Parkinson's disease in PC 12 cell lines, *Int. J. Phytomedicine*, 9(2) (2017) 219–222.

Ramanathan, M., B. Balaji, A. Justin, N. Gopinath, M. Vasanthi, R. Ramesh, Behavioural and neurochemical evaluation of Perment® an herbal formulation in chronic unpredictable mild stress induced depressive model, *Indian J. Exp. Biol.*, 49(4) (2011) 269–275.

Ramasamy, S., L.V. Kiew, L.Y. Chung, Inhibition of human cytochrome P450 enzymes by *Bacopa monnieri* standardized extract and constituents, *Molecules*, 19(2) (2014) 2588–2601.

Rani, A., S. Prasad, A special extract of *Bacopa monnieri* (CDRI-08)-restored memory in CoCl2-hypoxia mimetic mice is associated with upregulation of Fmr-1 gene expression in hippocampus, *Evid. Based Complement. Alternat. Med.*, 501 (2015) 347978.

Rastogi, S., R. Pal, D.K. Kulshreshtha, Bacoside A3-A triterpenoid saponin from *Bacopa monniera*, *Phytochemistry*, 36(1) (1994) 133–137.

Rauf, K., F. Subhan, M. Abbas, A. Badshah, I. Ullah, S. Ullah, Effect of bacopasides on acquisition and expression of morphine tolerance, *Phytomedicine*, 18 (2011) 836–842.

Rauf, K., F. Subhan, A. Al-Othman, I. Khan, A. Zarrelli, M. Shah, Preclinical profile of bacopasides from *Bacopa monnieri* (BM) as an emerging class of therapeutics for management of chronic pains, *Curr. Med. Chem.*, 20(8) (2013) 1028–1037.

Rauf, K., F. Subhan, R.D.E. Sewell, A bacoside containing *Bacopa monnieri* extract reduces both morphine hyperactivity plus the elevated striatal dopamine and serotonin turnover, *Phytother. Res.*, 26 (2011) 758–763.

Rehni, A.K., H.S. Pantlya, R. Shri, M. Singh, Effect of chlorophyll and aqueous extracts of *Bacopa monniera* and Valeriana wallichii on ischaemia and reperfusion-induced cerebral injury in mice, *Indian J. Exp. Biol.*, 45(9) (2007) 764–769.

Renukappa, T., G. Roos, I. Klaiber, B. Vogler, W. Kraus, Application of high-performance liquid chromatography coupled to nuclear magnetic resonance spectrometry, mass spectrometry and bioassay for the determination of active saponins from *Bacopa monniera* Wettst, *J. Chromatogr. A*, 847(1) (1999) 109–116.

Rohini, G., C. Devi, *Bacopa monniera* extract Induces apoptosis in murine sarcoma cells (S-180), *Phytother. Res.*, 22(12) (2008) 1595–1598.

Roodenrys, S., D. Booth, S. Bulzomi, A. Phipps, C. Micallef, J. Smoker, Chronic effects of Brahmi (*Bacopa monnieri*) on human memory, *Neuropsychopharmacology*, 27(2) (2001) 279–281.

Russo, A., F. Borrelli, *Bacopa monniera*, a reputed nootropic plant: An overview, *Phytomedicine*, 12(4) (2005) 305–317.

Russo, A., F. Borrelli, A. Campisi, R. Acquaviva, G. Raciti, A. Vanella, Nitric oxide-related toxicity in cultured astrocytes: Effect of *Bacopa monniera*, *Life Sci.*, 73(12) (2003) 1517–1526.

Sahoo, P.K., D. Pradhan, P. Behera, Neuroprotective effect of *Bacopa monnieri* leaf extract targeted at adenosine receptor in diabetic neuropathic pain, *J. Pharm. Res.*, 3(8) (2010) 1806–1809.

Saini, N., D. Singh, R. Sandhir, Neuroprotective effects of *Bacopa monnieri* in experimental model of dementia, *Neurochem. Res.*, 37(9) (2012) 1928–1937.

Sairam, K., M. Dorababu, R. Goel, S. Bhattacharya, Antidepressant activity of standardized extract of *Bacopa monniera* in experimental models of depression in rats, *Phytomedicine*, 9(3) (2002) 207–211.

Sairam, K., C.V. Rao, M.D. Babu, R. Goel, Prophylactic and curative effects of *Bacopa monniera* in gastric ulcer models, *Phytomedicine*, 8(6) (2001) 423–430.

Salvio Escandón, A., J.C. Hagiwara, L.M. Alderete, A new variety of *Bacopa monnieri* obtained by in vitro polyploidization, *Electron. J. Biotechnol.*, 9(3) (2006) 181–186.

Samiulla, D., D. Prashanth, A. Amit, Mast cell stabilising activity of *Bacopa monnieri*, *Fitoterapia*, 72(3) (2001) 284–285.

Sampathkumar, P., B. Dheeba, Z. Vidhyasagar, T. Arulprakash, R. Vinothkannan, Potential antimicrobial activity of various extracts of *Bacopa monnieri* (Linn.), *Int. J. Pharmacol.*, 4(3) (2008) 230–232.

Sandhya, T., J. Sowjanya, B. Veeresh, *Bacopa monniera* (L.) Wettst ameliorates behavioral alterations and oxidative markers in sodium valproate induced autism in rats, *Neurochem. Res.*, 37(5) (2012) 1121–1131.

Saraf, M., S. Prabhakar, A. Anand, *Bacopa monniera* alleviates N [omega]-nitro-l-arginine-induced but not MK-801-induced amnesia: A mouse Morris water maze study, *Neuroscience*, 160(1) (2009) 149–155.

Saraf, M., S. Prabhakar, P. Pandhi, A. Anand, *Bacopa monniera* ameliorates amnesic effects of diazepam qualifying behavioral-molecular partitioning, *Neuroscience*, 155(2) (2008) 476–484.

Saraf, M.K., A. Anand, S. Prabhakar, Scopolamine induced amnesia is reversed by *Bacopa monniera* through participation of kinase-CREB pathway, *Neurochem. Res.*, 35(2) (2010) 279–287.

Saraf, M.K., S. Prabhakar, A. Anand, Neuroprotective effect of *Bacopa monniera* on ischemia induced brain injury, *Pharmacol. Biochem. Behav.*, 97(2) (2010) 192–197.

Saraf, M.K., S. Prabhakar, K.L. Khanduja, A. Anand, *Bacopa monniera* attenuates scopolamine induced impairment of spatial memory in mice, *Evid. Based Complement. Alternat. Med.*, 2011 (2011) 1–10.

Saraphanchotiwitthaya, A., K. Ingkaninan, P. Sripalakit, Effect of *Bacopa monniera* Linn. extract on murine immune response in vitro, *Phytother. Res.*, 22(10) (2008) 1330–1335.

Sathiyanarayanan, L., A.R. Paradkar, K.R. Mahadik, In vivo and in vitro antioxidant activity of lipid based extract of *Bacopa monniera* Linn. compared to conventional extract and traditional preparation, *Eur J. Intern. Med.*, 2(2) (2010) 93–101.

Semphuet, T., A. Boongird, M.H. Tantisira, K. Tiloksakulchai, S. Tapechum, N. Pakaprot, The Neuroprotective Effect of *Bacopa monnieri* against pilocarpine induced status epilepticus in Rats, *Siriraj Med. J.*, 69(6) (2017) 345–350.

Sengupta, S., S. Ghosh, A. Das, Antimycotic potentiality of the plant extract *Bacopa monnieri* (L.) Penn, *Res. J. Bot.*, 3(2) (2008) 83–89.

Shahare, M., P. D'Mello, Standardization of *Bacopa monnieri* and its formulations with reference to Bacoside A, by high-performance thin-layer chromatography, *Tablet*, 2(4) (2010) 8–12.

Shahid, M., F. Subhan, N. Ahmad, R. Sewell, The flavonoid 6-methoxyflavone allays cisplatin-induced neuropathic allodynia and hypoalgesia, *Biomed. Pharmacother.*, 95 (2017a) 1725–1733.

Shahid, M., F. Subhan, N. Ahmad, I. Ullah, A bacosides containing *Bacopa monnieri* extract alleviates allodynia and hyperalgesia in the chronic constriction injury model of neuropathic pain in rats, *BMC Complement. Altern. Med.*, 17(1) (2017b) 293.

Shahid, M., F. Subhan, G. Ali, I. Ullah, J. Alam, S. Ullah, K. Rauf, Neuroprotective effect of *Bacopa monnieri* against morphine-induced histopathological changes in the cerebellum of rats, *Pak. J. Pharm. Sci.*, 30(6) (2017) 2067–2074.

Shahid, M., F. Subhan, I. Ullah, G. Ali, J. Alam, R. Shah, Beneficial effects of *Bacopa monnieri* extract on opioid induced toxicity, *Heliyon*, 2(2) (2016) e00068.

Shahid, M., F. Subhan, Protective effect of *Bacopa monniera* methanol extract against carbon tetrachloride induced hepatotoxicity and nephrotoxicity, *Pharmacologyonline*, 2(2) (2014) 18–28.

Sharath, R., B. Harish, V. Krishna, B. Sathyanarayana, H. Swamy, Wound healing and protease inhibition activity of Bacoside-A, isolated from *Bacopa monnieri* wettest, *Phytother. Res.*, 24(8) (2010) 1217–1222.

Sharma, S., B. Kamal, N. Rathi, S. Chauhan, V. Jadon, N. Vats, A. Gehlot et al., In vitro rapid and mass multiplication of highly valuable medicinal plant *Bacopa monnieri* (L.) Wettst, *Afr. J. Biotechnol.*, 9(49) (2010) 8318–8322.

Sheikh, N., A. Ahmad, K.B. Siripurapu, V.K. Kuchibhotla, S. Singh, G. Palit, Effect of *Bacopa monniera* on stress induced changes in plasma corticosterone and brain monoamines in rats, *J. Ethnopharmacol.*, 111(3) (2007) 671–676.

Shikha, S., M. Nidhi, M. Upama, *Bacopa monniera*-a future perspective, *Int. J. Pharm. Sci. Drug Res.*, 1(3) (2009) 154–157.

Shinde, R., S. Deshmukh, H. Vitekari, P. Kamble, Effect of Bacoside extract on H2O2 stressed lymphocytes, *Int. J. Pharm. Biol. Sci.*, 1(4) (2011) 567–571.

Shinomol, G.K., *Bacopa monnieri* modulates endogenous cytoplasmic and mitochondrial oxidative markers in prepubertal mice brain, *Phytomedicine*, 18(4) (2011) 317–326.

Shinomol, G.K., M.S. Bharath, Neuromodulatory propensity of *Bacopa monnieri* leaf extract against 3-Nitropropionic acid-induced oxidative stress: *In vitro* and *in vivo* evidences, *Neurotox. Res.*, 22(2) (2012) 102–114.

Shinomol, G.K., R.B. Mythri, M. Srinivas Bharath, *Bacopa monnieri* extract offsets rotenone induced cytotoxicity in dopaminergic cells and oxidative impairments in mice brain, *Cell. Mol. Neurobiol.*, 32(3) (2011) 455–465.

Shobana, C., R.R. Kumar, T. Sumathi, Alcoholic extract of *Bacopa monniera* Linn. Protects against 6-hydroxydopamine-induced changes in behavioral and biochemical aspects: A pilot study, *Cell. Mol. Neurobiol.*, 32(7) (2012) 1099–1112.

Shukla, O., S. Dubey, U. Rai, Preferential accumulation of cadmium and chromium: toxicity in *Bacopa monnieri* L. under mixed metal treatments, *Bull. Environ. Contam. Toxicol.*, 78(3) (2007) 252–257.

Siddique, Y.H., S.F. Mujtaba, M. Faisal, S. Jyoti, F. Naz, The effect of *Bacopa monnieri* leaf extract on dietary supplementation in transgenic *Drosophila* model of Parkinson's disease, *Eur. J. Integr. Med.*, 6(5) (2014) 571–580.

Simpson, T., M. Pase, C. Stough, *Bacopa monnieri* as an antioxidant therapy to reduce oxidative stress in the aging brain, *Evid. Based Complement. Alternat. Med.*, 501 (2015) 615384.

Singh, A., S.K. Singh, Evaluation of antifertility potential of Brahmi in male mouse, *Contraception*, 79(1) (2009) 71–79.

Singh, B., S. Pandey, S.K. Yadav, R. Verma, S.P. Singh, A.A. Mahdi, Role of ethanolic extract of *Bacopa monnieri* against 1-methyl-4-phenyl-1, 2, 3, 6-tetrahydropyridine (MPTP) induced mice model via inhibition of apoptotic pathways of dopaminergic neurons, *Brain Res. Bull.*, 135 (2017) 120–128.

Singh, H.K., Brain enhancing ingredients from Āyurvedic medicine: Quintessential example of *Bacopa monniera*, a narrative review, *Nutrients*, 5(2) (2013) 478–497.

Singh, M., V. Murthy, C. Ramassamy, Standardized extracts of *Bacopa monniera* protect against MPP+-and paraquat induced toxicity by modulating mitochondrial activities, proteasomal functions, and redox pathways, *Toxicol. Sci.*, 125(1) (2012) 219–232.

Singh, M., V. Murthy, C. Ramassamy, Neuroprotective mechanisms of the standardized extract of *Bacopa monniera* in a paraquat/diquat-mediated acute toxicity, *Neurochem. Int.*, 62(5) (2013) 530–539.

Singh, N.M., P. Jassal, R. V. Kumar, Comparative *In vitro* and *In vivo* study of antioxidants and phytochemical content in *Bacopa monnieri*, *Recent Res. Sci. Technol.*, 3(9) (2011) 78–83.

Singh, R., R. Rachumallu, M. Bhateria, J. Panduri, R.S. Bhatta, *In vitro* effects of standardized extract of *Bacopa monniera* and its five individual active constituents on human P-glycoprotein activity, *Xenobiotica*, (0) (2015) 1–9.

Sinha, S., R. Saxena, Effect of iron on lipid peroxidation, and enzymatic and non-enzymatic antioxidants and bacoside-A content in medicinal plant *Bacopa monnieri* L, *Chemosphere*, 62(8) (2006) 1340–1350.

Sivaramakrishna, C., C.V. Rao, G. Trimurtulu, M. Vanisree, G.V. Subbaraju, Triterpenoid glycosides from *Bacopa monnieri*, *Phytochemistry*, 66(23) (2005) 2719–2728.

Soni, K.K., P. Shrivastava, T. Jones, L. J Mahady, U. Patel, P. Mukherjee, B. Mahady, Extracts of *Bacopa monnieri* (L) Pennell down-regulate the expression of leukotriene C4 synthase mRNA in HL-60 cells and suppress OVA-induced inflammation in BALB/c mice, *Curr. Bioact. Comp.*, 10(1) (2014) 21–30.

Srimachai, S., S. Devaux, C. Demougeot, S. Kumphune, N.D. Ullrich, E. Niggli, K. Ingkaninan, N. Kamkaew, C.N. Scholfield, S. Tapechum, *Bacopa monnieri* extract increases rat coronary flow and protects against myocardial ischemia/reperfusion injury, BMC Complement. *Altern. Med.*, 17(1) (2017) 117.

Srivastava, P., H.N. Raut, H.M. Puntambekar, A.C. Desai, Stability studies of crude plant material of *Bacopa monnieri* and quantitative determination of bacopaside I and bacoside A by HPLC, *Phytochem. Anal.*, 23(5) (2012) 502–507.

Stough, C., J. Lloyd, J. Clarke, L. Downey, C. Hutchison, T. Rodgers, P. Nathan, The chronic effects of an extract of *Bacopa monniera* (Brahmi) on cognitive function in healthy human subjects, *Psychopharmacology*, 156(4) (2001) 481–484.

Stough, C., L.A. Downey, J. Lloyd, B. Silber, S. Redman, C. Hutchison, K. Wesnes et al., Examining the nootropic effects of a special extract of *Bacopa monniera* on human cognitive functioning: 90 day double-blind placebo-controlled randomized trial, *Phytother. Res.*, 22(12) (2008) 1629–1634.

Stough, C., A. Scholey, V. Cropley, K. Wesnes, A. Zangara, M. Pase, K. Savage et al., Examining the cognitive effects of a special extract of *Bacopa monniera* (CDRI08: Keenmnd): A review of ten years of research at Swinburne University, *J. Pharm. Pharm. Sci.*, 16(2) (2013) 254–258.

Subhan, F., M. Abbas, K. Rauf, A. Baseer, Anti GIT motility, toxicological and phytochemical studies on *Bacopa monnieri*, *Pharmacologyonline*, 3 (2010) 937–950.

Sudharani, D., Pharmacological profiles of *Bacopa monnieri*: A review, *Int. J. Pharm.*, 1(1) (2011) 15–23.

Sumathi, T., S. Devaraj, Effect of *Bacopa monniera* on liver and kidney toxicity in chronic use of opioids, *Phytomedicine*, 16(10) (2009) 897–903.

Sumathi, T., V. Nathiya, M. Sakthikumar, Protective effect of bacoside-A against morphine-induced oxidative stress in rats, *Indian J. Pharm. Sci.*, 73(4) (2011) 409–415.

Sumathi, T., M. Nayeem, K. Balakrishna, G. Veluchamy, S.N. Devaraj, Alcoholic extract of *Bacopa monniera* reduces the in vitro effects of morphine withdrawal in guinea-pig ileum, *J. Ethnopharmacol.*, 82(2) (2002) 75–81.

Sumathi, T., A. Nongbri, Hepatoprotective effect of Bacoside-A, a major constituent of *Bacopa monniera* Linn, *Phytomedicine*, 15(10) (2008) 901–905.

Sumathi, T., C. Shobana, J. Christinal, C. Anusha, Protective effect of *Bacopa monniera* on methyl mercury induced oxidative stress in cerebellum of rats, *Cell. Mol. Neurobiol.*, 32(6) (2012) 979–987.

Sumathi, T., G. Veluchamy, Inhibitory effect of *Bacopa monniera* on morphine induced pharmacological effects in mice, *Nat. Prod. Sci.*, 13(1) (2007) 46–53.

Sumathy, T., S. Subramanian, S. Govindasamy, K. Balakrishna, G. Veluchamy, Protective role of *Bacopa monniera* on morphine induced hepatotoxicity in rats, *Phytother. Res.*, 15(7) (2001) 643–645.

Tanveer, A., M. Khan, F. Shah, In vitro Micropropagation of Brahmi-*Bacopa monniera* (L.) Pennell – A step for conservation, *Nanobiotechnica Universale*, 1(2) (2010) 139–150.

Taur, D.J., R.Y. Patil, Some medicinal plants with antiasthmatic potential: A current status, *Asian Pac. J. Trop. Biomed.*, 1(5) (2011) 413–418.

Tiwari, K.N., J. Singh, Effective organogenesis from different explants of *Bacopa monniera* L. (Wettst.) – An important medicinal plant, *Biol. Forum*, 2(1) (2010) 18–22.

Tiwari, V., K.N. Tiwari, B. Deo Singh, Shoot bud regeneration from different explants of *Bacopa monniera* (L.) Wettst. by trimethoprim and bavistin, *Plant Cell Rep.*, 25(7) (2006) 629–635.

Tothiam, C., W. Phrompittayarat, W. Putalun, H. Tanaka, S. Sakamoto, I.A. Khan, K. Ingkaninan, An enzyme-linked immunosorbant assay using monoclonal antibody against bacoside A3 for determination of juju-bogenin glycosides in *Bacopa monnieri* (L.) Wettst, *Phytochem. Anal.*, 22(5) (2011) 385–391.

Uabundit, N., J. Wattanathorn, S. Mucimapura, K. Ingkaninan, Cognitive enhancement and neuroprotective effects of *Bacopa monnieri* in Alzheimer's disease model, *J. Ethnopharmacol.*, 127(1) (2010) 26–31.

Ullah, I., F. Subhan, Z. Lu, S.W. Chan, J.A. Rudd, Action of *Bacopa monnieri* to antagonize cisplatin-induced emesis in *Suncus murinus* (house musk shrew), *J. Pharmacol. Sci.*, 133(4) (2017) 232–239.

Ullah, I., F. Subhan, J.A. Rudd, K. Rauf, J. Alam, M. Shahid, R. Sewell, Attenuation of cisplatin-induced emetogenesis by standardized *Bacopa monnieri* extracts in the pigeon: Behavioral and neurochemical correlations, *Planta Med.*, 80(17) (2014) 1569–1579.

Vajpayee, P., A. Dhawan, R. Shanker, Evaluation of the alkaline comet assay conducted with the wetlands plant *Bacopa monnieri* L. as a model for ecogenotoxicity assessment, *Environ. Mol. Mutagen.*, 47(7) (2006) 483–489.

Vani, G., K. Anbarasi, C. Shyamaladevi, Bacoside A: Role in cigarette smoking induced changes in brain, *Evid. Based Complement. Alternat. Med.*, 501 (2015) 286137.

Verma, P., R.K. Gupta, B.S. Gandhi, P. Singh, CDRI-08 attenuates REST/NRSF-mediated expression of NMDAR1 gene in PBDE-209-exposed mice brain, *Evid. Based Complement. Alternat. Med.*, 501 (2015) 403840.

Vidya, S., D. Sravya, P. Neeraja, A. Ramesh, Evaluation of anti-inflammatory and analgesic activity of poly herbal formulation (PHF) in albino rats, *Int. J. Res. Pharm. Sci.*, 2(3) (2011) 444–449.

Vijayan, V., G. Shyni, A. Helen, Efficacy of *Bacopa monniera* (L.) Wettst in alleviating lysosomal instability in adjuvant-induced arthritis in rats, *Inflammation*, 34(6) (2011) 630–638.

Viji, V., A. Helen, Inhibition of lipoxygenases and cyclooxygenase-2 enzymes by extracts isolated from *Bacopa monniera* (L.) Wettst, *J. Ethnopharmacol.*, 118(2) (2008) 305–311.

Viji, V., A. Helen, Inhibition of pro-inflammatory mediators: role of *Bacopa monniera* (L.) Wettst, *Inflammopharmacology*, 19(5) (2011) 283–291.

Viji, V., S. Kavitha, A. Helen, *Bacopa monniera* (L.) wettst inhibits type ii collagen-induced arthritis in rats, *Phytother. Res.*, 24(9) (2010) 1377–1383.

Vohora, D., S. Pal, K. Pillai, Protection from phenytoin-induced cognitive deficit by *Bacopa monniera*, a reputed Indian nootropic plant, *J. Ethnopharmacol.*, 71(3) (2000) 383–390.

Vollala, V.R., S. Upadhya, S. Nayak, Effect of *Bacopa monniera* Linn. (brahmi) extract on learning and memory in rats: A behavioral study, *J. Vet. Behav.*, 5(2) (2010) 69–74.

Vollala, V.R., S. Upadhya, S. Nayak, Enhanced dendritic arborization of amygdala neurons during growth spurt periods in rats orally intubated with *Bacopa monniera* extract, *Anat. Sci. Int.*, 86(4) (2011a) 179–188.

Vollala, V.R., S. Upadhya, S. Nayak, Enhanced dendritic arborization of hippocampal CA3 neurons by *Bacopa monniera* extract treatment in adult rats, *Rom. J. Morphol. Embryol.*, 52(3) (2011b) 879–886.

Volluri, S.S., S.R. Bammidi, S.C. Chippada, M. Vangalapati, In-vitro anti-arthritic activity of methanolic extract of *Bacopa monniera*, *Pharm. Res.*, 2(2–3) (2011) 156–159.

Williams, R., G. Münch, E. Gyengesi, L. Bennett, *Bacopa monnieri* (L.) exerts anti-inflammatory effects on cells of the innate immune system in vitro, *Food Funct.*, 5(3) (2014) 517–520.

Yadav, R.S., R.K. Shukla, M.L. Sankhwar, A.B. Pant, V.K. Khanna, Modulating effect of *Bacopa monniera* against monocrotophos induced cholinergic and dopaminergic dysfunctions in rats, *Neurosci. Res.*, 71 (2011) e320.

Yamada, K., P. Hung, T.K. Park, P.J. Park, B.O. Lim, A comparison of the immunostimulatory effects of the medicinal herbs Echinacea, Ashwagandha and Brahmi, *J. Ethnopharmacol.*, 137(1) (2011) 231–235.

Zandar, N.A.M., M.M. Zain, Potential neuroprotective effect of commercial *Bacopa monniera* extract, *Signal Processing and Its Applications (CSPA), 2010 6th International Colloquium on*, 2010, pp. 1–5.

Zhou, Y., D.Y. Kong, L. Peng, W.D. Zhang, A new triterpenoid saponin from *Bacopa monniera*, *Chin. Chem. Lett.*, 20(5) (2009) 569–571.

Zhou, Y., Y.-H. Shen, C. Zhang, W.-D. Zhang, Chemical constituents of *Bacopa monnieri*, *Chem. Nat. Compd.*, 43(3) (2007) 355–357.

Zhu, S., K. Zou, H. Fushimi, S. Cai, K. Komatsu, Comparative study on triterpene saponins of Ginseng drugs, *Planta Med.*, 70(7) (2004) 666–677.

26 Natural Medicines
Categories, Comebacks and Catalysts

Ashok Vaidya, Hiteshi Dhami-Shah and Shobha Udipi

CONTENTS

26.1 INTRODUCTION

Natural medicines (NMs) have been all-pervasive in human civilisation for millennia (Petrovska 2012). These have tackled many health-related global problems, safely and with a reasonable efficacy, too. However, as microbiology, pharmacology, chemistry and pharmaceutical technology have developed over the last century, there has been a growing awareness and concern about the quality and potency of NM. Variability in efficacy and safety of NM could also result from such differences in quality (Handa and Kapoor 2015). In addition, the number of categories of NM and their immense diversity in world cultures, historical eras and climatic zones have also presented a formidable challenge to therapeutic research (Erah 2002).

The pharmaceutical renaissance in the twentieth century eclipsed the popularity of NM, primarily also due to the push of the drug industry. There was a general lack of awareness that even many modern drugs had their roots in NM (Vaidya and Vaidya 2010). The backlash of severe and sometimes fatal adverse drug reactions to modern drugs rekindled an interest in 'Green Medicine' (Malerba 2010). There was a comeback of NM, with more science, technology and regulations added to their sourcing, manufacture and marketing.

The emergence of reverse pharmacology (RP) in traditional medicine (TM) was a paradigm shift for NM, used from the bedside to the bench, for the discovery of novel phytopharmaceuticals, botanicals and nutraceuticals (Vaidya 2006). The vast potential of these molecules to serve as scaffolds for the synthesis of new chemical entities (NCEs) was realised as a catalytic force (Patwardhan et al. 2008). Reverse nutraceutics (RN) have also offered a novel approach to convert the unexpected therapeutic responses to macro- and micronutrients into NM by evolving robust evidence-based data. There is a need to evolve novel experimental, analytical and clinical methods and designs for testing safety, quality and efficacy of NM by both RP and RN. Such fast-track, innovative and economical approaches may usher in a research revolution in therapeutics due to research and development based on known bedside safety and the efficacy of NM sources via systematic and organised RP and RN.

26.2   NATURAL MEDICINES: CATEGORIES, COMEBACKS AND CATALYSTS

Natural medicines are defined by *Segen's Medical Dictionary* as 'Any substance (e.g. foxglove, menthol, peyote, etc.) used in an unadulterated state to manage a condition or evoke a desired change in person's physical or mental status' (2011). There are chances of confusion as natural medicine is also as a synonym of naturopathy.

In this digital age, the following definition is alarming: 'Natural Medicines is the combination of two of the leading evidence-based information databases in the field of complementary and alternative medicine: the Natural Medicines Comprehensive Database (NMCD) and Natural Standard'. In 2013, the Therapeutic Research Center merged with Natural Standard in order to create Natural Medicines, calling itself, "The most authoritative resource available on dietary supplements, natural medicines, and complementary alternative and integrative therapies" (Yakobucci 2016; Natural Medicines 2016). The ambitious goal of the database is daunting: 'to provide unbiased, evidence-based information and ratings for over 90,000 dietary supplements, natural medicines, and integrative therapies for healthcare professionals' (Therapeutic Research Center Natural Medicines 2016). The database is huge, with more than 1400 monographs (A–Z), having more than 50,000 scientific references (!). The database has five more searchable sources, besides food, herbs, supplements and commercial products. These also include health and wellness, sports medicine, comparative effectiveness, medical conditions and manufacturers!

Notwithstanding the evidence-based ratings in such a database, one has no clue as to the criticality and reliability of the evidence cited. It is unfortunate that currently apps are made available for people to check the effectiveness checker, nutrient depletion checker, natural product/drug interaction checker, and the grading! Yakobucci gloats over this a bit prematurely: 'It provides high-quality, evidence-based information on natural medicines and alternative therapies in an often-overlooked area of medicine. No other resources in this field seem to offer an equivalent amount of evidence-based rigor' (Yakobucci 2016). There is an urgent need to have a peer review of the quality of evidence in the database by a team of trans-disciplinary experts in medicinal chemistry, pharmacology, toxicology and traditional medicine. Such critical reviews can only build trust for the human use of NMs.

We feel that when one uses the term 'medicine', it has to have a clear dictionary meaning of 'a drug or other preparation for the treatment or prevention of disease' (Oxford Living Dictionaries: English n.d.). Dietary supplements (DS) and nutraceuticals, by the DSHEA Act (US National Institutes of Health 1994), are not supposed to claim to cure or prevent diseases. So categorising all DS as Natural Medicines is untenable. The claims for improvement with DS are permitted mainly for the structures, functions and health of organs. Unlike DS, the category of botanical drugs can be 'intended for use in diagnosing, curing, mitigating, or treating disease would meet the definition of a drug under section 201(g) (1)(B) of the FD&C Act and would be subject to regulation as such' (US FDA 2016). In India too, phytopharmaceutical and AYUSH medicines are distinct categories to be used as drugs, apart from DS/nutraceuticals meant for self-medication (Bhat 2016).

NMs are preventive or therapeutic products of mineral, plant or animal origin, used singly or in combination for defined medical indications. With this definition, the natural remedies used in the approved systems of medicine like Ayurveda, Siddha, Unani, Chinese Medicine, Tibetan Medicine, Kampo Medicine and Homeopathy can be considered under individual system categories. When these remedies are further investigated as per the efficacy at current therapeutic targets and for safety studies, the labels of botanical drugs and phytopharmaceuticals would create a new category of NM. These are indeed comebacks of herbal drugs in their new incarnations, with efficacy, safety and quality. The latter characteristics would make NM acceptable globally. The ethnobotany and ethnopharmacology of medicinal plants and certain mineral, plant or animal products have also provided several hits and leads that can offer opportunities for new NMs (Mukherjee et al. 2007; Gonzalez et al. 2016).

Current cultural conditioning does not permit Western nations to accept the Asian systems of medicine, with their unique epistemology that is alien to materialistic medicine. It is often forgotten that the very first wave of modern drugs arose from understanding of the mechanisms of actions of the medicinal and poisonous plants of the ancient world. Those phytomolecules provided impetus for drug discovery and development. A brief recapitulation of that history would convince us that NMs are still available for more research and development. Then the potential of NM would expand immensely, ranging from home remedies to semi-synthetic new drugs based on clinically active molecules as scaffolds (Patwardhan and Vaidya 2010).

26.3 ROOTS OF MODERN DRUGS IN NATURAL MEDICINES

It was stated by Aulus Cornelius Celsus (ca. 25 BCE to ca. 50 CE), 'That medicines and cures were first found out, and then after the reasons and causes were discoursed; and not the causes first found out, and by light from them the medicines and cures discovered'. Several major NM in the past were discovered at the bedside and from folklore usage. It has been stated in the *Oxford Textbook of Clinical Pharmacology and Drug Therapy*, 'Historically modern drug therapy has developed from the herbal and folklore medicine of the past with its mixture of magic, empirical pharmacology and faith of the patient in the doctor' (Grahame-Smith and Aronson 1984). Antimalarial, anticancer and antidiabetic drugs also have their roots in TM used in different countries, including artemisinin, vincristine and metformin. Ayurveda and traditional Chinese medicine still have a large repertoire of TM that could serve as initiatives for natural drug discovery through reverse pharmacology.

The most dramatic effects of plants were as poisons, observed and recorded for centuries in Asia, Africa and South America (Neuwinger 1996). Poisonous plants were also used in small non-toxic doses as drugs by the natives of these continents. Table 26.1 lists how the study of poisons led to the mechanisms of actions, which led to the discovery and development of new chemical entities (NCEs) as agonist and antagonist modern drugs (Neuwinger 1996).

Rauwolfia serpentina was shown to be anti-hypertensive, in India, by Gananath Sen and Kartik Bose, as early as 1931. They also reported some remarkable side effects (Sen and Bose 1931). After a gap of 18 years, Vakil confirmed its anti-hypertensive effect (Vakil 1949). Several astute observations and a record of the side effects such as depression, gynecomastia and galactorrhea, Parkinsonism, nasal congestion and hyperacidity eventually led to their mechanistic understanding of amine depletion and many NCEs and modern drugs were developed as spin-offs for these indications such as antidepressants, bromocriptine, L-dopa, oxymetazoline and cimetidine. The path to NM and NCEs can also be facilitated through the understanding the mechanisms of the side effects of widely used herbal or animal products used in the traditional systems of medicine.

TABLE 26.1
Poisons as Roots of Modern Drugs

Poisonous Plants Modern Drug	Human/Animal Effect	Mechanism
Curare tomentosum Tubocurarine	Conscious paralysis	Neuromuscular block
P venenosum Neostigmine	Ordeal poison	Anti-cholinesterase
Atropa belladonna Atropine	Fatal poisoning	Cholinergic blockage
Meliotus alba Dicumarol	Bleeding disease	Anti-vitamin K
Claviceps purpurea Ergotamine	St. Anthony's fire	Vasoconstrictor
Erythroxylon coca Procaine	Central stimulant	Local anaesthetic
Bothrops jaraca Captopril	Viper poison	ACE inhibitor

26.4 REVERSE PHARMACOLOGY FOR NATURAL MEDICINES

There are two nuances of the term 'reverse pharmacology': one meaning is the path of pharmacology from the bedside observations to bench experiments, and the second is the quest for drug-like molecules (endogenous or extrinsic) that dock with human macromolecules as receptors or enzymes. For the present chapter, our focus is on the first meaning of RP (Raut et al. 2016). RP can be pursued in three stages. First, the experiential stage covers robust documentation, by meticulous records, of clinical and laboratory observations of the effects of standardised natural drugs of traditional medicine. Second, the exploratory stage includes studies for safety, efficacy, interactions and dose-range finding in patients with defined therapeutic targets, besides paraclinical studies in relevant *in vitro* and *in vivo* models to evaluate pharmacological activities. The third stage consists of experimental studies, basic and clinical, at several levels of biological organisation, to investigate and identify the pharmacological correlates of the safety and efficacy of the NM. The RP path is economical, fast-track and productive (Figure 26.1). The scope of RP extends also to the unveiling of the molecular mechanisms of action and the use of active phytomolecules as scaffolds for synthetically modified novel candidates of NM (Patwardhan et al. 2008).

The path of RP was chosen for a nationwide major NM discovery endeavour by the Council of Scientific and Industrial Research under its New Millennium Indian Technology Leadership Initiative (NMITLI; India n.d.). The three major indications chosen were: (1) diabetes mellitus, (2) viral hepatitis and (3) osteoarthritis. The collective research and development led to very interesting hits, leads and candidates for NM for these conditions. The state-of-the-art targets were studied and showed significant activity with interventional NM. For diabetes, phytoactivity was detected on GLUT-4 translocation, inhibition of glycation, AKT phosphorylation and cataract formation. In osteoarthritis, chondrocyte protection, CTX reduction and increased muscle strength were observed. The effects of the NM as hepatoprotective was shown with a reduction in fatty infiltration, prevention of AKT/paracetamol liver damage and a reduction in pro inflammatory cytokines.

For malaria, medicinal plants have played a major role in the history as shown by *Cinchona officinale* and *Artemisia annua*. However, it was unfortunate that there was an inordinate delay of global use of the therapeutic wisdom of traditional medicine. RP has opened up fast-tracking NM for malaria, as shown by the studies with *Nyctanthes arbor-tristis* and *Argemone mexicana* (Karnik et al. 2008; Willcox et al. 2011; Godse et al. 2016). In view of the current challenges of drug-resistant malaria,

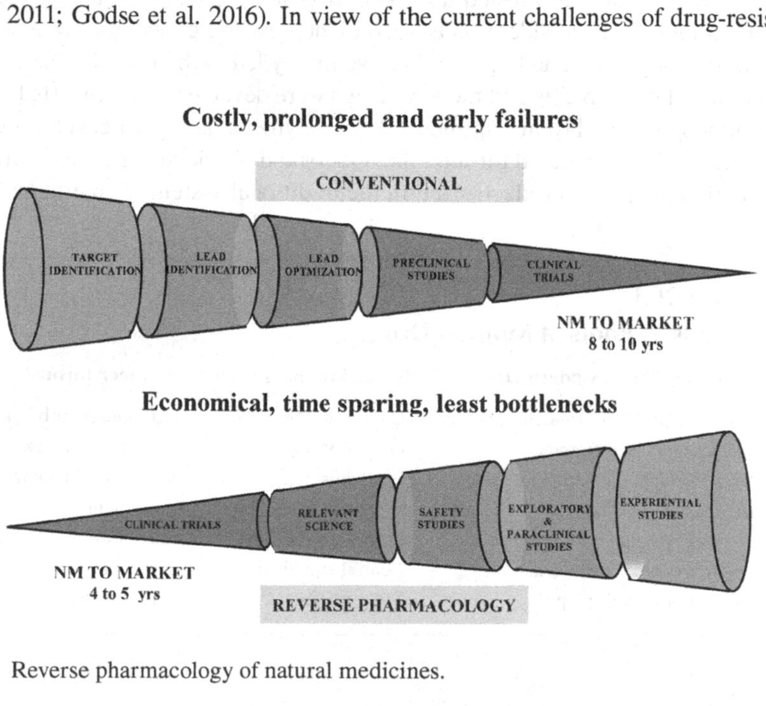

FIGURE 26.1   Reverse pharmacology of natural medicines.

TABLE 26.2

Reverse Nutraceutics

Experiential	Exploratory	Experimental
Case reports	Human nutra-dynamics	Models *in vitro, ex vivo*
Case series	Nutrakinetics	Models *in vivo*
Observational studies	$N = 1$ studies	Target markers
Nutra-epidemiology	Sequential design	Surrogate markers
Retrolective	Prospective	Controlled trails
Field studies	Open comparative	Double 'vision' studies

even disease-modifying NM have a significant potential in reducing severity and mortality in malaria (Gogtay et al. 2006). The fact that *Nyctanthes arbor-tristis* can significantly reduce TNF-α as well as the morbidity, NM do have a place in the management of malaria (Godse et al. 2006).

For hepatoprotective NM, there have been many clinical and experimental studies on plants and natural formulations (Antarkar et al. 1978, 1980; Vaidya et al. 1996; Shetty et al. 2010; Dhami-Shah et al. 2018). The entire story, starting with the double-blind trial of an Ayurvedic drug *Arogyavardhini* and leading to its active plant (50%) – *Picrorhiza kurroa* – and eventually to the phytoactive picroside II with molecular actions in HepG2 cell lines, illustrates how RP on traditional remedies can indeed be a paradigm-shifting path for NM discovery and development (Vaidya 2014).

26.5 REVERSE NUTRACEUTICS FOR NUTRIENTS AS NATURAL MEDICINES

There are innumerable books, monographs, journals, magazines, reviews and articles on nutraceuticals, functional foods and health foods with structure and function health claims (Wildman 2002; US FDA 2013; Gupta 2016; *Journal of Nutraceuticals and Food Science* n.d.). There are, however, relatively limited references for macro- and micronutrients that can be used or developed as NM, with preventive and curative efficacy in diseases other than deficiencies. Reverse nutraceutics (RN) is, like RP, a path for the development of NM from bedside to bench (Vaidya et al. 2013; Pathak et al. 2014; Vaidya and Shukla 2015). The stages of experiential, exploratory and experimental are also relevant to RN (Table 26.2).

RN can be applied to the individual proximate principles or their combinations. The basic constituents of proteins, fats and carbohydrates are also candidates as NM for the prevention or cure of diseases other than of nutritional nature. Vitamins and minerals, too, can be NM when used or developed for extra-nutritional medical indications. Sometimes the dividing line between NM and DS may be unclear. In view of many categories like functional foods, health foods and medical foods recognised in different regulatory nomenclature, however, NM needs its identity not as a generic term (*vide supra*) but as a specific class of natural products–derived medicines, with evidence of safety, efficacy and quality and with defined medical indications.

As early as in 1817, William Prout reported on the nature of what he then called the proximate principles of urine (Prout 1817, p. 538). He reported 'the striking effect produced by a common laxative, in restoring my own urine from an unnatural and turbid state to its proper colour and transparency'. He related the state of the digestion and bowels to kidney function. He prophetically said, 'Remedies, no matter of what description, that have a tendency to restore general health, must have a tendency to insure the due performance of all bodily function, and secretion among the rest' (Prout 1817, 539). The current claims of organ health improvements with DS were almost anticipated! Recent advances in understanding of the pathogenesis and its markers nudge us to correlate specific phytoactive compounds that reverse the disease and the mechanisms. Such an approach for

RN applied to amino acids, fatty acids, oligosaccharides, vitamins and minerals could be very useful for discovering and developing NM for several non-deficiency diseases.

The supply of L-dopa to restore dopamine levels in the corpus striatum of patients with Parkinson's disease, excitatory amino acids (AA) in Alzheimer's disease to facilitate neural transmission in hippocampus and increased brain availability of tryptophan in anorexia are some examples of the potential of AA-related NM (L-dopa; Timothy et al. 1889; Rossi-Fanelli and Cangiano 1991). DHA, α-linolenic acid, sciadonic acid and α-lipoic acid have been reviewed substantially (Huk-Kolega et al. 2011; Swanson et al. 2012; Balk and Lichtenstein 2017; Pedrono et al. 2018). However, there is a need to focus on specific indications of unmet medical needs rather than claim general coverage of multiple diseases. Among natural polysaccharides there has been a significant emphasis on oligosaccharides from soluble fibres as a prebiotic. There has been relatively less attention paid to polysaccharides of some of the widely used traditional plants like *Curcuma longa* and *Tinospora cordifolia* (Gonda et al. 1990; Gupta et al. 2017). The immunomodulatory activities of plant polysaccharides offer a significant potential for NM.

There is a controversy about the use of vitamins as nutraceuticals when persons are receiving a balanced diet, exposure to sunlight and adequate food intake. Indeed, a sub-segment of this industry – gummy vitamins – has been projected to reach $4.17 billion by the year 2025 in the United States (*Nutraceuticals World* 2017). Our emphasis is primarily on non-nutritional medical indications for vitamins. In chronic obstructive pulmonary disease, vitamin C has been observed to increase resistance to skeletal muscle fatigue (Rossman et al. 2013). It is worthwhile to explore whether large doses of vitamin C prove to be beneficial in chronic fatigue syndrome also. Recently, a cardiologist observed that there was an attenuation and disappearance of sore throat in common cold by dissolution of 1–2 tablets of 500 mg of vitamin C in the mouth (Mehta Akshay, personal communication). However, the systemic administration in well-designed trials for the common cold has not earlier reported any success. The entire story of vitamin C has been muddled with protagonists like Linus Pauling and Albert Szent-Gyorgyi, both Nobel laureates, and antagonists with double-blind trials (Pauling 1970; Edsall 1972). Szent-Gyorgyi reported how yeast and wheat germ at breakfast eliminated frequent colds in a Jamaica horseman and himself. He had added vitamin C to his breakfast (Szent-Gyorgyi 1932, 71–73). In Ayurveda, Chyavanprash (a jam with *Emblica officinalis* among its major constituents) is widely used for enhancing resistance to respiratory infections (Narayana et al. 2017). It may be worthwhile to explore the possibility of *Emblica officinalis* in the common cold, in view of the plant containing significant amounts of vitamin C and immunopotentiating polyphenols. Vitamin K for many years was primarily related to its impact on coagulation. It is only recently that its role in bone and cardiovascular health has emerged globally. Our group serendipitously discovered some novel effects of vitamin K_{2-7} – that is, its significant therapeutic effect in systremma (idiopathic muscle cramps) and relief in mild to moderate peripheral neuropathy (Mehta et al. 2010; Kulkarni et al. 2013).

26.6 CLINICAL STUDIES FOR ACTIVITY, EFFICACY AND COMPLEMENTARITY

India and China, being leaders in pluralistic healthcare, offer an immense scope to build bridges between modern medicine (MM) and TM (Vaidya and Vaidya 1998). Synergy between their diverse epistemology is not easy to achieve save through political will and a concerted effort. Starting at the TM bedside for therapeutic outcomes is a pragmatic way to detect leads for novel MM (Vaidya 1996a; Vaidya and Mehta 2002). The quest for therapeutic activity takes precedence over efficacy in RP. There is a need for sophisticated markers of therapeutic response during experiential and exploratory studies in RP. As an example, we had not only recorded malaria parasite clearance but also monitored the disappearance of the parasite DNA by PCR/RFLP in the exploratory study with *Nyctanthes arbor-tristis* in patients (Godse et al. 2016). Similarly for the exploratory study with *Tinospora cordifolia* as a bone marrow protective in cancer chemotherapy, Thatte et al. measured GM-CSF besides the white cell count (Thatte et al. 1994).

The designs of clinical trials for the efficacy of NM have a wide spectrum. These cover $n = 1$ studies, sequential trial design, dose-optimisation with kinetics, human pharmacodynamic sand controlled randomised/comparative studies. The advantage of knowledge gained on the activity and usage safety, from previous traditional text records, observational therapeutic (OT) data and Ayurvedic pharmacoepidemiology (AyPE) is immense. Hence the initial studies with NM, in open experiential manner, offer a major advantage over an NCE that has to be tested for the first time in humans (Mehta 1949; Vaidya et al. 2003; Vaidya 2011). The insistence on huge, randomised, placebo-controlled, multi-centric clinical trials as a gold standard of evidence is due to the bias for NCE experience in the past. NM, with ready-made knowledge base of prior human use, requires a different mode of generating evidence. As this has been lost sight of, we have lost many opportunities in India to discover new drugs based on robust clinical observations. This happened with *Rauwolfia serpentina* as so aptly described by Jain and Murthy (Jain and Murthy 2009). The need for not missing out on serendipitous clinical effects – beneficial or adverse – of natural remedies cannot be overemphasised. There has to be an organised database for such effects with ready access to physicians, for timely entries. The statistics to be used for the efficacy of NM also require novel approaches like falsifiability, consensual and other types of validity, and so forth (Bland and Altman 1986; Popper 2002). Age-old uses of NM by millions of people have to be looked at with an open mind and with more experiential and observational approaches in humans.

In the West, there is a widespread misconception about the safety of DS for self-medication or as complementary remedies. It is often forgotten that such over-the-counter available DS are most often age-old drugs from the traditional systems of other nations like China, India and the peoples of Africa. These drugs are used for clinical indications, as per the principles, dosage, practice and experience of practitioners in traditional systems. In Western nations there is in general a non-acceptance of physicians trained in the Asian traditional systems of practicing medicine. The very drugs TM practitioners use are, however, sold freely as DS and nutraceuticals. This situation is not only potentially hazardous, but also disrespectful of millennia-old Asian systems of healthcare and their training courses. Dropping such xenophobia, there is a need to permit well-trained healers to practice and use such DS as NM. This urgency cannot be overemphasised. The path of RP and RN can also be adopted in the West, for limited human studies for efficacy and safety, with the help TM physicians, as done in India. The current – often haphazard and relatively uninformed – use of NM for complementary and self-administration has to be corrected by training of the health personnel and community in rational uses of NM.

26.7 SAFETY AND TOXICITY OF NATURAL MEDICINES

It is a widespread myth that all the natural products are safe. Some of the products of mineral, plant and animal origin can be toxic even with very small doses, but considering all the natural remedies of other systems of medicine as toxic is equally irrational. For RP research based on remedies used clinically in traditional medicine, the records and observations on safety in patients are crucial. It has been reported that about 80% of people globally use herbal drugs for health (Zhang et al. 2015). This fact leads to the necessity of conducting pharmacoepidemiological studies of herbal/natural drugs in a systematic way. Despite the huge global market of herbal remedies, there are no regulations for post-marketing surveillance of tolerability. As a consequence, sudden surprises of adverse drug reactions are often encountered with DS usage. Applying OECD guidelines for toxicity, meant for NCEs, is an irrational approach when traditional usage safety and experiential record in TM are available.

As early as 2004, WHO published guidelines on safety monitoring of herbal medicines in pharmacovigilance systems (WHO 2004). The challenges in safety monitoring were highlighted vis-à-vis quality control. The diversity in national regulatory systems was also pointed out. There has been more stress on vigilance rather than on pharmacoepidemiology in traditional systems of medicine. Several pharmacovigilance programmes for herbal drugs have failed. The safety protocols needed for NM, used in its crude original source for centuries, will have to take into consideration the available reports on human safety data, the concomitant diet prescribed, the nature of prescribed dosage forms and the phytochemistry of the plants, as well as precautions noted in TM.

Semecarpus anacardium (Bhallataka) is traditionally given with milk in Ayurveda. When toxicity studies were carried out in animals there was mortality that was nullified when the plant was co-administered with milk. Similarly, in the traditional Chinese formulation, *Dichroa febrifuga* was always administered with other plants such as *Glycyrrhiza glabra*, *Ziziphus jujuba* and *Zingiber officinale* (Rasoanaivo et al. 2011). This was forgotten in clinical trials for malaria. There was good efficacy, but tolerability of the plant was considered unacceptable with a high incidence of the side effects nausea and vomiting. The additional plants effectively controlled such side effects. Such examples emerge time and again when dietary supplements are borrowed from other systems without any knowledge of the precise modes and limitations of their original drug use. The side effects of *Ephedra* and *Piper methysticum* (kava) led to their ban (National Institutes of Health 2004; FAO and WHO 2010). There are also risks of litigation when one nation's drug is sold as a DS in another nation.

Mucuna pruriens seed powder has been shown to be effective and safe in the management of Parkinson's disease (Vaidya et al. 1978; Manyam 1990; Katzenschlager et al. 2004). This is a drug in Ayurveda, but it is sold widely in the United States as a dietary supplement. The plant contains substantial amounts of L-dopa and indole alkaloids. The plant has been reported to cause toxic psychosis (Infante et al. 1990), and a concomitant administration of an MAO inhibitor with *Mucuna pruriens* can be hazardous (Sjoqvist 1965). Warnings for such side effects, although common in L-dopa drug leaflets, are hardly ever seen on the current DS packages of *Mucuna pruriens*. Unlike such *laissez-faire* approaches in DS, the usage of NM needs appropriate package inserts with precautions, contraindications, interactions and the detailed instruction on dosage and concomitant drugs and diet.

26.8   QUALITY ASSURANCE OF NATURAL MEDICINES

There are innumerable articles, reviews and books on the theme of quality control and assurance of herbal medicines. A Google Scholar search of the phrase 'quality of herbal medicines' on 12 April 2018 yielded around 256,000 results. At one end of the spectrum, there is an insistence that TM have the same level of QC as NCE and biotech drugs, and at the other end there is an insistence on retaining the simple criteria for QC as in TM. The middle path is more pragmatic. It insists on the identification and standardisation of the source, good agricultural collection and manufacturing practices, fingerprinting of the key phytomarkers, shelf-life and analysis for microbial contamination, fungal toxins, pesticides and heavy metals. There is currently no international harmonisation for the guidelines for these criteria. There are many herbal pharmacopoeias that have very divergent monographs on plants (Handa et al. 1998–1999; Brendler et al. 2010; Upton et al. 2011), but these volumes quite cursorily deal with human usage safety, pharmacology and clinical evidence. There is much more stress on pharmacognosy and analysis that helps QC but not therapy. There is a need to develop a critical volume of Natural Drug Formulary for the most widely used 100 remedies globally, with an orientation to RP and clinical usage safety and precautions. There are basic books and guidelines available that can guide such an endeavour (Alasalvar and Shahidi 2013; US FDA 2018). The unique ways to formulate traditional medicines has to be kept in mind while planning the pre-formulation research and development on TM.

26.9   CONCLUSIONS

NMs are derived from the natural products/drugs of the traditional systems of medicine and also from macronutrients and micronutrients that have non-nutritional medical indications. For the former, the RP path is suitable, economical and productive to assess efficacy and safety. For NMs derived from nutrients, the novel path of RN is highlighted. There is a need for substantial evidence on usage safety, efficacy with objective markers of response and standardisation for the quality control and batch to batch fidelity. There is immense scope for NM discovery and development from TM and nutritional sciences.

REFERENCES

Alasalvar, C. and Shahidi, F., eds. (2013). *Tree Nuts: Composition, Phytochemicals and Health Effects*. Boca Raton, FL: CRC Press.

Antarkar, D. S., Tathed, P. S. and Vaidya, A. B. (1978). A pilot phase II trial with Arogyawardhini and Punarnavadi-Kwath in viral hepatitis. *Panminerva Medica*, **20**(3), 157–560.

Antarkar, D. S., Vaidya, A. B., Doshi, J. C., Athavale, A. V., et al. (1980). A double-blind clinical trial of Arogya-Wardhini – an Ayurvedic drug – in acute viral hepatitis. *Indian Journal of Medical Research*, **72**, 588–593.

Balk, E. M. and Lichtenstein, A. H. (2017). Omega-3 fatty acids and cardiovascular disease: Summary of the 2016 agency of healthcare research and quality evidence review. *Nutrients*, **9**(8), 865. doi:10.3390/nu9080865.

Bhat, A. (2016). Phytopharmaceuticals: A new drug class regulated in India. *Perspectives in Clinical Research*, **7**, 59–61.

Bland, J. M. and Altman, D. G. (1986). Statistical methods for assessing agreement between two methods of clinical measurement. *Lancet*, **1**, 307–310.

Brendler, T., Eloff, J., Gurib-Fakim, A. and Phillips, D., eds. (2010). *African Herbal Pharmacopoeia*. Mauritius: Graphic Press.

Dhami-Shah, H., Vaidya, R. A., Udipi, S., Raghavan, S., Abhijit, S., Mohan, V., Balasubramanyam, M. and Vaidya, A. D. B. (2018). Picroside II attenuates fatty acid accumulation in HepG2 cells via modulation of fatty acid uptake and synthesis. *Clinical and Molecular Hepatology*, **24**, 77–87.

Edsall, J. T. (1972). Linus Pauling and vitamin C. *Science*, **178**(4062), 696.

Erah, P. O. (2002). Editorial: Herbal medicines: Challenges. *Tropical Journal of Pharmaceutical Research*, **1**, 53–54.

Food and Agriculture Organization of the United Nations (FAO) and World Health Organization (WHO). (2010). Discussion paper on the development of kava. Rome, Italy: Joint office of FAO and WHO. [Accessed 12 April 2018]. Available from: http://www.ikec.org/sites/default/files/Codex%20alimentarius%20kava_draft_0.pdf

Godse, C. S., Tathed, P. S., Talwalkar, S. S., Vaidya, R. A., Amonkar, A. J., Vaidya, A. B. and Vaidya, A. D. B. (2016). Antiparasitic and disease-modifying activity of *N. arbor-tristis* in malaria: An exploratory clinical study. *Journal of Ayurveda and Integrative Medicine*, **7**, 238–248.

Godse, C. S., Vaidya, A. B., Tathed, P. S. and Vaidya, R. A. (2006). Thrombocytopenia and TNF-α levels in malaria. *Journal of the Association of Physicians of India*, **52**, 1009.

Gogtay, N.J., Kshirsagar, N.A., Vaidya, A.B. (2006). Current challenges in drug-resistant malaria. *Journal of Postgraduate Medicine*, **52**, 241–242.

Gonda, R., Tomoda, M., Shimizu, N. and Kanari, M. (1990). Characterization of polysaccharides having activity on the reticuloendothelial system from the rhizome of *Curcuma longa*. *Chemical and Pharmaceutical Bulletin (Tokyo)*, **38**, 482–486.

Gonzalez, J. A., Amich, F., Postigo-Mota, S. and Vallejo, R. (2016). Therapeutic and prophylactic uses of invertebrates in contemporary Spanish ethno-veterinary medicine. *Journal of Ethnobiology and Ethnomedicine*, **12**, 36.

Grahame-Smith, D. G. and Aronson, J. K. (1984). *Oxford Textbook of Clinical Pharmacology and Drug Therapy*. Oxford, London, UK: Oxford University Press.

Greenamyre, J. T. and Young, A. B. (1989). Excitatory amino acid and Alzheimer's disease. *Neurobiology of Aging*, **10**, 593–602.

Gupta, P. K., Rajan, M. G. R. and Kulkarni, S. (2017). Activation of murine macrophages by G1-4A, a polysaccharide from *Tinospora cordifolia*, in TLR4/MyD88 dependent manner. *International Immunopharmacology*, **50**, 168–177. doi:10.1016/j.intimp.2017.06.025.

Gupta, R. C., ed. (2016). *Nutraceuticals–Efficacy, Safety and Toxicity*. Amsterdam, the Netherlands: Academic Press.

Handa, S. S. and Kapoor, V. K. (2015). *Textbook of Pharmacognosy*. Delhi, India: Vallabh Publications.

Handa, S. S., Mundkinajeddu, D. and Mangal, A. K. (1998–1999) Indian Herbal Pharmacopoeia, 2 vols. Jammu, India: Regional Research Library – Council of Scientific and Industrial Research & Indian Drug Manufacturers' Association.

Huk-Kolega, H., Skibska, B., Kleniewska, P., Piechota, A., Michalski, Ł. and Goraca A. (2011). Role of lipoic acid in health and disease. *Polski Merkuriusz Lekarski*, **31**(183), 183–185.

India. Government of India. (n.d.). New millennium Indian technology leadership initiative by CSIR. *National Portal of India*. [Accessed: 11 April 2018]. Available from: https://www.india.gov.in/ new-millennium-indian-technology-leadership-initiative-csir.

Infante, M. E., Perez, A. M., Simao, M. R., et al. (1990). Outbreak of acute toxic psychosis attributed to *Mucuna pruriens*. *Lancet*, **336**, 1129.

Jain, S. and Murthy, P. (2009). The other Bose: An account of missed opportunities in the history of neurobiology in India. *Current Science*, **97**, 266–269.

Journal of Nutraceuticals and Food Science. (n.d.). Nutraceuticals: High impact articles. *Journal of Nutraceuticals and Food Science* [Accessed 13 April 2018]. Available from: http://nutraceuticals.imedpub.com

Karnik, S. R., Tathed, P. S., Antarkar, D. S., Godse, C. S., Vaidya, R. A. and Vaidya, A. D. B. (2008). Antimalarial and clinical safety of traditionally used *Nyctanthes arbor-tristis* Linn. *Indian Journal of Traditional Knowledge*, **7**, 330–334.

Katzenschlager, R., Evans, A., Manson, A., et al. (2004). *Mucuna pruriens* in Parkinson's disease: A double blind clinical and pharmacological study. *Journal of Neurology, Neurosurgery, and Psychiatry*, **75**, 1672–1677.

Kulkarni, V. K., Upase, D. P., Dound, Y. A., Jadhav, S. S., Bhave, A. A., Mehta, D. S. and Vaidya, A. B. (2013). The effect of vitamin K2-7 in peripheral neuropathy due to vitamin B-12 deficiency and/or diabetes mellitus: A preliminary study. *Indian Practitioner*, **66**, 625–630.

Malerba, L. (2010). What is the 'green' medicine revolution? *Huffington Post*. [Accessed on 9 April 2018]. Available from: https://www.huffingtonpost.com/larry-malerba/what-is-the-green-medicin_b_679095.html.

Manyam, B. V. (1990). Paralysis agitans and levodopa in "Ayurveda": Ancient Indian medical treatise. *Movement Disorders*, **5**, 47–48.

Mehta, D. S., Vaidya, R. A., Dound, Y. A., Nabar, N. S., Pandey, S. N. and Vaidya, A. D. B. (2010). Therapeutic activity and safety of vitamin K 2-7 in muscle cramps: An interventional case-series. *Indian Practitioner*, **63**, 287–291.

Mehta, P. J. (1949). *Caraka Saṃhitā*. Jamnagar, India: Gulabkunvarba Ayurvedic Society.

Mukherjee, P. K., Maiti, K., Mukherjee, K. and Houghten, P. J. (2007). Leads from Indian medicinal plants with hypoglycemic potentials. *Journal of Ethnopharmacology*, **106**, 1–28.

Narayana, D. B., Durg, S., Manohar, P. R., Mahapatra, A. and Aramya, A. R. (2017). Chyawanprash: A review of therapeutic benefits as in authoritative texts and documented clinical literature. *Journal of Ethnopharmacology*, **197**, 52–60. doi:10.1016/j.jep.2016.07.078.

Natural Medicines. (2016). *TRC: Natural Medicines*. [Accessed 9 April 2018]. Available from: https://natural-medicines.therapeuticresearch.com.

Neuwinger, H. D. (1996). *African Ethnobotany–Poisons and Drugs: Chemistry, Pharmacology & Toxicology*. Weinheim, Germany: Chapman & Hall.

Nutraceuticals World. (2017). U.S. gummy vitamins market to reach $4.17 billion by 2025. *Nutraceuticals World*. [Accessed 14 April 2018]. Available from: https://www.nutraceuticalsworld.com/issues/2017-12/ view_breaking-news/us-gummy-vitamins-market-to-reach-417-billion-by-2025/1521.

Oxford Living Dictionaries: English. (n.d.). S.v. medicine. [Accessed 9 April 2018]. Available from: https:// en.oxforddictionaries.com/definition/medicine.

Pathak, N., Shah, H. and Vaidya, A. (2014). Clinical perspective of Ayurceuticals: Challenges and opportunities for global health and wellness. In D. Ghosh, D. Bagchi and T. Konishi, eds., *Clinical Aspects for Functional Foods and Nutraceuticals*. Boca Raton, FL: CRC Press. pp. 33–49.

Patwardhan, B. and Vaidya, A. D. (2010). Natural products drug discovery: Accelerating the clinical candidate development using reverse pharmacology approaches. *Indian Journal of Experimental Biology*, **48**, 220–227.

Patwardhan, B., Vaidya, A. D. B., Chorghade, M. and Joshi, S. P. (2008). Reverse pharmacology and systems approach for drug discovery and development. *Current Bioactive Compounds*, **4**, 1–12.

Pauling, L. (1970). Vitamin C and Common Cold. San Francisco, CA: Freeman.

Pedrono, F., Boulier-Monthean, N., Boissel, F., et al. (2018). The hypotriglyceridemic effect of sciadonic acid is mediated by the inhibition of Δ9-desaturase expression and activity. *Molecular Nutrition & Food Research*, **62**(4). doi:10.1002/mnfr.201700567.

Petrovska, B. B. (2012). Historical review of medicinal plants' usage. *Pharmacognosy Reviews*, **6**, 1–5.

Popper, K. (2002). *The Logic of Scientific Discovery*. London, UK: Routledge.

Prout, W. (1817). Observations on the nature of some of the proximate principles of the urine). with a few remarks upon preventing those diseases connected with the morbid state of that fluid. *Medico-Chirurgical Transactions*, **8**, 521–544.

Rasoanaivo, P., Wright, C. W., Willcox, M. L. and Gilbert, B. (2011). Whole plant extracts versus single compounds for the treatment of malaria: Synergy and positive interactions. *Malaria Journal*, **10**(Suppl 1), S4.

Raut, A. A., Chorghade, M. S. and Vaidya, A. D. B. (2016). Reverse pharmacology. In B. Patwardhan and R. Chaguturu, eds. *Innovative Approaches in Drug Discovery*. Amsterdam, the Netherlands: Elsevier. pp. 89–124.

Rossi-Fanelli, F. and Cangiano, C. (1991). Increased availability of tryptophan in brain as common pathogenic mechanism for anorexia associated with different diseases. *Nutrition*, **7**, 364–367.

Rossman, M. J., Garten, R. S., Groot, H. J., Reese, V., Zhao, J., Amann, M. and Richardson, R. S. (2013). Ascorbate infusion increases skeletal muscle fatigue resistance in patients with chronic obstructive pulmonary disease. *American Journal of Physiology-Regulatory, Integrative and Comparative Physiology*, **305**(10), R1163–R1170. doi:10.1152/ajpregu.00360.2013.

Segen's Medical Dictionary. (2011). S.v. Natural medicine. [Accessed 9 April 2018]. Available from: https://medical-dictionary.thefreedictionary.com/Natural+medicine.

Sen, G. and Bose, K. (1931). *Rauwolfia serpentina* & new Indian drug industry and high blood pressure. *Indian Medical World*, **2**, 194.

Shetty, S. N., Mengi, S., Vaidya, R. and Vaidya, A. D. (2010). A study of standardized extracts of *Picrorhiza kurroa* Royle ex Benth in experimental non-alcoholic fatty liver disease. *Journal of Ayurveda and Integrative Medicine*, **1**(3), 203–210.

Sjoqvist, F. (1965). Psychotropic Drugs (2) Interaction between monoamine oxidase (MAO) inhibitors and other substances. *Proceedings of the Royal Society of Medicine*, **58**, 967–978.

Swanson, D., Block, R. and Mousa, S. A. (2012). Omega-3 Fatty Acids EPA and DHA: Health Benefits Throughout Life. *Advances in Nutrition*, **3**(1), 1–7. doi:10.3945/an.111.000893.

Szent-Gyorgyi, A. (1932). *The Living State–With Observation on Cancer*. New York: Academic Press.

Thatte, U., Rao, S. G. and Dahanukar, S. A. (1994). *Tinospora cordifolia* induces colony stimulating activity in serum. *Journal of Postgraduate Medicine*, **40**, 202–203.

Therapeutic Research Center. (2016). Natural medicines. *Therapeutic Research Center*. [Accessed 9 April 2018]. Available from: http://trchealthcare.com/solutions/natural-medicines.

Upton, R., Graff, A., Jolliffe, G., Langer, R. and Willamson, E., eds. (2011). *American Herbal Pharmacopoeia: Botanical Pharmacognosy*. Boca Raton, FL: CRC Press.

US FDA (Food and Drug Administration). (2013). Food labeling guide. [Accessed 13 April 2018]. Available from: https://www.fda.gov/food/guidanceregulation/guidancedocumentsregulatoryinformation/labelingnutrition/ucm2006828.htm.

US FDA. (2016) Botanical drug development: Guidance to industry. Washington, DC: US FDA.

US FDA (2018). Label claims for conventional foods and dietary supplements. US FDA. Available from: https://www.fda.gov/food/labelingnutrition/ucm111447.htm.

U.S. National Institutes of Health. (1994). *Dietary supplement health and education act of 1994, Public Law 103-417, 103rd Congress*. [Accessed 9 April 2018]. Available from: https://ods.od.nih.gov/About/DSHEA_Wording.aspx.

U.S. National Institutes of Health. (2004). FDA prohibits sales of dietary supplements containing ephedra. National Institutes of Health: Office of Dietary Supplements. [Accessed 12 April 2018]. Available from: https://ods.od.nih.gov/Health_Information/Ephedra.aspx.

Vaidya, A. and Vaidya, R. (1998). Healing through pluralistic medicine. *Journal of the National Integrated Medicine Association*, **40**, 5–9.

Vaidya, A. and Vaidya, R. (2010). Roots of modern drugs in reverse pharmacology. *Association of Physicians of India: Medicine Update*, **20**(1), 871–873.

Vaidya, A. B., Antarkar, D. S., Doshi, J. C., et al. (1996). *Picrorhiza kurroa* Royle Ex Benth is a hepatoprotective agent – Experimental and clinical studies. *Postgraduate Medical Journal*, **42**, 105–108.

Vaidya, A. B., Rajagopalan, T. G., Mankodi, N. A., et al. (1978). Treatment of Parkinson's disease with the cowhage plant—*Mucuna pruriens* Bak. *Neurology India*, **26**, 171–176.

Vaidya, A. B., (2006). Reverse pharmacological correlates of Ayurvedic Drug Actions. *Indian Journal of Pharmacology*, **38**, 311–315.

Vaidya, A. D. B., Dhami, H. and Shukla, N. (2013). Nutraceuticals, naturals and nutritionals – A discovery path from Ayurveda. *NuFFooDS Spectrum*, **1**(1), 16–17.

Vaidya, A. D. B. and Mehta, D. S. (2002). Synergy of different systems of medicine: The Sevagram declaration. *Journal of the Association of Physicians of India*, **50**, 618–619.

Vaidya, A. D. B. and Shukla N. (2015). Ayurceuticals-Nutraceuticals from India. *Ingredients South Asia*, **8**(15), 66–68.

Vaidya, A. D. B. (1996a). Therapeutic potential of medicinal plants – A global perspective. In S. S. Handa, ed. *Supplement to Cultivation & Utilization of Medicinal Plants*. Jammu Tavi, India: Regional Research Laboratory (C.S.I.R.). pp. 1–12.

Vaidya, A. D. B. (2014). Reverse pharmacology-A paradigm shift for drug discovery and development. *Current Research in Drug Discovery*, **1**, 39–44.

Vaidya, R. A. (2011). Observational therapeutics: Scope, challenges and organization. *Journal of Ayurveda and Integrative Medicine*, **2**, 165–169.

Vaidya, R. A., Vaidya, A. D. B., Patwardhan, B., Tillu, G. and Rao, Y. (2003). Ayurvedic Pharmacoepidemiology: A proposed new discipline. *Journal of the Association of Physicians of India*, **51**, 528.

Vakil, R. J. (1949). A clinical trial of *Rauwolfia serpentina* in essential hypertension. *British Heart Journal*, **11**, 350–355.

Wildman, R. E. C. (2002). *Handbook of Nutraceuticals and Functional Foods*. Boca Raton, FL: CRC Press.

Willcox, M., Graz, B., Falquet, J., Diakite, C., Giani, S. and Diallo, D. (2011). "Reverse Pharmacology" approach for developing an anti-malarial phytomedicine. *Malaria Journal*, **10**(Suppl 1), 1–10.

World Health Organization (WHO). (2004). *Guidelines on Safety Monitoring of Herbal Medicines in Pharmacovigilance Systems*. Geneva, Switzerland: WHO.

Yakobucci, K. L. (2016). Natural medicines. *Journal of the Medical Library Association*, **104**, 371–374.

Zhang, J., Onakpoya, I. J., Posadzki, P. and Eddouks, M. (2015). The safety of herbal medicine: From prejudice to evidence. *Evidence-Based Complementary and Alternative Medicine*, **2015**, 316706.

27 Management of Diabetes and Hyperlipidaemia by Natural Medicines

Kalpana Bhaskaran, Ong Jing Ting and Tan Tengli

CONTENTS

27.1 INTRODUCTION

The alarming rate of increase in the number of new cases of diabetes worldwide is akin to the 'modern plague' of this century. Approximately 425 million adults (20–79 years) were living with diabetes; by 2045 this will rise to 629 million (IDF 2017). The increased prevalence places an undue stress on many fronts, as it is well known that the complications related to diabetes cause considerable morbidity and mortality worldwide. They also negatively affect the quality of life in individuals with diabetes, with an increase in disability and death. The economic burden of caring for diabetes and its related complications are staggering. Diabetes caused at least $727 billion in health expenditure in 2017 – 12% of total spending on adults (IDF 2017).

27.2 DIABETES AND ITS COMPLICATIONS

Diabetes mellitus is a chronic condition that can lead to complications over time. There are a wide range of complications that could arise from just diabetes alone, mostly cardiovascular diseases, kidney failure and loss of limbs (American Diabetes Association 2018).

The two main complications in type 2 diabetes mellitus (T2DM) are impaired insulin action through insulin resistance and insulin secretion with an abnormal pancreatic β-cell. Insulin resistance is characterized in many ways, one of which is where the free fatty may initiate the phosphorylation of serine of IRS proteins, which ultimately leads to the reduction of IRS-tyrosine phosphorylation and decreased IRS-1-associated P13-kinase activity. This then results in decreased insulin-stimulated glucose transport activity (Yu et al. 2002). Hyperlipidaemia is characterized by excess lipids such as free fatty acids (FFA), low-density lipoprotein (LDL), triglycerides (TG) in the bloodstream. The increasing amount of excess lipids in the blood contributes to increased production of serum pro-inflammatory cytokines (e.g. IL-1β, TNF-α), which then leads to insulin resistance.

27.3 HYPERLIPIDAEMIA

Hyperlipidaemia is considered one of the major risk factors causing cardiovascular diseases (CVDs). Hyperlipidaemia is an increase in one or more of the plasma lipids, including triglycerides, cholesterol, cholesterol esters and phospholipids and or plasma lipoproteins such as very low-density lipoprotein (VLDL) and low-density lipoprotein (LDL), and reduced high-density lipoprotein levels (HDL; Shattat 2014). One of the most common causes of hyperlipidaemia in poorly controlled diabetes is the decrease of activity of the lipoprotein lipases due to insulin deficiency (Taskinen et al. 1982). Type 1 diabetes (T1DM) is also known as insulin-dependent diabetes mellitus (IDDM), where there is the absence of endogenous insulin, which leads to hyperglycaemia and eventually ketoacidosis and pronounced hypertriglyceridemia due to the insufficient activation of the lipoprotein lipase system (Garcia et al. 1974). In T2DM, also known as non-insulin-dependent diabetes mellitus (NIDDM), hyperinsulinaemia is present, which leads to the overproduction of VLDLs and triglycerides, and this is associated with metabolic consequences for the lipoproteins (Tilly-Kiesi et al.1996). To manage diabetes, both the blood glucose levels and lipid concentration have to be regulated.

27.4 HISTORICAL USE OF NATURAL MEDICINES

The use of plants as therapeutic agents is culturally ubiquitous, and there is archaeological evidence to suggest that plants have been thus used since prehistoric times. In Europe, the earliest evidence of prehistoric peoples' use of plants as natural medicine comes from a mummified body of a man who lived about 5300 years ago (Heinrich et al. 2012). It is estimated that 70–95% of the populations in developing countries depend on traditional medicine to meet their primary healthcare needs, and most traditional treatments make use of plants and crude extracts (Robinson and Zhang 2011). Another change is the paradigm shift in herbal medicine towards a more scientific, evidence-based medicine model (the application of the best available evidence to aid clinical decision making), as opposed to a model based on traditional knowledge (anecdotal knowledge gained from folklore or tradition). This paradigm shift is due to the influence of modern medicine and can be credited to the researcher-physicians of the eighteenth century, notably William Withering (1741–1799), who as a botanist and physician used extensive clinical trials to assess the effects and toxicity of digitalis, the drug produced from the dried leaves of foxglove (*Digitalis purpurea* L.). In addition, improved analytical techniques in the nineteenth century enabled active principle extraction and isolation of specific chemicals from plants, which were tested for their pharmacological and toxicological effects (Heinrich et al. 2012). Societies from both the developed and developing world often have a pluralistic approach to medicine, employing both mainstream medicine and alternative treatments.

27.5 NATURAL MEDICINES AND THEIR USE IN THE TREATMENT OF DIABETES

One of the major objectives in the therapeutic management of diabetes is to design a regimen that will improve the metabolic factors associated with the development and progression of complications. As such, it is well recognised that a primary strategy is to achieve the target levels recommended for blood pressure, lipids and glycaemia. This strategy may consist of lifestyle modification alone, but more commonly it consists of lifestyle management – that is, dietary modification and enhanced physical activity – combined with pharmacological intervention from agents in multiple classes (Riddle 2005). However, as providers caring for patients with diabetes, we recognise that patients are very interested in alternative (complementary) strategies that consist of dietary supplementation with over-the-counter agents. Supplementing conventional approaches to medical care with alternative means is extensively practiced by a large number of patients. Interestingly, more times than not, these practices appear to be undertaken without consultation with a medical provider. Herbs have been reported as one of the remedies used for treatment by patients with diabetes in many countries, and it has been reported that the market size for this segment is reported to grow exponentially. The global herbal medicine market size was valued at $71.19 billion in 2016 and is expected to exhibit profitable growth over the forecast period. The increase is attributed to the increasing preference of consumers for traditional medicines (Ayurveda, Unani and traditional Chinese medicine), which do not cause overdose toxicity and have fewer side effects. In addition, increasing substantial research investments and funding will support the market growth in the near future (Hexa Research 2017). Herbal plants with several medicinal properties are used to treat a variety of disease conditions. Interestingly, a single plant may contain many chemical constituents such as phenols, glycosides, polysaccharides, alkaloids, resins and terpenoids that demonstrate therapeutic activities in more than one medical condition. However, the efficacy of traditional herbs in the treatment of diabetes is still mixed. Some studies have demonstrated that herbs can delay the progress of diabetic complications (Jung et al. 2006), while other studies have shown that certain herbs used in the management of diabetes are not efficacious. Using herbs that have no proven clinical benefit to patients may lead to delays in seeking appropriate treatment, leading to severe diabetes-related complications and associated disability and mortality.

27.6 NATURAL MEDICINES AND THEIR MECHANISM OF ACTION

These are significant limitations, and in large part these limitations explain why there is considerable scepticism regarding the effectiveness of natural remedies in Western medicine. However, there is growing evidence in this area, and if a botanical is demonstrated to have a favourable effect on a given mechanism, that will provide the rationale for further and more definitive studies on a particular botanical.

To exert an effect, botanicals may theoretically modulate glucose at several different levels in multiple tissues (Figure 27.1). Thus, based on reported abnormalities for T2DM, botanicals could be proposed to affect whole-body metabolism by modulating adipocyte function and thus, regulating endocrine secretions that play a role in enhancing the skeletal muscle insulin action. In addition, based on the known abnormalities, botanicals may regulate hepatic processes – that is, hepatic gluconeogenesis – and may affect whole-body glucose levels.

27.6.1 *Gymnema sylvestre* (Gurmar)

Gymnema sylvestre is a herb belonging to the class dicotyledonous of the family Asclepiadaceae. It has been used to treat conditions like diabetes and snakebites in the Ayurvedic system of medicine. It can be served in tea bags, tablets, supplements or in confectioneries. Gymnemic acids, gymnemasaponins and gurmarin present in the herb are phytoconstituents that are responsible for the sweet repression activity and thus, this particular herb becomes an effective natural remedy for diabetes. This herbal extract has been proven to be able to reduce triglyceride levels and blood cholesterol (Tiwari et al. 2014).

The mechanism of action of *Gymnema sylvestre* is through stimulation in insulin secretion from the pancreas. In the intestine, the gymnemic acids attaches itself to the receptors lined at the external layer of the intestine, which prevents the absorption of sugar, leading to a decrease in blood sugar levels. The hypoglycaemic effect of gymnemic acids leads to series of events, triggering insulin secretion. Pancreatic islet cells start to regenerate to enhance enzyme- mediated uptake of glucose, decreasing the FA and glucose absorption in the small intestines and interfering with the ability of receptors in the mouth to sense sweetness. Gymnemic acid present in the herb was found to interact with glyceraldehyde-3-phosphate dehydrogenase (G3PDH), an enzyme involved in glycerol metabolism, suggesting that gymnemic acid may have antidiabetic activity and lipid-lowering effects through their interaction (Ishijima et al. 2007).

In a study done by Rachh, it was found that hydroalcoholic extract of gymnemic acids fed to rats induced with high cholesterol diet showed a significant reduction in total serum cholesterol, triglycerides and low-density lipoproteins after 7 days (Rachh et al. 2010). In a different study, 22 patients with

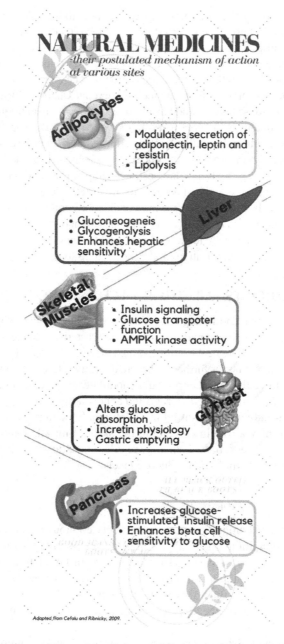

FIGURE 27.1 **(See color insert.)** Natural medicines and their postulated mechanism of action.

T2DM were administered with 400 mg/day of GS4, a water soluble extract of the leaves of *Gymnema sylvestre*, who showed a significant decrease of blood glucose, glycosylated haemoglobin and glycosylated plasma proteins. Some participants were even able to halt their conventional drug and maintain blood glucose homeostasis with just GS4 supplementation alone. However, there was no significant reduction in serum lipids, HbA1c or glycosylated plasma proteins (Baskaran et al. 1990).

To further investigate the effects of *G. sylvestre* on the control of blood glucose in insulin-dependent diabetes (IDDM) patients, 27 patients with IDDM were administered 400 mg/day of GS4 for 18–20 months while concurrently taking their conventional oral anti-hyperglycaemic drugs. The study has shown that the patients showed no reduction in glycosylated plasma proteins, HbA1c and serum lipids (Shanmugasundaram et al. 1990).

27.6.2 SALACIA (*SALACIA OBLONGA; SALACIA RETICULATA*)

Salacia reticulata is a plant native to India, and it is known as a traditional Ayurvedic medicine. The roots and stems are used for glycaemic control and weight loss. The active ingredients include kotalanol, salacinol, kotalagenin-16 acetate and mangiferin, and these are known to slow down carbohydrate breakdown. The two compounds salacinol and kotalanol inhibit the action of enzymes such as sucrose, maltase, and isomaltase in the small intestines, so it was deduced that it might be a powerful herb to treat DM by lowering postprandial blood glucose (Matsuda et al. 2002). *Salacia* species contain different active components that target diabetes by modulating PPAR-α-mediated lipogenic gene transcription and inhibiting α-glucosidase and pancreatic, lipase as well as aldose reductase. Most studies have shown that this herb can target diabetes and obesity, although most of the trials are done in animal models.

Serasinghe et al. showed that *S. reticulata* was able to inhibit hyperglycaemia in rats. To induce diabetes in Sprague-Dawley rats, they were injected with streptozotocin. After 7 days, the animals fasted for 16 hours and were divided into control and test group. The test group were fed with *S. reticulata* as a single-point intervention, while the control group received only water. The results showed that the *S. reticulata* group had a decrease of blood glucose from 420 mg/dL at baseline to 156 mg/dL by the end of 4 hours (Serasinghe et al. 1990).

A study done by Radha and Amrithaveni (2009) showed that *S. reticulata* is effective in reducing glycosylated haemoglobin, all lipids and blood glucose. Sixty T2DM patients (30 for the experimental group and 30 for the control group) participated in the study; the experimental group were given 2 g of *S. reticulata* (powdered form) every day for 90 days, while the control group did not take any supplements. It was found that the experimental group showed a decrease in total cholesterol (262 mg/dL–255.13 mg/dL) and a decrease in fasting blood glucose (161.73 mg/dL–153.47 mg/dL) with a statistical significance level ($P < 0.001$ and $P < 0.01$, respectively). The outcome may be even more evident when it is taken for extended periods of time.

27.6.3 *ALOE VERA* L

Aloe barbadensis is the most widely used species of aloe in the world. It is a plant that belongs to the *Liliaceae* family. *Aloe vera* contains several chemical constituents such as glucomannans, alkaloids, flavonoids, phenols, vitamins, minerals, anthraquinones, saponins, phytosterols and lignins. The aloe leaf contains two major parts, the outer green rind and the inner colourless parenchyma (which contains the aloe gel). This medicinal plant has been shown to lower blood glucose levels and high blood pressure and reduce serum cholesterol and triglycerides in diabetic patients (Yongchaiyudha et al. 1996). The phytosterols present in aloe vera helps to reduce the absorption of cholesterol from the gut, which reduces serum concentrations of cholesterol. Although there are many benefits of aloe vera, there are also potential adverse effects, one of which is that it may cause laxative effects due to the anthraquinones present in latex, as it stimulates mucus secretion and intestinal peristalsis (Ishii et al. 1994), abdominal discomfort, itching, rash or even cardiac dysrhythmias. Further studies were done to investigate the hypoglycaemic and hypolipidaemic effect of *Aloe vera* L. in T2DM (Choudhary et al. 2011).

In a study done by Misawa E. et al. 6-week-old male Zucker diabetic rats were fed with a high-fat diet for 3 weeks. The experimental rats were fed with lophenol and cycloartanol, which are minor phytosterols of aloe vera gel, at 25 μg/(kg day) consecutively for 44 days. The control rats were fed with distilled water containing 0.1%DMSO. It was demonstrated that the two constituents were able to reduce blood glucose, serum FFA, TG levels and visceral fat accumulation in the Zucker diabetic fatty rats (Misawa et al. 2008).

In another study done by Yongchaiyudha et al. (1996), the effect of aloe vera juice in combination with glibenclamide was investigated in 15 diabetic patients (nine males and six females) and it was found that the aloe vera juice greatly reduced levels of blood glucose within 2 weeks and triglycerides in 4 weeks.

To further investigate the effects of blood glucose and lipid levels in dyslipidaemic T2DM, a randomised, double blind, placebo-controlled clinical trial was carried out in 30 hyperlipidaemic (hypercholesterolaemic and/or hypertriglyceridaemic) T2DM patients aged 40–60 years (Huseini et al. 2011). They were administered with one 300 mg capsule every 12 hours for 2 months, concurrently taking the drugs, two 5 mg of glyburide and two 500 mg metformin tablets, and were compared to the placebo group ($n = 30$). The fasting blood glucose, HbA1c, total cholesterol and LDL levels reduced significantly ($p = 0.036$, $p = 0.036$, $p = 0.006$ and $p = 0.004$, respectively). There were no adverse effects reported.

Similar to another study done by Yagi et al. (2009), blood glucose level and triglyceride levels were significantly reduced however, it also showed that the cholesterol levels remained the same compared to before the treatment. In this study, 0.05 g of aloe vera gel high molecular weight fractions (AHM) were administered orally to T2DM patients three times daily for 12 weeks along with the oral hypoglycaemic drugs. AHM is a high molecular weight natural polysaccharide that promotes vasodilation and maintenance of homeostasis within the vascular endothelium. Triglycerides level was reduced 35% from before treatment with AHM ($P < 0.001$). Blood glucose levels were significantly reduced after 12 weeks of treatment ($p < 0.001$).

27.6.4 Ginseng

Ginseng has been used in herbal medicine as a general tonic for the promotion of health in Asian countries for centuries. The roots of two different forms are used for diabetes – Chinese ginseng (*Panax ginseng*) and American ginseng (*Panax quinquefolius*). *Panax ginseng* has the highest therapeutic potency.

The pharmacological properties of ginseng are attributed to ginsenosides that are found in extracts of ginseng (Kim 2012). It has been reported that there are effects of ginseng on obesity and metabolic disease, such as hypertension, diabetes and hyperlipidaemia (Song et al. 2014). The ginseng and its components affect hyperglycaemia by enhancing pancreatic β-cell function and reducing insulin resistance (Luo and Luo 2009).

Based on Li and Ji (2018), there is limited evidence supporting the suggestion that ginseng exerts an anti-obesity effect in humans. Out of seven papers on humans that associated ginseng with obesity, only one of the papers had a positive result. A study conducted in Korea investigated the influence of *Panax ginseng* on obesity and gut microbiota in obese middle-aged Korean women. The participants were given 4 g of freeze-dried granulated extracts to take twice a day for a duration of 8 weeks. Ginseng exerted a weight loss effect and slight effects on gut microbiota in all participants. They noted that the anti-obesity effects differed between individuals depending on the composition of their gut microbiota prior to ginseng intake (Song et al. 2014).

On the effects of ginseng on glucose levels, a study was conducted in 10 T2DM patients where they were administered with placebo, 3, 6 or 9 g of ground American ginseng root in capsules at 120, 80, 40 or 0 minutes before a 25-g oral glucose challenge. It was found that the treatment and not the time of administration significantly affected the postprandial glucose. They concluded that American Ginseng reduces postprandial glucose irrespective of dose and time of administration (Vuksan et al. 2000).

In a randomised, double-blinded study of *Panax ginseng*, 36 newly diagnosed T2DM patients were assigned to placebo, 100 mg/day or 200 mg/day of *Panax ginseng* for 8 weeks. The 200 mg dose improved glycated haemoglobin and reduced body weight (Sotaniemi et al. 1995).

The most commonly experienced adverse events are headache, sleep and gastrointestinal disorders (Coon and Ernst 2002). Serious adverse effects may occur when ginseng is one of the constituents of a combination product or when it is taken with other medications. Ginseng may induce diuretic resistance and may also decrease the anticoagulant activity of warfarin (Shane-McWhorter 2009). The recommended dosage of ginseng application is 1–3 g of root or 200–600 mg of extract (Vuksan et al. 2000).

27.6.5 MOMORDICA CHARANTIA (BITTER MELON)

Bitter melon is a flowering vine in the family Cucurbitaceae, also known by other names such as bitter gourd, karela, balsam pear, or Ampalaya tea. *M. charantia* is one of the plants that have been investigated thoroughly for the treatment of diabetes (Hasan and Khatoon 2012).

Bitter melon extract from the fruit, seeds and leaves contains several bioactive compounds that have hypoglycaemic activity in both diabetic animals and humans. The fruit of the bitter melon has a more pronounced hypoglycaemic effect as it contains a high amount of hypoglycaemic chemicals that include a mixture of steroidal saponins known as charantins, insulin-like peptides and alkaloids. Studies have shown that the fruit has shown the ability to enhance cellular uptake of glucose, promote insulin release (as supported by Jeevathayaparan et al. 1995) and potentiate the effect of insulin (Taylor 2002).

Dosage forms include juice, powder, vegetable pulp suspensions, injections and capsules. In powder form, a dosage of 18 g/day has been shown to reduce blood glucose (Chen, 1981). In a study conducted in Thailand, they compared the hypoglycaemic effect of three different doses (200 mg, 1000 mg or 2000 mg/day) of bitter melon to metformin in newly diagnosed T2DM patients for 4 weeks. Dried powder of fruit pulp of bitter melon was used. It was found that 2000 mg/day of bitter melon has a modest hypoglycaemic effect and significantly reduced fructosamine levels from baseline, but it is not as effective as 1000 mg/day of metformin (Fuangchan et al. 2011). When comparing the bitter gourd tablets (BGT)-treated group to the diabetic group for 12 weeks, there were significant differences of glucose, cholesterol, HDL, LDL and triglyceride. It was concluded that bitter gourd tablets have beneficial effects on glucose tolerance (Hasan and Khatoon 2012).

An injectable 'plant insulin' preparation was studied in patients with type 1 or type 2 diabetes and compared to a control group with diabetes. The dosage was based on blood glucose levels. They found that type 1 diabetic patients have significant decrease of mean fasting glucose 4 hours after injection and the effect as maintained at the 6th and 8th hours. On the other hand, the T2DM patients did not have a significant decrease of mean fasting glucose, but it was lower compared to the control group at 1 and 6 hours (Khanna et al. 1981).

In a randomised, double blind, placebo-controlled trial in the Philippines, 40 newly diagnosed or poorly controlled T2DM patients were randomised to either treatment or control group. The treatment group were given two capsules of *M. charantia* three times a day after meals for 3 months, while the control group was given a placebo. The difference in mean change in A1c between the two groups was only 0.22%, resulting in them being unable to make a definite conclusion on the effectiveness of *M. charantia* in capsule form (Dans et al. 2007).

Bitter melon can be used as a dietary supplement herbal medicine for the management of diabetes and/or metabolic syndromes (Cefalu et al. 2008). Some of the adverse effects that have been reported are hypoglycemic coma, convulsions in children, a favism-like syndrome and headaches. Bitter melon may also have an additive effect with other glucose-lowering agents (Basch et al. 2018).

27.6.6 CINNAMOMUM CASSIA

Cinnamomum (cinnamon) is a genus of the Lauraceae family. Cinnamon comes from the inner bark of tropical evergreen tree. There are two major types of cinnamon, *Cinnamomum verum* also known as *Cinnamon zeylanicum* (true cinnamon), and *Cinnamomum cassia*, also known as *Cinnamomum aromaticum*. There are studies that found that the cassia extract was superior to the zeylanicum extra in terms of the antidiabetic effect (Verspohl et al. 2005). *In vivo* and *in vitro* studies have shown that cinnamon in dried powder or aqueous extracts can help to improve the glucose metabolism by increasing GLUT-4 receptor synthesis, glycogen synthesis and phosphorylation of the insulin receptor (Khan et al. 2003; Medagama 2015).

The consumption of cinnamon on T1DM was not very effective, as a double-blinded study found that there was no significant difference between treating T1DM adolescents with 1 g of cinnamon or placebo per day for 90 days in improving glycaemic control (Altschuler et al. 2007).

However, the effect of cinnamon on T2DM subjects provided some interesting findings. In a study conducted in Pakistan, 60 patients on sulphonylurea with poorly controlled T2DM found that cinnamon in dosages of 1, 3 or 6 g/day improved fasting glucose, triglycerides, LDL and total cholesterol levels after 40 days (Khan et al. 2003). The change in HDL was not significant. There was a 20-day washout period after the 40 days of consumption, and they found that the levels were still lower compared to baseline. In a randomised, double-blinded, placebo-controlled trial in 79 German patients with well-controlled T2DM, 112 mg of aqueous cinnamon or placebo was taken three times a day with meals for 4 months (Mang et al. 2006). There was a decline in fasting glucose by 10.3% in the cinnamon group compared to 3.4% in the placebo group, but there was no significant difference in the HbA1c or the lipid profiles.

In the United States, a double-blinded, placebo-controlled trial was conducted in 57 subjects with T2DM. They received 1 g of cinnamon or placebo daily for 3 months, but there was no significant change in fasting glucose, lipid, A1c or insulin levels. They concluded that the effects of cinnamon differ by population (Blevins et al. 2007). The outcome was supported by a nonrandomised, non-blinded, placebo-controlled study in the Netherlands, where they evaluated 25 postmenopausal women with stable T2DM on oral medications; 1.5 g of cinnamon or a placebo was given once a day for 6 weeks and no significant differences were found between groups in A1c or fasting glucose (Vanschoonbeek et al. 2006).

The side effects for cinnamon are rare, however additive hypoglycaemia may occur if it is consumed with secretagogues (Jellin et al. 2009).

27.6.7 Ginger

Ginger (*Zingiber officinale* Roscoe, Zingiberaceae) is one of the most widely consumed spices and/or medicinal herbs worldwide. Ginger contains various phytochemicals and biologically active compounds, such as phenolics and flavonoids. They have shown numerous pharmacological benefits, including improvement of blood glucose tolerance, enhancement of lipid profile and modulation of inflammatory factors (Wang et al. 2017).

A study was conducted on 80 obese women where they were randomly assigned to 2 g of ginger powder or placebo (cornstarch) for 12 weeks. Based on the results, ginger consumption significantly decreased BMI, serum insulin and HOMA-IR index as well as increasing QUICKIs compared to the placebo (Attari et al. 2015).

In another study, 70 T2DM patients were enrolled to assess the effect of ginger consumption on glycaemic status, lipid profile and some inflammatory markers. They were randomly allocated to ginger or control group, where they consumed 1600 mg of either ginger or wheat flour daily for 12 weeks. It was found that ginger reduced fasting plasma glucose, HbA1c, insulin, HOMA, triglyceride, total cholesterol, CRP and PGE2 significantly compared with placebo group. They concluded that ginger could be considered an effective treatment for prevention of diabetes complications (Arablou et al. 2014).

In another study with 41 T2DM patients, oral administration of 2 g per day of ginger powder supplement for 12 weeks improved fasting blood sugar, haemoglobin A1c, apolipoprotein B, apolipoprotein A-I and malondialdehyde (Khandouzi et al. 2015).

On the effect of ginger powder supplementation on insulin resistance and glycaemic indices in patients with 2TDM, 88 patients with at least 10 years of T2DM participated and were given 3 g of ginger powder or placebo to consume daily for 8 weeks. There was a significant decrease of fasting blood sugar mean (10.5%) in the ginger group compared to the placebo group. The mean variation of HbA1c was similar to the fasting blood sugar. There was a significant decrease in the fasting insulin and HOMA-IR index, and significant increase in insulin sensitivity in both groups. There was a significantly higher QUICKI index in the ginger group. However, there was no significant difference in the mean BMI mean (Mozaffari-Khosravi et al. 2014). A systemic review found that prolonged daily intake of ginger powder preparations would lead neither to serious adverse effects nor to complications that normally occurred in the administration of hypoglycaemic or hypolipidaemic drugs (Zhu et al. 2018).

Please refer to the tables below for the studies related to the different types of natural medicine.

Bittergourd

	Study Design	Subjects	Duration	Dosage	Form	Results/Outcome
Akhtar et al. (1982)	Case series	8 with DM	1 week	Not specified	Powdered dried fruit	(1) Fasting glucose level, (2) Qycosuria, (3) OGTT
Welihinda et al. (1986)	Not placebo controlled	18 newly diagnosed type 2 diabetic patients without antidiabetic drugs		100 mL orally	Clear juice from the flesh of Sri Lankan bitter gourd variety/distilled water as control	Improved glucose tolerance in oral tolerance test after bitter gourd treatment; indication for possible nonresponders
Srivastava et al. (1993)	Not placebo controlled	Diabetic patients (7 patients tested extract/5 patients tested tablets)	7 weeks (extract) or 3 weeks (tablet)	100 mL (extract) or three times a day 5 g (tablet) orally	Aqueous extract/fruit powder as tablet	Lower postprandial blood glucose levels and lower HbA1C after treatment with bitter gourd extract; no significant effect after treatment with bitter gourd tablets
		6 type 2 diabetics	7 weeks	100 mL/day	Bitter melon decoction	After 3 weeks, their fasting blood glucose dropped by 54%. After 7 weeks, all six were at or near the normal glucose limit, urinary sugar was no longer detectable, and glycosylated hemoglobin dropped nearly 2 mg%;
Rosales and Fernando (2001)	Randomised unblinded cross-over clinical trial	27 type 2 diabetics with suboptimal glycemic control	24 week study	200 mL bitter melon tea after meals; Placebo consisted of tea made from leaves of *Camellia sinensis*		$\downarrow$HbA1c (63% reduction, $p = 0.005$), $\downarrow$Fasting serum glucose ($p = 0.403$)
John et al. (2003)	Randomised single-blind placebo controlled, clinical trial	50 type 2 diabetic patients	4 weeks	6 g per day orally	Dried whole fruit powder pressed to tablets/riboflavin as placebo	No statistically significant results in regard to fasting plasma glucose, postprandial glucose, or fructosamine levels
Tongia et al. (2004)	Not placebo controlled	15 type 2 diabetic patients	7 days	200 mg/day orally in addition to metformin, glibenclamide or both	Methanolic fruit extract	Bitter gourd lowered fasting and postprandial glucose levels compared to the drug treatment alone

(Continued)

Bittergourd

	Study Design	Subjects	Duration	Dosage	Form	Results/Outcome
Dans et al. (2007)	Randomised double blind placebo controlled, Intent-to-treat	40 newly diagnosed type 2 diabetic patients or patients with poor blood glucose control	3 months	3 g per day orally in addition to standard therapy	Charantia Ampalaya Capsules and placebo	No statistically significant differences compared to placebo group concerning fasting blood glucose, HbA1c, total cholesterol, or body weight; ↓Fasting plasma glucose ($p = 0.5862$); Achieved study power was only 11%
Lim et al. (2010)	Double-blind, placebo-controlled trial	40 newly diagnosed type 2 diabetes mellitus (18 males, 22 females)		Single oral dose; 3 treatment groups of 60, 80, 100 mg/kg/day	Tablets containing dried bitter melon leaves	↑Insulin levels at 15 min ($p = 0.0402$) ↓Average plasma glucose levels at 15 min ($p = 0.0121$), 100 mg/kg/day dose of bitter melon was more effective than lower doses and placebo in reducing mealtime glycemic excursions within 4-hour postdose, with more rapid return to baseline levels
Fuangchan et al. (2011)	Randomised double-blind active controlled, dosage was placebo controlled, Intent-to-treat	143 newly diagnosed type 2 diabetic patients	4 weeks	500/1000/2000 mg per day or 1000 mg metformin per day orally	Capsules of dried fruit pulp powder or metformin/roasted rice powder and lactose as placebo	2000 mg per day significantly reduced fructosamine levels; ↓Mean fructosamine levels (-10.2 μmol/L; 95% CI $= -19.1$ to -1.3)
Kochhar et al. (2011)	Not placebo controlled	60 type 2 diabetic patients free from serious complications	90 days	45 days 1 g per day orally + 45 days 2 g per day orally	Mixed powder of bitter gourd fruit, fenugreek seeds, and jambu seeds in either capsule (raw) or biscuit (cooked) form	Lower fasting and postprandial blood and urine levels; reduced intake of oral hypoglycemic drugs; raw powder was more effective
Zanker et al. (2012)	Double-blind placebo controlled	97 type 2 diabetic patients without insulin treatment	4 months	1 g per day orally	Water soluble bitter gourd extract (Glucokine®) with or without chromium and zinc supplements	HbA1C dropped significantly after bitter gourd treatment without chromium and zinc supplementation

(Continued)

Bittergourd

	Study Design	Subjects	Duration	Dosage	Form	Results/Outcome
Tsai et al. (2012)	Open-labeled single-arm study	42 patients diagnosed with the metabolic syndrome	3 months	4.8 g per day orally	Whole fruit powder capsules (lyophilized wild type bitter gourd powder)	Decreased incidence rate of metabolic syndrome among study population; lower waist circumference; the trend of increased insulin sensitivity was not significant
Hasan et al. (2012)	Random design	26 subjects	4 weeks	2 tablets thrice daily, after meals (each tablet contained 1 gm of dried fruit)	Bitter gourd (BG) tablets from shade dried powdered fresh whole fruit	Reduced the cholesterol, VLDL and triglyceride levels in diabetic patients and increased the HDL-cholesterol levels
Ooi et al. (2012)		127 Thai men and women with DM2	4 weeks	Form of 500 mg, 1 g, or 2 g of dried fruit pulp powder (standardized to 0.04%–0.05% charantin) or 1 g of metformin per day		Only the highest dose of bitter melon or of metformin lowered serum fructosamine levels significantly
Trakoon-osot et al. (2013)	Clinical trial	38 Thai men and women with DM2	16 weeks	Either 6 g of deseeded, unripe, dried fruit pulp of bitter melon (standardized to contain 420 mcg of charantin per capsule) or placebo		Serum HgbA1c and total advanced glycation end product (AGE) levels fell significantly in the bitter melon group, compared to in the placebo group. No serious adverse effects occurred in either group. Diarrhea and flatulence were significantly more common in the bitter melon group, compared to the placebo group
Today's Dietitian	Clinical trial	100 patients with type 2 diabetes			Aqueous suspension of bitter melon pulp	They evaluated bitter melons effect 1 hour after administration and then 2 hours later with a 75-g oral glucose tolerance test. After the 2-hour glucose tolerance test, subjects average blood glucose was 222 mg/dL. This was 14% lower than the previous days value of 257 mg/dL. Regardless, researchers measured bitter melons effects after only 2 hours; whether there is any long-term benefit to using bitter melon is unknown

Gymnema

	Study Design	Subjects	Duration	Dosage	Form	Results/Outcome
Khare et al. (1983)			15 days	2 g 3 times a day	Aqueous extracts of the plant	Significantly reduced FBG values and improved the tolerance to an oral glucose loads
Okabayahi et al. (1990)				1 g/kg BW	GS4 extract	Administration of 1 g/kg BW of GS4 extract to 18-h fasted rats significantly attenuated the serum glucose response to oral administration of 1 g/kg glucose
Shanmugasundaram et al. (1990)		27 patients with insulin-dependent diabetes mellitus (IDDM) on insulin therapy	10–12 months	400 mg daily	Water-soluble extract of the leaves of *Gymnema sylvestre*	IDDM patients on insulin therapy only showed no significant reduction in serum lipids, HbAlc or glycosylated plasma proteins when followed up after 10–12 months. GS4 therapy appears to enhance endogenous insulin, possibly by regeneration/revitalisation of the residual beta cells in insulin-dependent diabetes mellitus
	open-label trials	27 patients with type 1 diabetes	6–30 months		Gymnema extract	Compared with baseline data, gymnema significantly reduced glycosylated plasma protein ($p < 0.001$) in the first 6–8 months, and serum amylase ($p < 0.001$) at 16–18 months. In comparison to conventional therapy (insulin, $n = 37$), gymnema significantly increased serum C-peptide levels within 16–18 months (p 0.001). The conventional treatment group, on the other hand, demonstrated no significant improvement in glycemic control during the treatment period
Baskaran, Kizar et al. (1990)		22 type 2 diabetic patients	18–20 months	400 mg per day	Extract from the leaves of *Gymnema sylvestre*	A significant reduction in blood glucose, glycosylated haemoglobin and glycosylated plasma proteins, and conventional drug dosage could be decreased. Five of the 22 diabetic patients were able to discontinue their conventional drug and maintain their blood glucose homeostasis with GS4 alone

(Continued)

Gymnema

	Study Design	Subjects	Duration	Dosage	Form	Results/Outcome
Joffe (2001)	Open-label trial	65 patients with type 1 and type 2 diabetes	90 days	400 mg b.i.d. (twice a day)	*G. sylvestre* leaf extract	Preprandial blood glucose level(BGL), postprandial BGL and HbA1c decreased by 11%, 13%, and 0.6%, respectively
Paliwal et al. (2009)		20 non-insulin-dependent diabetic female subjects	1 month	6 gm of gurmar leaf powder per day		Fasting blood glucose level was significantly lowered at 1% ($p < 0.01$), mean postprandial blood glucose level is also significant at 1% ($p < 0.01$)
Al-Romaiyan et al. (2010)		T2D patients	2 months	1 g/day	*G. sylvestre*-based product	Led to significant decreases in FBG and PPBG levels which were accompanied by increases in circulating insulin and C-peptide. Moreover, it stimulated insulin secretion from isolated human islets of Langerhans
Pandey et al.		22 patients with type 2 diabetes	18–20 months	400 mg daily	*G. sylvestre* extract along with their oral	All patients demonstrated improved blood sugar control. Twenty-one out of the twenty-two were able to reduce blood glucose level
Mahajan et al. (2015)		32 human subjects with type 2 diabetes mellitus	6 months	50 mL of aqueous extract derived from 10 g of "GSPF kwath" daily	GSPF kwath: A *Gymnema sylvestre*-containing polyherbal formulation	Significant reductions of blood glucose and glycosylated hemoglobin levels. There was also a significant increase in high-density lipoprotein cholesterol levels and concomitant decreases in total cholesterol, triglyceride, low-density lipoprotein cholesterol, and very-low-density lipoprotein levels

Salacia Reticulata (SR)

	Study Design	Subjects	Duration	Dosage	Form	Results/Outcome
Shimoda et al. (1998)	Single-point sucrose tolerance test	7 healthy adults	Single-point intervention	200 mg	Aqueous extracts from the stem of the plant	Significant suppression of postprandial glucose values
Kajimoto et al. (2000)	Placebo-controlled crossover trial	20 type 2 diabetes patients	6 weeks	240 mg/day	Aqueous extracts from the stem of the plant	Significant reductions in fasting plasma glucose, HbA1C and BMI in treatment groups compared to the control-diet groups where no changes were observed
Jayawardena et al. (2005)	Double-blind randomised placebo-controlled crossover trial	51 type 2 diabetes patients	3 months	Not mentioned	Herbal tea containing *Salacia reticulata* (Kothala Himbutu tea)	Treatment groups demonstrated a reduction in HbA1C of $0.54 \pm SD$ 0.93 compared to a decrease of $0.3 \pm SD$ 1.05 in the placebo group ($P < 0.001$)
Shivaprasad et al. (2013)	Double-blind randomised placebo-controlled trial	29 prediabetes (IFG & IGT)	6 weeks	500 mg/day	Leaves and root bark extracts of the plant	Administration of SR at dosage of 500 mg/day in prediabetic patients showed significant reduction in fasting blood glucose at the end of 6 weeks. (leaf extract, $P < 0.05$ and root extract, $P < 0.01$) Thus, Salacia extracts may be benefical towards prediabetic patients with mild to moderate hyperlipidemia
Ofner et al. (2013)	Randomised open-label study	40 healthy adults	4 weeks	600 mg/day	Root powder (Exadipin)	Healthy volunteers that were treated with SR and vitamin D showed 6.1% of weight loss and 4.5% decrease of body fat compared to the controls

Ginger

	Study Design	Subjects	Duration	Dosage	Form	Results/Outcome
Mahluji et al. (2013)	Randomised clinical trial	64 type 2 diabetes patients	8 weeks	1000 mg	Ginger powder capsule	Significant decrease levels of insulin while no significant effect on fasting plasma glucose and HbA1c
Khandouzi et al. (2015)	Randomised, double-blind, placebo-controlled clinical trial	64 type 2 diabetes patients	12 weeks	1 g, twice daily	Ginger powder capsule	Administration of ginger capsules greatly reduces the levels of fasting blood glucose, HbA1c. Ginger seems to be able to improve apolipoprotein B and A-I
Moaffari-Khosravi et al. (2014)	Randomised, double-blind, placebo-controlled clinical trial	88 type 2 diabetes patients	8 weeks	1000 mg, taken with 3 meals	Ginger powder capsule	Ginger lowered fasting blood glucose, HbA1c and showed improvement of insulin resistance indices
Arablou et al. (2014)	Randomised, double-blind, placebo-controlled clinical trial	70 type 2 diabetes patients	12 weeks	1600 mg	Ginger powder capsule	There were no significant differences in the HDL, LDL, and TNF-α ($P > 0.05$), however, levels of insulin in patients with T2DM decreased
Andallu et al. (2001)	Randomised clinical trial	32 type 2 diabetes hypercholesterolemic patients	30 days	3 g/day	Ginger powder capsule	Effective in lowering blood glucose levels and serum lipids

Cinnamon

	Study Design	Subjects	Duration	Dosage	Form	Results/Outcome
Akilen et al. (2010)	Double-blind randomised controlled trial	58 type 2 diabetic patients treated only with hypoglycemic agents	12 weeks	2 g daily	*C. cassia* powder	Intake of 2 g of cinnamon for 12 weeks significantly reduces the HbA1c, SBP and DBP among poorly controlled type 2 diabetes patients
Anderson et al. (2016)	Randomised placebo-controlled trial	137 people with elevated serum glucose.	2 months	500 mg daily	Water extract of cinnamon	Supplementation with 500 m of water-extract of cinnamon for 2 months reduced fasting insulin, glucose, total cholesterol, and LDL cholesterol and enhanced insulin sensitivity of subjects with elevated blood glucose
Blevins et al. (2007)	Double-blind RCT	77 people with type 2 diabetes	3 months	1 g daily	*C. cassia* powder	Cinnamon taken at a dose of 1 g daily for 3 months produced no significant change in fasting glucose, lipid, A1C, or insulin levels
Crawford (2009)	Randomised placebo-controlled trial	109 type 2 diabetics	90 days	1 g daily	*C. cassia* powder	Cinnamon lowered HbA1C 0.83% (95% CI, 0.46–1.20) compared with usual care alone lowering HbA1C 0.37% (95% CI, 0.15–0.59)
Khan et al. (2003)	Single-blind randomised controlled trial	60 people with type 2 diabetes	40 days followed by a 20-day washout period	1, 3, or 6 g daily	Powder in capsules	All three levels of cinnamon had reduced mean fasting serum glucose (18%–29%), triglyceride (23%–30%), LDL cholesterol (7%–27%), and total cholesterol (12%–26%) levels after 40 days. The serum glucose and lipid levels maintained low after the washout period of 20 days
Mang et al. (2016)	Double-blind randomised controlled trial	79 patients with type 2 diabetes not on insulin therapy	40 days	3 g daily	*C. cassia* aqueous extract	There was a significant reduction of fasting plasma glucose level in the cinnamon group (10.3%) than in the placebo group (3.4%) but there were no significant differences in HbA1c, lipid profiles. There is significant decrease in plasma glucose with the baseline concentrations, indicating that subjects with a higher initial plasma glucose level may benefit more from cinnamon intake
Suppapitipom et al. (2006)	Single-blind randomised controlled trial	60 people with type 2 diabetes	12 weeks	1.5 g daily	*C. cassia* powder	There was no significant difference in reducing fasting plasma glucose, HbA1c and serum lipid profile when 1.5 g of cinnamon cassia powder was consume daily
Vanschoombe et al. (2006)	Double-blind RCT	25 postmenopausal patients with type 2 diabetes	6 weeks	1.5 g daily	*C. cassia* powder	Cinnamon supplementation of 1.5 g daily does not improve whole-body insulin sensitivity or oral glucose tolerance and does not modulate blood lipid profile in postmenopausal patients with type 2 diabetes

Ginseng

	Study Design	Subjects	Duration	Dosage	Form	Results/Outcome	References
Vuksan et al. (2000)	Single-blinded RCT	10 type 2 diabetic patients	3, 6, or 9 g at 120, 80 or 40 min before 25 g glucose challenge	3, 6, or 9 g at 120, 80 or 40 min before 25 g glucose challenge	Ground American ginseng root in capsules	There was improved postprandial glycemia however there was no differences between the 3, 6, or 9 g doses and any of the times of administration.	Vuksan, V., Stavro, M., Sievenpiper, J., Beljan-Zdravkovic, U., Leiter, L., Josse, R., & Xu, Z. (2000). Similar postprandial glycemic reductions with escalation of dose and administration time of American ginseng in type 2 diabetes. *Diabetes Care, 23*(9), 1221–1226. doi:10.2337/diacare.23.9.1221
Vuksan et al. (2008)	Randomised double-blind placebo-controlled crossover trial	19 type 2 diabetic patients	12 weeks	6 g/day	Korean red ginseng preparation (rootlets)	The treatment decreased 75 g-OGTT-plasma glucose indices by 8%–11% and fasting plasma insulin (PI) and 75 g-OGTT-PI indices by 33%–38% and increased fasting-ISI (homeostasis model assessment [HOMA]) and 75 g-OGTT-ISI by 33%, compared with placebo (P < 0.05)	Vuksan, V., Sung, M., Sievenpiper, J., Stavro, P., Jenkins, A., & Di Buono, M. et al. (2008). Korean red ginseng (*Panax ginseng*) improves glucose and insulin regulation in well-controlled, type 2 diabetes: Results of a randomised, double-blind, placebo-controlled study of efficacy and safety. *Nutrition, Metabolism And Cardiovascular Diseases, 18*(1), 46–56. doi:10.1016/j.numecd.2006.04.003
Ma et al. (2008)	Randomised double-blind placebo-controlled crossover trial	20 diabetic patients	4 weeks	2 × 369 mg 3 times daily	Capsules	There was a significantly lower fasting plasma glucose (p < 0.05) and reduced fasting insulin level (P > 0.05) after ginseng treatment compared with after placebo. This led to the significant decrease in HOMA-IR after ginseng treatment (45%) compared to the placebo (12%). There were no significant changes in antioxidant biomaricers	Ma SW, Benzie IF, Chu TT, Fok BS, Tomlinson B, Critchley LA. (2008) Effect of *Panax ginseng* supplementation on biomarikers of glucose tolerance, antioxidant status and oxidative stress in type 2 diabetic subjects: Results of a placebo-controlled human intervention trial. *Diabetes Obesity and Metabolism* 10. 1125–1127. doi:10.1111/j. 1463-1326.2008.00858.x

(Continued)

Ginseng

	Study Design	Subjects	Duration	Dosage	Form	Results/Outcome	References
Reeds et al. (2011)	Randomised double-blind placebo-controlled trial	15 overweight / obese with impaired glucose tolerance or type 2 diabetic	4 weeks	3 g/day for 2 weeks and then 8 g/day for 2 weeks 250 mg/day × 2 weeks followed by 500 mg/day × 2 weeks	Korean red ginseng extract ginsenoside Re	Korean red ginseng and ginsenoside Re therapy do not improve oral glucose tolerance, P-cell function, or insulin sensitivity	Reeds, D., Patterson, B., Okunade, A., Holloszy, J., Polonsky, K., & Klein, S. (2011). Ginseng and Ginsenoside Re Do Not Improve-Cell Function or Insulin Sensitivity in Overweight and Obese Subjects with Impaired Glucose Tolerance or Diabetes. *Diabetes Care*, 34(5), 1071–1076. doi:10.2337/dc10-2299
Bang et al. (2014)	Randomised, double-blinded, placebo-controlled	Sixty patients with IFG, IGT, and T2DM impaired fasting glucose (IFG) and impaired glucose tolerance (IGT)	12 weeks	500 mg per day	Korean red ginseng (KRG)	5 g of KRG capsules per day attained significant decrease in serum glucose at 30 min during a 75-g OGTT over the intervention period relative to the placebo group. There was significant improvements or trends toward improvements in fasting glucose, glucose at 60 min, and glucose AUC in the test group relative to the placebo group. There were also significant decrease or tendencies to decrease in both serum insulin and C-peptide concentrations at most time intervals in the test group	Bang, H., Kwak, J., Ahn, H., Shin, D., & Lee, J. (2014). Korean Red Ginseng Improves Glucose Control in Subjects with Impaired Fasting Glucose, Impaired Glucose Tolerance, or Newly Diagnosed type 2 diabetes Mellitus. *Journal of Medicinal Food*, 17(1), 128–134. doi:10.1089/jmf.2013.2889
Mucalo et al. (2014)	Double-blind, randomised, placebo-controlled, parallel design	74 type 2 diabetes	12 weeks	3 g/day	American ginseng extract	American ginseng did not alter any of the studied markers: hepatic (aspartate aminotransferase (AST) and alanine aminotransferase (ALT)), renal (serum urates and serum creatinine), and haemostatic (prothrombin time (PT) and international normalized ratio (INR)) functions	Mucalo, I., Jovanovski, E, Vuksan, V., Bozikov, V., Romic, Z., & Rahelic, D. (2014). American Ginseng Extract (*Panax quinquefolius* L.) Is Safe in Long-Term Use in Type 2 Diabetic Patients. *Evidence-Based Complementary And Alternative Medicine*, 2014, 1–6. doi:10.1155/2014/969168

(Continued)

Ginseng

	Study Design	Subjects	Duration	Dosage	Form	Results/Outcome	References
Oh et al. (2014)	A randomised, double-blind, placebo-controlled clinical trial	42 impaired fasting glucose or type 2 diabetes	4 weeks	2.7 g/day	Fermented red ginseng extract (FRG)	FRG supplementation significantly reduced the 2-h postprandial glucose level and increased the 2-h postprandial insulin level. There were no significant differences in total cholesterol, HDL-cholesterol, LDL-cholesterol, or triglyceride levels between the FRG and placebo groups	Oh, M., Park, S., Kim, S., Baek, H., Kim, M., & Jeon, J. et al. (2014). Postprandial glucose-lowering effects of fermented red ginseng in subjects with impaired fasting glucose or type 2 diabetes: a randomised, double-blind, placebo-controlled clinical trial. *BMC Complementary And Alternative Medicine*, 14(1). doi:10.1186/1472-688214-237
Park et al. (2014)	Randomised, double-blind, placebo-controlled clinical trial	23 impaired fasting glucose participants	8 weeks	960 mg per day	Hydrolyzed ginseng extract (HGE) (*Panax ginseng* Meyer)	Fasting plasma glucose and postprandial glucose were significantly decreased in the HGE group compared to the placebo group. No clinically significant changes in any safety parameter were observed	Park, S., Oh, M., Choi, E., Kim, M., Ha, K., & Lee, S. et al. (2014). An 8-wk, randomised, double-blind, placebo-controlled clinical trial for the antidiabetic effects of hydrolyzed ginseng extract. *Journal of Ginseng Research*, 38(4), 239–243. doi:10.1016/j.jgr.2014.05.006
Yoon et al. (2011)	Double-blind, placebo-controlled	72 diabetic patients without any antidiabetic medication for more than 3 months	8 weeks	1500, 2000 or 3000 mg	Ginsam (Vinegar extraction from P. ginseng that is enriched with ginsenoside Rg3)	Change in HbA1c level significantly differed between the placebo and 1500mg ginsam groups. TNF-α and IL-6 concentrations were decreased after ginsam treatment and there was a correlation analysis between the changes in HbA1c level and these makers. The change in HbA1c level of ginsam treatment correlated positively and significantly with the changes in TNF-α and IL-6 concentrations	Yoon, J., Kang, S., Vassy, J., Shin, H., Lee, Y., & Ahn, H. et al. (2011). Efficacy and safety of ginsam, a vinegar extract from *Panax ginseng*, in type 2 diabetic patients: Results of a double-blind, placebo-controlled study. *Journal Of Diabetes Investigation*, 3(3), 309–317. doi:10.1111/j.2040-1124.2011.00185.x

REFERENCES

Ad Hoc Committee on Diagnostic Criteria for Diabetes Mellitus, Clinical and Scientific Section, Canadian Diabetes Association. (1986). Acceptance of new criteria for diagnosis of diabetes mellitus and related conditions by the Canadian Diabetes Association. *Canadian Medical Association Journal*, **126**, 473–476.

Altschuler, J., Casella, S., MacKenzie, T. and Curtis, K. (2007). The effect of cinnamon on A1C among adolescents with Type 1 diabetes. *Diabetes Care*, **30**(4), 813–816. doi:10.2337/dc06-1871.

American Diabetes Association. (2018). Diabetes basics. Available at: http://www.diabetes.org/about-diabetes.jsp [Accessed 31 May 2018].

Arablou, T., Aryaeian, N., Valizadeh, M., Sharifi, F., Hosseini, A. and Djalali, M. (2014). The effect of ginger consumption on glycemic status, lipid profile and some inflammatory markers in patients with type 2 diabetes mellitus. *International Journal of Food Sciences and Nutrition*, **65**(4), 515–520. doi:10.3109/09637486.2014.880671.

Attari, V. E., Ostadrahimi, A., Jafarabadi, M. A., Mehralizadeh, S. and Mahluji, S. (2015). Changes of serum adipocytokines and body weight following *Zingiber officinale* supplementation in obese women: A RCT. *European Journal of Nutrition*, **55**(6), 2129–2136. doi:10.1007/s00394-015-1027-6.

Bang, H., Kwak, J., Ahn, H., Shin, D., and Lee, J. (2014). Korean red ginseng improves glucose control in subjects with impaired fasting glucose, impaired glucose tolerance, or newly diagnosed type 2 diabetes mellitus. *Journal of Medicinal Food*, **17**(1), 128–134. doi:10.1089/jmf.2013.2889.

Basch, E., Gabardi S. and Ulbricht C. (2018). Bitter melon (*Momordica charantia*): A review of efficacy and safety. *American Journal of Health-System Pharmacy*, **60**(4), 356–359.

Baskaran, K., Ahamath, B., Shanmugasundaram, K. and Shanmugasundaram, E. (1990). Antidiabetic effect of a leaf extract from *Gymnema sylvestre* in non-insulin-dependent diabetes mellitus patients. *Journal of Ethnopharmacology*, **30**(3), 295–305. doi:10.1016/0378-8741(90)90108-6.

Blevins, S., Leyva, M., Brown, J., Wright, J., Scofield, R. and Aston, C. (2007). Effect of cinnamon on glucose and lipid levels in non insulin-dependent type 2 diabetes. *Diabetes Care*, **30**(9), 2236–2237. doi:10.2337/dc07-0098.

Cefalu, W., Ye, J. and Wang, Z. (2008). Efficacy of dietary supplementation with botanicals on carbohydrate metabolism in humans. *Endocrine, Metabolic & Immune Disorders-Drug Targets*, **8**(2), 78–81. doi:10.2174/187153008784534376.

Chen, K. (1981). Understanding and treatment of diabetes mellitus by traditional Chinese medicine. *American Journal of Chinese Medicine*, **9**(1), 93–94. doi:10.1142/s0192415x81000123.

Choudhary, M., Kochhar, A. and Sangha, J. (2011). Hypoglycemic and hypolipidemic effect of *Aloe vera* L. in non-insulin dependent diabetics. *Journal of Food Science and Technology*, **51**(1), 90–96. doi:10.1007/s13197-011-0459-0.

Coon, J. and Ernst, E. (2002). *Panax ginseng. Drug Safety*, **25**(5), 323–344. doi:10.2165/00002018-200225050-00003.

Daily, J. W., Zhang, X., Kim, D. S. and Park, S. (2015). Efficacy of ginger for alleviating the symptoms of primary dysmenorrhea: A systematic review and meta-analysis of randomized clinical trials. *Pain Medicine*, **16**(12), 2243–2255. doi:10.1111/pme.12853.

Dans, A., Villarruz, M., Jimeno, C., Javelosa, M., Chua, J., Bautista, R. and Velez, G. (2007). The effect of *Momordica charantia* capsule preparation on glycemic control in type 2 diabetes mellitus needs further studies. *Journal of Clinical Epidemiology*, **60**(6), 554–559. doi:10.1016/j.jclinepi.2006.07.009.

Fuangchan, A., Sonthisombat, P., Seubnukarn, T., Chanouan, R., Chotchaisuwat, P. and Sirigulsatien, V. et al. (2011). Hypoglycemic effect of bitter melon compared with metformin in newly diagnosed type 2 diabetes patients. *Journal of Ethnopharmacology*, **134**(2), 422–428. doi:10.1016/j.jep.2010.12.045.

Garcia, M., McNamara, P., Gordon, T. and Kannell, W. (1974). Morbidity and mortality in diabetics in the Framingham population: Sixteen year follow-up study. *Diabetes*, **23**(2), 105–111. doi:10.2337/diab.23.2.105.

Hasan, I. and Khatoon, S. (2012) Effect of *Momordica charantia* (bitter gourd) tablets in diabetes mellitus: Type 1 and type 2. *Prime Research on Medicine*, **2**(2), 72–74.

Heinrich, M., Barnes, J., Gibbons, S. and Williamson, E. (2012). *Fundamentals of Pharmacognosy and Phytotherapy*. 2nd ed. Churchill Livingstone, London, UK.

Hexa Research. (2017). *Herbal medicine market size and forecast, by product (tablets & capsules, powders, extracts), by indication (digestive disorders, respiratory disorders, blood disorders), and trend analysis, 2014–2024*. Felton, CA: Hexa Research.

Hu, F., Manson, J., Stampfer, M., Colditz, G., Liu, S., Solomon, C. and Willett, W. (2001). Diet, lifestyle, and the risk of type 2 diabetes mellitus in women. *New England Journal of Medicine*, **345**(11), 790–797. doi:10.1056/nejmoa010492.

Huseini, H., Kianbakht, S., Hajiaghaee, R. and Dabaghian, F. (2011). Anti-hyperglycemic and anti-hypercholesterolemic effects of *Aloe vera* leaf gel in hyperlipidemic Type 2 diabetic patients: A randomized double-blind placebo-controlled clinical trial. *Planta Medica*, **78**(04), 311–316. doi:10.1055/s-0031-1280474.

International Diabetes Federation (IDF). (2017). About diabetes. Available from: https://www.idf.org/about-diabetes/what-is-diabetes/facts-figures.html.

Ishii, Y., Tanizawa, H. and Takino, Y. (1994). Studies of aloe. IV. Mechanism of cathartic effect.(3). *Biological & Pharmaceutical Bulletin*, **17**(4), 495–497. doi:10.1248/bpb.17.495.

Ishijima, S., Takashima, T., Ikemura, T. and Izutani, Y. (2007). Gymnemic acid interacts with mammalian glycerol-3-phosphate dehydrogenase. *Molecular and Cellular Biochemistry*, **310**(1–2), 203–208. doi:10.1007/s11010-007-9681-5.

Jeevathayaparan, S., Tennekoon, K. H. and Karunanayake, E. H. (1995). A comparative study of the oral hypoglycaemic effect of *Momordica charantia* fruit juice and tolbutamine in streptozotocin induced graded severity diabetes in rat. *International Journal Diabetes*, **13**, 99–108.

Jellin, J. M., Gregory, P. J. et al. (2009). *Pharmacist's Letter/Prescribers Letter Natural Medicines Comprehensive Database*. 11th ed. Stockton, CA: Therapeutic Research Faculty.

Johansen, K. (1990). Hyperlipidemia in diabetes mellitus: Pathogenesis, diagnosis, and pharmacological therapy. *Annals of Saudi Medicine*, **10**(2), 194–201. doi:10.5144/0256-4947.1990.194.

Jung, M., Park, M., Lee, H. C., Kang, Y. H., Kang, E. S. and Kim, S. K. (2006). Antidiabetic agents from medicinal plants. *Current Medicinal Chemistry*, **13**(10), 1203–1218. doi:10.2174/092986706776360860.

Khan, A., Safdar, M., Ali Khan, M., Khattak, K. and Anderson, R. (2003). Cinnamon improves glucose and lipids of people with type 2 diabetes. *Diabetes Care*, **26**(12), 3215–3218. doi:10.2337/diacare.26.12.3215.

Khandouzi, N., Shidfar, F., Rajab, A., Rahideh, T., Hosseini, P. and Mir Taheri, M. (2015). The effects of ginger on fasting blood sugar, hemoglobin A1c, apolipoprotein B, apolipoprotein A-I and malondialdehyde in type 2 diabetic patients. *Iranian Journal of Pharmaceutical Research*, **14**(1), 131–140.

Khanna, P., Jain, S., Panagariya, A. and Dixit, V. (1981). Hypoglycemic activity of polypeptide-p from a plant source. *Journal of Natural Products*, **44**(6), 648–655. doi:0.1021/np50018a002.

Kim, D. (2012). Chemical diversity of *Panax ginseng*, *Panax quinquifolium*, and *Panax notoginseng*. *Journal of Ginseng Research*, **36**(1), 1–15. doi:10.5142/jgr.2012.36.1.1.

Li, Z. and Ji, G. E. (2018). Ginseng and obesity. *Journal of Ginseng Research*, **42**(1), 1–8. doi:10.1016/j.jgr.2016.12.005.

Luo, J. Z. and Luo, L. (2009). Ginseng on hyperglycemia: Effects and mechanisms. *Evidence-Based Complementary and Alternative Medicine*, **6**(4), 423–427. doi:10.1093/ecam/nem178.

Ma SW, Benzie IF, Chu TT, Fok BS, Tomlinson B, Critchley LA. (2008) Effect of *Panax ginseng* supplementation on biomarkers of glucose tolerance, antioxidant status and oxidative stress in type 2 diabetic subjects: Results of a placebo-controlled human intervention trial. *Diabetes Obesity and Metabolism*, **10**,1125–1127. doi:10.1111/j. 1463- 1326.2008.00858.x.

Mang, B., Wolters, M., Schmitt, B., Kelb, K., Lichtinghagen, R., Stichtenoth, D. and Hahn, A. (2006). Effects of a cinnamon extract on plasma glucose, HbA1c, and serum lipids in diabetes mellitus type 2. *European Journal of Clinical Investigation*, **36**(5), 340–344. doi:10.1111/j.1365-2362.2006.01629.x.

Matsuda, H., Morikawa, T. and Yoshikawa, M. (2002). Antidiabetogenic constituents from several natural medicines. *Pure and Applied Chemistry*, **74**(7), 1301–1308. doi:10.1351/pac200274071301.

Medagama, A. B. (2015). The glycaemic outcomes of cinnamon: a review of the experimental evidence and clinical trials. *Nutrition Journal*, **14**, 108. doi:10.1186/s12937-015-0098-9.

Misawa, E., Tanaka, M., Nomaguchi, K., Yamada, M., Toida, T. and Takase, M. et al. (2008). Administration of phytosterols isolated from *Aloe vera* gel reduce visceral fat mass and improve hyperglycemia in Zucker diabetic fatty (ZDF) rats. *Obesity Research & Clinical Practice*, **2**(4), 239–245. doi:10.1016/j.orcp.2008.06.002.

Mozaffari-Khosravi, H., Talaei, B., Jalali, B., Najarzadeh, A. and Mozayan, M. (2014). The effect of ginger powder supplementation on insulin resistance and glycemic indices in patients with type 2 diabetes: A randomized, double-blind, placebo-controlled trial. *Complementary Therapies in Medicine*, **22**(1), 9–16. doi:10.1016/j.ctim.2013.12.017.

Mucalo, I., Jovanovski, E, Vuksan, V., Bozikov, V., Romic, Z., and Rahelic, D. (2014). American ginseng extract (*Panax quinquefolius* L.) is safe in long-term use in type 2 diabetic patients. *Evidence-Based Complementary and Alternative Medicine*, **2014**, 1–6. doi:10.1155/2014/969168.

Nikkila, E. (1985). Are plasma lipoproteins responsible for the excess atherosclerosis in diabetes? *European Journal of Endocrinology*, **110**(4 Suppl), S27–S30. doi:10.1530/acta.0.110s027.

Oh, M., Park, S., Kim, S., Back, H., Kim, M., Jeon, J. et al. (2014). Postprandial glucose-lowering effects of fermented red ginseng in subjects with impaired fasting glucose or type 2 diabetes: A randomized, double-blind, placebo-controlled clinical trial. *BMC Complementary And Alternative Medicine*, **14**(1). doi:10.1186/1472-688214-237.

Park, S., Oh, M., Choi, E., Kim, M., Ha, K., Lee, S. et al. (2014). An 8-wk, randomized, double-blind, placebo-controlled clinical trial for the antidiabetic effects of hydrolyzed ginseng extract. *Journal of Ginseng Research*, **38**(4), 239–243. doi:10.1016/j.jgr.2014.05.006

Rachh, P., Rachh, M., Ghadiya, N., Modi, D., Modi, K., Patel, N. and Rupareliya, M. (2010). Antihyperlipidemic activity of gymenma sylvestre R. Br. Leaf extract on rats fed with high cholesterol diet. *International Journal of Pharmacology*, **6**(2), 138–141. doi:10.3923/ijp.2010.138.141.

Radha, R. and Amrithaveni, M. (2009). Role of medicinal plant *Salacia reticulata* in the management of type II diabetic subjects. *Ancient Science of Life*, **29**(1), 14–16.

Reeds, D., Patterson, B., Okunade, A., Holloszy, J., Polonsky, K., and Klein, S. (2011). Ginseng and ginsenoside re do not improve cell function or insulin sensitivity in overweight and obese subjects with impaired glucose tolerance or diabetes. *Diabetes Care*, **34**(5), 1071–1076. doi:10.2337/dc10-2299.

Riddle, M. C. (2005). Glycemic management of type 2 diabetes: An emerging strategy with oral agents, insulins, and combinations. *Endocrinology and Metabolism Clinics*, **34**, 77–98.

Robinson, M. M. and Zhang, X. (2011). *The World Medicines Situation 2011. Traditional Medicines: Global Situation, Issues and Challenges*. Geneva, Switzerland: World Health Organization.

Serasinghe, S., Serasinghe, P., Yamazaki, H., Nishiguchi, K., Hombhanje, F. and Nakanishi, S. et al. (1990). Oral hypoglycemic effect of *Salacia reticulata* in the streptozotocin induced diabetic rat. *Phytotherapy Research*, **4**(5), 205–206. doi:10.1002/ptr.2650040511.

Shane-McWhorter, L. (2009). Dietary supplements for diabetes: An evaluation of commonly used products. *Diabetes Spectrum*, **22**(4), 206–213. doi:10.2337/diaspect.22.4.206.

Shanmugasundaram, E., Rajeswari, G., Baskaran, K., Kumar, B., Shanmugasundaram, K. and Ahmath, B. (1990). Use of *Gymnema sylvestre*: leaf extract in the control of blood glucose in insulin-dependent diabetes mellitus. *Journal of Ethnopharmacology*, **30**(3), 281–294. doi:10.1016/0378-8741(90)90107-5.

Shattat, G. (2014). A review article on hyperlipidemia: Types, treatments and new drug targets. *Biomedical and Pharmacology Journal*, **7**(2), 399–409. doi:10.13005/bpj/504.

Song, M.-Y., Kim, B.-S. and Kim, H. (2014). Influence of *Panax ginseng* on obesity and gut microbiota in obese middle-aged Korean women. *Journal of Ginseng Research*, **38**(2), 106–115. doi:10.1016/j.jgr.2013.12.004.

Sotaniemi, E., Haapakoski, E. and Rautio, A. (1995). Ginseng therapy in non-insulin-dependent diabetic patients: Effects on psychophysical performance, glucose homeostasis, serum lipids, serum amino-terminalpropeptide concentration, and body weight. *Diabetes Care*, **18**(10), 1373–1375. doi:10.2337/diacare.18.10.1373.

Taylor, L. (2002). *Herbal Secrets of the Rainforest*. 2nd ed. Thousand Oaks, CA: Sage Publications.

Taskinen, M., Nikkil, E., Kuusi, T. and Harno, K. (1982). Lipoprotein lipase activity and serum lipoproteins in untreated type 2 (insulin-independent) diabetes associated with obesity. *Diabetologia*, **22**(1), 46–50. doi:10.1007/bf00253869.

Tilly-Kiesi, M., Knudsen, P., Groop, L. and Taskinen, M. R. (1996). Hyperinsulinemia and insulin resistance are associated with multiple abnormalities of lipoprotein subclasses in glucose-tolerant relatives of NIDDM patients. *The Journal of Lipid Research*, **37**, 1569–1578.

Tiwari, P., Mishra, B. and Sangwan, N. (2014). Phytochemical and pharmacological properties of *Gymnema sylvestre*: An important medicinal plant. *Biomed Research International*, **2014**, 1–18. doi:10.1155/2014/830285.

Vanschoonbeek, K., Thomassen, B., Senden, J., Wodzig, W. and van Loon, L. (2006). Cinnamon supplementation does not improve glycemic control in postmenopausal type 2 diabetes patients. *Journal of Nutrition*, **136**(4), 977–980. doi:10.1093/jn/136.4.977.

Verspohl, E., Bauer, K. and Neddermann, E. (2005). Antidiabetic effect of *Cinnamomum cassia* and *Cinnamomum zeylanicum* in vivo and in vitro. *Phytotherapy Research*, **19**(3), 203–206. doi:10.1002/ptr.1643.

Vuksan, V., Stavro, M., Sievenpiper, J., Beljan-Zdravkovic, U., Leiter, L., Josse, R. and Xu, Z. (2000). Similar postprandial glycemic reductions with escalation of dose and administration time of American ginseng in type 2 diabetes. *Diabetes Care*, **23**(9), 1221–1226. doi:10.2337/diacare.23.9.1221.

Vuksan, V., Sung, M., Sievenpiper, J., Stavro, P., Jenkins, A., and Di Buono, M. et al. (2008). Korean red ginseng (*Panax ginseng*) improves glucose and insulin regulation in well-controlled, type 2 diabetes: Results of a randomized, double-blind, placebo-controlled study of efficacy and safety. *Nutrition, Metabolism and Cardiovascular Diseases*, **18**(1), 46–56. doi:10.1016/j.numecd.2006.04.003.

World Health Organization. (2016). Global report on diabetes. WHO, Geneva, Switzerland.

Yagi, A., Hegazy, S., Kabbash, A. and Wahab, E. (2009). Possible hypoglycemic effect of *Aloe vera* L. high molecular weight fractions on type 2 diabetic patients. *Saudi Pharmaceutical Journal*, **17**(3), 209–215. doi:10.1016/j.jsps.2009.08.007.

Yoon, J., Kang, S., Vassy, J., Shin, H., Lee, Y., Ahn, H. et al. (2011). Efficacy and safety of ginsam, a vinegar extract from *Panax ginseng*, in type 2 diabetic patients: Results of a double-blind, placebo-controlled study. *Journal of Diabetes Investigation*, **3**(3), 309–317. doi:10.1111/j.2040-1124.2011.00185.x.

Yongchaiyudha, S., Rungpitarangsi, V., Bunyapraphatsara, N. and Chokechaijaroenporn, O. (1996). Antidiabetic activity of *Aloe vera* L. juice. I. Clinical trial in new cases of diabetes mellitus. *Phytomedicine*, **3**(3), 241–243. doi:10.1016/s0944-7113(96)80060-2.

Yu, C., Chen, Y., Cline, G., Zhang, D., Zong, H., Wang, Y. et al. (2002). Mechanism by which fatty acids inhibit insulin activation of insulin receptor substrate-1 (IRS-1)-associated phosphatidylinositol 3-kinase activity in muscle. *Journal of Biological Chemistry*, **277**(52), 50230–50236. doi:10.1074/jbc.m200958200.

Zhu, J., Chen, H., Song, Z., Wang, X. and Sun, Z. (2018). Effects of ginger (*Zingiber officinale* Roscoe) on type 2 diabetes mellitus and components of the metabolic syndrome: A systematic review and meta-analysis of randomized controlled trials. *Evidence-Based Complementary and Alternative Medicine*, **2018**, 1–11. doi:10.1155/2018/5692962.

28 Globalisation of Traditional Medicine under the Modern Medicine Portfolio

Pulok K. Mukherjee, Subhadip Banerjee and Amit Kar

CONTENTS

28.1   TRADITIONAL MEDICINE IN GLOBAL HEALTHCARE

Traditional medicine alludes to health practices, methodologies, learning and convictions incorporating plant, animal and mineral based medications, spiritual treatments, manual strategies and activities, connected independently or together to treat, analyse and counteract ailments or look after prosperity (Mukherjee et al. 2010a). Nations in Africa, Asia and Latin America use traditional medicine (TM) to meet some of their essential health needs. In Africa, up to 80% of the populace uses traditional drugs for essential medicinal healthcare. In industrialised nations, traditional medicine prescriptions are called 'complementary' or 'alternative' medicine (CAM).

TM is the sum total of the learning, aptitudes and practices in view of the hypotheses, convictions and encounters indigenous to various societies, regardless of whether logical or not, used as a part of the support of well-being, and additionally in management or treatment of physical and psychological sicknesses. The terms complementary/alternative/non-traditional medicine are used, conversely, with TM in a few nations. The World Health Organization (WHO) perceives that traditional and complementary medicine (T&CM) are a key piece of the worldwide social global healthcare framework. Considering this, the WHO prescribes that legislatures bridle the potential commitment of T&CM health and wellness and advance the sheltered and powerful use of T&CM by controlling frameworks. In October 2013, the WHO discharged the WHO Traditional Medicine Strategy 2014–2023 (hereafter, the Strategy) to give direction to nations as they work to oversee the needs, controls and administration of T&CM inside their own particular locale (WHO 2013).

28.2   GLOBAL STATUS OF TRADITIONAL MEDICINE

TM has kept up its prominence in all areas of development and its use is quickly spreading in industrialised nations. In China, herbal TM represents 30%–50% of the total medicine use. In Europe, North America and other industrialised areas, more than half of the populace have used complementary and alternative drugs at least once. In San Francisco, London and South Africa, 75% of individuals living with HIV/AIDS use TM/CAM drugs. In Canada, 70% of the populace has used integral medicine at least once. In Germany, 90% of the populace has used an alternative cure at some point (WHO 2013). In the United States, 158 million people from the adult populace uses CAM solutions, and as indicated by the US Commission for Alternative and Complementary solutions, billions of US dollars are spent on TM cures. In the United Kingdom, yearly consumption of alternative medication is more than $200 million. The worldwide market for herbal medicines presently remains at over $100 billion yearly and is developing consistently (WHO 2013). Scientific evidence from randomised clinical trials is strong for the use of medicinal plants in several therapies including acupuncture, while further research is needed to ascertain the safety and efficacy of several other practices and uses of medicinal plants.

Unregulated or incorrect use of traditional medicine prescriptions and practices can have negative or perilous impacts. Notwithstanding persistent security issues, there is the hazard that a developing herbal market and its awesome business advantage may represent a risk to biodiversity through over-collection of the crude material for herbal medicines. These practices, if not controlled, may prompt the annihilation of threatened species and the reduction of environmental assets. Another related issue is the necessity for TM-related international standards for patent law, as most national TM patent laws are insufficient to ensure traditional information and biodiversity.

While India, China, Korea, Vietnam and some other countries have incorporated traditional medicine into their medicinal healthcare frameworks, numerous nations have yet to gather and incorporate institutionalised proof on this kind of healthcare. Traditional systems of medicine in different countries have a national direction on herbal prescriptions, yet the administrative control of medicinal plants has not developed around an organised model (Mukherjee et al. 2015a). This is because therapeutic items or herbs are characterised distinctively in various nations, and assorted methodologies have been embraced as to licensing, dispensing, manufacturing and trading. The restricted logical confirmation about TM/CAM's security, adequacy and other considerations make it imperative for governments to detail national approaches and controls for the correct use of TM/CAM and its amalgamation into national healthcare frameworks in accordance with the arrangements of the WHO methodologies on TM (WHO 2013).

28.3   AYURVEDA AND INDIAN SYSTEMS OF MEDICINE

India has a rich heritage of TM and the traditional healthcare system has been practiced for many centuries. It mainly consists of three major systems, namely Ayurveda, Siddha and Unani. The *Materia Medica* of India provides much information on the folklore practices and traditional aspects of therapeutically important natural products. These traditional systems of Indian medicine have their uniqueness no doubt, but there is a common thread running through these systems in their fundamental principles and practices. With the emerging global interest to adopt and study traditional systems and to exploit their potential based on different healthcare systems, the evaluation of the rich heritage of the TM is essential. The government and private sectors are trying their best to explore all possibilities for the evaluation of these systems to bring out therapeutic approaches available in the original system of medicine as well as to help in generating data to put these products on a national healthcare programme. In almost all TM, medicinal plants play a major role and constitute the backbone of the TM. Indian *Materia Medica* includes about 2000 drugs of natural origin, almost all of which are derived from different traditional system and folklore practices. Out of these drugs derived from the traditional system, 400 are of mineral and animal origin, while the rest are of plant origin (Mukherjee et al. 2012).

Archaeological evidence reveals that drug taking is an extremely old human phenomenon. By necessity, the drugs used in ancient civilisation were extracts of plants or animal products, with a few inorganic salts. In India, the Ayurvedic system of medicine developed an extensive use of medicines from plants dating from at least 1000 BCE. The earliest Chinese records give descriptions of diseases, but not medicines; illnesses were thought to be godly punishments and they were treated by prayers and offerings. The earliest recorded Chinese prescriptions after about 500 BCE show the beginning of the use of natural products as drugs. The first classic texts in Chinese medicine appeared in 25–220 CE, and some of their formulae remains in use (Mukherjee et al. 2010b). Similarly, the Egyptian Ebers papyrus (around 1550 BCE) contains descriptions of several active ingredients (notably purgatives) that are still used today. Western medicine continues to show the influence of ancient practices. Current examples are the use of cardiac glycosides from the purple foxglove *Digitalis purpurea* and related plants, opiates from the opium poppy *Papaver somniferum*, reserpine from Rauwolfia species and quinine from Cinchona species. More recently, there has been interest in other products from traditional systems of medicine; artemisinin is an active antimalarial compounds isolated from *Artemisia annua*, a constituent of the Chinese antimalarial preparation *qinghaosu*, and forskolin was isolated from *Coleus forskohlii*, a species used in Ayurvedic preparations for cardiac disorders. A new standardised preparation, artemether, has recently been introduced for treatment of drug-resistant malaria, and new analogues of forskolin are being tested for a variety of uses (Mukherjee et al. 2015b).

Much effort has been taken by the government and private sectors in India for the development of the traditional systems. The Government of India had established the Department of Indian Systems of Medicine and Homoeopathy (ISM&H) under the Ministry of Health & Family Welfare in March

1995 for the growth and development of Ayurveda and other systems of Indian Medicine. It was re-named the Department of Ayurveda, Yoga & Naturopathy, Unani, Siddha and Homoeopathy (AYUSH) in November 2003. Each letter of the acronym AYUSH represents an officially recognised system of medicine other than allopathic medicine. In 2014, a conscious decision was further taken to upgrade the Department of AYUSH to a full-fledged Ministry of AYUSH, with an independent Minister. The mandate for change was for systematic development in all spheres of Indian Medicine and to bridge the prevailing gaps in healthcare delivery and outreach of healthcare. The Ministry is responsible for policy formulation, planning and implementation of schemes and programme for augmenting the domain, quality and outcomes of the AYUSH sector in inclusive terms. Sowa Rigpa, traditional medical system of the people of Himalayan region, has also been given recognition and added into AYUSH (India 2011). The objectives of the Ministry of AYUSH are multifaceted and include the following:

- Upgrading of educational standards of teaching and training institutions
- Strengthening of research and development institutions and time-bound execution of prioritised research programmes
- Implementation of schemes for promotion, cultivation, conservation, sustainable development and resource augmentation of medicinal plants used in AYUSH systems
- Standardisation and quality control of drugs as per global trends
- Mainstreaming and integration of AYUSH healthcare in the national health delivery network
- Awareness building and propagation of AYUSH through information, education and communication

The significance of Indian Systems of Medicine and Homoeopathy was first brought in the National Health Policy (India 1983), and later emphasised in the National Population Policy, 2000, and National Health Policy (India 2002), and ultimately in comprehensive terms in the National AYUSH Policy, 2002. It was envisaged in the policy statements that Ayurveda would have a substantial role because of its advantages, such as diversity, modest cost and the growing popularity of natural plant–based products, especially in the under-served, remote and tribal areas (India 2002). The policy envisaged the consolidation of documentary knowledge of Ayurveda to protect it from commercial exploitation, piracy and misappropriation by foreign entities. It promotes measures to ensure affordable healthcare and drugs that are safe and efficacious. Integration of AYUSH in the healthcare delivery system and national programmes to ensure optimal use of the vast infrastructure of hospitals, dispensaries and physicians were a focus of the policy (Samal 2015). Optimal use of Ayurveda has been taken up for mainstreaming in healthcare through the National Rural Health Mission, which is now upgraded into a flagship programme called the National Health Mission (Shrivastava et al. 2015). As a result of this initiative, the public perception is evolving, and increased opportunities are emerging in AYUSH, including development of Ayurveda in various aspects.

The Central Council of Indian Medicine (CCIM) is a statutory body constituted under the Indian Medicine Central Council Act, 1970. The Council is envisioned to be a dynamic regulatory body that will regulate the practice of Ayurveda and also guide, develop and sustain a network of 'institutions of excellence' in education to meet the national needs considering the global trends. The mission of the council is to establish, guide, develop and sustain for the conservation of standards and quality of academic study programmes as well as practice of Ayurveda to meet national as well as global standards through resource allocation, good governance and management (Katoch 2017).

28.3.1 Ayurveda – The Ancient Indian System

Ayurveda is accepted to be the oldest medical system, as it came into existence in about 900 BC. The Sanskrit word 'Ayurveda' is comprised of two words – 'Ayus', meaning life and 'Veda', meaning learning or science. Accordingly 'Ayurveda' in totality signifies 'Knowledge of life'.

The Ayurveda is said to be an Upaveda (part) of Atharva Veda, and the *Charaka Samhita* (1900 BCE) is the first recorded treatise fully devoted to the concept of practice of Ayurveda. This describes 341 plants and plant products for use in medicine. The next landmark of Ayurvedic literature was the *Sushruta Samhita* (600 BCE), which has special emphasis on surgery. It describes 395 medicinal plants, 57 drugs of animal origin, 64 minerals and metals as therapeutic agents. Sushruta, the father of surgery as claimed by Indian traditional medicine, lived and practiced surgery in Varanasi, India, approximately 2500 years ago. Another important authority of Ayurveda was Bagbhatta of Sind (present-day Pakistan), who practiced Ayurveda in around seventeenth century CE, and his work *Ashtanga Hridaya* is considered unrivalled for the principles and practice of medicine. The *Madhava Nidana* (800–900 CE) was the next important milestone and is the most famous work on the diagnosis of diseases as per Ayurvedic concept. Bhava Mishra of Magadha is the last writer on Hindu medicine whose treatise *Bhava Prakasha*, written around 1550 CE, is held in high esteem by modern Ayurvedic practitioners for its description of approximately 470 medicinal plants (Debnath et al. 2015).

In India, the historical backdrop of healthcare spans back 5000 years, when human healthcare needs and sicknesses were noted in antiquated literary works like the *Rig Veda* and *Atharva Veda*. Afterward, writings like *Charaka Samhita* and *Sushruta Samhita* were reported in around 1000 BCE, where the use of plants and polyherbal formulations was featured for human healthcare. Development of Ayurveda and plant-based solutions for human healthcare through everyday beneficial encounters is a piece of the social legacy of India. Indian *Materia Medica* incorporates around 2000 medications of common source derived from various traditional systems and folklore practices (Mukherjee et al. 2017).

The old Vedic content *Atharva Veda* was recorded around 5000 years ago and contains different references to Ayurvedic medication and united parts of human healthcare. It incorporates each feature of presence including physical, mental, profound and social. It clarifies what is useful and what is destructive for life, how an upbeat life can be accomplished and a hopeless life defrosted, and all these imperative inquiries and life expectancy unified issues are extravagantly and fervently presented in Ayurveda (Mukherjee et al. 2012). According to Indian Hindu mythology, there are four Veda written by the Aryans – *Rig Veda*, *Sham Veda*, *Yajur Veda* and *Atharva Veda*. Amongst these the *Rig Veda*, the oldest one, was written later than 1500 BCE. Ayurveda depends on involvement from time immemorial, some of which has been demonstrated tentatively. For the most part Ayurvedic details are multi-segment blends, containing plant and animal items, minerals and metals. Old writings like the *Rig Veda*, *Atharva Veda* and official compendia like the Ayurvedic Pharmacopeia and Ayurvedic Formulary have shown the strength of plant-derived items (Katoch 2017). The *Charaka Samhita* (900 BC) is considered the main recorded treatise of the ideas and routine with regard to Ayurveda; its essential concentration was therapeutics. This work recorded 341 plants and plant items for use in medication (Mukherjee et al. 2015b).

Ayurveda is said to be an Upaveda (part) of Atharva Veda whereas the Charaka Samhita (1900 BC) is the first recorded treatise fully devoted to the concept of practice of Ayurveda. This describes 341 plants and plant products for use in medicine. The next landmark of the Ayurvedic literature was the Sushruta Samhita (600 BC), which has special emphasis on surgery. It described 395 medicinal plants, 57 drugs of animal origin, 64 minerals and metals as therapeutic agents. Sushruta, the father of surgery as claimed by Indian traditional medicine lived and practiced surgery in Varanasi, India approximately 2500 years ago. Another important authority of Ayurveda was Bagbahtta of Sind, the present-day Pakistan, who practiced Ayurveda in around seventeenth century AD and his work Astanga Hridaya is considered unrivaled for the principles and practice of medicine. The Madhab Nidana (800–900 AD) was the next important milestone and is the most famous work on diagnosis of diseases as per Ayurvedic concept. Bhava Mishra of Magadha is the last writer on Hindu medicine whose treatise Bhava Prakasha, written around 1550 is held in high esteem by modern Ayurvedic practitioners for its description of approximately 470 medicinal plants.

The historic point in Ayurvedic writing was the Sushruta Samhita (600 BC), which has unique accentuation on surgery. It portrayed 395 medicinal plants, 57 medications of animal sources and 64 minerals and metals as remedial specialists. Sushruta, the father of surgery, lived and rehearsed surgery in Varanasi, India, roughly 2500 years back. Another essential specialist in Ayurveda was Vagbhata, who honed around the 700 AD. His work Ashtanga Hridaya is viewed as unrivaled for the standards and routine with regard to medicine. The Madhava Nidana (800–900 AD) was the following critical point of reference; it is the most well-known Ayurvedic text for finding of illnesses. The praised essayist on traditional Indian medicine was Bhava Mishra of Magadha, whose treatise Bhava Prakasha, composed around 1550. This is highly regarded by current Ayurvedic experts for its portrayals of roughly 470 therapeutic plants.

Other than these amazing treatises, more than 70 'Nighantu Granthas' (drug store vocabularies) were composed, for the most part between the seventh and sixteenth century CE. The 'Raj Nighantu' by Narhari Pandit and 'Madanpala Nighantu' by Madanpala are considered gems on medicinal plants. The *Charaka Samhita* ordered plant drugs into 50 bunches in light of their Sanskrit name. Subsequently, Ayurveda from its source experimentally sorted out knowledge. Ayurvedic writings are tremendously regarded in neighbouring nations and were translated into Greek (300 BCE), Tibetan and Chinese (300 CE) and a few other Asian dialects (Mukherjee 2001). Among the Indian Systems of medicine, other than Ayurveda there are a few other integral and elective frameworks of medication like homeopathy, Siddha and Unani, which are additionally honed and created over the course of time in India, where plants and plant-based details are used for healthcare.

Based on the Ayurvedic writings detailed above, Ayurveda introduces broad information on the counteractive action of maladies, the advancement of well-being and its safeguarding and administration of infections, too, in all encompassing terms (Mukherjee and Wahile 2006). Way of life administration or *Swasthyavritta* is a noteworthy zone of centre specified in Ayurvedic writing, which in TM practice manages solid status. Ayurveda can effectively oversee way of life related infections, medicate manhandling, degenerative ailments, immune system illnesses and metabolic and hypersensitive disarrangements with its special treatments, body–mind constitution based way of life rules and medicaments. It has the multidimensional scope of treatment viability in ailment conditions like headache, Parkinsonism, neurological scatters and musculoskeletal infections, which are not all that adequately sensible with ordinary treatment (Mukherjee et al. 2010a). Plenty of the therapeutic herbs in Ayurveda have been deductively approved for their indicated impacts as against convulsions, hostile to malignancy and against maturing specialists. Ayurveda is known as a productive method of treatment for the vast majority of illnesses identified with different frameworks of the body with its novel treatments known as *Panchakarma* (Debnath et al. 2015). The all-encompassing methodology and reasonableness of Ayurvedic human healthcare has been built up in a way that individuals have begun using it as an adjuvant with the progressing treatment and for individualised way of life adjustments. In India, Ayurveda is the generally rehearsed and culture bound custom of healthcare, and its learning is accessible in both systematised and non-classified structures.

28.4   GLOBALISATION OF AYURVEDA

India has an ancient system of Ayurvedic medicine that gives an abundance of data on old folklore and traditional aspects of remedially vital natural products. One of the significant difficulties of Ayurvedic medicine is the issue of quality, safety and adequacy and these things should be more underlined (Mukherjee et al. 2016). Globalisation and improvement of Ayurvedic medicine is important for the foundation of the confirmation of healthcare claims. There is a growing acceptance of Ayurveda among consumers in the domestic and global market. It is growing as a crucial component of the pluralistic healthcare system in India and throughout the world. The Ministry has decided to identify and promote through reputed Ayurvedic knowledge centres engaged in drug development and research, education, clinical research both within the government or in non-government, non-profit centres to support them to enhance their functions and facilities to the levels of excellence (Mukherjee et al. 2017).

For globalising the system and its products, the Ministry of AYUSH has focused its attention on standardisation and quality control of Ayurvedic drugs. Good manufacturing practices (GMPs) have been notified under 'Schedule T' of the Drugs & Cosmetics Rules, 1945, and testing for heavy metals such as mercury, arsenic, lead and cadmium in all purely herbal Ayurvedic drugs is mandatory for export purposes (Anonymous 2013). All these measures have been introduced to give greater impetus to consumer awareness, consumer and doctor benefit, acceptance in the globalised markets and to ensure safety, which is of utmost concern while using Ayurveda medicines. Clinical safety and efficacy documentation proof for Ayurvedic medicine has been a persistent and increasing demand globally (Singh 2010). The history of 'good clinical practice' (GCP) statutes traces back to one of the oldest enduring traditions in the history of medicine – Ayurveda. Therefore clinical trials in Ayurveda need to be guided by the principle of GCP. The safety and therapeutic efficacy of the AYUSH drugs can be readdressed to assure their quality. Thus clinical research in these lines helps us to generate quality data acceptable to regulatory authorities. Research has focused more on ethical guidelines while treating a patient with medical/surgical interventions. The requirement for proof of effectiveness in licensing on the patent or proprietary AYUSH medicine for the enactment of Drugs & Cosmetics Rule 158 B since August 2010 has necessitated the development of present guidelines of GCP. These guidelines have been prepared by a comprehensive consultative process and are fine-tuned to the best interest of Ayurveda (Katoch 2017).

Global promotion and propagation of Ayurveda has been an important thrust area of the Department of Ministry over the past few years. It has adopted a strategy for the signing of Country to Country Memorandum of Understanding (MoU) on cooperation in TM. It has established AYUSH academic chairs in foreign universities and institutes. The AYUSH Information Cell has been opened in the premises of the India Missions/ICCR Cultural Centre to disseminate authentic information about AYUSH. The significant achievements of international cooperation have been tremendous, which have resulted in Ayurveda emerging at the global level. Globally, TM regained its prestige when traditional Chinese medicine (TCM) earned the Nobel Prize in Medicine for the discovery of an anti-malarial drug in 2015 and the UN decided to celebrate 21 June as World Yoga Day. It is a matter of triumph when 'Traditional Medicine: Delhi Declaration' was adopted as the resolution of the WHO Regional Committee for South-East Asia SEA/RC67/R3 as proposed by AYUSH, and it has now been adopted by the countries of whole southeast Asia region.

The people bear a strong faith in AYUSH and are also convinced of its effectiveness. However it requires genuine need for developing awareness and ease of access to traditional medical systems in India. Interdisciplinary research, standardisation, quality control and validation of Ayurvedic medicine is needed to establish a knowledge base to meet global standards. The AYUSH industry also needs mentoring from the government to flourish in India and abroad. The Ministry of AYUSH is taking a huge step towards the promotion and development of Ayurveda nationally and internationally (Katoch 2017).

28.5 TRADITIONAL KNOWLEDGE DIGITAL LIBRARY

The Traditional Knowledge Digital Library (TKDL; http://www.tkdl.res.in) deals with the documentation of existing knowledge on Ayurvedic systems of medicine. It is imperative to safeguard the sovereignty of traditional Ayurvedic knowledge to protect it from being misused in patenting on non-patentable inventions. Although this knowledge is in the public domain, the patent office does not have a mechanism to access this information to deny patenting rights. Obtaining patents for all such medicinal uses is impossible. It is also extremely costly and time-consuming to fight patents granted to others. Thus, bringing such knowledge into an easily accessible format to forestall wrongful patents was actualised through the TKDL, which is an original proprietary database that is fully protected by national and international laws on intellectual property. The core of the project is the innovative approach in the form of Traditional Knowledge Resource Classification (TKRC) that enables conversion of 140,000 pages of information, containing 36,000 formulations described in 14 texts of Ayurveda, into the patent-compatible format in various languages, including translation of Sanskrit *shlokas* not only into Hindi but also into English, French, German, Spanish and Japanese, among other languages. The information includes names of plants, Ayurvedic description of diseases under their modern names, therapeutic formulations, and so on (Mukherjee et al. 2010b). The Ministry of AYUSH, Government of India, has launched the National AYUSH Mission (NAM) during 12th Plan for implementing through States/UTs. It envisages better access to healthcare, strengthening educational institutions, enforcement of quality control of drugs and continuous availability of raw materials in the States/UTs during 12th Plan (India 2015). The new initiatives under NAM include school health programmes through AYUSH. The public health outreach activity has been taken up to focus on increasing awareness regarding the strength of Ayurveda in managing community health problems.

28.6   VALIDATION OF TRADITIONAL MEDICINE

In most countries today, practices of allopathic and traditional systems of medicine crop up side by side in a complimentary way. So the efforts are made to harmonise the process of their evaluation and quality control for optimum use of the botanicals in relation with drug discovery and development. In order to ensure the accurate identification and authentication of the herbs the first crucial step is to avoid confusion, admixtures or adulterations in the botanicals (Mukherjee et al. 2015b). With regard to quality assurance, plant identification is crucial to guarantee that raw material of the right medicinal plant has been used and to detect possible admixtures, adulterations and confusions. Identification should be carried out combining various methods, including macroscopic and microscopic examination or chemical fingerprinting and DNA-based characterisation. The useful active compounds in plants for medicinal preparation are amongst the huge diversity of secondary plant products that are often specific for certain plants or plant groups (Mukherjee 2009). These are some vital aspects that should be considered for the correct identification and authentication of traditional medicine herbs (Mukherjee 2002). There are several important processes and integrated strategies that need to be considered for validation in traditional medicine like Ayurveda at each and every step (Mukherjee et al. 2015). Global implementation of evidence-based validation is required for TM that would transform healthcare for all (Mukherjee et al. 2014). The development of TM requires the convergence of modern techniques and integrated approaches related to their evidence-based research in various fields. Botanicals are standardised based on the presence of a known active ingredient or specific markers when the active markers are not yet recognised, but this can help in establishing the product's quality depending on the characteristic fingerprints. Plants contain several active substances in certain ratios and in standardised extracts. This ratio must be kept constant, within narrow limits, from one preparation to another. The unique processing methods followed for the manufacturing of TM products turn herbal ingredients into very complex mixtures, through which the separation, identification and estimation of chemical components become more challenging in some cases. Moreover, herbals are known to contain several components and in many cases the absolute compound responsible for the pharmacological activity is unknown (Mukherjee et al. 2016).

In spite of the considerable synthetic variety got from the improvement of combinatorial sciences and high-throughput screening strategies in the course of recent years, natural products and related structures keep on being critical components of pharmacopoeias. Looking forward, natural products and related structures are probably going to end up considerably more essential for the advancement of enhanced and new medicines, because of the assortment of practically applicable secondary metabolites of microbial and plant species whose concoction and hereditary decent variety are being uncovered by ultra-fast DNA sequencing and related genomics and bioinformatics apparatuses (Mukherjee et al. 2017).

Until now, strategies for recognising and describing the exercises of optional metabolites have been wasteful and frequently dreary, but recent advances in genomics, informatics and related twenty-first century 'omics' innovations are drastically quickening the pace of disclosure and investigation. Refined fractionation techniques hyphenated to current spectrometries and spectroscopies can characterise the metabolomes of cells, tissues and even life forms. Multivariate investigations and network modelling empower complete distinguishing proof and assessment of natural products of assorted variety and usefulness, and when incorporated with network approaches, it is conceivable to profile molecular changes caused by transformation and by pathogens and other ecological stressors, and accordingly to anticipate the objectives and mode(s) of activity and toxicities of natural products and its derivatives. This commitment of natural products appears to be moving, particularly against a background of where interest in natural products by the significant pharmaceutical organisations has been unimportant. This absence of excitement by business has a few reasons. The United Nations Convention on Biological Diversity has concerns regarding the regulation of natural products and worldwide access. This can be managed by following regular best practices.

28.7   QUALITY ASSURANCE OF TRADITIONAL MEDICINE

Herbal drugs have turned out to be an important part of new generation health system in many countries. It has been observed in recent times that herbal products are being substituted for traditional medicines in many countries. Increased demand for herbal products has led to growing demand in global market (Mukherjee et al. 2015a), with the increase in the use of herbal medicine there is also an increase in the reports of toxicity and adverse reactions. Such undesirable reactions can be due to:

1. Side effects (usually these are predictable in nature)
2. Reactions which are resultant of overdose, over-duration, tolerance, dependence-addiction
3. Hypersensitivity, allergic and idiosyncratic reactions
4. Mid-term and long-term toxic effects including liver, renal, cardiac and neurotoxicity also genotoxicity and teratogenicity

The herbal products being marketed are generally not thoroughly tested for their pharmacological and toxicological effects. In addition there has been a problem related to the quality of herbal products due to unexpected toxicity, which occurs due to use of poor quality raw materials, misidentified herbs, adulterations and contaminations. With the help of GMP, these quality issues can be addressed properly, and manufacturing of herbal medicine can be improved. Although there are some issues, which cannot be neglected – like the herbs that come from different countries and areas have different standards and regulations – these matters will remain a problem. Due to reports of serious effects like hepatotoxicity, renal failure and allergic reactions, the regulatory authorities are facing questions regarding the safety of marketed herbal medicines. The World Health Organization has developed guidelines for the monitoring of herbal safety within the existing pharmacovigilance framework (Shaw et al. 2012).

28.8   MODERN DRUGS INSPIRED FROM TRADITIONAL MEDICINE

The natural product compilation uncovers a broad scope of pharmacophores with a high level of stereochemistry. These benefits can add to the capacity to give hits – even contrary to the new disease screening targets, for example, protein–protein interaction. Be that as it may, natural products may demonstrate some extra advantage over synthetic by being natural metabolites: aggregates that are prospering as medications have been found to demonstrate the property of metabolite resemblance. This implies natural products can be organically dynamic and furthermore liable to be substrates for at least one of the numerous transporter frameworks that can convey the mixes to their intracellular site of activity. These focal points roused a re-developing enthusiasm for natural product research in drug discovery (Mukherjee et al. 2017).

The traditional medicine inspired development of new novel drugs, improved significantly the quality of healthcare. Virtually, expedition of natural product discovery was started in 1785, with the English physician Withering. He published his observations on the use of the foxglove, *Digitalis purpurea*, for the treatment of heart disorders, and this eventually led to the isolation of the cardiotonic agent, digoxin, which inhibited sodium-potassium ATPase. Later, isolation of morphine from *Papaver somniferum* by Sertürner in 1806 opened a new era for the use of pure chemicals as painkillers for cancer patients suffering from terminal pain. In 1875, salicylic acid was isolated from willow bark and its acetyl salt known as aspirin is an important milestone in drug discovery. Starting from the discovery of molecules like aspirin as analgesic in 1842 to longer molecules like taxol for anticancer has been a long journey of drug discovery and development (Mukhejee et al. 2017). Malaria still continues to be one of the extreme health challenges threatening humankind. In the history of anti-malarial medication, the important success stories have been attributed to natural products. After its serendipitous discovery, quinine maintained its position as a vital anti-malarial drug for almost 400 years since its effectiveness was first documented (Achan et al. 2011). In 1820, it was first isolated from the bark of Cinchona species (e.g. *C. officinalis*) by two pharmacists from France (Buss and Waigh 1995). In the mid-twentieth century its synthetic counterparts chloroquine and mefloquine replaced quinine. However they became resistant soon, so another plant from traditional Chinese medicine, *Artemisia annua* (*quinghaosu*), came to prominence in anti-malarial therapy. This discovery in 1971 by Chinese researchers using ethnopharmacological information from antiquated messages in traditional Chinese medicine gave an energizing new characteristic item lead compound, now known as artemisinin (Cragg and Newman 2013). Its account of disclosure is extremely whimsical yet moving. They began working with more than 2000 Chinese herb arrangements and distinguished 640 hits with conceivable antimalarial exercises. After a long hit and trial, they recognised *qinghao* (the Chinese name of *Artemisia annua* L.) to be powerful against plasmodium parasites. However their outcomes were not reproducible. At that point in the wake of looking through the traditional Chinese literature they discovered its exclusive reference in Ge Hong's *A Handbook of Prescriptions for Emergencies,* which stated 'A modest bunch of qinghao inundated with 2 Liters of water, wring out the juice and drink everything'. This sentence gave them the key thought of its extraction that the warming associated with the traditional medicine extraction step must be maintained at a strategic distance. They got a superior outcome at a lower temperature extraction process. Subsequent to getting great preclinical outcomes without clinical trial offices, the researchers fearlessly volunteered to be the primary individuals to take the concentrate. At that point they led clinical trials in Hainan region to test its clinical viability with patients tainted with both *Plasmodium vivax* and *P. falciparum*. It was disconnected in 1971 and distributed in 1982. The WHO has taken artemisin in based blend treatments (ACTs) to control intestinal sickness with critical impact. This critical revelation from a characteristic item brought acknowledgment, as Tu Youyou received the Noble Prize in physiology or medicine for it in 2015. In this manner the historical backdrop of research into a regular item points towards its wonderful future (Mukherjee et al. 2017).

28.9 GLOBAL HARMONISATION OF TRADITIONAL MEDICINE

For most of mankind's history data and learning have been transmitted orally and by perception and direct duplicating. With the coming of composing frameworks a more exact duplicating and learning transmission was conceivable and the transmission of information identified with material medica over wide spatial and temporal areas was conceivable. Oral and composed learning transmission is in steady trade, and composed information may bring about changes to conventions, which are then passed on orally – and the other way around – and taking this as a dichotomisation has neither rhyme nor reason. In any case, there exists a reasonable quantitative distinction in learning transmission exuded by writings used as aides and references over a drawn out stretch of time, over expansive land augmentations and various social foundations. By and large, content permits a more preservationist information transmission and may prompt a homogenisation of learning.

That products and related learning from Indian and Chinese *Materia Medica* were traded along the Silk Road coming to and affecting early Mediterranean medicinal customs can be followed in writing managing *Materia Medica* from the fifth to the fourth century BCE onwards. An accumulation of 51 birch-bark leaves known as the Bower Manuscript is viewed as the most established content managing Hindu prescription. It was found in Kucha (Chinese Turkestan) on the Silk Road in 1889, interpreted by the German-British orientalist Rudolf Hoernlé (1841–1918) and dated to the fifth century CE. Not by any means was opium, which around then was a standout amongst the most imperative medications in the Mediterranean and the Near East, specified in the Bower Manuscript. Despite the fact that earlier – and now lost – therapeutic contents managing antiquated Hindu medication existed, such medicinal information inside India has principally been passed on by specialists and through the individual preparing of replacements (Mukherjee et al. 2012). Medicinal practices on the Indian subcontinent started to mix with the Arab medical system (Unani-Tibb) from the twelfth century onwards, and towards the end of the eighteenth century the British started to present the Western arrangement of medicine. The principal European therapeutic school in India, the Calcutta Medical College, opened in 1835. This recorded advancement prompted the present circumstance that, while the Sanskrit works of art thoroughly depict somewhere in the range of 700 medicinal plant species, contingent upon the source, more than 10,000 plant species are related with Ayurvedic prescription.

On account of worldwide commercialisation and intercultural learning and data trade, patients progressively have the decision among various therapeutic frameworks for their healthcare needs with access to doctors concentrated inside various medicinal frameworks. In view of the authentic and monetary advancement in a nation or area, a country's traditional medicine system(s) are frequently supplemented with biomedicines. Alternately, in different areas, close by biomedicine, diverse traditional medicine frameworks of medicine and choices (correlative prescription) are built up. How elective treatments ought to be incorporated and secured by national healthcare administrations and what is a reasonable cost for singular treatments and solutions remain open questions, and human healthcare by and large is the matter of consistent verbal confrontations. However, Khan (2006) contends that although medicinal pluralism is at present notable reality in numerous social orders, there is a need to bring the dialogue past the pluralist and liberal arguments – including components, for example, 'mastery and dominion' – and extend the verifiable, social and political setting of the discourse (Ngo et al. 2014). With regard to India, while Western culture and drugs are applied over indigenous science and medicine amid the pilgrim stage, it was the national pioneer boats and governments that combined this advancement. Then again, the interest in indigenous choices, albeit successful, did not receive sufficient reaction from the national experts. In like manner, nearby healthcare and solutions are subjected to worldwide corporate greed, which continuously impacts singular helpful decisions and inclinations.

A recent illustration comes from a cutting edge group medical facility in Thailand, where Thai traditional medicine is closely coordinated with biomedicine into advanced human healthcare benefits. The recognised key elements for the effective mix are information transmission from Royal Thai traditional medicine and privately practised herbal medicine among the clinic experts and a healthcare group consisting of individuals with various foundations, together with an efficient supply of natural drugs. Coordinating therapeutic frameworks is not just a test for doctor's facility offices, but also for well-being informatics (Health Information Systems), which is at present firmly connected to the measurements of Western biomedicine. Because the pattern toward concurrence of various medicinal frameworks will undoubtedly expand, it is suitable to outline well-being informatics applications consistent with the qualities of various therapeutic frameworks. There is an absence of clinical examinations concentrating on the similar adequacy of traditional herbal drug and sustenance products. Traditional medicines will just be considered important and accepted by essential healthcare frameworks when exploratory and clinical information sets up a confirmation base. Elevated expectations consider that affirming well-being and the adequacy of traditional medicine drugs are, in this way, required. Because co-prescription of therapeutic plants and biomedicine is as often as possible watched, experts and clinicians are urged to keep an eye out for antagonistic and also useful communications. Clinical investigations – as opposed to concentrating only on viability – could concentrate additionally on adequacy by including a more heterogeneous example of members and embracing research settings that broadly reflect the regular heath–mind circumstances. The changing worldwide monetary scene and changing worldview in medical improvement may display leverage in the endeavour to authoritatively enrol traditional medicines with legislative offices (Leonti and Casu 2013).

There has been increasing interest in and mainstream use of traditional and complementary medicine (T&CM) around the world. In some nations, local healers remain the sole or principle well-being suppliers for many individuals living in rustic territories. For example, the proportion of traditional well-being professionals to residents in Africa is 1:500, while the proportion of therapeutic specialists to natives is 1:40,000. In the Lao People's Democratic Republic, 80% of the populace lives in provincial territories, with every town being attended by maybe a couple traditional well-being professionals. More than 100 million Europeans are right now clients of T&CM, with one-fifth being traditional medicine clients; comparative extents pick human healthcare that incorporates T&CM. As per a national study in China, professionals of traditional Chinese medicine received 907 million visits from patients in 2009, which represents 18% of all single medicinal visits to studied foundations. Further, the quantity of traditional Chinese medicine inpatients was 13.6 million, or 16% of the aggregate in all clinics overviewed. In several nations, certain kinds of traditional medicine (TM) have been totally incorporated into the healthcare framework, including China, the Democratic People's Republic of Korea (North Korea), the Republic of Korea (South Korea), India and Vietnam. In China, for example, traditional Chinese medicine and regular medicine are kept close by each other at each level of the human healthcare administration, and open and private protection cover the two types of treatment. In numerous different nations, T&CM is in part coordinated into the national well-being framework, while in a few nations there is no joining by any stretch of the imagination.

Late changes, rising difficulties and needs have changed significantly since the last World Health Organization (WHO) worldwide strategy document was published in 2002. An ever-increasing number of nations are coming to acknowledge the commitment that T&CM can make to the well-being and prosperity of people and the completeness of their healthcare systems. In the period 1999–2012, the quantity of partner conditions of WHO with national arrangements covering TM have expanded entirely. This incorporates nations better controlling natural medicines or making national research organisations think about T&CM. Governments and shoppers are ending up more open to more extensive parts of T&CM and to considering them as an incorporated piece of well-being administration conveyance. In Africa, the quantity of national administrative systems expanded from one in 1999/2000 to 28 in 2010. Across the Atlantic, the Ministry of Health in Brazil has built up a national arrangement on integrative and complementary and alternative practices. Materials that show up in this segment were not inspected or surveyed by Science Editorial staff, but rather have been assessed by a worldwide publication group consisting of specialists in traditional medicine research. In the Mediterranean area, five partner states report having directions particularly for T&CM experts. Partner states in the southeast Asia are currently seeking after a fit way to deal with training, practice, research, documentation and control of TM (5); in Japan, 84% of Japanese doctors use Kampō (Japanese traditional medicine) in every day practice. In Switzerland, certain correlative treatments have been re-established into the essential medical coverage accessible to every Swiss subject.

Regardless of noteworthy advances, the control of TM items, practices and specialists is not happening at an equivalent pace. Partner states report that speedier advance is being made in the direction of herbal medicines, while T&CM practices and professionals are slacking. Of concern is that the well-being, quality and viability of T&CM administrations cannot be guaranteed if there is not proper control of practices and specialists. This circumstance exhibits a genuine test for some partner states, where an absence of information and experience exists with respect to the planning of national strategy, prompting frail or missing direction and an absence of legitimate joining of T&CM administrations into the well-being administration conveyance framework. It additionally mirrors the need of all partner states to push WHO to refresh its worldwide technique on TM. The WHO Traditional Medicine Strategy: 2014–2023, responds to the necessities and difficulties recognised by member states and expands on the work done under the WHO Traditional Medicine Strategy 2002–2005; the refreshed procedure for the period 2014–2023 dedicates more consideration than its forerunner to well-being administrations and frameworks, items, practices and specialists (Burton et al. 2015).

28.10 REGULATORY STATUS OF TRADITIONAL MEDICINE

Countries across the globe have different approaches towards the regulatory controls over herbal drugs. In the herbal drug sector, licensing, manufacturing and trading of products are not universal and some countries have well-laid policies to control them, whereas in a few countries the control is either very lax or non-existent. The main concern of authorities today is documentation of safety and efficacy of herbal drugs.

This is a major hindrance in the way of recognition of herbal products as medicines, as only a few plant species have been scientifically studied for their medicinal applications. Safety and efficacy data is available for an even smaller number of medicinal plants and their active ingredients (Mukherjee et al. 2017).

There exists a difference across the globe in the legal status of herbal medicines owing to the difference in legal frameworks. In some countries like India and China, plant-based medicines are recognised as established systems of medicine, whereas in some other countries like the United States and Canada, they are regarded as foods or supplements. It is mostly in the developing countries where herbal medicines are used in folklore but they do not have legislative procedures to include these remedies as drugs. Some of the factors that influence the classification of herbal drugs are inclusion of monographs in pharmacopoeias, claims of therapeutic effects, prescription status and period of use (Sharma 2012).

28.10.1 SOUTHEAST ASIA

28.10.1.1 India

The Drugs and Cosmetics Act (1940) and the Drug and Cosmetics Rules (1945) of India are the main regulatory law of Ayurveda, Unani and Siddha medicines. They are regulated by Schedule T of the rules, which establishes the Good Manufacturing Practices for Ayurvedic, Siddha, and Unani medicines. Poisonous substances are listed under Schedule E1. Any product containing detoxified toxic ingredient(s) needs to be taken under medical supervision. The Ayurvedic Pharmacopoeia of India (API), published by the Ministry of AYUSH, has monographs giving information regarding identity, purity, constitution, quality specifications, properties, actions, dosage, and so forth of drugs and their testing methods. API, part I has seven volumes providing 540 monographs on individual Ayurvedic herbs; API, part II has three volumes providing 152 monographs on Ayurvedic formulations. Ayurveda, Unani and Siddha are all recognised as established systems of medicine by the government of India. The Ministry of AYUSH regulates the practice of herbal system of medicine and homoeopathy through the Central Council of Indian Medicine and the Central Council of Homoeopathy. The Ayurveda, Siddha or Unani drugs include all medicines intended for internal (except injectable) or external use for, or in the diagnosis, treatment, mitigation or prevention of disease or disorder in human beings or animals (Patwardhan 2015).

Regulations of the Ministry of Health of the Government of India cover all the formulations manufactured according to the formulae and methods described in the textbooks included in first schedule; patent, or proprietary medicines including the formulations for health promotion; cosmetic formulations and medicinal extracts. Recently, the Ministry of AYUSH has made pilot clinical trials mandatory for proprietary medicines for licensing of Ayurveda, Siddha and Unani products in certain cases (Katoch et al. 2017).

28.10.1.2 Bangladesh

In Bangladesh, the Board of Unani and Ayurvedic Systems of Medicine, controls the standardisation of Unani and Ayurvedic medicines. Other functions controlled by the board are registration of traditional medicines, recognition of teaching of the International Regulatory Status of Herbal Drugs' 339 institutions, holding qualifying examinations and publication of textbooks, pharmacopoeias, and formularies. The National Formularies, one for Unani and the other for Ayurvedic drugs, published by the board are approved by the government. They are used as official guides for the manufacture of all recognised Unani and Ayurvedic medicinal preparations.

28.10.1.3 Indonesia

Traditional medicine regulates Indonesia's Health Law Act in the country. Articles 1, 2 and 3 of Indonesia's Health Law Act guide various aspects of the practice of traditional medicine. Article 1 places traditional medicine as an integral part of curative and nursing care. Article 2 emphasises the supervision of traditional medicine to ensure its safety and efficacy. Article 3 deals with further development and improvement of forms of traditional medicine.

The Health Law Act classifies traditional medicines into two groups: (1) those produced by individuals and (2) those produced and packaged on a commercial scale. In the former, the Ministry of Health permits the use of only 54 plants in these medicines. These plants are accepted as safe by virtue of their history of safe use in the country. The traditional medicines produced and packaged on a commercial scale require mandatory registration and a license to sell.

In order to be registered, traditional medicines not indigenous to Indonesia must have undergone scientific study to ensure their safety, efficacy, rationality of composition, dosage form and justification of claims. For use in formal healthcare, the medicines must have gone through structured clinical trials for scientific evaluation of their safety and efficacy in human subjects. The Ministry of Health of Indonesia has published Guidance for Clinical Trial of Traditional Drugs to guide the manufacturers. The National Agency for Drug & Food Control (NADFC) issues the registration number to foreign drugs that are registered that have undergone quality and safety evaluation.

28.10.1.4 Myanmar

Ayurveda is the traditional medicine of Myanmar where the production and sale of traditional medicines is regulated by the Traditional Medicine Drug Law to control the production and sale of traditional medicine drugs systematically. The registered and manufacturers must have licenses to produce their products following good manufacturing practice standards. The production of traditional medicines is controlled by the Department of Traditional Medicine according to the national formulary in two of its own facilities. Private organisations are engaged in the manufacture of traditional medicines. The Myanmar Traditional Medicine National Formulary contains 57 traditional medicine formulations; each monograph gives information on therapeutic uses, caution and dosage. These traditional medicines were standardised and evaluated for safety and efficacy between 1984 and 1989. The published monograph of 120 Myanmar medicinal plants provides basic information related to their use in primary healthcare.

28.10.1.5 Nepal

Nepal has a rich history of use of Ayurvedic herbal drugs in traditional medicine as an integral part of the national health system. The Institute of Medicine of Tribhuvan University supervises education in the Ayurvedic system. The Council of Ayurvedic Medicine regulates the practice of Ayurveda in Nepal. The Ministry of Health of Nepal has established a focal unit, the Ayurveda and Alternative Medicine Section, which section plays a vital role in coordination, providing direction and monitoring progress under the ministry. It is responsible for establishing the necessary policies, rules and regulations for all the systems of traditional medicine existing in the country.

28.10.1.6   Sri Lanka

The National Institute of Traditional Medicine, which is a government establishment, imparts educational courses in Ayurveda and traditional medicine. Ayurveda is widely practiced as a traditional system of medicine. Traditional medicine is an integral part of healthcare in Sri Lanka. There is an education and training institute that is under the Department of Ayurveda. The Institute of Indigenous Medicine, University of Colombo, offers postgraduate study courses. The Ministry of Indigenous Medicine regulates the registration of Ayurvedic practitioners. The Ayurvedic Medical Council Act advocates a code of ethics for Ayurvedic practitioners. Prior approval for the sale of Ayurvedic medicine products is required from the Ayurvedic Formulary Committee.

28.10.2   Eastern Mediterranean

28.10.2.1   Egypt

Herbal medicines are regulated as prescription medicines, over-the-counter medicines, self-medication and dietary supplements. The law permits medical, health and nutrient content claims on herbal medicines. The Egyptian pharmacopoeia (1972, 1980) is the national pharmacopoeia and contains monographs on herbal medicines. The safety of the herbal products is reviewed by the National Organization for Drug Control and Research (NODCAR). The manufacture of herbal medicines has to be as per GMP norms. There is a post marketing surveillance system and a national system to monitor adverse events for herbal medicines. Both registration and quality control of herbal drugs must be performed in the laboratories of NODCAR.

Herbal preparations and herbal products must be manufactured in a licensed medicine plant in compliance with the local and international GMP. They must be registered with the Central Administration of Medicine Affairs.

28.10.2.2   Iran

Traditional medicine and Islamic medicine are practiced in Iran through hokama who prepare, recommend and sell the medicines. The Shahid Beheshti University of Medical Sciences has done a lot of research on medicinal plants, but most of it has been preclinical. Although all the students of pharmacy must study pharmacognosy, in a few universities pharmacy students are required to do research related to a medicinal plant. Traditional medicine practitioners are neither supported nor banned by the government. The Food and Drug Control Agency has been working in the field of herbal medicines. In 1991, the National Academy of Traditional Medicine in Iran and Islam was established. Its area of activity involves research and preservation of traditional Iranian medicine. As per the recommendation of the academy, medical students should be trained in the field of Iranian traditional medicine. The Council Committee of Medicinal Herbs and Products regulates the safety and efficacy of herbs and herbal products and the packaging of herbal medicines.

28.10.2.3   Kuwait

In the year 1978, the Islamic Medicine Centre was established and the regulation of traditional medicine was started in Kuwait. The Islamic Medicine Centre also serves as a research institute in herbal medicine. In 1984, a national programme on traditional medicine was created, and in 1989, laws and regulations were laid down for the same. Kuwait began regulation of herbal medicine in 1989 with the introduction of a separate law on herbal medicines.

The laws in Kuwait prohibit traditional medicine providers from practicing medicine. However, herbal medicines are not banned. Herbal medicines are regulated as over-the-counter medicines, self-medication, dietary supplements, health foods, and functional foods. Medical and health claims may legally be made. A document and guidelines have been issued on the safety and quality assurance of herbal medicines.

28.10.2.4   Pakistan

Herbal medicine is practiced in Pakistan following the Ayurveda and Unani systems of medicine. There are institutions offering 4-year diploma courses in Pakistani traditional Unani and Ayurvedic systems of medicine that follow the prescribed curriculum and conditions set in the regulations. Unani Tibb and Ayurveda have been accepted and integrated into the national health system in Pakistan. The Unani, Ayurvedic and Homoeopathy Practitioners Act of 1965 regulates the qualifications and registration of practitioners of the systems.

28.10.2.5   Saudi Arabia

Traditional medicine in Saudi Arabia is based on herbal remedies and spiritual healing, and is widespread. Herbal, nutritional and health food products are very popular. Paragraph 13A of the special provisions on registration regulations for medicine companies and their products requires the registration of medicines and all products having medical claims, including herbal preparations containing active ingredients that possess medicinal effects. The License Committee under the Ministry of Health is responsible for approving the marketing and use of herbal products, health food products and natural health products, mainly based on their safety and efficacy.

28.10.2.6   United Arab Emirates

The Ministry of Health's Zayed Centre for Herbal Research and Traditional Medicine was established in Abu Dhabi to conduct research on medicinal plants. There is high consumer demand for herbal preparations and herbal products in the United Arab Emirates. Section 1 of Federal Law 7 of 1975 regulates the licensing and registration requirements for the practice of medicine. In order to provide a legal framework, registration criteria for herbal medicines were published in January 1998. Priority is given to single-ingredient products. Products containing more than one herb must have a rationale for the combinations beyond traditional uses and are not accepted unless scientifically validated as the therapeutic claims.

28.10.3   WESTERN PACIFIC

28.10.3.1   Australia

Australia has a history of usage of herbal medicine owing to the Chinese migration. Regulatory Status includes regulatory control over the sale of complementary medicine in Australia. The Australian Regulatory Guidelines for Complementary Medicines (ARGCM) provides guidance for the registration of complementary medicines to manufacturers or traders. The Therapeutic Goods Act (TGA) contains general provisions relating to all the therapeutic products to control this registration or cancellation of existing registrations of medicines.

The safety and efficacy of the raw material and finished product is a major determining factor for permitting the registration. The TGA maintains a list of substances that may be used as active ingredients in listed medicines in Australia. The active ingredients that can be included in complementary medicine are listed in Schedule 14. Medicines that are composed of only approved ingredients and make only general or medium-level indications are eligible to be entered in the Australian Register of Therapeutic Goods. Traditional herbal medicines have a special mention in complementary medicine and are defined as 'those therapeutic goods which are, or contain as the major active ingredient(s), herbal substances'. For registration purposes in Australia, the traditional herbal medicine should have an established and acknowledged use of an herbal preparation well-established efficacy, dosage, and usage established botanical identity of the herbal ingredient.

28.10.3.2 China

China has a long history of herbal medicine. Chinese *Materia Medica* has listed a large number of herbal drugs. There has been continuous support to the herbal system of medicine from the constitution resulting in the integration and simultaneous development of an herbal system of medicine. The Chinese pharmacopoeia has the listing of herbal drugs and the monographs provide information about identification, indications, and dosage. For marketing an herbal preparation, there is the requirement of a dossier having data on the quality, safety and efficacy. A new drug is given an approval number, and thereafter it is permitted to be placed in the market. The Drug Administration Law of the People's Republic of China regulates the drugs.

28.10.3.3 Fiji

Fiji has a history of practice of herbal medicine. In addition to traditional Fijian medicines, traditional herbal medicines from other countries like India and China are also marketed in Fiji. The Pharmacy and Poisons Act controls the import of herbal medicines into the country. If there is a therapeutic claim on the label of a product, the marketer has to provide the scientific evaluation data for the efficacy before it is permitted to be sold in the market. The national drug policy of Fiji encourages research in the area of herbal medicine; however, the safety and efficacy of the products are major areas of concern.

28.10.3.4 Japan

The per-capita consumption of herbal medicine in Japan is one of the highest in the world. The traditional medicine is known as Kampo medicine. New Kampo drugs are regulated in the same way as Western drugs in Japan. Chronic toxicity studies (including carcinogenicity, mutagenicity, and teratogenicity studies) and three-phase clinical studies are required depending upon the duration of usage and indications. There is a three-way pharmacovigilance system in Japan for collecting adverse drug reaction data.

28.10.4 AFRICA

28.10.4.1 South Africa

The traditional healers and herbal medicines are used by *significant* number of people However, non-regulated trade in the herbal medicines. However, health-related claims on any finished products have to go through the medicine evaluation procedure in the Medicine Control Council before marketing.

28.10.5 THE AMERICAS

28.10.5.1 United States

In the United States, complementary and alternative medicine is gradually gaining recognition however herbal drugs play a substantial part in alternative medicine. The Food and Drug Administration (FDA) regulates and controls access to treatments. Licensing, practice, and malpractice are regulated by state laws. Legal rules are made to safeguard consumers' interest. Any products that claim to treat, cure, mitigate, or prevent a disease are treated as a drug by the FDA. Thus, for claims on any herbal medicine to be allowed, the same procedures must be followed as for a chemical drug. For the standards of some herbal drugs, the US Pharmacopeia has given quality specifications of crude raw materials extracts and dosage forms of herbs. Although many herbal products are used by consumers as folk medicines, most natural products in the United States are regulated as foods, supplements, or food additives. The main concern of the regulatory authorities is safety of the consumers, and the sale of a product containing a herb that is categorised as generally recognised as safe (GRAS) is permitted. Natural products have GRAS status, so long as qualified experts confirm this and are not contradicted by other experts. Herbs that are commonly used in food or as food are permitted to be used in food products. The requirement of 'common use in food' is not restricted to herbs used in the United States alone, but applies also to herbs that are alien to the United States. Dietary Supplements law provides that a dietary supplement is considered to be a food that does not need premarket approval by the FDA and not as a food additive, which needs premarket approval from an authority. The FDA requires that randomised controlled trials should be done to evaluate the efficacy of an herbal product to market it as a drug or to give it medicinal claims. The trials should be conducted as per good clinical practice (GCP) to be accepted as valid scientific data by the FDA.

28.10.5.2   Argentina

In Argentina, herboristerias, pharmacies, and the medicine industry sell herbal drugs controlled by pharmacists. The people cultivating medicinal plants need permission from the Ministry of Health. Under the Drug Law, mixtures of vegetable drugs are controlled, together with preparations made by industry. A regulation for registration and commercialisation of medicinal plants by the Health Ministry of the Provincia de Buenos Aires has made the registration of medicinal herbs mandatory.

28.10.5.3   Canada

In Canada, private institutes, universities, and community colleges provides training programme on complementary and alternative medicine. But there is no universal accreditation and validation of these programmes. Health Canada, the regulatory body, has given legal status to natural health products and has defined a provision for registration of these products. The system ensures safe and quality natural products reaching the population and there is a recall provision in case of an adverse event being reported or a quality issue associated with a product. Natural health products are regulated by the Natural Health Products Regulations of the Food and Drugs Act.

28.10.5.4   Chile

The Unidad de Medicina Tradicional looks after the regulation for the control of the practice of alternative medicines in Chile. It was established for integrating traditional medicine with validated efficacy into health programmes. A registration for marketing authorisation is needed for herbal products. Natural products are acknowledged as medications suggested to cure, alleviate, or prevent diseases, food products for medicinal use and with therapeutic properties, food products for nutritional purposes. The pharmacies and drug stores require a special authorisation from the Ministry of Health.

28.10.5.5   European Union

Safety, efficacy, and lack of reliable information, and quality of some unlicensed herbal products is a growing concern around the globe. Although many unlicensed herbal medicines on the market are already manufactured under good manufacturing practice (GMP) standards, it is impossible for consumers to identify which products are made to acceptable standards. All of these concerns have caused the establishment of the European Union (EU) directive on traditional herbal medicinal products (THMPD). The directive requires each EU member state to set up its own traditional herbal registration scheme. A provision has thus been made to market herbal medicinal products as medicines, instead of foods or supplements through the THMPD. The THMPD is therefore the main regulatory approval process for traditional herbal medicines in the EU. If a medicine is registered under this directive, the manufacturers are permitted to make restricted medicinal claims on the label and the patient information leaflet.

For providing guidelines, European pharmacopoeia has given standards of certification in medicinal herbs. In addition, European Scientific Cooperative on Phytotherapy International Regulatory Status of Herbal Drugs 351 (ESCOP) monographs have been published on several medicinal herbs. Presently, the EU is developing community herbal monographs on medicinal herbs that are traditionally used to facilitate inclusion in THMPD.

REFERENCES

Achan, J., Talisuna, A.O., Erhart, A., Yeka, A., Tibenderana, J.K., Baliraine, F.N., Rosenthal, P.J. et al. (2011). Quinine, an old anti-malarial drug in a modern world: Role in the treatment of malaria. *Malaria Journal,* **10**, 144. doi:10.1186/1475-2875-10-144.

Burton, A., Smith, M. and Falkenberg, T. (2015). Building WHO's global strategy for traditional medicine. *European Journal of Integrative Medicine,* **7**(1), 13–15. doi:10.1016/j.eujim.2014.12.007.

Buss, A. D. and Waigh, R. D. (1995). Natural products as leads for new pharmaceuticals. In: M. E. Wolff, Ed., *Burger's Medicinal Chemistry and Drug Discovery, Principles and Practice,* 4th ed. New York: Wiley.

Cragg, G. M. and Newman, D. J. (2013). Natural products: A continuing source of novel drug leads. *Biochimia et Biophysica Acta,* **1830**(6), 3670–3695.

Debnath, P. K., Banerjee, S., Debnath, P., Mitra, A. and Mukherjee, P. K. (2015). Ayurveda: Opportunities for developing safe and effective treatment choices for the future. In: P. K. Mukherjee, Ed., *Evidence-Based Validation of Herbal Medicines.* Amsterdam, the Netherlands: Elsevier. pp. 427–454.

India. Ministry of Health and Family Welfare. (1983). *National health policy.* New Delhi, India: Ministry of Health and Family Welfare. Available from: http://www.mohfw.nic.in.

India. Ministry of Health and Family Welfare. (2002). *National health policy.* New Delhi, India: Ministry of Health and Family Welfare. Available from: http://www.mohfw.nic.in.

India. Ministry of Health and Family Welfare. (2011). *Report of the Working Group on AYUSH for 12th Give-Year Plan (2012–2017).* [Accessed 4 July 2016]. Available from: http://planningcommission.nic.in/aboutus/committee/wrkgrp12/health/WG_7_ayush.pdf.

India. Ministry of Health and Family Welfare. (2015). *Framework for Implementation of National AYUSH Mission (NAM).* New Delhi, India: Department of AYUSH, Ministry of Health and Family Welfare, Government of India. Available from: http://ayush.gov.in/sites/default/files/4197396897-Charakasamhita%20ACDP%20%20english_0.pdf.

Katoch, D., Sharma, J. S., Banerjee, S., Biswas, R. et al. (2017). Government policies and initiatives for development of Ayurveda. *Journal of Ethnopharmacology,* **197**, 25–31. doi:10.1016/j.jep.2016.08.018.

Leonti, M. and Casu, L. (2013). Traditional medicines and globalization: Current and future perspectives in ethnopharmacology. *Frontiers in Pharmacology,* **4**, 1–13.

Mukherjee, P. K. (2001). Evaluation of Indian traditional medicine. *Drug Information Journal,* **35**, 631–640.

Mukherjee P. K. 2002. *Quality Control of Herbal Drugs.* New Delhi, India: Business Horizons.

Mukherjee, P. K., Bahadur, S., Chaudhary, S. K., Kar, A. and Mukherjee, K. (2015a). Quality related safety issue-evidence-based validation of herbal medicine farm to pharma. In: P. K. Mukherjee, Ed., *Evidence Based Validation of Herbal Medicines.* Amsterdam, the Netherlands: Elsevier. pp. 1–28.

Mukherjee, P. K., Bahadur, S., Harwansh, R. K., Biswas, S. and Banerjee, S. (2017). Paradigm shift in natural product research: Traditional medicine inspired approaches. *Phytochemistry Reviews,* **16**(5), 803–826. doi:10.1007/s11101-016-9489-6.

Mukherjee, P. K., Bahadur, S., Harwansh, R. K. and Chaudhary, S. K. (2014). Shifting paradigm for validation of medicinal plants in Indian traditional medicine. *Indian Drugs,* **51**(8), 5–14.

Mukherjee, P.K., Chaudhary, S.K., Bahadur, S. and Debnath, P.K. (2015b). Ethnopharmacology and integrative medicine: An Indian perspective. In: M. Heinrich and A. K. Jäger, Eds. *Ethnopharmacology – A Reader.* Chichester, UK: John Wiley & Sons. pp. 277–292.

Mukherjee, P. K., Harwansh, K., Bahadur, R. Banerjee, S. and Kar, A. (2016). Evidence based validation of Indian traditional medicine: Way forward. *World Journal of Traditional Chinese Medicine,* **2**, 48–61.

Mukherjee, P. K., Harwansh, R. K., Bahadur, S., Banerjee, S., Kar, A., Chanda, J., Biswas, S., Ahmmed, S. M. and Katiyar, C. K. (2017). Development of Ayurveda tradition to trend. *Journal of Ethnopharmacology,* **197**, 10–24.

Mukherjee, P. K., Nema, N. K., Venkatesh, P. and Debnath, P.K. (2012). Changing scenario for promotion and development of Ayurveda: Way forward. *Journal of Ethnopharmacology,* **143**, 424–434.

Mukherjee, P. K., Venkatesh, M. and Gantait, A. (2010a). In comprehensive natural products II. In: L. Mander and H.W. Lui, eds., *Chemistry and Biology.* Oxford, UK: Elsevier. pp. 479–507.

Mukherjee, P. K., Venkatesh, P. and Ponnusankar, S. (2010b). Ethnopharmacology and integrative medicine: Let the history tell the future. *Journal of Ayurveda and Integrative Medicine,* **1**, 100.

Mukherjee, P. K. and Wahile, A. (2006). Integrated approaches towards drug development from Ayurveda and other Indian system of medicines. *Journal of Ethnopharmacology,* **103**, 25–35.

Ngo, L. T., Okogun, J. I. and Folk, W. R. (2014). 21st century natural product research and drug development and traditional medicines. *Natural Product Reports,* **30**, 584–592.

Patwardhan, B. (2015). Public perception of AYUSH. *Journal of Ayurveda and Integrative Medicine,* **6**, 147–149.

Samal, J. (2015). Role of AYUSH workforce, therapeutics, and principles in health care delivery with special reference to National Rural Health Mission. *Ayush,* **36**, 5–9.

Sharma, S. (2012). International regulatory status of herbal drugs. In: C.P. Khare and C.K. Katiyar, Eds., *The Modern Ayurveda.* Boca Raton, FL: CRC Press. pp. 337–345.

Shaw, D., Graeme, L., Pierre, D., Elizabeth, W. and Kelvin C. (2012). Pharmacovigilance of herbal medicine. *Journal of Ethnopharmacology,* **140**(3), 513–518. doi:10.1016/j.jep.2012.01.051.

Shrivastava, S. R., Shrivastava, P. S. and Ramasamy, J. (2015). Mainstreaming of Ayurveda, Yoga, Naturopathy, Unani, Siddha, and Homeopathy with the health care delivery system in India. *Journal of Traditional and Complementary Medicine,* **5**, 116–118.

Singh, R. H. (2010). Exploring larger evidence-base for contemporary Ayurveda. *International Journal of Ayurveda Research,* **1**(2), 65–66.

World Health Organization (WHO). (2013). *WHO Traditional Medicine Strategy 2014–2023: World Health Systems Should Be Explored.* Geneva, Switzerland: World Health Organization. pp. 15–56.

29 Cannabis and Cannabinoids
A Journey from an Ancient Belief to the Fore

Dilip Ghosh

CONTENTS

29.1 INTRODUCTION

The Cannabis plant, which may be of different species (principally *Cannabis sativa* and *Cannabis indica*) or variants of the same species, is a dioecious entity that contains a number of unique resorcinol metabolites (van Bakel et al. 2011), although the estimated number may vary from 60–110. The most recognisable cannabinoid metabolite is Δ9-tetrahydrocannabinol (THC). Recent published data described the pharmacology of two of these agents, cannabidiol (CBD) and Δ9-tetrahydrocannabivarin (THCV) and concluded that these compounds exhibited complex interactions with the human endocannabinoid system. Apart from these three compounds, other cannabinoids showing pharmacological affects include cannabigerol, cannabidivarin, cannabidiolic acid and cannabichromene.

Cannabis is perhaps one of the oldest plants cultivated for human use. Archaeological evidence suggests that it was grown for use as fibre and rope as early as 12,000 BCE in central Asia (Schultes 1973) and in many parts of China (Booth 2005). The use of cannabis for the treatment of human disease first appeared in Chinese pharmacopoeia from the second century BCE, and the Emperor Shen Nung is recognised as the father of Chinese medicine for his systematic exploration of herbal remedies, particularly cannabis (Aldrich and Mathre 1997). The use of a medicinal plant that is most likely cannabis for a host of ailments including nocturnal convulsions around 1800 BCE is also found in the Middle East, in Ancient Sumerian and Akkadian references (Russo 2007). Ancient Egyptian papyri also described its use for numerous afflictions including infections, analgesia and vaginal contractions from approximately this same time period (Russo 2007). Around 1500 BCE, Vedic texts from India documented the anxiolytic effects of cannabis (Russo 2014). By the first and second century CE, cannabis is noted in medical texts of civilisations throughout Asia and North Africa for many different ailments. Specific mentions of the treatment of epilepsy are found in the eleventh century writings of the Arabic physician al-Majusi who advocated the use of extracts of cannabis through the nose (Lozano 2001).

Since the exploration in the ancient world, there have been wide variations in the use and acceptance of cannabis as a drug therapy in Western medicine. In 1999, California was the only state that allowed patients to access cannabis for medicinal purposes. By 2016, there were 24 states where cannabis was available as a therapeutic agent and three that had approved cannabis for recreational use. The National Academies of Sciences, Engineering and Medicine (NASEM) in collaboration with many federal, state and independent agencies such as the US Centers for Disease Control and Prevention, the Food and Drug Administration, the National Institute on Drug Abuse, the National Cancer Institute and the National Highway Traffic Safety Administration are working on for updating the 1999 report (NASEM 2017).

29.2 CANNABIS PLANT

Cannabis is one of the most complicated challenging plants to taxonomists and arboriculturists. Cannabis is predominantly dioecious, with male and female flowers, which means flowers develop on separate plants if grown naturally from seed. However, occasionally it exhibits a monoecious (hermaphrodite) nature. Cannabis is normally a so-called 'short-day plant'. At the end of summer, when the plant detected increase in night length, they commence flowering. After decades of research, scientists were able to develop 'auto flowering' cannabis plants that instead of being day-length sensitive, start commencing flowering when only approximately 2 weeks old. For the production of cannabinoids, all-female crops are preferred, because male plants produce much lower quantities of cannabinoids. The cannabinoids are predominantly, if not entirely, synthesised and sequestered in small structures called glandular trichomes and these appear in the female flower.

29.3 TERMINOLOGY AND PRODUCTS

Raw herbal (botanical) cannabis – Any part of any plant of the genus Cannabis. The genus Cannabis belongs to the Cannabaceae family. Some people believe cannabis is a single species with *C. indica*, *C. sativa* and *C. ruderalis* as three different subspecies and some describe them as three different species of cannabis.

Hemp – Plants grown for fibre and seed are commonly referred to as hemp.

Cannabis extract – Any extract, usually by organic solvents to produce oil, which is extracted from the plant, and any preparation consisting mainly of it.

Cannabinoids – A class of chemical compounds that have the typical cannabinoid skeleton in common and affect the cannabinoid receptors. Other than naturally occurring cannabinoids, a few synthetic cannabinoids are manufactured today as approved drugs or cannabinoid-based medicines.

29.4 USES OF CANNABIS

29.4.1 COMMON USAGE

The hemp plant has also been used across the globe for centuries in the production of rope, sail, cloth and paper (for a review, see Russo 2007). There is strong anecdotal evidence of medicinal use of hemp from ancient China, India and Egypt for centuries. The term 'cannabis abuse' is a relatively recent used phrase. In the 1970s, cannabis extract was widespread available in Europe and North America as a 'recreational drug'. The leaves (variously referred to as marijuana or herbal cannabis, among other names) or resin derived mostly from the buds (known as hashish, among other names) is typically mixed with tobacco and rolled into a cigarette (known as a joint, among other names). Smoking involves measures of volatilisation and pyrolysis, and results in a relatively poor delivery of metabolites. Please refer to Table 29.1 for better understanding of different administration routes with health effects.

29.4.2 THERAPEUTIC/MEDICINAL USE

Currently, there are only three cannabinoid-based medicines available for marketing in different countries: *nabiximols* (Sativex®), which is an oromucosal spray formulated from extracts of the

TABLE 29.1
Cannabis Route of Administration

Smoking	Vaporisation	Oral	Other Routes
• Most common route	• Heats cannabis at 160°C–230°C, reducing some toxicity	• Oils, capsules and other PO routes	• Topical cream
• Combustion at 600°C 900°C producing toxic by-products, such as tar, PAH, CO, NH_3	• Decreased pulmonary symptoms compared to smoking	• Edibles (brownies, cookies) but difficult to dose	• Suppositories for special medical purpose
• Chronic use associated with respiratory symptoms but not lung cancer and COPD		• Juicing and tea are feasible but problem of decarboxylation	• Recreational routes include 'shatter', 'dads', concentrates
• 30%–50% of cannabis is lost to 'side-stream' smoke		• Oromucosal spray (Nabiximols) with 1:1 ration of THC/CBD dosing	
		• Tinctures and lozenges are candidates	

Source: MacCallum, C.A. and Russo, E.B., *Eur. J. Inter. Med.*, 49, 2018.

C. sativa plant that contains the cannabinoids THC and CBD; *nabilone* (Cesamet® or Canemes®) in oral capsules containing a synthetic cannabinoid similar to THC; and *dronabinol* (Marinol® or Syndros), taken via oral capsules or an oral solution containing synthetic Δ9-THC.

29.4.3 Nutraceutical/Lifestyle/Cosmetics/Skin Care Use

The market for more peripheral cannabis products such as cosmetics, food supplements, edible, oil and smoking recreational drug use and to provide fibre and biofuel may become a more immediate market than as a medicinal drug, given the shorter path to market (see Table 29.1). Functional beverages containing cannabis are one of the best delivery mechanisms. Plantine Holdings Limited, Gibraltar, is one of the leading manufacturers of water-soluble hemp products. Donny Christian Mistarz, CSO, and co-founder of Plantine has said that 'we can in this way produce a fully neutral and water-soluble product with increased bioavailability, giving the formulators back the full control over the taste experience of their final products' (Vitafoods Europe 2018). Plantine is a large vertically integrated producer, manufacturer and distributor of hemp products. There are a few other producers of cannabis-based consumer products around the world.

29.5 CHEMISTRY OF CANNABIS

Cannabis contains many unique resorcinol metabolites, but the exact number is still debatable. The best estimate is around 60–110. The most recognisable cannabinoid is Δ9-tetrahydrocannabinol (THC). Many recent studies have identified and described the pharmacology of three of these agents, cannabidiol (CBD), Δ9-tetrahydrocannabivarin (THCV), cannabigerol (CBG) and concluded that these compounds exhibited complex interactions with the endocannabinoid system (Mechoulam et al. 2014; McPartland et al. 2015).

In fresh plant material, these cannabinoids all exist in the cannabinoid acid forms, such as Δ9-tetrahydrocannabinolic acid (THCA) and cannabidiolic acid (CBDA). As the plant material ages or is heated, the acid molecules lose carboxyl moiety. Decarboxylation results in the conversion of the cannabinoid acids into their neutral forms (e.g. CBDA→CBD).

29.6 HOW THEY WORK IN THE HUMAN BODY?

The major cannabinoids have multiple targets within the central nervous system (CNS) and can modulate activity of neurons, glia and microglia, but it is still not absolute clear which mechanism(s) are critical for therapeutic actions. It has long been known that Δ9-THC has partial agonist activity at the endocannabinoid receptors CB1 and CB2, although it also binds to other targets that may modulate neuronal excitability and neuroinflammation (Mitchell 1995). The actions of Δ9-THCV and Δ9-THCA are less well understood. In contrast to Δ9-THC, CBD has low affinity for CB1 and CB2 receptors, but their anticonvulsant property is linked to regulation of voltage-gated potassium and sodium channels and GPR55. There are selective agonists and antagonists available that are able to define pharmacologically the involvement of CB1 or CB2 cannabinoid receptors. HU210, WIN55212-2 and CP55940 are all high potency (nanomolar) agonists at both CB1 and CB2 cannabinoid receptors (Felder et al. 1995).

29.7 ADVERSE EFFECTS AND DRUG INTERACTIONS

Cannabis has a superior safety profile in comparison to many other medications, with no reported deaths due to overdose. This may be due to a lack of CB1 receptors in brain stem cardiorespiratory centres (Herkenham et al. 1990). THC-mediated side effects are most pertinent and rate limiting and are dose-dependent. Using a 'start low and go slow' dosing strategy mitigates most adverse

---

TABLE 29.2

Adverse Events Associated with Cannabis-Based Medicines

Side Effects	Most Common	Common	Rare
Drowsiness/fatigue/dizziness	√		
Dry mouth	√		
Anxiety	√		
Nausea	√		
Cognitive effects	√		
Euphoria		√	
Blurred vision		√	
Headache		√	
Toxic psychosis			√
Depression			√
Ataxia/lack of coordination			√
Diarrhoea			√

Source: MacCallum, C.A. and Russo, E.B., *Eur. J. Inter. Med.*, 49, 2018.

---

events of THC. Also, combining CBD with THC can further reduce those effects. A recent large review of herbal cannabis in Canada revealed no increase in serious adverse events in chronic administration, no harm on cognitive function, pulmonary function tests, biochemistry such as creatinine, liver function test and CBC (Ware et al. 2015), confirming patterns seen in decades-long usage in the United States (Russo et al. 2002). Common adverse events are listed in Table 29.2.

Most drug interactions are associated with concurrent use of other CNS depressants with cannabis. Clinically, significant drug interactions have proven rare (Russo 2016). Existing studies have not demonstrated toxicity or loss of effect of concomitant medications, but pertinent drug interaction studies are few.

29.8 THE SCIENCE BEHIND THE EFFICACY OF CANNABIS

The use of cannabis and cannabinoids for medical conditions has become more popularised in recent years around the world. There is growing evidence that cannabis and cannabinoids are efficacious for several health conditions, such as chronic pain, spasticity, nausea and vomiting associated with chemotherapy (Goldenberg et al. 2017). However, effect sizes are typically small, the quality of evidence is moderate to low, and there is no conclusive evidence for which either cannabis or cannabinoids have been recommended as first line therapeutic agents (Table 29.3).

The largest 2015 meta-analysis (Whiting et al. 2015) revealed moderate quality proofs in favour of nabiximols, nabilone, dronabinol or THC/CBD in treating spasticity from multiple sclerosis. The same level of proof was shown for nabiximols or smoked THC in the treatment of chronic cancer pain and neuropathic pain. Very recently, Abrams (2018) published a comprehensive report on the therapeutic effects of cannabis and cannabinoids from the report published by NASEM. Most of the quality studies involved trials of isolated cannabinoids, most frequently pharmaceutical preparations of THC and, less frequently, CBD. An oromucosal whole plant extract, nabiximols, is also increasingly being investigated and generating published results. Quality data on inhaled cannabis are rare and there were no published reports found that used any of the increasingly available oral edibles, tinctures and oils that US patients currently have access to in dispensaries across the nation.

TABLE 29.3

Health Benefits from Cannabis and Cannabinoids

Health Area	Conclusion	Level of Evidence
Chronic pain is one of the most often cited reasons that patients are accessing medicinal cannabis where it is available	There are five fair-to-good quality systematic reviews that contributed to the conclusion that there is substantial evidence that cannabis is an effective treatment for chronic pain in adults.	Convincing evidence
Chemotherapy-induced nausea and vomiting	From 23 trials it was concluded that cannabinoids were highly effective, being more efficacious than the placebo and similar to conventional anti-emetics in treating chemotherapy-induced nausea and vomiting.	Convincing evidence
Spasticity associated with multiple sclerosis	Pooled clinical data concluded that there is substantial evidence that oral cannabinoids are effective for improving patient-reported multiple sclerosis spasticity symptoms.	Convincing evidence
Sleep disturbance	Many clinical trials, systematic review meta-analysis revealed greater improvement in sleep quality and sleep disturbance, but the improvements were deemed to be small.	Moderate evidence
Post-traumatic stress disorder	There are frequent anecdotal reports of remarkable success, but not many clinical trials support this claim.	Moderate evidence
Anxiety	One good study demonstrated that cannabidiol was associated with a significantly greater improvement in the anxiety factor of a 100-point visual analogue mood scale compared to placebo.	Moderate evidence
Cancer	There is only one published clinical trial in the anticancer area. The bulk of the substantial literature is preclinical and heavily focused on the effect of cannabinoids on gliomas.	Insufficient evidence
Epilepsy	Two systematic reviews assessing the effect of cannabinoids or Cannabis for reducing seizures in patients with epilepsy and no pre-specified endpoint of freedom from seizures.	Insufficient evidence

Source: Abrams, D.I., *Eur. J. Intern. Med.*, 49, 7–11, 2018.

29.8.1 CONVINCING EFFICACY

29.8.1.1 Chronic Pain

Chronic pain is one of the most often cited reasons that patients are accessing medicinal cannabis in states where it is available (Sexton et al. 2016). There were five fair-to-good quality systematic reviews that have contributed to the conclusion that there is substantial evidence that cannabis is an effective treatment for chronic pain in adults. The comprehensive review by Whiting et al. published in 2015 provided the basis for many of the conclusions reached in the NASEM report and included 28 randomised controlled trials in patients with chronic pain involving 2454 patients.

29.8.1.2 Chemotherapy-Induced Nausea and Vomiting

Several reports, including Whiting et al. (2015) and Cochrane reviews, concluded that all trials suggested a greater benefit for cannabinoids and their being more efficacious than the placebo and similar to conventional anti-emetics in treating chemotherapy-induced nausea and vomiting. The Δ9-THC pharmaceutical agents, dronabinol and nabilone, were both initially approved in 1985 for use in treating nausea and vomiting associated with cytotoxic chemotherapy. The American Society for Clinical Oncology Expert Panel on Anti-emetics recently issued updated guidelines and recommended 'FDA-approved cannabinoids dronabinol or nabilone to treat nausea and vomiting that is resistant to standard antiemetic therapies. Evidence remains insufficient to recommend marijuana in this setting' (Hesketh et al. 2017).

29.8.1.3   Spasticity Associated with Multiple Sclerosis

In 2010 nabiximols was first approved in the United Kingdom for the treatment of spasticity associated with multiple sclerosis (Tanasescu et al. 2011). In a pooled analysis of three trials investigating nabiximols or nabilone, Whiting et al. (2015) found that the cannabinoids decreased the patient self-reported spasticity score and improvement of a global impression of change score also favoured nabiximols over placebo. In the previous year, Koppel et al. (2014) also concluded that nabiximols and oral THC were 'probably effective' and oral cannabis extract was 'established as effective' in reducing patient reported spasticity scores. Considering these two favourable systematic reviews, the NASEM report concluded that there is substantial evidence that oral cannabinoids are effective for improving patient reported multiple sclerosis spasticity symptoms.

29.8.2   Moderate Efficacy

29.8.2.1   Sleep Disturbance

It has been hypothesised that the endocannabinoid system may have a role in sleep and it has been recognised that cannabis may have effects on sleep latency. A 22-patient study with a high risk of bias found that dronabinol was better than placebo in patients with obstructive sleep apnoea. A crossover trial in 32 patients with fibromyalgia comparing nabilone to amitriptyline reported that nabilone was more effective in treating insomnia and producing greater sleep restfulness (Whiting et al. 2017). The conclusion was that there is moderate evidence that cannabinoids, predominantly nabiximols, are effective in improving the short-term sleep outcomes in individuals with sleep disturbances associated with obstructive sleep apnoea, fibromyalgia, chronic pain and multiple sclerosis.

29.8.3   Limited Efficacy

29.8.3.1   Anxiety

Another condition for which many have been using cannabis is anxiety. The Whiting review included one 24-participant trial of cannabidiol in individuals with social anxiety disorder. No other studies were identified addressing the condition leading to the conclusion of limited evidence.

29.9   PROMISING TARGET: EPILEPSY

Another area of high promise for cannabinoid-related medicines is epilepsy (Alexander 2017; Gaston and Friedman 2017). Cannabis has been associated with the treatment of epilepsy throughout history. A tradition of usage continued in Arabic medicine and Ayurvedic practice in India, which led, in turn, to early experiments in Europe and North America with 'Indian hemp'. In several US states, cannabis is approved for use as an anti-epilepsy therapy. A recent meta-analysis of published data suggested that there were not many high-quality data available at the time of review on clinical efficacy, in particular of cannabidiol, although there appeared to be an absence of adverse effects (Gloss and Vickrey 2014). The future for cannabinoid-related medicines in epilepsy indication is very promising in the absence of effective medications to treat intractable forms of epilepsy, together with anecdotal evidence of the efficacy of cannabidiol in these patients (Devinsky et al. 2014). Multiple ongoing randomised, adequately powered, controlled trials of specific cannabinoids (e.g. NCT02224560, NCT02224690, NCT02318537, NCT02091375, NCT02369471), once completed, could hopefully provide the highest levels of evidence regarding the antiseizure effects of cannabis constituents and determine if they will benefit the one-third of people with epilepsy who cannot get adequate seizure control with currently available treatments (Friedman and Sirven 2017).

29.10   EPIGENETIC EFFECT OF CANNABIS USE

The reduced risk perception associated with marijuana (*C. sativa*, *C. indica*), as well as the sudden outburst of the cannabis industry around recreational and medical usage, has led to its increased popularity and use, particularly among young people. It is the first time in the United States' history that adolescents smoke marijuana more than cigarettes, an increasing tendency since 2010. The relationship between cannabis use and neuropsychiatric vulnerability is clearly complex. Based on the theoretical assumption, there is a possibility of epigenetic memory mark due to early exposure during one's lifetime. It will be important to investigate how different cannabinoids or other components of the cannabis plant and even their interactions (e.g. THC and CBD) influence behavioural, physiological and epigenetic effects in long-term users (Szutorisza and Hurd 2018). Overall, expanding technological advancement and strong genomic knowledge about the protracted neurobiological signature marker of epigenetic memory associated with marijuana and various cannabinoids will identify novel targets to develop preventive strategies and treatments for neuropsychiatric risks.

29.11   CANNABIS CULTIVATION AND MEDICAL-GRADE PRODUCTS

Generally, plant-based drugs represent unusual challenges in the pharmaceutical world with respect to large-scale cultivation, processing, quality, consistency and standardisation. Additionally, considerable complexity derives from regulatory perspectives, depending on the countries of production and marketing. The major complexity and challenges of working with cannabis or interpreting data obtained from human studies using the plant or its extracts is its quality and authenticity. A considerable amount of variability in genetic background, growth conditions, harvesting times, preparation handling and so on has been identified. The alleles purported to control THC or CBD synthesis are codominant. As a result, landrace populations consist of homozygous plants dominant in THC or CBD (and referred to as being of the THC or CBD chemotype) alongside heterozygous 'mixed chemotype' individuals synthesising a more even balance of both THC and CBD (Chandra et al. 2017).

In recent years, the production of CBD-based medicinal materials for research has come into greater focus because of its potential therapeutic opportunities in childhood epilepsy syndromes and other disorders. Many companies optimised methods for growing cannabis chemotypes indoors in a tightly controlled growing environment. All female cannabis crops with high-CBD have also been grown outdoors. When the plant ages, the amount of cannabinoid has been found to generally increase, reaching the highest level at the budding stage and achieving a plateau before the onset of senescence. Because the whole plant does not mature at the same time, mature upper buds are harvested first (visual confirmation) and other branches are given more time to achieve maturity. Table 29.4 describes the essential steps of selection and propagation of high-quality plant material (adapted from Chandra et al. 2017).

CBD is the main cannabinoid found in hemp floral tissue. The concentration of CBD in the dry floral tissue would typically be 2% weight for weight (w/w) or less. One (ECs315) of the leading extracts from Swiss company Linnea's CM5 (5% CBD) from cloned plant (chemotype) using a patented extraction process. Cannabis grown for recreational use, however, is dominated by the presence of THC. The THC content of floral tissue in modern varieties typically exceeds 20% w/w. Because of the extensive breeding programme at GW Pharmaceuticals, USA, the materials used to produce CBD for Epidiolex® contain a similar cannabinoid concentration to the most potent THC varieties, with floral material typically containing over 20% CBD.

TABLE 29.4

Essential Steps of Selection and Propagation of High-Quality Cannabis Plant Material

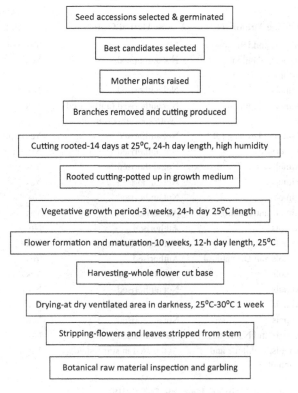

Seed accessions selected & germinated

Best candidates selected

Mother plants raised

Branches removed and cutting produced

Cutting rooted-14 days at 25°C, 24-h day length, high humidity

Rooted cutting-potted up in growth medium

Vegetative growth period-3 weeks, 24-h day 25°C length

Flower formation and maturation-10 weeks, 12-h day length, 25°C

Harvesting-whole flower cut base

Drying-at dry ventilated area in darkness, 25°C-30°C 1 week

Stripping-flowers and leaves stripped from stem

Botanical raw material inspection and garbling

Source: Chandra, S. et al., *Epilepsy Behav.*, 70, 302–312, 2017.

29.12 REGULATORY AND LEGAL STATUS IN RECENT YEARS

In 1937, the United States criminalised the use of cannabis and as a result its consumption decreased rapidly. In recent decades, there has been growing interest in the wide range of medical uses of cannabis and its constituents; however, the laws and regulations are substantially different between countries (Table 29.5). Laws differentiate between raw herbal cannabis, cannabis extracts and cannabinoid-based medicines. Both the European Medicines Agency (EMA) and the US Food and Drug Administration (FDA) do not approve the use of herbal cannabis or its extracts. The FDA approved several cannabinoid-based medicines, as did 23 European countries, Australia and Canada. In Australia, cannabis possession and use are currently illegal, but in several states and territories (South Australia, ACT and Northern Territory) a small amount for personal use is decriminalised. That means that it is illegal, but not a criminal offence. Very recently, the Canadian Senate voted to legalise recreational marijuana.

However, only four of the reviewed countries have fully authorised the medical use of herbal cannabis – Canada, Germany, Israel and the Netherlands, together with more than 50% of the states in the United States. Most of the regulators allow the physicians to decide what specific indications they will prescribe cannabis for, but some regulators dictate only specific indications.

TABLE 29.5

Regulatory Status of Cannabis Use Country-Wise

Country	Medicine Authorised	Raw Herbal Cannabis	Magistral Preparation (Patient-Specific) Authorised
Australia	Nabiximols and Dronabinol	No	Yes, with restrictions
Austria	Nabiximols, Nabilone and Dronabinol	Not authorised	Yes
Belgium	Nabiximols	Not authorised	No
Canada	Nabiximols, Nabilone	Not authorised (authorised with special permission)	Yes
Croatia	Nabilone and Dronabinol	Not authorised	Yes (drugs containing THC)
Cyprus	Not authorised	Not authorised	No. Oil approved on a named basis
Czech Republic	Nabiximols	Not authorised	Yes
Denmark	Nabiximols	Not authorised	Yes
France	Nabiximols	Not authorised	No
Germany	Nabiximols and Nabilone	Authorised	Yes
Israel	Nabiximols	Authorised	No
Italy	Nabiximols	Not authorised	Yes
The Netherlands	Nabiximols and Dronabinol	Authorised	Yes
Norway	Nabiximols	Not authorised	Yes
Spain	Nabiximols	Not authorised	No
Sweden	Nabiximols	Not authorised	No
Switzerland	Nabiximols	Not authorised	Yes
United Kingdom	Nabiximols and Nabilone	Not authorised	No
USA	Nabiximols, Nabilone and Dronabinol	Authorised in some states	Yes

Source: Abuhasira, R. et al., *Eur. J. Inter. Med.*, 49, 2–6, 2018.

29.13 MARKET SIZE POTENTIAL/ESTIMATES

The gradual legalisation of cannabis has led to an amazing flurry of activity – much of it on share markets including Canada and Australia – as companies move to address the huge markets for cannabis products.

In the United States, cannabis is not legal at a federal level but it is legal in many states. As a result, sales grew by a staggering 30% in 2016 to reach US$6.7 billion. There have been realistic estimates that US cannabis sales will reach US$20.2 billion by 2021 and even a staggering US$50 billion by 2026. The combined world consumption is estimated to be as high as $500 billion by 2029. Big companies outside their core business are getting involved, as for example, Constellation Brands – the parent company behind Corona, Modelo, Svedka and many other alcoholic drinks – recently bought a 9.9% stake in leading Canadian cannabis company Canopy Growth for US$191 million and plans to experiment with cannabis infused drinks. The Gibraltar-based company, Plantine Holdings Limited, had recently introduced a fully neutral and water-soluble hemp powder with increased bioavailability for functional beverage formulations. It is not hard to envisage several blockbuster cannabis-based drugs reaching massive global sales in markets such as pain, nausea, appetite and convulsion or muscle spasm reduction. For example, the Australian cannabis company AusCann is researching a drug to treat chronic and neuropathic pain – a market that is greater than $5 billion a year in Australia alone. Blackmores, one of the Australian complementary and vitamin manufacturers, is likely to move into the medical cannabis sector and in the third week of November they confirmed that the company is to 'partner with the leaders in the research and cultivation of medicinal cannabis', the likely outcome being commercial agreements to manufacture and sell cannabis-related products that could be popular with consumers. More specifically, the company plans to 'seek authorisation to launch medical cannabis products through general practitioners and medical specialists' via its fast-growing Bioceuticals alternative and herbal therapies healthcare business.

29.14   CANNABIS IS GOING MAINSTREAM

A few months ago, Canada took a key step towards legalising recreational marijuana after senators voted in favour of new legislation permitting nationwide use of the drug. Canada is not the first nation to consider making recreational cannabis legal. Uruguay, in 2014, became the first country to legalise the sale and distribution of cannabis. In 2012, Washington State and Colorado were just two US states that have legalised the recreational use of cannabis. Many industrialised countries are also considering making cannabis legal for recreational purposes. In more than 11 European countries, including the Netherlands, Belgium and Spain, cannabis is legalised for medicinal use or is decriminalised. Australia joined the list of countries where medicinal cannabis became legal in 2016. As cannabis-based medicines return to mainstream use, it is essential that clinicians gain a greater understanding of their pharmacology, dosing and administration to maximise therapeutic potential and minimise associated problems.

29.15   CANNABIS: DARLING OF THE STOCK MARKET

In the last few years more than 30 companies dealing with cannabis have been listed in the Australian stock exchange; a few major players are:

AusCann (ASX: AC8) is fully licenced for growing and researching medicinal cannabis and has a strong relationship with Canada's largest player, Canopy Growth, which holds AusCann shares.

Bod Australia (ASX: BDA) is working with the Swiss herbal extract company Linnea to extract a full spectrum of compounds (ECs315) from cannabis plants, which it thinks will be more effective and reliable in treating patients than current extraction methods.

Cann Group (ASX: CAN) was the first company in Australia to secure its necessary licences and permits to cultivate and research cannabis for human medicinal purposes and was subsequently Australia's first company to harvest a medicinal cannabis crop.

Creso Pharma (ASX: CPH) has strong exposure to medicinal cannabis markets in Australia, Latin America, Canada and China. Creso also plans to access Canada's edible and recreational cannabis demand, with its growing facility in the country due for completion mid-year.

Medlab Clinical (ASX: MDC) has created the world's most advanced CBD and THC-based drug, NanaBis, for treating cancer patients with intractable pain.

MMJ Phytotech (ASX: MMJ), through acquisition of Weed Me, has become a licenced cannabis producer by developing unique lower cost cultivation techniques.

Zelda Therapeutics (ASX: ZLD) is developing a range of cannabinoid-based formulations to treat medical conditions with perhaps the most exciting an observation autism trial in Chile.

29.16   THE WAY FORWARD

Cannabis is the most widely used illicit drug in the developed world and its use has long been associated with negative social and economic outcomes. It is estimated that more than 170 million people worldwide consume cannabis daily in different forms (Ghosh 2018).

The unique challenges scientific and business communities are experiencing for using cannabinoids as therapeutic agents include low bioavailability and potentially erratic absorption in oral formulations, significant accumulation in adipose and other tissues, and interactions with other drugs metabolised by the cytochrome P450 system. Some of these problems may be overcome by advance novel delivery systems (oromucosal, transdermal) or through synthesis of related compounds with optimised properties.

Clinicians are still in the dark as to how to advise patients pursuing such treatment because of legal prohibition, biochemical complexity and variability, quality control issues, lack of appropriately powered randomised controlled trials and pertinent education.

We stand at an interesting crossroads for cannabis-related drugs from both scientific and political perspectives. At the current moment, there is strong consumer hype in translating the promise of the drug, particularly for multiple sclerosis and epilepsy, but there is still not convincing evidence to support these claims. We all agree that 'the absence of evidence is not necessarily indicative of evidence of the absence of effectiveness'. Investigators must take on these challenges and undertake further additional trials so that clinicians can be informed on how to best use this versatile medicine in future practice.

REFERENCES

Abuhasira, R., Shbiro, L. and Landschaft, Y. (2018). Medical use of cannabis and cannabinoids containing products – Regulations in Europe and North America. *European Journal of Internal Medicine*, **49**, 2–6.

Abrams, D. I. (2018). The therapeutic effects of Cannabis and cannabinoids: An update from the National Academies of Sciences, Engineering and Medicine report. *European Journal of Internal Medicine*, **49**, 7–11.

Aldrich, M. and Mathre, M. L. (1997). History of therapeutic cannabis. In: M. L. Mathre, Ed. *Cannabis in Medical Practice*. Jefferson, NC: McFarland & Co. pp. 35–55.

Alexander, S. (2017). Therapeutic potential of cannabis-related drugs. *Progress in Neuro-Psychopharmacology & Biological Psychiatry*, **64**, 157–166.

Booth, M. (2005). *Cannabis: A History*. 1st ed. New York: Picador.

Chandra, S., Lata, H., El-Sohly M. A., et al. (2017). Cannabis cultivation: Methodological issues for obtaining medical-grade product. *Epilepsy Behavior*, **70**, 302–312.

Devinsky, O., Cilio, M. R., Cross, H., et al. (2014). Cannabidiol: Pharmacology and potential therapeutic role in epilepsy and other neuropsychiatric disorders. *Epilepsia*, **55**, 791–802.

Felder, C. C., Joyce, K. E., Briley, E. M., et al. (1995). Comparison of the pharmacology and signal transduction of the human cannabinoid CB1 and CB2 receptors. *Molecular Pharmacology*, **48**, 443–450.

Friedman, D. and Sirven, J. I. (2017). Historical perspective on the medical use of cannabis for epilepsy: Ancient times to the 1980s. *Epilepsy Behavior*, **70**, 298–301.

Gaston, T. E. and Friedman, D. (2017). Pharmacology of cannabinoids in the treatment of epilepsy. *Epilepsy Behavior*, **70**, 313–318.

Ghosh, D. (2018). The science of cannabis & cannabinoids. *Nutraceuticals World*, 54–57.

Gloss, D. and Vickrey, B. (2014). Cannabinoids for epilepsy. *Cochrane Database of Systemic Reviews*, **3**, CD009270.

Goldenberg, M., Reid, M. W., IsHak W. W., et al. (2017). The impact of cannabis and cannabinoids for medical conditions on health-related quality of life: A systematic review and meta-analysis. *Drug and Alcohol Dependence*, **174**, 80–90.

Herkenham, M., Lynn, A. B., Little, M. D., et al. (1990). Cannabinoid receptor localization in brain. *Proceedings of the National Academy of Sciences of the United States of America*, **87**, 1932–1936.

Hesketh, P. J., Kris, M. G., Basch, E., et al. (2017). Antiemetics: American Society of Clinical Oncology clinical practice guideline update. *Journal of Clinical Oncology*, **35**, 3240–61.

Koppel, B. S., Brust, J. C., Fife. T., et al. (2014). Systematic review: Efficacy and safety of medical marijuana in selected neurologic disorders: Report of the guideline development Subcommittee of the American Academy of Neurology. *Neurology*, **82**, 1556–1563.

Lozano, I. (2001). The therapeutic use of *Cannabis sativa* L. in Arabic medicine. *Journal of Cannabis Therapeutics*, **1**, 63–70.

MacCallum, C. A. and Russo, E. B. (2018). Practical considerations in medical cannabis administration and dosing. *European Journal of Internal Medicine*, **49**, 12–19.

Mechoulam, R., Hanuš, L. O., Pertwee, R., et al. (2014). Early phytocannabinoid chemistry to endocannabinoids and beyond. *Nature Reviews Neuroscience*, **15**, 757–764.

McPartland, J. M., Duncan, M., Di Marzo, V., et al. (2015). Are cannabidiol and Δ9 tetrahydrocannabivarin negative modulators of the endocannabinoid system? A systematic review. *British Journal of Pharmacology*, **172**, 737–753.

Mitchell, R. L. (1995). Comparison of the pharmacology and signal transduction of the human cannabinoid CB1 and CB2 receptors. *Molecular Pharmacology*, **48**, 443–450.

National Academies of Sciences, Engineering and Medicine (NASEM). (2017). The health effects of cannabis and cannabinoids: The current state of evidence and recommendations for research. US National Academy of Sciences. Available from: http://www.nationalacademies.org/hmd/Reports/2017/health-effects-of-cannabis-and-cannabinoids.aspx

Russo, E. B. (2007). History of cannabis and its preparations in saga, science, and sobriquet. *Chemistry and Biodiversity*, **4**, 1614–1648.

Russo, E. B. (2014). The pharmacologic history of cannabis. In: R. G. Pertwee, Ed. *Handbook of Cannabis*. Oxford, UK: Oxford University Press. pp. 23–43.

Russo, E. B. (2016). Current therapeutic cannabis controversies and clinical trial design issues. *Frontiers of Pharmacology*, **7**, 309.

Russo, E. B., Mathre, M. L., Byrne, A., et al. (2002). Chronic cannabis use in the compassionate investigational new drug program: An examination of benefits and adverse effects of legal clinical cannabis. *Journal of Cannabis Therapeutics*, **2**, 3–57.

Sexton, M., Cuttler, C., Finnell, J. S., et al. (2016). A cross-sectional survey of medical Cannabis users: patterns of use and perceived efficacy. *Cannabis and Cannabinoid Research*, **1**, 131–138.

Schultes, R. E. (1973). Man and marihuana. *Journal of Natural History*, **82**, 59.

Szutorisza, H., and Hurd, Y. L. (2018). High times for cannabis: Epigenetic imprint and its legacy on brain and behaviour. *Neuroscience & Biobehavioral Reviews*, **85**, 93–101.

Tanasescu, R., Rog, D., and Constantinescu, C. S. (2011). A drug discovery case history of 'delta-9-tetrahydrocannabinol, cannabidiol'. *Expert Opinion on Drug Discovery*, **6**, 437–52.

van Bakel, H., Stout, J. M., Cote, A. G., et al. (2011). The draft genome and transcriptome of *Cannabis sativa*. *Genome Biology*, **12**, R102.

Whiting P., Wolff, R. F., Deshpande, S., et al. (2015). Cannabinoids for medical use: A systematic review and meta-analysis. *JAMA*, **313**, 2456–2473.

Ware, M. A., Wang, T., Shapiro, S., et al. (2015). Cannabis for the management of pain: assessment of safety study (COMPASS). *Journal of Pain*, **16**, 1233–1242.

30 Shifts in Global Healthcare

R.B. Smarta

CONTENTS

30.1 INTRODUCTION

Irrespective of not being a path-breaking scientist, Andy Gove created an association with Gordon Moore's philosophy of technological development. Andy Gove was neither a household name like famous scientists or socialists, nor a genius who could perhaps overwhelmingly change customer sentiments, but nobody like Andy Gove has much to do with enabling third industrial revolution.

All of us are aware of the first industrial revolution with the mechanisation of the textile industry. The second industrial revolution was an era of mass production. The third industrial revolution, which we are currently experience, has been with the gestation of Silicon Valley scientists empowered by communication technology in the era of Internet and digitalisation. What we are looking at now is the IoT – Internet of Things!

Health perspectives have been dramatically changed from the 'not being healthy' to the 'want to be healthy' perspective. Diseases, therapies and all those specific medicines that we use to make ourselves healthy from sickness has been replaced by doing in advance something that will prevent one from falling ill. What a dramatic change from illness to wellness!

In this paradigm shift from illness to wellness, pro-action, correction and prevention stages have been observed when the shift was taking place. Countries with a legacy of traditional medicines are trying to go back to those alternatives to treat themselves from a different therapy angle. 'Pathy'-agnostic thought processes have started taking a lead, and at least those who are suffering from lifestyle diseases tried to shift their focus and treat themselves with traditional medicines along with modern medicines and other systems of medicines.

From a scientific point of view, the quality, safety, efficacy and other gaps of standardisation along with the changing dynamics of regulatory mechanisms have provided a boost to re-think this 'pathy'-agnostic process. In order to take care of the on-going environment and demographic changes, the emphasis on natural products for treatment becomes significant for remaining healthy.

Irrespective of having quality and the delivery of the product in a scientific way, it was still an enigma of how to convert this science into business. A number of models have been tested and more precisely, the marketing-revenue model ranked at the top to create value in business terms. On the basis of the risk and returns of this health progression, consumers looked at health and living a full life throughout the age pyramid as a synchronised process, even from the World Health Organization's (WHO) earlier definitions of health, where mind, body and soul remain in healthy position surmounted minds of new generation. Obviously people look for something beyond prevention, treatment and all other aspects of part of health – they look for wellness that needs to be redefined yet the path is towards wellness.

30.2   EVEN IN HEALTH PERSPECTIVES

The emergence of technology-driven diagnostics through digitalisation, computerisation and bio-informatics even before treating patients has become a way of life today in technology-driven society. Those who are not even in health and health domains but having a deeper understanding of the Internet and technology in Internet of Things (IOT) have become important stakeholders in healthcare. Google and all other information sources have impacted patients, making them aware and helping them to understand their own health from different perspectives (Figure 30.1).

In fact, gadgets have come in handy to measure day-to-day health and making individuals conscious about their health. A few examples include the following:

* Mobile health (m-Health) technology
* Offsite patient monitoring
* Mobile (moving) health clinics
* Home healthcare
* e-Diagnostics
* e-Medicines
* Genomics
* Hospital practice
* Community pharmacy
* Technological impact
* Digital drugs

As technology is rampantly available and has created an access economy, it is also equally important for herbal medicines as well as alternate medicines to ensure that they are being accessed by

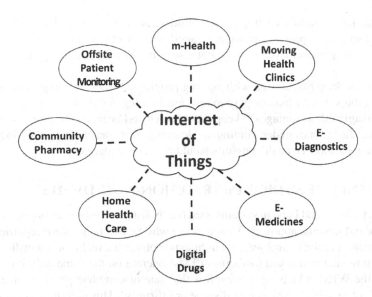

FIGURE 30.1 Internet of Things. (From Interlink Knowledge Cell.)

everybody who needs them. An essential aspect of ensuring access to all these herbals as well as alternate medicines in any form – whether it is digital or not – is that it should provide patient safety.

This can happen through plant-to-patient journey, safety, efficacy, quality, standardisation and dosage of medicines, along with digitisation for awareness in the upcoming millennium for those who have already become conscious about health and have a new paradigm of remaining healthy through prevention, even if they want to take any form of medicine, they feel safe and effective as per promise of the medicines. This needs to be monitored so that this belief is preserved.

Scientists are working all over the world on gut politics that encompasses the essential, critical space of gut health in the arena of health and healing. In order to understand gut health – which encompasses lifestyle diseases and also acute and chronic areas of aliment – deeper study of micro-biomes is needed to complete the circle of healing to health as it completes its journey in the body.

30.3 A JOURNEY FROM 'HEALING-HEALTHY-HEALING'

Healing and being healthy is perhaps the most crucial centre point for all those who are seeking the journey from illness to wellness, as well as a cornerstone of a newer healthier society. Coincidently, the journey of medicines as it happened and would happen is really a journey from healing to medicines to once again 'healing'! Hippocrates (460–375 BCE), the father of modern medicine, long ago declared that one should 'let food be thy medicine'. How poignant was and is this basic direction of life. Chinese and Indian healers, as well as experts, have also expressed themselves during those centuries that perhaps living plants and herbs are the lifesaving medicines available for human beings, along with variety of food.

Advances through modern medicines along with the life cycle of human beings have shown that certain lifestyle diseases and their effects on health need to be treated differently. Those who have been advocating alternate medicines along with modern medicines have shown that it is time for human beings to look at integrated medicines.

Technological innovations and the upsurge of knowledge among medical consumers through the Internet have created further awareness of plant life biology and organic aspects of food, as well as any supplement to be taken inside the body. Further knowledge of drug–food interactions and the safety and efficacy of plant based medicines and the toxicity of herbals and other drugs has created higher expectations from common medical consumers.

Even beyond that, natural catastrophes, calamities, air pollution, global warming, terrorism, chemical wars and atomic pressure provide an another class of psycho-centric issues that need to be handled not at the physical level or body, but also at the mental level or spiritual level of human beings.

As observed, the loop that started with healing progressed towards being healthy and environmental effects grouped with human psychology are looking for those 'timeless medicines' that could have all imaginable advantages to keep them healed and healthy. The journey is very fascinating and revealing. Just to start understanding and learning from ancient Indian, Chinese and Persian systems and end with modern health pursuits would be a rich experience.

30.4   A JOURNEY OF MEDICINES: TRADITIONAL TO TIMELESS

Ancient Indian, Chinese and Persian systems used the 'holistic' approach, as opposed to the present-day scientific or reductionist approach. Hence, those who healed many were regarded as 'miracle-generating' humans and their cures were thought to be outside the realm of scientific reasoning. It is interesting to know that traditional medicines (TMs) operate on the same definition of health that is accepted by the WHO, which says: 'Health is the state of complete physical, mental and social well-being and not merely the absence of disease or infirmity'. This definition broadens the role of physicians today.

In the seventeenth century, the progress of medical science closely followed the progress of biology and other natural sciences. It was Descartes who introduced the theory of separation of 'mind' and 'body'. In fact, the Cartesian model is well known for its reductionist approach, which regarded the human body as a machine and in which disease was seen as a malfunction of the biological mechanism. The Cartesian paradigm has greatly influenced even today's medical thought.

In the eighteenth century, medical science progressed towards cellular and structural changes. Rudolf Virchow postulated that all illness involved structural changes at a cellular level. At about the same time, Louis Pasteur, working on microorganisms, demonstrated the relationship between bacteria and disease. The focus of the physician for the first time moved from the individual organ to mechanical and biological interventions. It then moved further to the structural aspects of cells, and finally it focused on the control of invading bacteria. With this change, the major shift in the direction of treatment and therapy took place, with physicians aiming to 'kill' bacteria to provide relief to patients.

In the nineteenth century, while Pasteur continued his work on bacteria, Bernard studied the environmental factors related to disease. The concept of a specific aetiology for disease was formed by Robert Koch. At the same time the medical technology improved and the stethoscope, sphygmomanometer and other surgical instruments were invented. The pathologists helped physicians to locate, diagnose and label diseases. Hospitals were transformed from 'houses of mercy' to 'centres for diagnosis, therapy and teaching'. The availability of diagnosis tools and the gradual shift in the focus from the 'patient' to the 'disease' led to specialisation, with separate roles for general practitioners and specialists (Figure 30.2).

The twentieth century witnessed progress towards a more specific understanding of biological phenomena and invention of newer medicines. The first major advance was the development of vaccines for typhoid, tetanus and diphtheria. The invention of other vaccines led to virtually a conquest of the three major tropical diseases – malaria, yellow fever and leprosy.

Twenty-first century technology promises to continue changing the nature, complexity and cost of healthcare. As knowledge is evolving about the genetic bases of disease, the healthcare industry has started using gene therapies and is developing ways to prevent genesis of disease. The impact of new technologies such as surgical advances and advancement in diagnosis like functional pathology testing has changed early and mid-twentieth-century medicine socially and scientifically.

Irrespective of all advancements, the biomedical model has now begun working in a different direction. Physicians started facing the side effects of the medicine they prescribed. The existing

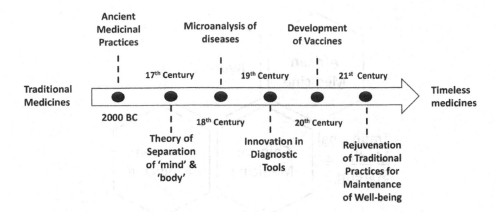

FIGURE 30.2 Journey of medicines: Traditional to timeless. (From Interlink Knowledge Cell.)

medicines were not strong enough to provide 'rest' to the patient, and the role of tranquilisers became important, along with curative medicines. This brought about a change in bacteria like *Mycobacterium tuberculosis* with stronger drugs, and the prescribed rest, while making use of tranquilisers to provide relief from continuous coughs at nights, preventing sleep and disallowing rest. The effects and side effects of these different medicines were analysed, and physicians gradually adopted the use of different therapies to provide complete treatment inclusive of treating the psyche.

O. Carl Simonton's approach to cancer is the most recent example of this, and it is likely to further change the pattern of treatment, care and the attitude of physicians. Today, patients are treated through chemotherapy, radiation, surgery or a combination of these. In fact such treatment is drastic, negative and causes further injury to the body. The Simontonian approach affirms that the development of cancer involves a number of interdependent psychological and biological processes; it views the problem as involving the whole person and does not view the tumour in isolation.

Simonton's approach and other similar techniques have brought about the concept of 'energy medicine'. Bioenergy, according to Wilhelm Reich, flows in wave movements and its basic dynamic characteristic is pulsation. This concept comes very close to the Indian concept of *nadi* and the Chinese concept of *chi*, and the basic premise is that the human body consists of chemicals, bones, muscles and also 'waves'. 'Waves' were regarded as the scientific form of 'spirit' to complete the whole – mind, body and spirit!

So in the amidst of the increase in lifestyle diseases, the fear of side-effects of allopathic treatment, microbe resistance to modern medicines and 'out of pocket payments' for healthcare services, people around the globe are resorting to traditional knowledge of medicines for various health challenges.

30.4.1 FOUR NICE THREADS OF TRADITIONAL SYSTEMS OF MEDICINES

30.4.1.1 Indian Traditional Medicines: *Ayurveda*

Traditionally preserved Indian *Upanishads* proclaim that human beings should be conscious of five different aspects of life (Figure 30.3).

1. Consciousness about matter and lives around you
2. Consciousness about matter and lives within you
3. Consciousness about your body
4. Consciousness about all sensory organs (five physical and five perceptible)
5. Consciousness about your mind

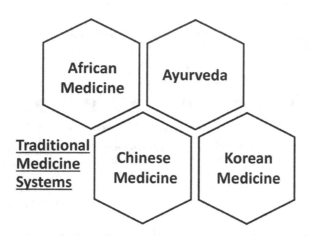

FIGURE 30.3 Four nice threads of traditional systems of medicines. (From Interlink Knowledge Cell.)

How important it is even today when we are talking about healing and being healthy – especially when we talk about herbal and natural products or medicines, they are nothing but matter and lives around us in natural form. When we talk about medicines, we are talking about matter and lives that we take within us for better healing and being healthy. Other consciousness aspects are more philosophical, but in totality they all need to be in one cluster when it comes to healing. Healing is not only physical but also emotional. Many individuals suffer and need emotional healing, even before physical healing takes place in their body, mind and well-being.

Ayurveda – meaning 'the science of life' – is an ancient Indian system of medicine that even today believes in a synergy of mental, physical and spiritual factors. A crucial difference between the scientific approach and the holistic *Ayurvedic* approach lies in the fact that in the former approach the physician 'attacks' the disease or ailment, while in the latter the 'vaidya' (physician) develops strength in the host (patient) and builds up his immunity to fight the disease or ailment. This is basically achieved through a combination of different herbs, which counterbalance each other's toxic effects along with proper regulation of diet and sleep pattern, and self-control.

Ayurveda is considered an *Upaveda* (accessory Veda) of *Atharva* Veda, which is known to be the first Hindu literature on medicine. *Ayurveda* as a system of medicine has historical roots in the Indian subcontinent. Beyond India, *Ayurveda* have been known as an alternative therapy and is integrated in general wellness applications. *Ayurveda* emphasising *Dosha* balance and suppressing natural urges is considered unhealthy and is claimed to lead to illness. In *Ayurveda*, three elemental *Doshas* – namely *Vata*, *Pitta* and *Kapha* – are given importance. It is stated that, the equality (*samyatva*) of these *Doshas* results in health, while inequality (*visamatva*) results in disease.

30.4.1.2 Traditional Chinese Medicines

Traditional Chinese medicine (TCM) is a medical system with a history of around 5000 years in China. The basic principle of TCM holds the belief that life is just a result of equilibrium between *yin* and *yang*, where yin is the inner and negative principle and yang is positive energy. These two energies are called *chi* or *qi*, which are thought to circulate through different channels in the body.

The most astonishing thing is that TCM practitioners could cure patients without any assistant apparatus. The methodology of diagnosis is based only on examination, which is divided into four parts: observation, auscultation and olfaction, interrogation, pulse taking and palpation.

In the first step of observation doctors directly watch the appearance of the patient to know the condition; auscultation and olfaction is a way to collect messages through listening and smell. In next step, they interrogate the patient and his relatives, to know the symptoms, and the last step of taking the pulse and palpation finds the doctors noting the pulse condition of patients on the radial artery, and then determining the inner change of the symptoms.

Once the diagnosis is over, then patient is treated using different techniques, including herbal medicine, acupuncture, massage, exercise and dietary therapy. The raw materials used to prepare medicines in this therapy include plants and their parts, animal parts and even human organs such as placenta.

30.4.1.3   Korean Medicines

The origin of Korean medicine dates to ancient and prehistoric times in 3000 BCE. It includes herbalism, acupuncture and moxibustion.

Moxibustion is a technique in which heat is applied to the body with a stick or a cone of burning mugwort. The tool is placed over the affected area without burning the skin. The cone or stick can also be placed over a pressure point to stimulate and strengthen the blood.

30.4.1.4   African Medicines

There is an ancient African discipline of medicine involving herbal medicines and African spirituality. Practitioners of traditional African medicine claim that they can cure various chronic diseases such as cancers, psychiatric disorders, high blood pressure and even acute diseases like cholera and fever.

30.5   LIMITATIONS OF TM AS PART OF THE NATURE

According to the WHO, there are three major challenges for TM to be a viable business – lack of information sharing, lack of safety monitoring and lack of methods to evaluate safety and efficacy. The growing use of TM by the public and increasing health consciousness is forcing the TM industry to evaluate its health claims through the standards of quality, safety and efficacy.

30.5.1   Gap in Plant-to-Patient Control

The cultivation, production and primary processing of the plant/herb have a direct impact on the quality of the active components. In the current TM system, a robust quality assurance system for the collection, harvest, storage and primary processing of the plant/animal material is lacking as a foundation to ensure consistent composition of the active compound. Another problem is that there is the lack of information transfer from manufacturers to people. Composition is not well-documented enough to obtain reproducible results. Hence, people tend to rely more on testimonials on the benefits of herbal products than solid, scientific evidence.

30.5.2   Lack of Standardisation

In spite of the widespread usage of TM, there is a lack of proper standardisation and quality control of TM drugs. Therefore, TM needs to be regarded as rational drugs – hence the need for standardisation and approved pharmaceutical quality. The problems associated with standardisation of TM drugs are often due to its association with the drug's plant origin.

For plants, generally, the active constituents of herbal drugs are not well established; stability and quality control testing are relatively time consuming, tedious and expensive. Similarly, TMs are mixtures of many herbs, metals and other ingredients, so the genuine raw materials are not easily found. Due to natural variation and lack of reference compounds, the active principle is also hardly known.

30.5.3 Issues with Quality, Safety and Efficacy

All those who are committed to excellence because they want to pleases their customers and increase profits. For them this can be a good motive. But as followers of Divine the motive that drives everybody to excellence should be a desire to please the One who gives us our final reward. Everything should be done with conscious awareness and realization of Somebody is watching for the benefit and wellness of the society......Colossians 3/23/24...Bible

The most important question regarding any drug to be used is how safe it is for clinical use. Pharmaceutical products used as medicines are usually single chemical entities with specific actions at receptors, enzymes and other cellular sites. As pharmaceuticals, drugs are marketed after vigorous preclinical and clinical trials, but unfortunately pharmacological and toxicological studies are not addressed clearly and not transparent to the consumer who wants to use TM.

Generally TM is thought to be 'natural', so many people believe that TMs are safe. However, well-controlled randomised clinical trials have revealed TMs can be as toxic as or even more toxic than prescription medicines. They can cause drug interactions and can create surgical problems. The Journal of the American Medical Association has reported that roughly 15 million adults are at risk of possible adverse interactions between prescription medicines and herbs. This substantiates the need for development of TM and also provides understanding of their limitations.

TMs sold as over-the-counter (OTC) remedies have different protocol regarding preparation, acquiring licenses and marketing. The active principles of such OTC drugs are not often well defined. Similarly, regulations regarding safety and efficacy are also not known to stakeholders or consumers.

At present, it is considered that TM consists of practices, approaches, knowledge and beliefs not based on scientific evidence that are applied to treat, diagnose and prevent illness within society. When modern society adopts such folk medicinal practices, however, it becomes 'non-conventional or alternative medicines'. If we want to capture the untapped potential in TM, it is necessary for us to change the lens through which we are looking at it.

30.6 REGULATORY REFORMS

In countries like China and Germany, traditional medicines are considered drugs, while some countries like the United States and the Netherlands consider TMs as nutritional supplements and have framed definite legislation. In the United States, under the Dietary Supplement Health and Education Act (DSHEA), TMs are considered dietary supplements, whereas in the UK market, licensed or unlicensed herbal products are sold as food supplements.

Being the birthplace of Ayurveda, the Indian marketplace for Ayurvedic products is more established compared to other parts of the world. Any product based on the classical Ayurvedic Formulary can be sold in the Indian market without any prior approval. TMs are, however, being classified as a drug, so health and disease claims are permitted. There are many products not tied down by DSHEA-like structure/function claims that are sold OTC. There are regulatory authorities like Ayurvedic, Yoga and Naturopathy, Unani, Siddha and Homeopathy (AYUSH) and Food Safety and Standards Authority of India (FSSAI) that have established guidelines to control the quality of TMs. Although standards for medicines are mentioned in the Drugs and Cosmetics Act of 1940, there are still some grey areas in the status of traditional medicines, and there are no definite policies about their status as food supplements. Recently the Government of India has published the Food Safety Act to resolve this problem, under which the FBO are compelled to show science-based evidence of specialty foods containing ingredients based on *Ayurveda*, *Unani* and *Siddha* and other traditional health systems. AYUSH has made GMP mandatory for the manufacturing of ASU medicines since the incorporation of revised Schedule T.

In the United States, under the DSHEA of 1994, any herb, botanical and natural concentrate, metabolite and constituent of extract, is classified as a dietary supplement.

As the Food and Drug Administration considers dietary supplements as safe, TM do not have to be approved for safety and efficacy before they enter the market.

Herbal products are available on the UK market as licensed herbal medicines, herbal medicines exempt from licensing or unlicensed herbal products sold as food supplements. In several cases, the same herb is available in all three legal categories. Potentially hazardous plants are controlled as prescription-only medicines (POM) and certain others are subject to dose (but not duration of treatment) and route of administration restrictions, or can be supplied only via a pharmacy and by, or under the supervision of, a pharmacist.

In Canada, herbal remedies must comply with the Natural Health Products Regulations (Health Canada 2003). According to these regulations, all natural products require a product license before they can be sold in Canada.

In addition to health and safety concerns, there has also been a substantial increase in the demand for 'Kosher' or 'Halal' certification for traditional medicines to fulfil the scrupulous religious standards among consumers.

If we look at the present scenario, the major threat is the change in product patterns of TM and the importance given to nutraceuticals and phytopharmaceuticals. The reason behind this is nothing but the failure of regulation systems, which may hamper the spread of TM and its clinical value in the future. Conscious efforts are needed to promote the therapeutic aspects of TM as a system towards wellness, so that it can emerge as a distinct branch of medicine in the versatile healthcare market, rather than just a supplier of some 'safe' herbal remedies for the international market.

Uniformity in regulations of different country is unlikely to happen, as such things are dependent upon different aspects of the country, ranging from their practices to the availability of such medicines. However a group needs to be formed to try to normalise and harmonise all regulatory aspects, keeping the uniqueness of each regulatory focus. It would thereby be easier for players to ensure that this harmonisation facilitates innovation and business, as well as use of TMs.

30.7   THE SITUATION TODAY

Experts at the WHO have identified and enlisted more than 100 types of TM practices that are in use throughout the world. These forms of medicine are globally known as 'traditional medicine' (as most of these are practiced from time immemorial), 'complementary medicine' (as these medicines supplement the allopathic medicines in many cases, or as they differ from orthodox medicine) and 'holistic medicine' (most of the alternative medical systems consider the human body as a complete being comprised of physical mental, social and spiritual dimensions).

Ethnomedicines (as these traditional healthcare systems are closely associated with the life and culture of the masses) and NM (as these methods of treatments are based on the laws of nature and natural substances are used to treat the patients) are also part of these forms available in the world.

Around the globe TM has been practiced differently. In China, it includes acupuncture where in France they use magnetic healing. Germans call it *Heilpraxis* and in Sweden it is known as herbalism. India – one of the countries with a prolonged history – has the traditions of Ayurveda, Siddha, Unani and Yoga as medical practices.

In some cases, TMs are summarised and available in written form (Ayurveda India) or in other cases it is a body of knowledge and techniques that are held by the community and transmitted orally. These are further classified as the traditional medicine systems (TMSs) and traditional folk practices (TFPs). We should understand that TMs are not a stagnant science, but are evolving through the ages as communities find new techniques for the betterment of humanity.

Developed countries like the United Kingdom, United States and Australia have also embraced traditional medicines as complementary and alternative medicine (CAM), which is mainstream in the healthcare sector now. CAM is an umbrella term for a collection of different approaches to diagnosis and treatment. Over 50 diverse complementary therapies have been listed, from homoeopathy (which involves the use of infinitely dilute preparations) to herbal medicine (which involves the use of chemically rich preparations of plant material), and from acupuncture (which involves the insertion of needles into specific points on the body) to spiritual healing (including 'distant' healing, which does not require the laying on of hands). The global traditional market is booming because of the belief that traditional medicine will promote healthier living and because of its 'easy availability', not only through drug stores but also through food markets and supermarkets.

30.8 STRATEGIC BUSINESS PERSPECTIVES

In order to make the TM business viable, the initiative steps should be taken by governments and other stakeholders.

30.8.1 SCIENCE PERSPECTIVES – SCIENCE TO BE SUBSTANTIATED

Government should identify existing standards, policies and regulations to ensure product quality and safety. It can increase credibility by supporting the TM business with an appropriate regulatory framework that underpins quality, safety and effectiveness. The guarantee in the regulatory framework will support the market needs and its growth.

Similarly, stakeholders should create evidence-based claims as per guidelines to encourage the awareness in customers. To build this trust, the industry should adopt the standards as a quality culture. In addition, the industry should participate in a surveillance system after product launches (Figure 30.4).

30.8.2 MARKET PERSPECTIVE

The global TM market is expected to generate revenue of $196.87 billion by 2025, and the major growth contributors are the increasing support by the masses, increased usage of traditional

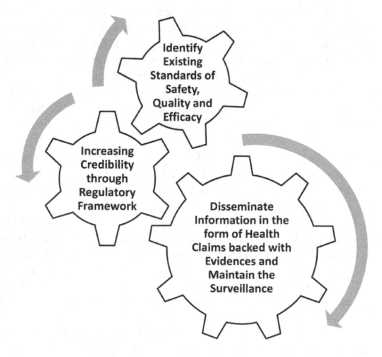

FIGURE 30.4 Strategic business perspectives. (From Interlink Knowledge Cell.)

therapeutic methods and increased percentage of disposable income being spent on health care. TM has the scope for considerable growth in the coming decade.

TM encompasses the traditional methods of diagnosis and the products derived from herbs, elements and animals. Similarly, it focuses on mind and body healing techniques, which are mostly based on faith and belief.

The TM market is therefore segmented into magnetic intervention, acupuncture and botanicals and animal extracts. However, most of these TM practices and medicines are not supported by regulatory approval, so many countries are putting effort to build evidence-based data to support regulatory efforts to improve the market and treatment methods.

Out of all four segments, herbal medicine is booming today. Global Industry Analysts, Inc., based in the United States, have stated that the global herbal medicine market was valued at $71.19 billion in 2016 and is projected to reach *$115 billion by the year 2020.* The industry is *led by Europe* and followed closely by the fast-growing *Asia-Pacific region with, 9.1% CAGR.* Interestingly, *multi-herb supplements* are taking the lead with *7.7% CAGR* compared to single herb supplements. Western herbalism is still in *the lead with 50.9%, followed by traditional Chinese medicine (34.6%),* home-opathy (8.2%) *and Ayurveda (6.3%).* Let us explore the key trends, market dynamics and forecast of herbal medicines.

30.8.3 GEOGRAPHY WISE

The global herbal medicine/supplement market is divided among Germany (28%), Asia (19%), Japan (17%), France (13%), the rest of Europe (12%) and North America (11%).

India and China being the major markets for herbal medicinal products in their region, these countries have a strong background. India being the mother country for Ayurveda supports the use of TM. Similarly growing disposable income, increasing healthcare costs and increased awareness for well-being has powered the growth in the Ayurvedic market, which has reached an estimated market size of *$2 billion.*

In 2016, *Europe* dominated the global herbal medicine market with 45% share and is expected to retain this share during the forecast period as well (Figure 30.5).

30.8.4 SEGMENT WISE

The global herbal pharmaceutical industry revenue is $44 billion. Herbal dietary supplements ($11 billion) and herbal functional foods ($14 billion) make up over a third of the market, where herbal beauty products make up the remaining $14 billion of the market.

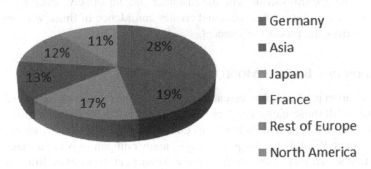

FIGURE 30.5 Market dynamics: Geography wise. (From https://www.nutraceuticalsworld.com/issues/2008-07 /view_features/the-global-herbs-amp-botanicals-market/.)

30.8.5 GALENIC FORMULATIONS

The *extracts segment* generated revenue of $27.1 billion in 2016 and is expected to reach $44.6 billion by 2024. The higher rate of absorption in extract form in comparison with others is driving the TM market over the forecast period.

The *tablets and capsules segment* is expected to grow fastest, as tablets are easy to carry, which gives them an advantage over other formulations. Now traditionally made powders are being made available in the form of tablets and capsules, which provide higher dose accuracy.

30.8.6 SCIENCE TO BUSINESS PERSPECTIVE

Patient consciousness of community has been increased by the Internet as well IoT. Considering that decisions have to be made on their own, patients have become aware, conscious and looking for better natural alternatives and trying to shy away from chemical products.

Consumers consider plant-based medicines, as well natural medicines, to be harmless and safe. They are not aware of the side effects that even those plant-based medicines can cause. However, the approach science has taken to overcome this is a conscious journey of plant to patient, which provides safety, efficacy, quality, standardisation and all other aspects which would have caused side effects.

Usually it is understood that herbal-based medicines are not as useful as chemical medicines in acute cases and preference is always given to such medicines to treat chronic disease, as well as life-style diseases. Knowing the population of entire world tilts towards Asian and emerging markets, almost all countries are looking at remedies for lifestyle diseases. The present situation is such that chemical products through pharmaceuticals and natural and herbal products through nutraceuticals, 'Ayurceuticals', phytopharmaceuticals will co-exist.

Earlier NMEs (new medical entities) were not as important as NCEs (new chemical entities), but these are now moving towards NNEs (new natural entities). These NNEs are designed within a safety, quality, clinical efficacy and clinical output format. As these entities are regulated, as evident from regulatory reforms, it is essential to consider interactions between such entities and regular food that patients take. Similarly, those patients who are taking drugs must be aware that these entities do not interfere and yet remain effective in the gut. Technologies have proven that they can do this through different techniques. All these perspectives put together will help to create a viable business model for TMs.

30.9   IS A BUSINESS MODEL NECESSARY?

Yes, a business model provides models for the interactions between all components of the business that interact with each other in the market place from identifying the right target customer, the value proposition, the value, the transaction with the customer and, ultimately, revenue. This process in a model from provides a design for business and creates confidence in those who operate, fund and derive satisfaction from the product or concept.

30.9.1 CREATION OF A BUSINESS MODEL

To create an innovation platform, it is essential to look at trends and at the gaps and work out what needs to be done to fill those gaps. The forces responsible for these trends include demographics, psychographics and environmental changes. To understand the way ahead, we need to scrutinise the marketing process. Possibly the biggest failing of many companies is the unilateral decision and procedure they follow in trying to successfully place products in the market. Brainstorming sessions and rudimentary market research is carried out and the product ideas are discussed. Democratic consensus may lead to shortlisting and a further narrowing of a path to follow.

While building a business model, we need to consider how the belief in our products, services or ideas will be conveyed to potential buyers. In this regard, it is important to look at the core capabilities of the organisation and the existing infrastructure. In the case of 'timeless medicine', the traditional structures and infrastructures are already available in every country. However, the core capabilities required for plantation, processing, technology and research and development, as well as a suitable combination of academia and industry need to be properly chosen to develop the right product. Similarly, in order to make the business healthy, we need to ensure that the knowledge of TM is converted into business with the proper steps – and only then will business and revenue go hand in hand.

The heart of any industry is the value it offers to consumers through its products or services. To convert knowledge and insights of TM into a viable business, it has become now a need to bridge the gap between knowledge and business through the value proposition. Let us explore the business models that emphasise value propositions where knowledge-based science gets converted into business.

As we discussed earlier, a business model is necessary to convey belief in our product effectiveness to buyers. First we have to struggle to identify the niche in the market and, as the inside-out approach following Chandler is providing us the product, what needs to be done is to also work on an outside-in approach. The present model is inside out, which involves discovery to development to availability. It focuses on prevention and cure for diseases or ailments for their customers. Where the needs and trends in the environment are changing, thought, the focus of the business model will have to shift from an inside-out to outside-in approach (Figure 30.6).

The outside-in model works on three layers, the first of which is the origin of the idea could have grown from social and medical issues that could have economic, technological and political dimensions. Mounting on this first layer of trends, industry must look at 'Ayureconomics'. Changing disease challenges, health consciousness and health costs provide enough insight on the needs of Ayureconomics, and the third layer covers interfaces with all stakeholders.

The stepping-stone for any business is innovation and it should be measured by what it contributes to market and the customer. Research and development is the tool to find out what needs your customers wants fulfilled today. For that we should analyse market trends to build competencies and capabilities to satisfy stakeholder needs.

The value of the product can be made only when it is differentiated from other products. Nowadays, the demand to demonstrate superiority – not just non-inferiority – is increasing.

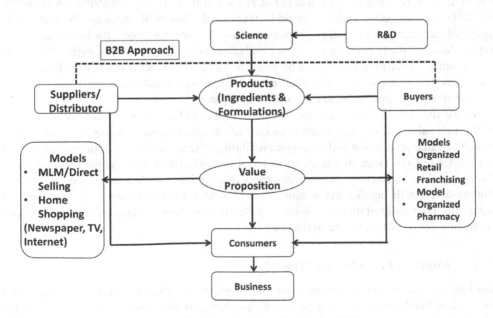

FIGURE 30.6 Outside-in business model. (From Interlink Knowledge Cell.)

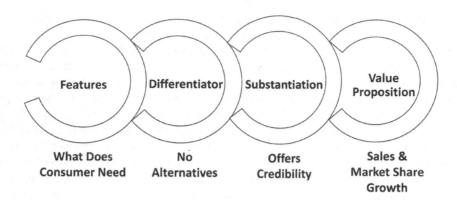

FIGURE 30.7   Value proposition. (From Interlink Knowledge Cell.)

It is therefore important to make an offer to the consumer that has to be very specific. We have to remember that creating value propositions is about communicating why our product is worth paying for, in quantitative terms that later establish the relationship with the customer (Figure 30.7).

The flow of information about the products is of primary importance to the consumer in the market place. As it makes long-term impact on health, global legislation to regulate the type of health claims (e.g. the value proposition) and their scientific substantiation has become the need of the hour. Today, the TM industry recognises the functional and health-promoting benefits of its constituents with the use of health claims and reduction-of-disease health claims. These claims support the value proposition, through 'features' of the product like how it can serve the consumer. Features are nothing but the differentiator that makes the product unique.

The gap between TM and the consumer can be bridged only with perceptual imagery along with substantiation of claims. Thus, the TM industry needs to provide scientific narration in such a way that the results can be statistically and clinically significant and substantiated. This would create a different perception of TM in the minds of consumers.

Once the product has made it all the way through the new product development stage, the next step is to make it available to the consumer at any given time. For this, distribution channels are required. These distribution channels could be traditional – like B2B where one business makes a commercial transaction with another – or non-traditional – like B2C where the business or transaction is conducted directly between a company and consumers who are the end users of its products. The intermediate governing factors that propose the value of product is marketing. Marketing can be done directly by the means of direct selling or through organised/unorganised hospital pharmacies, home shopping, franchising and organised /unorganised retail.

Here, we realised that to create the revenue for the TM industry, credibility in customers' mind through value propositions needs to be created. Biomarkers have the potential to fill the gap between the value proposition and customer credibility. The word biomarker describes a traceable and characterised substance that is an indicator of biological morphology, process and function. The concept of biomarkers for drug development is no unique. FDA is as taking an initiative to support research in the application of biomarkers. Biomarkers can be used for many applications including the assessment of disease condition, differentiating between benignancy and malignancy and detecting progress as response to the drug.

30.9.2   Biomarker as a 'Quality Marker'

Biomarkers are specifically intertwined with major excretions from the body that result from its normal or abnormal functioning (e.g. saliva). Biomarkers provide a bridge between all dimensions of science and are essential for facilitating as well as identifying milestones during treatment.

As we have seen earlier, quality control is critical for ensuring the safety and effectiveness of TM. Current quality control methods for botanical drugs are mainly based on chemical testing. However, chemical testing alone may not be sufficient, as it may not capture all constituents of botanical drugs. Therefore, it is necessary to establish a bioassay correlating with the drug's known mechanism of action to ensure its potency and activity.

Biomarkers offer the potential to bridge the gap between quality control metrics and clinical efficacy by detecting the presence of a compound in a given product. In the traditional medicine industry, biomarkers play an important role in identifying herbs and chemical constituents, given the respective herb activity. In traditional medicine, it is also sometimes useful to identify adulterated and spurious components.

The biological stability of herbs with reference to their chemicals relating to medicinal efficacy offers a special advantage in the standardisation and quality control of heterogeneous botanical products. *Piper nigrum* is a well-known example from natural product standardization program which is cited frequently for validation standard and also to determine the efficacy of the drug.

There are various detection methods for identification of biomarkers such as ultraviolet visible spectra, high-performance thin-layer spectroscopy, high-performance liquid chromatography and infrared spectra. The simpler the method, the faster and more cost effective it is. In the course of development of technology, multiple biomarker assays have been used to assess the quality of botanicals.

A recent advancement is 'microfluidics', where enzyme inhibition is employed to indicate the drug's activity and thereby evaluate biological consistency. This technique was exemplified on QiShenYiQi (QSYQ) pills, a Chinese medicine composed of *Astragalus membranaceus* (Huangqi, HQ), *Salvia miltiorrhiza* (Danshen, DS), *Panax notoginseng* (Sanqi, SQ), and essential oil of *Dalbergia odorifera* (Jiangxiang, JX). This polyherbal preparation is widely prescribed for cardiac dysfunction, and related mechanisms have been well investigated. Two enzymes – thrombin and angiotensin-converting enzyme (ACE) – were chosen as quality biomarkers for QSYQ.

In the above experiment, a dual-channel microfluidic chip was designed to perform the bioassay, where one channel allowed for the formation of the enzymatic complex, and the subsequent enzymatic reaction takes place in the other channel. Magnetic beads were employed both as an efficient surface to immobilise the enzyme and as a controllable solid support to enhance on-chip mixing and transport.

30.9.3 Move towards Business

Connecting value propositions with biomarkers and understanding customers' unmet needs to provide desired value from the product is an intricate and core part of the business model. Once this process brings out the value proposition for a product, as a business it is important to consider the route to engaging and influencing the target customer such as through B2B, B2C, pharmacies or over the counter. Knowing these routes and their implications, as well as their requirements, the supply side chain needs to be established so that consumers are properly serviced. This brings a major transaction between customer and company or product with the sweet smell of revenue.

30.10 COMMERCIALISATION AND CUSTOMISATION PROCESS

In developed countries it is easy for people to go recurrently to the private sector for healthcare, but for developing and underdeveloped nations, healthcare has become a matter of 'out of pocket payments'. Commercialising the TM that could potentially be accessed across the range of socio-economic status has become the need of the hour. So, commercialisation has become potentially important to turn sustainable development goals (SDG) 2013 into reality.

Commercialisation is the process of bringing new innovations to market, that is, the market-based scaling-up of production from pilot to mass market that transforms new knowledge to wealth.

The commercialisation process starts with overlapping aspects of product innovation, marketing innovation and the commercial process based on the business model.

Although TMs do not have therapeutic evidence like pharmaceutical drugs, this has become a necessity for the industry to focus on innovation and value creation. So in short, we can say that TM product manufacturing has better prospects with the present growth provided that there are higher incentives for research and development to add value to cater to the health of the consumer. Later, the product stems towards acceptance and is diffused in the market for better market shares. When we want to commercialise the TM, we have to understand how a buyer adopts and engages with new products or technologies over time. The first step towards engaging the consumer is portraying products to highlight their best value in the best possible way.

30.10.1   DIFFUSION OF INNOVATION MODEL

This model explains how the product can be adopted by five different customer types and what can be done to engage them (Figure 30.8).

The consumers are divided as follows:

- *Innovator*: These are a small group of people exploring new ideas and technologies.
- *Early Adopters*: These people are considered to be opinion leaders who help to share positive testimonials about new products and services. Engagement requires little persuasion, as they are receptive to change.
- *Early Majority*: These are followers who will read reviews by earlier adopters about new products before making the decision to purchase. They can be engaged with reviews and via YouTube, where they can assess products.
- *Late Majority*: These are critics who not willing to change, but can only adopt a new product or service if there is a strong feeling of being left out. They can be engaged with marketing material, evidence, reviews from opinion leaders and case studies to show how the product works.
- *Laggards*: These people will only adopt new products or service if there are no alternatives. Laggards will come on board when other consumers have praised the products.

30.10.2   RISKS AND REWARDS

Any new idea, concept, product or service comes with inherent risks in its commercialisation. This risk needs to be evaluated on different parameters. One of the most important parameters is the need of the particular product or product portfolio. We need to further examine whether such needs are latent or obvious, where there are substitutes or similar products available.

If such products are available, risk is reduced as we can recognise and factor price points. In cases where there is no substitute or competition, understanding price points becomes an important factor for that product. It is equally important to map the market and arrive at macro as well as micro

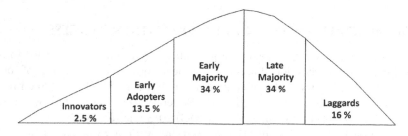

FIGURE 30.8   Diffusion of the innovation model. (From Essential Market Model.com.)

level specifics in terms of size, dynamics, growth and relative price. Once a certain level of comfort has been reached, the basic attitude towards taking that risk remains positive. From an outside-in perspective, as well as inside-out perspective, it is important to work out the investment in overall marketing, as well as infrastructure development in the market and along the entire value chain. This perspective provides the investment requirements.

On the basis of potential and investment – along with marketing capabilities – it is important to take an informed decision about capturing specific market share. In doing so, revenue is mapped along with the investment essential to procure that revenue, so the investor can definitely make an informed call as to whether to invest or not, depending on the return on investment – which could be staggered from 1 to 3 years on the basis of acceptance, consumption, repeat purchases, competitive edge and the revenue performance. At the end, it is important to understand that if there is no pain there is no gain.

30.11 TOWARDS WELLNESS

There is a reason why the TM system is considered a holistic science – it focuses towards attaining complete health. In recent years, there has been rising awareness among consumers about the health benefits of foods and their nutritional benefits for disease prevention and health enhancement. As we have seen earlier, TM is a pure natural science that advocates optimum health should be attained and maintained with the help of a balanced mind, body and soul. To attain this harmony in all TM practices, importance has been given to particular diet. There is evidence that, people around the globe who follow the TM on regular basis have taken these formulations as a part of their daily food supplements for quite some time.

In recent years the pharmaceutical product 'nutraceuticals' have drawn special attention among health professionals and people for their nutritional supplementation. The collaboration of nutraceuticals with TM brings the consumer acceptance. Although the term nutraceutical has recently become popular, we can trace its origin back in the plantation and perhaps traditional medicines. Ayurveda places great emphasis on the quality of nutritious food, including *Rasayana* (preventing degenerative changes), *Balya* (post-illness nutrition), *Brihan* (providing deficient nutrients), *Jeevaniya* (maintaining longevity), *Vyadhikshamatva* (enhancing the immunity) and *Vajikaran* (maintaining vitality and vigour). The science of food and nutrition in Ayurveda has been well-developed.

Similarly, phytopharmaceuticals have also been considered as an important alternative medicine to modern allopathic treatment. Phytopharmaceuticals are nothing but the purified and standardised fraction with a defined minimum of four bioactive or phytochemical compounds (qualitatively and quantitatively assessed) of an extract of a medicinal plant or its part, for internal or external use of human beings or animals for diagnosis, treatment, mitigation or prevention of any disease or disorder, but does not include administration by parenteral route. The new studies in this sector encourage the development of plant-based drugs using advanced techniques like solvent extraction, fractionation, potentiating steps and modern formulation development.

From the above examples, we can say that TM is a powerful instrument in maintaining health and acting against nutritionally induced acute and chronic diseases, thereby promoting optimal health, longevity and quality of life. The association of the wellness industry with TM is bound to bring long-lasting consumer acceptance, but the acceptance will be whole-hearted only if the TM industry can build trust regarding safety, efficacy and quality in the mind of consumer.

As society has changed with knowledge exposure through the use of technology, the new diagnostic methods coupled with genetics has empowered each individual to look at and be responsible for his or her own health. Genetics and genomics along with other DNA fingerprinting would further accelerate social decision making for health benefits. In the flux of newer technology, precise diagnostics, genetic fingerprinting awareness about body, body shops and also deep understanding of mechanism of body and life would become a reality for each individual of new society.

Responsible health behaviour would be the next step for remaining healthy, much as fashion diets, diet restrictions and other behaviours surrounding diet are seen in society especially with new millennium even today. Obesity and other lifestyle health discrepancies are creeping in due to work habits, as well as aspirations of the new generation resulting in a lack of more than necessary availability of essential nutrients and other disorders.

Environmental effects from global warming, tsunamis, volcanoes and other climatic black swans would further make each individual of the new society aware of mental health, robustness and a willingness to survive and be productive in the new society would become essential. The market is already occupied by the wellness industry on different platforms from yoga, meditation, spas, chiropody, rejuvenation centres, naturopathy, to Chinese therapies like acupuncture. In this environment of wellness, traditional or timeless medicines will have to look beyond usual therapies and create a beautiful mix of products and services. So that fascinating value proposition of product with the added proposition of service and willingness to undergo this service included with product would be the reality of tomorrow.

REFERENCE

Natural Health Product Regulation in Canada. Available from: https://www.canada.ca/en/health-canada/services/drugs-health-products/natural-non-prescription/regulation.html.

31 Ayurveda
Evidence-Based Approach for Drug Development

Subhadip Banerjee, Sayan Biswas and Pulok K. Mukherjee

CONTENTS

31.1   INTRODUCTION

The philosophy of treating a system or body as a whole is gaining relevance as we look back or evolve towards a 'systems' approach in this post-genomic era. After so much technological boom, our understanding of Ayurveda is only at its beginning. What seems a philosophy in common sense may be found to have in-depth scientific nuances on exploration. Chemical standardisation like bio-marker analysis and metabolomic profiling has unfolded a diverse chemical space of safe and thera-peutically relevant drugs. Research on Ayurgenomics is adding evidence regarding the genomic correlates of *Vata*, *Pitta* and *Kapha,* the three principle bio-factors termed as *Tridosha* (bodily humours; Govindaraj et al. 2015). Exploring molecular the pharmacology of intelligent synergistic traditional formulations to elucidate and validate safety, toxicity, pharmacokinetics, metabolic sta-bility like herb–drug interactions is gaining importance. Next-generation approaches like 'network or systems pharmacology' are the tools of these efforts. Deciphering the novel mechanism to ensure harmony inside a system's signalling (*Vata*), metabolism (*Pitta*) and storage (*Kapha*) – called the balance of the *doshas* – presents a real challenge (Hopkins 2008; Chandran et al. 2015). However, we still need to focus on the validation of traditional claims and practices mentioned in Ayurveda like Panchakarma, Agnikarma, Rasayana, which require in-depth scientific exploration (Debnath et al. 2015).

Ayurveda delights us with its perception of healthy living. Its knowledge is enriched with every aspect, right from choosing the correct food and lifestyle to live healthy while combating diseases using drugs and formulations developed from natural resources in ancient times. Crossing the barrier of time, its relevance is continuing in spite of changes in the environment, lifestyle and culture and also disease patterns. Four Vedas, considered to be the oldest Indian literature (5000–1000 BCE) contain information about natural remedies. Ayurveda was established as a fully grown medicinal system. *Charaka Samhita* mainly highlighted internal medicine and *Sushruta Samhita* concen-trated on surgery both documented scientifically and are considered classical texts of Ayurveda. The vibrant particulars of *Charaka Samhita* and *Sushruta Samhita* were assembled and updated to write the *Ashtanga Sangraha* and *Ashtanga Hridaya*. The minor works of ancient literature in Ayurveda includes *Madhava Nidana*, dealing with diagnosis of disease, *Bhava Prakasha,* on addi-tional information related to plants and diet, while *Sarngadhara Samhita* enumerated formulation and dosage forms (Sen and Chakrabarty 2017).

The basic principle of Ayurvedic treatment – the world's most ancient medical science – consists of two essential parts: (i) to prevent the cause of disease, and (ii) to make the patient more aware about the cause of the disease and method of its prevention. Ayurveda treats a patient as a whole and not the disease alone. This holistic medicine emphasises the uniqueness of each person with regard to bio-identity, socioeconomic status and biochemical and physiological conditions, which may lead to a particular type of illness. Ayurveda needs further exploration under the light of modern scientific approaches for addressing various healthcare issues (Mukherjee et al. 2017a). The Ayurvedic system adopts a holistic approach towards healthcare by balancing the physical, mental and spiritual functions of the human body. The science of Ayurveda is unique, as it provides opportunity to provide a healthy, harmonious and long life. Over the past few decades, research on Ayurveda through various endeavours has given rise to interdisciplinary research programmes employing several disciplines in this field. Several lead molecules and ready-to-use products and processes are emerging. Ayurveda is quite popular among people due to their practical benefits, traditional beliefs, economical advantage and easy access and other reasons, which have a regional, religious and social basis. India certainly needs to generate a sufficient evidence base for Ayurveda with the help of modern science and experimental rigour (Mukherjee and Houghton 2009).

The development of Ayurvedic medicine (AM) is gaining momentum in keeping with the per-spectives of safety, stability, efficacy and quality for the betterment of human health. Medicinal plants serve as a most valuable source for the remedy of many diseases. The increasing search for therapeutic agents derived from plant species is justified by the emergence of new diseases. Bioactive compounds from different medicinal plants have a major role in the management and improvement of human health (Mukherjee et al. 2012). Ayurvedic medicines are used as a raw, crude powder, extracts and preparations for therapeutic purposes. Authentication, quality control, standardisation, chemo-profiling, validation processes, regulatory aspects, clinical risk assessment, consumer awareness and post-marketing surveillance are the key points that could ensure the quality, safety and effectiveness of AM. These are critical and essential matters that need to be considered for assuring the therapeutic efficacy, safety and justify their use in the healthcare (Mukherjee et al. 2014, 2015a). Development of standardised, synergistic, safe and effective traditional herbal formulations with robust scientific evidence can also offer faster and more economical alternatives. For instance, Ayurvedic texts include thousands of single or polyherbal formulations (Anonymous 2002a, 2002b). Systematic data mining of the existing formulations' huge database can certainly help the drug discovery processes to identify safe candidates and synergistic formulations.

31.2 IDENTIFICATION AND AUTHENTICATION OF AYURVEDIC HERBS

The accurate identification and authentication of Ayurvedic herbs is the first crucial step to avoid confusion, admixtures or adulterations in the botanicals. With regard to quality assurance, plant identification is crucial to guarantee that the right plant raw material has been used and to detect possible admixtures, adulterations and confusions. Identification should be carried out combining various methods, including macroscopic and microscopic examination, chemical fingerprinting and DNA based characterisation. The useful active compounds in plants for medicinal preparation are amongst the huge diversity of secondary plant products that are often specific for certain plants or plant groups. These are some vital aspects that should be considered for the correct identification and authentication of Ayurvedic herbs (Mukherjee 2002; Franz et al. 2011).

31.2.1 PHYTOCHEMICAL SCREENING AND CHARACTERISATION

Qualitative phytochemical tests of individual herbs and formulation to be followed by fingerprint profile of all the compounds is usually characteristic for individual plant or part of plant. The analysed compounds may or may not be the bioactive substances, but quite often characteristic marker substances only. Chemical and metabolite fingerprinting is required for validation of medicinal plants used traditionally. These should be properly documented for further study. The chemical characterisation of Ayurvedic plants should be made through modern technologies like HPTLC, HPLC, LC-MS/MS GC-MS/MS and NMR-MS.

31.2.2 AYURGENOMICS

The better understanding of the scientific basis of individual variations is eased by our understanding of the human genome. Nearly 5800 clinical signs and symptoms are obtainable in Ayurvedic texts. The effects of season, time and environmental conditions in line with the principles of Ayurvedic chronobiology ought to be thought of to advise lifestyle modifications followed by dietary recommendation. Over 1200 species of plants, nearly 100 minerals and over 100 animal products comprise the Ayurvedic pharmacopeia. Thousands of single, multiple mixtures and processed formulations are represented in the Ayurvedic literature, together with details of drug actions. The extent of this information is giant and it will be best managed for the treatment of human healthcare (Patwardhan and Vaidya 2010).

For years, researchers have noted these variations, but have had no way to predict them. Pharmacogenetics is the study of the hereditary basis for variations in the response of populations to a drug. The constant dose of a drug can end in elevated plasma concentrations for a few patients and low concentrations for others. Some patients can respond well to the medicine, whereas others will not. A drug may show adverse effects in some patients, but not in others. These variations have an effect on the condition of people with varied types of cancer. Numerous earlier studies indicated that the variations in response to disease and medicines differ from population to population, and actually from individual to individual. Ayurgenomics describes the idea of individual variation and its clear similarities with pharmacogenomics is expected to become the premise of designer drugs. Understanding the doable relationship between *Prakruti* (nature) and genome are going to be vital. Functionally, this may involve the creation of three organised databases that are capable of showing intelligent communication with one another to provide tailor-made prescriptions (Patwardhan and Vaidya 2010).

31.2.3 DNA Barcoding

Authentication of medicinal plants by molecular markers and DNA-based markers that are based on analysis of the unique genetic structure are undoubtedly higher level markers and have the upper hand over other marker systems, because these are not affected by age, environmental factors and physiological conditions. Moreover, these markers are not tissue-specific and thus can be detected at any stage of plant development. Compared with phenotypic and chemical markers, DNA-based technology can provide an efficient, accurate and cheaper means of testing the authenticity of hundreds of samples simultaneously as these can be amenable to automation (Mukherjee et al. 2017b).

Medicinal plants can be identified by DNA-based authentication as a tool for quality control and safety monitoring of herbal pharmaceuticals and nutraceuticals and will significantly add to the medical potential and commercial profitability of herbal products. A genetic marker may be defined as gene or a nucleotide sequence on a chromosome that has the potential to differentiate cells, individuals or species. The DNA sequences are very precise; they can be recognised with the help of the identified molecular markers, which can find out a particular sequence of DNA from a group of unknown. The prime cause of the problems associated with the standardisation of medicinal plants is due to the complex composition of drugs used in the form of whole plants, plant parts or extracts obtained therefrom. Therefore, a principal stride is to ensure reproducibility and negligible batch-to-batch variation in an anticipated quality of any herbal remedy, and side-by-side initiating steps towards use of authentic starting material. Many researchers have examined a number of market samples of crude drugs used in Indian systems of medicine and observed that the prevalence of adulteration is such that quite unrelated plants are being sold in the crude drug markets in place of genuine ones (Hussain et al. 2015). DNA markers that fill the maximum gap in solving the problem of identification, off-course is a boom to the molecular biology, but is dependent over two other markers because one cannot find the efficiency of an authentic drug without chemical analysis. In future, DNA markers can be used to build a reference library of AM (such as DNA sequences and fingerprints), in order to get rid of adulterants and spurious materials that have ruined AM (Li et al. 2015).

Herbal genomics has appeared as an efficient segment in chemical and biological analysis of complex herbal products that may contain more than one active component. An herbal gene bank is now being applied to many areas of herb-related biological research to help identification of the quality of the herb. Further, model herb research platforms, DNA barcoding and a gene bank of medicinal plants can nourish by functional herbal genomics research. Therefore, herbal genomics is emerging as a novel approach for maintaining quality control of medicinal plants (Chen et al. 2015). To define the molecular identity of herbs, illustration of the highly diverse core biosynthetic pathways of secondary metabolites formation is needed. This information helps us to understand the mechanisms underlying natural variation of secondary metabolite formation due to genetic difference of dissimilar cultivars of medicinal plants. In this context, medicinal plants like *Ganoderma lucidum*, *Salvia miltiorrhiza* and *Catharanthus roseus* are used as valuable models for studying the genetic activities of herbs. These plants synthesise active medicinal components like triterpenes, diterpene, quinone and indole alkaloids. In addition, similar models can also used to identify novel biosynthetic pathways for convergent secondary metabolites in closely related herb species (Chen et al. 2015).

31.3 QUALITY EVALUATION AND VALIDATION OF AYURVEDIC MEDICINE

Quality control and standardisation of raw materials and Ayurvedic formulation are the major criteria for their acceptability in modern medicine. These ensure the consumer's right to get pure, safe, potent and effective medication. The bioactive extract should be standardised on the basis of active principle or major compound(s) with chromatographic and spectroscopic techniques. The next important step is to make a stable Ayurvedic product with maximum shelf-life. It is a well-known fact that at large doses, herbal drugs (in association with conventional medicines) may cause unwanted side effects (Mukherjee et al. 2008). Phytochemistry plays an important and indispensable role in the implementation of each of these steps. Quality control of AM requires knowing what is in chemical constituents of the plant, what happens during its processing, chemical analysis and biological evaluation until the finished product reaches the consumers (Cordell and Colvard 2012). There are serious concerns being expressed all over the world with respect to contamination and adulteration of traditional medicines. Contaminants may include various pesticides, herbicides, insecticides, heavy metals (arsenic, cadmium, lead and mercury), microbial species and radiation. Adulterants may include other cheaper plant materials with similar biological effects or synthetic drugs (Mukherjee et al. 2012). All the adequate information about the botanical derived products should be considered with appropriate deliberation for analytical and batch to batch variability in the medicinal preparation. Identification, analytical specification and pharmacopoeial standard of Ayurvedic formulation should be evaluated based on the pharmacopoeial parameters as mentioned in the standard Ayurvedic Pharmacopoeia (Lavekar 2006). The different parameters for quality evaluation of AM are given in Table 31.1. There are the several important processes and integrated strategies that need to be considered for the careful validation of AM at each and every step.

TABLE 31.1
Quality Evaluation of Ayurvedic Medicine

Tests	Ayurvedic Terminology
Description	*Darshana pareeksha*
Colour	*Darshana pareeksha*
Odour	*Ghrana pareeksha*
Taste	*Rasana pareeksha*
Loss on drying at 11°C, total ash acid, insoluble ash, total solid, pH, volatile oils	*Bahya/rasayanika parikasha*
Particle size, bulk density, tap density	*Darshana* and *Sparshana pareeksha*
Heavy/toxic metal analysis	*Bahya/rasayanika parikasha*
• Lead, cadmium, mercury, arsenic	
Microbial analysis	*Krimi/desha pariksha*
• Total viable aerobic count	
• Total Enterobacteriaceae	
• Total fungal count	
Test for specific pathogen	*Krimi/desha pariksha,*
• *E. coli*	*Panchgyanendriya pariksha*
• *Salmonella* sp.	
• *S. aureus*	
• *Pseudomonas aeruginosa*	

(Continued)

TABLE 31.1 (*Continued*)
Quality Evaluation of Ayurvedic Medicine

Tests	Ayurvedic Terminology
Pesticide residue analysis	*Desha pariksha*
• Organo-chlorine pesticide	
• Organoposphorous pesticide	
• Synthetic pyrethroids	
Test for Aflotoxins	*Prabhava karakas*
• (B1 + B2 + G1 + G2)	
TLC/HPLC/HPTLC-Profile with marker	*Darshana pareeksha*
Tablets/Capsules	*Mana pariksha*
• Uniformiy of weight/content	
Disintegration time	*Darshana pareeksha*
Friability (if tablet)	*Darshana pareeksha*
Hardness	*Darshana pareeksha*
Lethal dose	*Vishakta matra*
Optimum effective dose	*Prabhava sheela matra*
Shelf life	*Saviryata avadhi*
Preservative	*Prakshipta dravyas*
Active compound	*Virya*
Binders	*Sandhana karakas*

Global implementations of evidence-based foundation are required for AM that would transform healthcare for all. Major strategies towards the quality evaluation and validation of Ayurvedic products include the following:

1. Phytochemical and pharmacological screening
2. Chemo-profiling
3. Metabolomics and target compound analysis
4. Phyto-informatics
5. High-throughput screening
6. Phyto-equivalence
7. System biology
8. Reverse pharmacology
9. Value added delivery systems
10. Safety profile
11. Clinical study and pharmacovigilance (Mukherjee et al. 2014)

The development and validation of AM requires the convergence of modern techniques and integrated approaches related to their evidence-based research.

31.4 SYSTEM BIOLOGY

System biology intends to understand biological complexity by indifferent measurements of as many parameters as possible, which could be a helpful approach to determine the effects of a drug in an extensive way. The focus of the rising area of systems biology is to inquire into the dynamics of all genetic, regulatory and metabolic processes in a cell and to understand the complexity of cellular networks. Its technological platforms, such as genomics, proteomics and metabolomics, provide powerful tools for study of the essence of TM syndrome and the function of herbal compound recipe (Mukherjee et al. 2010). Scientifically and technologically validated botanical products may be explored on a fast track using innovative approaches like reverse pharmacology and systems biology, which are based on knowledge of TM. Technologies such as genomics, proteomics, and metabolomics are high-throughput technologies called 'omic' technologies. Proteomics is the large-scale study of proteins, particularly their structures and functions. The term was coined to create an analogy with genomics. It was revealed by the Human Genome Project that there are fewer protein-coding genes in the human genome than there are proteins in the human proteome. Proteomics-based approaches can examine the expressed proteins of a tissue or cell type or they may complement the genome initiatives (Mukherjee et al. 2015a). The approaches are increasingly being used to answer biomedical questions in more detail. Proteins are the main functional output, and the genetic code cannot always indicate that proteins are expressed, in what quantity and in what form (Banks et al. 2000). The application of 'omic' technologies may lead to a change of paradigms towards the application of complex mixtures in medicine and open the new field of phytogenomics, proteomics, and metabolomics in medicinal plants and traditional medicine.

31.5   TOXICOKINETICS OF AYURVEDIC DRUGS

Generally the public believes that modern drugs are dangerous foreign chemicals with side effects while herbs are natural and safe. In fact, some herbs can also be dangerous and even cause serious diseases leading to death if used inappropriately. Unfortunately, at the present time, the fundamental sciences of botany, chemistry, and biology behind the marketed of products that could protect the patient – who rightfully expects safety, efficacy, and consistency in TMs as a result of a strong evidence base – remain essentially absent in some cases. The major sciences supporting TM are currently in the midst of dynamic change, so opportunities to improve this appalling healthcare situation are certainly available. Adequate funding as well as corporate and regulatory commitment to a significantly higher ethical standard for TMs need to be made. The complexity of herbal medicine preparations and the interpretation of bibliographic data on safety and efficacy reflecting the experience gathered during long-term use are best addressed by involving specific expertise and experience. Further, without the knowledge of the prescriber, consumers tend to consume herbal products, along with prescription medicine, which may lead to herb–drug interaction, *via* cytochrome P450 enzymes. The evaluation of herb–drug interactions is also essential because the concomitant oral administration of natural products and prescription drugs or over-the-counter products may affect human drug metabolism and significantly increase the risk for serious (clinical) adverse reactions. The most common cause of clinically significant drug–drug or herb–drug interaction is CYP450 inhibition (Mukherjee et al. 2011; Harwansh et al. 2014).

The cytochrome P450 isoenzymes (CYPs) predominantly present in the liver but are also found in the intestines, lungs, kidneys and brain. Several isoforms, such as CYP1A2, CYP2C9, CYP2D6 and CYP3A4 appear to be most relevant for the metabolism of clinically significant drugs. The medical literature is replete with reports suggesting that the concomitant use of these phytomolecules along with prescription medicines or over-the-counter products, which may alter human drug metabolism and pharmacokinetics, may cause serious clinical adverse reactions. Manufacturers' evaluations of these supplements for toxicology, preclinical and clinical data is not compulsory, and is not subject to standard pharmaceutical criteria for safety (Mukherjee et al. 2008).

The regulatory agencies require documentation on the interactions of herbal medicine involving CYP isoforms before licensing. Using *in vitro*, *in vivo* and *in silico* techniques, several phytoconstituents have been identified as inhibitors or inducers of cytochrome resulting in herb–drug interaction. Similarly, drug interactions between phytoconstituent and conventional medicines have also been reported. A few examples of such interactions of active compounds including allicin, quercetin and silymarin compounds have also been reported. Conventional pharmacokinetic literature generally deals with drug–drug interactions, but recently such interactions between phytoconstituents and prescription drugs have drawn attention, because of increasing physician awareness of the widespread adverse effects of undisclosed herbal use by patients. Establishing the safety of herbs using cytochrome modulating enzymes will attract TM manufacturers' attention to the potential marketing benefits (Mukherjee et al. 2010).

Herbal toxicokinetics deal with the prediction of toxicity due to pharmacokinetic disposition of an herb, or purified xenobiotics derived from it, due to genetics or from potential herb–drug interactions. Testing usually begins with assays using human liver microsomal Cytochrome P450 isoforms to identify metabolites that are known to cause toxicological modulation at any level of cellular organisation. Modulation of cytochrome P450 has great significance, as this largely affects drug biotransformation to active or inactive forms. For a drug that is dependent on these enzymes for inactivation via conjugation to chemical polar groups prior to elimination, any herb that induces these enzymes would lead to rapid inactivation and clearance of such a drug. Conversely, an herbal medicine that inhibits enzyme activity will lead to high concentrations of a drug whose inactivation relies on the inhibited enzyme. From findings in a recent survey (Bush et al. 2007), potential adverse drug–herb interactions were observed in 40% of patients receiving conventional therapy and taking an herbal product. Clinically significant drug–herb interactions may occur when a herb interacts with the metabolism of a co-administered drug and either reduces its efficacy due to decreased formation of an active metabolite or increases its toxicity due to reduced metabolic elimination. The latter type of interaction potentially predisposes human consumers to adverse reactions or toxic drug effects, especially if the drug has a narrow therapeutic range. Some herbs, notably St John's Wort (*Hypericum perforatum*), ginkgo (*Ginkgo biloba*), ginseng (*Panax ginseng*), kava (*Piper methysticum*) and garlic (*Allium sativum*) reportedly show significant interaction with some co-administered drugs by modulation of Cytochrome P450. In order to predict clinically significant effects that can occur when an herbal product inhibits or induces these enzymes, *in vitro* metabolic data can be used to correlate metabolic disposition of a test substance *in vivo*. From the early 1990s onwards, new techniques for generating as much information as possible from one experiment were developed, including DNA sequencing, microarrays to study gene expression, protein and metabolite profiling. Further structure-activity relationship of metabolites or pure compounds can be extrapolated from computer-based models and simulation studies. Thereafter, a pattern database of tissue/organ responses to drugs that allows for the parallel sequencing of all the relevant genes, measurement of genome transcription, protein expression and quantitation of metabolites produced by direct or indirect actions of the expressed protein is created. A final screening category for the compound or metabolite uses an integrative system biology approach, consisting of databases of metabolic pathways, genes, regulatory networks and protein interactions.

31.6 STABILITY STUDY OF AYURVEDIC FORMULATIONS

Ayurvedic medicine has been well explored for its diverse therapeutic potential, although lacks a complete study of its constituents, due to its complex nature. Evaluation of constituents is necessary to ensure the efficacy, quality, purity and stability of the finished product (Mukherjee et al. 2016). The stability study provides evidence of how the quality of a drug substance or product varies with time under the influence of a variety of environmental factors such as temperature, humidity, pH and light to establish a shelf life period for the Ayurvedic products at recommended storage conditions. Therefore, stability studies are very crucial aspects as an assessment of product quality (Patgiri et al. 2014). Ayurvedic formulations consist of more than one compound, so it is quite difficult to determine the single active compound that creates a problem in predicting the shelf life, because it is impossible to perform the Arrhenius equation and fix the rate of reaction that is taking place in the formulation for the estimation of shelf life or expiry periods. The marker analysis has been proved as a fruitful tool to check the quality and stability of Ayurvedic formulation (Gupta et al. 2011). Herbal medicine is still a challenge for developing into suitable dosage forms for promotion and development of human health. There are several challenges for developing an appropriate delivery system, due to their limited stability, as much as their low therapeutic efficacy and bioavailability. Research is now being concurrently conducted on basic as well as applied fields of herbal medicines, and this has led to the need for research in the delivery system of herbal drugs for maximum concentration as well as bioavailability (Mukherjee et al. 2015b).

The therapeutic efficacy of any Ayurvedic medication is dependent on delivery of an effective level of the bioactive constituents. Many herbal products demonstrated low therapeutic action due to solubility problems, which finally resulted in low bioavailability despite their extraordinary potential. However, a stark constraint exists in their bioavailability while administered orally. To overcome these limitations of absorption, developing novel drug delivery systems (NDDSs) with better absorption profiles is of premier importance. The therapeutic indices of the associated drugs are improved by increasing the drug concentration at the site of action. On the other hand, their bio-distribution is altered in favour of the diseased tissue. Value-added formulation, as its name suggests, is a formulation with supplementary value that provides better therapeutic efficacy of its main chemical constituents inside the body. The improvement of value-added herbal formulations having better absorption and uptake profiles in our body is the main goal. To lessen drug degradation and loss during the consumption of Ayurvedic drugs and to enhance their bioavailability, various drug delivery and drug targeting systems are being explored continuously (Mukherjee and Houghton et al. 2009).

31.7 REVERSE PHARMACOLOGY APPROACH IN AYURVEDA

Reverse pharmacology is a transdisciplinary approach based on observations of traditional practice, integrating traditional knowledge, clinical experiences and experimental observations with the aim of reversing from the classical laboratory to clinical practice. This reverse pharmacology approach can be used in Ayurveda-based drug discovery, in which drugs are first identified based on large-scale use in the population and validated in clinical trials. Time and cost are reduced for drug discovery from TM by reverse pharmacology. The Ayurvedic knowledge database allows drug researchers to start from a well-tested and safe botanical material and by using this knowledge, the conventional drug discovery begins from patients instead of laboratories. The reverse pharmacology approach first confirms the activity of a drug (like an Ayurvedic drug), after which further studies should link the activity to bioactive components. This method can emphasise the safety and efficacy and this is an alternative path for drug discovery. Drugs like reserpine, obtained from *Rauwolfia serpentina*, emerged only after 20 years of work although its antihypertensive property was demonstrated long ago. There is a need to document unknown, unintended and desirable novel prophylactic and therapeutic effects in observational therapeutics (Patawardhan and Vaidya 2010).

31.8 AYURINFORMATICS

There is a requirement of libraries for compounds present in Ayurvedic preparations. Although some institutions already have small plant extract libraries, they are not in the public domain. These libraries can serve as a powerful tool and source of extracts to be screened for biological activities using high-throughput assays. In recent years, a considerable body of information has accumulated on the chemical constituents of Ayurvedic herbs (Debnath et al. 2015). This is reflected in the appearance of a number of new electronic databases that contain both structural details of several thousand herbal constituents and accompanying information on their uses in Ayurveda. Although obscure at first, many of the therapeutic categories found in Ayurveda *Materia Medica* are interpretable in Western terminology and a variety of texts are now available in English. All the main classical works on Ayurveda, such as *Charaka Samhita*, *Sushruta Samhita*, *Ashtanga Sangraha* and *Ashtanga Hridaya*, deal with drugs with their composition and action in addition to the other aspects of the medical system (Mukherjee et al. 2015a).

31.9   CLINICAL STUDY AND PHARMACOVIGILANCE

The clinical study of classical Ayurveda is rare although huge knowledge resources and wisdom are available from many Ayurveda classic books and systematic data. Systematic documentation and reliable data on pharmacoepidemiology and pharmacovigilance related to the clinical practice, safety and adverse drug reactions are less available. As per present drug regulations in India, there are no scientific or clinical data required for manufacture and sale of classical Ayurvedic medicines. Good manufacturing practices (GMPs), quality control and pharmaceutical technologies for Ayurvedic medicine are evolving now. Issues related to appropriate research methodologies or treatment protocols for Ayurveda have also not been properly addressed. The status of Indian medicine and folk healing indicates the need to strengthen research and (Mukherjee 2003) use of Ayurveda, yoga, Unani, Siddha, homeopathy (AYUSH) systems in national healthcare. The evidence-based supports of scientific data are a prerequisite for good clinical practice, proper guidelines and documentation in Ayurvedic medicine. Recent efforts to develop robust clinical protocols for comparing the effectiveness of complex Ayurvedic and conventional treatments are laudable. Evidence-based validation needs good scientific research to support various theories in AM. Clinical practice and scientific research on AM is very necessary (Patwardhan and Vaidya 2010).

Pharmacovigilance is the practice of monitoring, evaluating and communicating drug safety with insightful suggestions that is subject to the reliability and cooperative responsibility of all parties, such as consumers, health professionals, researchers, academic, media, pharmaceutical industry, drug regulators, governments and international organisations. The main aim of pharmacovigilance is to spread the safety monitoring and detection of any adverse drug reactions that have previously been unrecognised in the evaluation of a clinical trial. These quality issues can be addressed to some degree by improved regulation requiring GMP standards for manufacturing. Pharmacovigilance is an indispensable tool for increasing reliable information on the safety of AM. The existing systems were developed for synthetic medicines and require some modification to address the specific differences of AM. Organised pharmacovigilance is indispensable to gather reliable information on the safety of herbal medicines for the development of appropriate guidelines for their safe and effective use (Mukherjee et al. 2010).

31.10   SUSTAINABILITY AND GLOBAL PROSPECTIVE OF AYURVEDIC MEDICINE

India has an ancient system of AM that provides a wealth of information on the folklore practices and traditional aspects of therapeutically important natural products. One of the major challenges of AM is quality, safety and efficacy issues and these things need to be more emphasised. The Ministry of AYUSH, Government of India, has taken several initiatives for the promotion and development of AM and ethnopharmacology at different levels, which consists of teaching institutions, government-funded research institutes, registered medical practitioners, hospitals, dispensaries and drug manufacturing units. Different national policies has been made to increase awareness about these systems by upgrading educational standards at national and international levels, keeping a vision to provide quality and standard of AM (Mukherjee et al. 2016).

Globalisation and reinforcement of AM is necessary for the establishment of evidence-based healthcare based on AM in consideration of its quality, safety, efficacy, therapeutic and clinical evidence. Science and technology has developed many techniques for the core disciplines including ethnomedicine, ethnobotany, ethnopharmacology and medical anthropology to raise AM to global awareness (Mukherjee et al. 2010). Establishment of global and regional regulatory harmonisation is obligatory for its promotion through scientific validation. The development of AM requires the convergence of modern techniques and integrated approaches related to their evidence-based research in various fields of science through worldwide coordination and cooperation. The question is raised: 'What are the global healthcare needs for medicinal agents?' The answer is hidden in the basic pillars, which are the foundation of global healthcare through natural resources. The pillars include information systems, botany, chemistry and system biology with well-designed and reported clinical studies. Thus, the systematic approach of AM is not about a single science or technique, but also amalgamation of these concomitant areas, which are mutually interrelated (Mukherjee 2001).

In order to address the growing market demand, there is a need of expeditious utilisation and scientific validation of medicinally useful plants globally, which requires 'globalising local knowledge and localising global technologies' through international collaboration and co-operation. Various approaches and technology to find out the perspective on globalisation of the traditional medicine and multiple objectives underlying efforts to develop, protect and promote traditional medicine are necessary for the betterment of the healthcare system. Development of effective guidelines for safety, efficacy and quality is regarded as a fundamental requirement in order to establish a solid evidence base for AM (Mukherjee et al. 2013).

31.11   KNOWLEDGE BASE FOR DRUG DEVELOPMENT IN AYURVEDA

There has been a development in the education and communication to disseminate the sources of Ayurvedic knowledge interpretable in Western terminology, and a variety of texts are now available online. The National Institute of Indian Medical Heritage (http://niimh.nic.in/) under the CCRAS, Ministry of AYUSH, has published e-Samhitas of all the main classical works on Ayurveda, such as *Charaka Samhita, Sushruta Samhita, Ashtanga Sangraha, Ashtanga Hridaya* and *Bhava Prakasha Nighantu* that are available online. The Pharmacopoeial Laboratory of India (PLIM, http://www.plimism.nic.in/) has published monographs for 326 single drugs of plant origin and 83 compound formulations of Ayurveda in several volumes as the Ayurvedic Pharmacopoeia of India (Anonymous 2008). The Ayurvedic Formulary of India deals with drugs, their composition and action in addition to the other aspects of the medical system. The Essential Drug List of Ayurveda has also been published by the Ministry of AYUSH, which contains 277 essential medicines of Ayurveda for familiar diseases in a tabular, readily available form. The *Materia Medica* of Ayurveda consists of an extremely rich armamentarium of natural drugs, derived from the plant, mineral, animal and marine sources. These drugs are used as monotherapies or in simple combinations, which are otherwise referred to as polypharmaceuticals. The forms in which these are used are varied, including extracted juices, decoctions, infusions, distillates, powders, tablets, pills, confections, syrups, fermented liquids, medicated oil, *bhasmas* (resulting from incineration) and many more. The *Materia Medica* of Ayurveda is an exhaustive publication that describes simple, safe and proven remedies, including remedies for common ailments. The *Treatise on Indian Medicinal Plants*, edited by A. Chatterjee and S. C. Pakrashi (1991), is a five-volume treatise, with each volume containing 180–325 pages. These volumes contain over 800 medicinal plants. This book also serves as a search engine for many scientific studies and clinical trials conducted on Ayurvedic therapies during the last 5 decades. A recent book on the scientific basis of Ayurvedic therapies, edited by L. C. Mishra, also summarises many of these findings. The *Compendium of Indian Medicinal Plants*, edited by R. Rastogi and B. N. Mehrotra, has published five volumes so far, with 518–1016 pages per volume. (Balachandran and Govindarajan 2007). The AYUSH Research Portal (http://ayushportal.nic.in/) presents evidence-based research data on AYUSH systems at a global level and is also a significant source of scientific knowledge. Some of the Ayurvedic books called *Nighantu Granthas* (lexica) – such as *Dhanvantari-Nighantu, Kaiyadeva-Nighantu, Bhava Prakasha Nighantu, Raja-Nighantu* – deal mainly with a single drug, describing its habitat, characteristics and therapeutic action.

Ayurvedic drugs are derived from different vegetable, animal and plant sources. Ayurvedic formulations, which are predominantly derived from plants, are known as *kasthausadhi*, where the formulations are made from the extract or juice of plants' parts. These include several Ayurvedic formulations like *aristra*, *avleha*, *grafa*, *churna* and *taila*. Formulations that are predominantly derived from metal and minerals are known as '*rasausadhi*'; these are made mainly from minerals and in combinations of minerals and plants, including *bhasma*, *pishti*, *lauha*, *kapibadkva* and *rasayana* (Mukherjee et al. 2010). A detailed description of all these formulations has been provided elsewhere in this chapter. The Ministry of AYUSH has launched many authentic books on both groups of compound formulations. While *Sarngadhara Samhita*, *Cakradatta*, *Bhaisajya Ratnavali*, *Sahasrayogam*, *Bharat Bhaisajya Ratnakara* and so on deal with both groups of formulations, others like *Rasendra Sara Sangraha*, *Rasaratna Samuccaya*, *Rasa Prakasha Sudhakara*, *Ayurveda Prakasha*, *Rasa Tarangini*, *Rasa Yogasagara* and so on deal only with the *rasausadhi* group of formulations. However, globally, there is a need to build molecular libraries for Ayurvedic phytoconstituents along with their probable mechanism of action and other databases regarding systems pharmacology, gene and target protein network and disease network.

Although some institutions have small plant extract libraries, they are not in the public domain. Such books could serve as a powerful tool and source of extracts to be screened for biological activities using high-throughput assays. However in recent years, a considerable volume of information has accumulated on the chemical constituents of Ayurvedic herbs. The development of suitable dosage forms of Ayurvedic or herbal drugs is still a challenging task. Some primary constraints for developing an appropriate delivery system are the limited solubility and permeability of herbal drugs through biological membranes. The herbal medicine therefore shows little therapeutic efficacy and bioavailability. Research is now being concurrently conducted on basic as well as applied fields of herbal medicines, and this has created the need for studies in the delivery system of herbal drugs for maximum bioavailability (Mukherjee and Houghton et al. 2009). The biological half-life ($t_{1/2}$) has an immense role in the therapeutic efficacy and potency of drug molecules at the site where it administered. If the drugs have shorter $t_{1/2}$, then it possesses low bioavailability compared to higher $t_{1/2}$. Biological membrane permeability offers more activity for lipophilic drugs. Hence, its chances of availability in the blood/plasma are greater in comparison to the hydrophilic drug. However, a number of the active pharmaceutical ingredients (API) obtained from high-throughput screening are poorly soluble molecules. Lower bioavailability results from poor solubility and incomplete dissolution *in vivo*. These are often holding back continuous development and coming into the market with some promising new chemical entities (NCEs), or elicits insufficient therapeutic effects from certain drugs. Hence, innovative formulation approaches are gaining attention for acquiring better bioavailability levels after oral administration (Rahman et al. 2013). In this context, novel drug delivery systems (NDDS) efficiently overcome some of the drawbacks associated with herbal drugs.

31.12   TRADITIONAL AYURVEDIC FORMULATIONS

Ayurvedic treatments are enriched by accepting and adopting the outcomes of experience. There are several formulations available from the Ayurvedic Formulary and Pharmacopoeia of India, which have been explored to a wide extent for treatment of several disorders and have a potential market as well. A list of the most important Ayurvedic formulations available in the Indian market has been produced in Table 31.2 (Mukherjee et al. 2010).

Drug delivery systems for Ayurvedic drugs are classified according to their method of preparation. They are described in the Ayurvedic Formulary of India (AFI), an official publication of the Government of India.

TABLE 31.2
Several Ayurvedic Formulations Used Extensively in Present-Day Practice as Prescribed in the Ayurvedic Formulary of India

Name of Formulation	Intended Use
Triphala	Increased frequency and turbidity of urine, diseases of eye, diseases of skin, dyspepsia, loss of sense of taste, intermittent fever
Chawanprash	Cough, asthma, debility due to chest injury, hoarseness of voice, heart disease, digestive impairment, urinary disease, diseases of semen, boosts immunity, ageing problems
Aswagandha aristha	Syncope, epilepsy, psychosis, cachexia, piles, digestive impairment
Asokaristha	Dysmenorrhea pain in female genital tract, leucorrhea, fever, bleeding disorder, piles, loss of sense of taste, excessive flow of urine, inflammation
Bhaskar lavan	Digestive impairment, pain/colic, malabsorption syndrome, spleen disease, diseases of abdomen, piles, constipation, anal fistula, oedema, rheumatism, angina pectoris
Draksharistha	Cough, digestive impairment, chest wound, laxative, weakness, disease of throat
Baiswanar choorna	Flatulence with gurgling sound, abdominal lump, duodenal ulcer, rheumatism, heart disease, diseases of urinary bladder, spleen disease, anorectal disease, constipation, disease of the limbs
Chandraprava vati	Constipation, distension of abdomen due to obstruction to passage of urine and stools, cyst, anaemia, jaundice, dysuria, piles, urinary obstruction, lower backache, itching, splenomegaly, loss of sense of taste
Sankha vati	Digestive impairment, malabsorption syndrome, loss of sense of taste, duodenal ulcer, phthisis
Dasamularista	Loss of sense of taste, emesis, malabsorption syndrome, abdominal lump, tissue wasting, piles, anal fistula, anaemia, excessive flow of urine, gravel in urine, infertility, emaciation, weakness
Punarnavasava	Hyperacidity, abdominal lump, inflammation, diseases of liver
Trikatu	Improves digestion strength, balances *kapha dosha*, burns fat, reduces cholesterol levels, useful in skin, diseases, running nose, allergic rhinitis, relieves anorexia, relieve indigestion, diabetes, abdominal tumour, bloating, throat infection and diseases
Yograj Guggul Tablet	Treatment of rheumatoid arthritis, gout, worm infestation. Infected wounds, splenomegaly, and abdominal tumours

31.12.1 CLASSICAL PREPARATIONS OF AYURVEDA

31.12.1.1 Asavas and Arishtas

These preparations are made by soaking the herb in a sugar solution for a specified period. Thus, it undergoes fermentation, producing alcohol, which extracts active principles and acts also as a preservative. Examples include *draksharishta* containing *Vitis vinifera* Linn. as a major ingredient, and *devadarvarista* with *Cedrus deodara* Loud as a major ingredient (Anonymous 2002a).

31.12.1.2 Arka

A liquid preparation obtained by distillation of certain liquids or herbs soaked in water using the distillation apparatus. For example, *ajamodarka*, which is used as a digestive, contains *Apium graveolens* as the main ingredient.

31.12.1.3 Avaleha or Leha and Paka

These are semisolid preparations, prepared with the addition of sugar or sugar candy and boiled with the prescribed juice of the herbs or its decoction. *Kutajavaleha* consist of *Holarrhena antidysenterica* used in treating hyperacidity, anaemia and diarrhoea.

31.12.1.4 Churna

Powder of herb(s), where a single herb or combinations of herbs are made into a coarse powder (*javkut*); for example, *narasimha churna* is used in the treatment of cough and fever and contains *Tinospora cordifolia* Miers and *Semecarpus anacardium* Linn. as the main ingredients.

31.12.1.5 Guggulu

A resinous material obtained from the plant *Commiphora wightii*. Preparations containing guggul as the main effective ingredient are known as *guggulu*. Among five different varieties, *Mahisaksa* and *Kanaka* guggulu are usually preferred for medicinal preparation. Examples include *Kaishore* guggulu (contains mainly *T. cordifolia* Miers) and *Kanchanar* guggulu (contains mostly *Bauhinia purpurea* Linn.).

31.12.1.6 Ghritas (Snehakalpa)

Preparation in which ghee (clarified butter derived from milk) is boiled with the prescribed decoction of drugs according to the formula as prescribed in the Ayurvedic text. This process ensures absorption of the active therapeutic principles of the ingredients used. For example, *Asoka ghrita* is used in the treatment of pelvic pain, lower backache and anaemia and contains *Saraca asoca* de Wilde as the major herb.

31.12.1.7 Taila

Preparations in which oil is boiled with the prescribed decoction of drugs according to the formula. This process ensures incorporation of the active therapeutic principles of the ingredients of the plant. Examples are *Prasarini* taila (principal part, *Paederia foetida* Linn.) and *Bhringaraja* taila (primary component, *Eclipta alba* Linn.).

31.12.1.8 Dravakas

Liquid preparations obtained from *lavanas* (rock salts) and *ksaras* (alkaline) by a distillation process with or without any addition of fluids. *Ksaras* are alkaline substances derived from the ash of drugs. The drugs are cut into small pieces, dried, kept in an earthen pot and burnt to ash. *Shankha dravaka* is used in treating diseases of the abdomen and spleen and contains *Calotropis procera* R. Br. and *Euphorbia neriifolia* Linn. along with other ingredients.

31.12.1.9 Lepa

Lepa is used for topical applications in the form of a paste. The drugs are made into a fine powder. Before use on the body, it is mixed with a liquid or any other medium indicated for each preparation to make a soft paste. Water, cow's urine, oil and ghee are some of the media used for mixing. *Avalgujadi lepa* (contains *Psoralea corylifolia* Linn.) and *Pathyadi lepa* (contains *Terminalia chebula* Retz. along with other ingredients) are some of the examples of this category.

31.12.1.10 Vati and Gutika

Vati and *gutika* are medicinal preparations in the form of tablets or pills. They are made of one or more drugs of plant, animal, or mineral origin. *Khadiradi gutika* is one example that contains *Acacia catechu* Willd. and is used in the treatment of halitosis, diseases of the teeth and dental cavities (caries).

31.12.1.11 Vartti, Netra Bindu and Anjana

Preparations used externally for the eye. *Nalikeranjana* (containing *Berberis aristata* DC and *Glycyrrhiza glabra* Linn.) and *Tamradi gutika* (containing *Glycyrrhiza glabra* Linn. and *Saussurea lappa* C.B. Clarke, along with other ingredients) are examples of this category.

31.12.1.12 Bhasma and Pishti

In Ayurveda, use of both *bhasma* (residue after incineration or calcined preparation), as well as pishti (powdered gems or metal) along with appropriate herbs is recommended for treatment of critical ailments. The procedures for preparing these medicines are time-consuming and complicated. *Bhasma* is a calcined preparation in which the gem or metal is converted into ash. Gems or metals are purified to remove impurities and treated by triturating and macerating in herbal extracts. The dough so obtained is then calcinated to obtain the ashes through *bhasmikaran*. *Bhasmikaran* is the process by which a substance that is otherwise bio-incompatible is made biocompatible by certain *samskaras* or processes. The objectives of *samskara* include the elimination of harmful matters from the drug and modification of undesirable physical properties to enhance the therapeutic action. For example, *loha bhasma* (ash made from iron) is the main ingredient of preparations like *lauha kalpas* (Anonymous 2002b).

31.12.1.13 Rasa Yoga

Rasa yoga contains mineral drugs as the main components and may be in pill or powder form. Examples are *Amlapittantaka rasa* (contains *T. chebula* Retz.) and *Ananda Bhairava rasa* (includes *Piper nigrum* Linn. and *Piper longum* Linn. (Anonymous 2002b)).

31.13 CONCLUSION

Traditional knowledge and heritage is currently assumed as a knowledgebase of time-tested concepts that may inspire novel scientific discovery. However we need to find a balance between evidence and belief. In this discourse, it may occur that the traditional practice bears some extraordinary technologies that need appreciation and proper validation ahead of time. Ayurveda-inspired discoveries present a similar scenario, where evidence-based approaches to develop new healthcare solutions are crucial to address the rising interest globally. However there are several challenges of translating ancient knowledge to the lab and then to the market. Future discoveries should make this process easier as more evidence is being generated – as of now it is not even the tip of iceberg.

REFERENCES

Anonymous. (2002a). *The Ayurvedic Formulary of India, Part 1*, 2nd ed. New Delhi, India: The Controller of Publications.

Anonymous. (2002b). *The Ayurvedic Formulary of India, Part II*. New Delhi, India: Department of Indian System of Medicine and Homeopathy.

Anonymous. (2008). *API (The Ayurvedic Pharmacopoeia of India)*, Part I, Vol. I. New Delhi, India: Government of India, Ministry of Health and Family Welfare, Department of AYUSH.

Balachandran, P. and Govindarajan R. (2007). Ayurvedic drug discovery. *Expert Opinion on Drug Discovery*, **2**, 1631–1652.

Banks, R., Dunn, M., Hochstrasser, D., Sanchez, J., Blackstock, W., Pappin, D. and Selby, P. (2000). Proteomics: New perspectives, new biomedical opportunities. *Lancet*, **356**, 1749–1756.

Bush, T. M., Rayburn, K. S., Holloway, S. W. et al. (2007). Adverse interactions between herbal and dietary substances and prescription medications: A clinical survey. *Alternative Therapies in Health and Medicine*, **13**, 30–35.

Chandran, U., Mehendale, N., Tillu, G. and Patwardhan, B. (2015). Network pharmacology: An emerging technique for natural product drug discovery and scientific research on Ayurveda. *Proceedings of the Indian National Science Academy*, **81**, 561–568.

Chatterjee, A. and Pakrashi, C.S. (1991). *The Treatise on Indian Medicinal Plants*, 1st ed. New Delhi, India: Publications & Information Directorate.

Chen, S., Song, J., Sun, C., Xu, J., Zhu, Y., Verpoorte, R. and Fan, T. (2015). Herbal genomics: Examining the biology of traditional medicines, The art and science of traditional medicine: Part 2: Multidisciplinary approaches for studying traditional medicine. *Science*, **347**(6219), S27–S29.

Cordell, G. A. and Colvard, M. D. (2012). Natural products and traditional medicine: Turning on a paradigm. *Journal of Natural Products,* **75**, 514–525.

Debnath, P. K., Banerjee, S., Debnath, P., Mitra, A. and Mukherjee, P. K. (2015). Ayurveda – Opportunities for developing safe and effective treatment choices for the future. In P. K. Mukherjee, ed., *Evidence-Based Validation of Herbal Medicines.* Elsevier. pp. 427–454.

Franz, C., Chizzola., R., Novak, J. and Sponza, S. (2011). Botanical species being used for manufacturing plant food supplements (PFS) and related products in the EU member states and selected third countries. *Food & Function,* **2**, 720.

Govindaraj, P., Nizamuddin, S., Sharath, A., et al. (2015). Genome-wide analysis correlates Ayurveda Prakriti. *Scientific Reports,* **5**, 15786, 1–12. doi:10.1038/srep15786.

Gupta, A., Jaiswal, M. and Prajapati, P. K. (2011). Shelf life of Ayurvedic dosage forms-traditional view, current status and prospective need. *Indian Journal of Traditional Knowledge,* **10**(4), 672–677.

Hopkins A. (2008). Network pharmacology: The next paradigm in drug discovery. *Nature Chemical Biology,* **4**, 682–690.

Hussain, G. S., Upadhyay, P., Das, S. and Sharma, M. P. (2015). Authentication of medicinal plants by DNA markers. *Plant Gene,* **4**, 83–99.

Lavekar, G. S. (2006). Scientific validation of drug development and clinical research in Ayurveda. *AYU,* **20**, 66–85.

Li, X., Yang, Y., Henry, R. J., Rossetto, M., Wang, Y. and Chen, S. (2015). Plant DNA barcoding: From gene to genome. *Biological Reviews of the Cambridge Philosophical Society,* **90**(1), 157–166.

Mukherjee, H., Ojha, D., Bag, P., Chandel, H. S., Bhattacharyya, S., Chatterjee, T. K., Mukherjee P. K., Chakraborti, S. and Chattopadhyay, D. (2013). Anti-herpes virus activities of *Achyranthes aspera*: An Indian ethnomedicine, and its triterpene acid. *Microbiological Research,* **168**, 238–244.

Mukherjee, P. K. (2001). Evaluation of Indian traditional medicine. *Drug Information Journal,* **35**, 623–631.

Mukherjee, P. K. (2003). Exploring botanicals in Indian systems of medicine-regulatory perspectives. *Clinical Research and Regulatory Affairs,* **20**, 249–263.

Mukherjee, P. K. (2002). *Quality Control of Herbal Drugs: An Approach to Evaluation of Botanicals,* 1st ed. New Delhi, India: Business Horizons.

Mukherjee, P. K., Bahadur, S., Chaudhary, S. K., Kar, A. and Mukherjee, K. (2015a). Quality related safety issue-evidence-based validation of herbal medicine – Farm to pharma. In P. K. Mukherjee, Ed. *Evidence-Based Validation of Herbal Medicine.* Amsterdam, the Netherlands: Elsevier Science. pp. 1–27.

Mukherjee, P. K., Bahadur, S., Harwansh, R. K. and Chaudhary, S. K. (2014). Shifting paradigm for validation of medicinal plants in Indian traditional medicine. *Indian Drugs,* **51**(8), 5–14.

Mukherjee, P. K., Bahadur S., Harwansh, R. K., et al. (2017b). Paradigm shift in natural product research: Traditional medicine inspired approaches. *Phytochemistry Reviews,* **16**, 803.

Mukherjee, P. K., Harwansh, R. K., Bahadur, S., Banerjee, S. and Kar, A. (2016). Evidence based validation of Indian traditional medicine – Way forward. *World Journal of Traditional Chinese Medicine,* **2**, 48–61.

Mukherjee, P. K., Harwansh, R. K., Bahadur, S., Banerjee, S., Kar, A., Chanda, J., Biswas, S., Ahmmed, S. M. and Katiyar, C. K. (2017a). Development of Ayurveda – Tradition to trend. *Journal of Ethnopharmacology,* **197**, 10–24.

Mukherjee, P. K., Harwansh, R. K. and Bhattacharyya, S. (2015b). Bioavailability of herbal products: Approach toward improved pharmacokinetics. In P. K. Mukherjee, Ed. *Evidence based Validation of Herbal Medicine.* Amsterdam, the Netherlands: Elsevier. pp. 217–245.

Mukherjee, P. K. and Houghton, P. J. (2009). The worldwide phenomenon of increased use of herbal products: Opportunity and threats. In *Evaluation of Herbal Medicinal Products – Perspectives on Quality, Safety and Efficacy,* 1st ed. London, UK: Pharmaceutical Press. pp. 3–12.

Mukherjee, P. K., Kumar, V., Kumar, N. S. and Heinrich, M. (2008). The Ayurvedic medicine *Clitoria ternatea* – From traditional use to scientific assessment. *Journal of Ethnopharmacology,* **120**(3), 291–301.

Mukherjee, P. K., Nema, N. K., Venkatesh, P., Debnath, P. K. (2012). Changing scenario for promotion and development of Ayurveda way forward. *Journal of Ethnopharmacology,* **143**, 424–434.

Mukherjee, P. K. and Ponnusankar, S. (2010). Exploring pharmacovigilance for traditional herbal medicines. In V. K. Gupta, S. C. Taneja and B. D. Gupta, Eds., *Comprehensive Bioactive Natural Products: Quality Control & Standardization,* Vol. 8. New Delhi, India: Studium Press LLC. pp. 248–280.

Mukherjee, P. K., Ponnusankar, S. and Venkatesh, M. (2011). Synergy in herbal medicinal products: Concept to realization. *Indian Journal of Pharmaceutical Education and Research,* **45**(3), 210–217.

Patgiri, B., Soni, H. and Bhatt, S. (2014). Evaluation of stability study of Ayurvedic formulation – Rasayana Churna. *Journal of Pharmacognosy and Phytochemistry,* **2**(5), 126–130.

Patwardhan, B. and Vaidya, A. D. (2010). Natural products drug discovery: Accelerating the clinical candidate development using reverse pharmacology approaches. *Indian Journal of Experimental Biology,* **48**(3), 220–227.

Rahman, M. A., Hussain, A., Iqbal, Z., Harwansh, R. K., Singh, L. R. and Ahmad, S. (2013). Nanosuspension: A potential nanoformulation for improved delivery of poorly bioavailable drug. *Micro and Nanosystems,* **5**, 273–287.

Sen, S. and Chakraborty, R. (2017). Revival, modernization and integration of Indian traditional herbal medicine in clinical practice: Importance, challenges and future. *Journal of Traditional and Complementary Medicine,* **7**, 234–244.

32 Natural Medicine
Potential in Public Healthcare and Research with Specific Focus on Ayurveda

Ajay George Varghese

CONTENTS

Nature has provided amazing resources for the treatment and cure of diseases for centuries. Mankind have always been dependant on nature for its primary healthcare and wellness solutions. Nature offers immense resources in terms of flora and fauna that are increasingly being explored by human society to provide solutions for its ever-increasing needs. However, the challenges posed in the healthcare arena are also increasing.

32.1 RISING HEALTHCARE THREATS AND CHALLENGES

Lifestyle diseases are posing an ever-increasing challenge owing to the unhealthy sedentary lifestyle and habits. Epidemic outbreaks are becoming a larger threat with mutant pathogens creating challenges to healthcare and public healthcare systems. Diseases such as cancer and

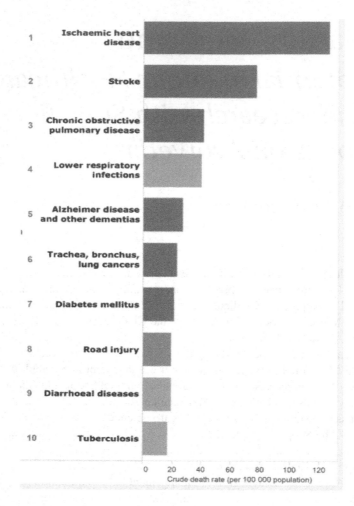

FIGURE 32.1 Top 10 causes of death—both ages and all sexes. (From World Health Organization, 2018.)

HIV are posing serious threats to human society, in spite of major developments in medical science (Figure 32.1). Antibiotic-resistant pathogens are posing a serious threat in containing infectious diseases.

32.2 HEALTHCARE EXPENDITURE AND PUBLIC HEALTHCARE

Public healthcare management across the world is a serious challenge owing to larger outlays required and the wide gaps in effective healthcare delivery. Healthcare spending today is a major responsibility for the government, and the outlay required for every country is a major economic challenge (Figure 32.2).

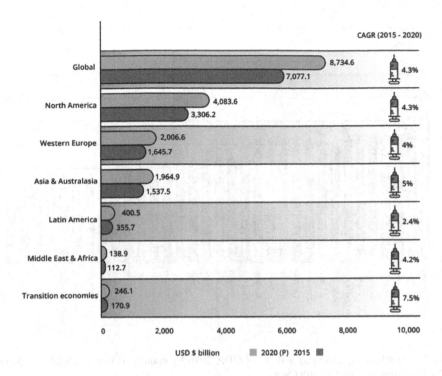

FIGURE 32.2   Healthcare spending, 2015–2020. (From 2018 Global healthcare outlook, The evolution of smart healthcare.)

32.3   NEW DRUG DEVELOPMENT – CHALLENGES

New drug development is another challenge area owing to the high cost of development of new molecules. The discovery and launch of new blockbuster drugs in the recent past was paltry in the last few decades. The risk in the area of new drug development has significantly escalated and has mostly witnessed abbreviated versions of existing patents or repurposing of erstwhile blockbusters.

The scenario is quite critical and needs to be evaluated from a perspective of future healthcare management and policy. The current state of affairs in the healthcare sector calls for a critical review of the existing systems, policy and possible approaches for the effective management of future healthcare challenges. Healthcare costs are significant and cannot be ignored at any cost in the current and future scenario. Figure 32.3 demonstrates the heath care expenditure as a share of country GDP.

Public healthcare calls for new approaches and interventions for effective management of diseases and disease control. The emphasis laid on primary healthcare management may need to shift towards preventive healthcare and wellness, which may be less costly to manage than to control and to cure.

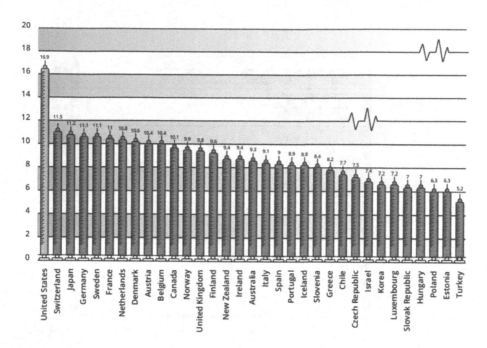

FIGURE 32.3 Healthcare spending as a share of GDP, 2016 by country. (From 2018 Global Health Care Outlook: The Evolution of Smart Health Care.)

The Kerala (an Indian state with a high track record of healthcare management) model of healthcare can be a good case to evaluate the effective management of healthcare. Kerala has a strong network of public specialised hospitals, hospitals and primary healthcare centres – both in modern medicine, Ayurveda and other systems of medicine, which offer highly subsidised medical care for the population. The dependence of people on both systems is chosen by patients on the basis of the effectiveness of the medical system. One of the recent mass healthcare intervention during floods has provided insights that the rural population of the state had a marked inclination towards Ayurveda for primary healthcare. However, people relied on modern medicine for the management of infectious diseases and acute conditions.

Therefore, it is quite important to review the various effective healthcare management approaches worldwide to develop a novel and cost-effective medical system.

32.4 TRADITIONAL MEDICINE – SCOPE FOR RESEARCH AND CHALLENGES

Traditional medicine is widely followed worldwide, especially in two major populous countries – India and China. Traditional medicine was always part of the healthcare management process in these countries for many centuries. Billions of people in these economies still follow their traditional health systems alongside the modern system of medicine.

A vast majority of the population in Africa still follows their local health tradition, which was followed generations ago. The local health traditions were followed in their respective regions for thousands of years, as compared with the modern medical science, which is in use for a few hundreds of years. The fact is most of these sciences were well documented, and the phytochemistry of the herbs, parts, processing, purification and even drug interactions were fairly well documented for many centuries.

32.5 HEALTHCARE – THE KERALA SCENARIO

The Kerala healthcare model is a case in point for the relevance of traditional medicine in public healthcare management. The State of Kerala, India, is rated one of the most evolved in terms healthcare indicators and can compare its health parameters with many developed nations. Kerala state has over 898 dispensaries and 126 hospitals with over 4037 beds and 16,639 registered practitioners in the Ayurveda public healthcare system according to AYUSH Ministry data. The average life expectancy in the state is 74.9 years (2016). The state has a very high penetration of state-run traditional medicine primary health centres in almost every *panchayat* (the smallest administrative unit of the government) and most its rural population relies on these centres as their primary healthcare option.

32.6 AYURVEDA IN PUBLIC HEALTHCARE MANAGEMENT

It would further be interesting evaluate the healthcare scenario in the State of Kerala, India, to understand the significant contribution of Ayurveda to healthcare management. Kerala is one of the top-ranking states in India on healthcare management and delivery. Kerala has one of the highest life expectancy and the lowest child mortality rates in India, which are comparable to developed countries. The bed to patient ratio is definitely better compared to rest of India, although it may not be comparable to the developed world.

The achievement in terms of public healthcare delivery vis-à-vis the cost may be substantially low compared to the developed economies. A significant point to be noted in this context in the Kerala scenario is the emphasis provided on Ayurveda in healthcare management. Kerala is one of the states in India that has an Ayurveda primary healthcare centre in every village. The preventive healthcare system is part of the public healthcare system and this could have contributed to the improved healthcare parameters in the state.

If the above parameters and cases are critically evaluated, a few pertinent points are often raised. The major deficiency cited in the case of traditional systems of medicine is the lack of data on clinical efficacy, safety and toxicology.

This necessitates some thought on the compilation of safety and effectiveness data. Ayush (the Ministry of Ayurveda, Yoga, Unani, Siddha and Homeopathy) has recently introduced Ayur Grid to capture and compile data of clinical outcomes done in various hospitals, clinics and health centres in India.

India has a large network of Ayurveda hospitals and clinics, and more specifically in Kerala, all panchayats (the basic governing unit) have an Ayurvedic public healthcare unit. Typically innumerable patients use medical services at these centres. If the clinical documentation is enabled on a computerised grid, the outcome could provide extensive data on clinical outcomes and intervention methodologies. This could lead to huge insights into drug development and identification of potential active molecules.

Clinical protocols and scientific validation often thrust upon traditional medicines and systems are guidelines followed by the modern systems of medicine. Each system of medicine must be studied in its own context, framework and as per the guidelines laid down or developed for the specific system, as against the protocols followed in other systems. A more objective and integrated understanding is required for the evaluation of the safety and efficacy of each system than the current system of comparing one system with the other on the basis of the research framework evolved by one.

This approach always results in outcomes that are not always acceptable and are questionable. However, the interest generated on such research outcomes carries more importance than the objective evaluation of the systems for public healthcare management or research. Therefore lot of time is wasted in defending or in establishing the validity of traditional medicinal systems, rather than assessing the appropriateness of the same for healthcare management. Traditional medicines certainly offer sustainable solutions, especially in preventive healthcare, NCD management and also in lifestyle modification for better health outcomes at substantially lower costs.

Traditional medicinal systems across the world, if studied in depth, can offer solutions for health conditions and can offer significant leads in drug development. Safety and efficacy are often the most projected concern, but this is probably a mirage when objectivity is brought into the assessment of safety and efficacy. Countries such as India have already embarked on clinical documentation programmes that have commenced capturing data on the various clinical interventions in the traditional medicine programmes.

32.7   TRADITIONAL MEDICINE INTERVENTION IN DISASTER MANAGEMENT IN KERALA FLOOD RELIEF

The State of Kerala was affected by a massive flood, which caused widespread damage and displacement of people and created havoc in the state. It is interesting to observe there the intervention of the traditional medicine department with the private sector in the post-flood relief measures. The medical teams were able to effectively offer medical support and post-flood relief using traditional medicinal knowledge to many flood-affected victims. The above initiative was also well documented and is at present being compiled to assess the outcomes of traditional medicine in disaster management (Thomas and James 2014).

32.8   AYURVEDA – THE INDIAN SYSTEM OF TRADITIONAL MEDICINE: SCOPE AND CHALLENGE

Ayurveda – an age-old healthcare science that has defied time – holds huge potential in healthcare management both in terms of its approach and its delivery mechanism. The term *Ayur* means life and *Veda* means science.

Ayurveda is an age-old science known to be in existence and practiced for over a few thousand years in India. It served as a sustainable healthcare system and was the solution for a large population for many generations. Ayurveda served as the source and the means for healthcare management for one of the largest demographics in the world today. The shift towards modern medicine in a country like India can be traced back only a few centuries.

32.9   AYURVEDA – POTENTIAL IN HEALTHCARE MANAGEMENT

This system of science has often been misunderstood and misinterpreted as an alternative system and was also often labelled as unscientific, which should be considered far from true. It is invariably a very scientific and advanced science in terms of its approach and has quite a well documented and codified knowledge base. The utility of this system is not derived owing to it being classified as an alternate healthcare system that is not validated. However, world is overlooking to assess its significance and potential in addressing the healthcare issues and problems worldwide.

32.10   AYURVEDA AS A SUSTAINABLE MODERN HEALTHCARE SCIENCE

Ayurveda holds tremendous potential as a healthcare science both in preventive healthcare and delivery. It holds significant leads for the development of potential new drug candidates. Primarily, it is a well-codified, documented science based on a huge database of herbal and non-herbal substances. The formulation process is well defined and based on principles that parallel current scientific thought, approaches and principles. The texts of Ayurveda clearly define the pre-processing of herbal raw materials, which optimises the herbal active ingredients such that they can equate to the current thoughts in modern pharmacology. Modern science would have to apply scientific methodology and protocols to validate the results and scientifically substantiate the science.

Modern science and technology certainly enable us to define and enumerate the pharmacological outcomes of herbs and herbal combinations. It also allows quantification of clinical outcomes and enables us to validate the qualitative aspects of the process at all stages. However, the status of the evaluation and assessment of pharmacological outcomes is limited or has not matched the potential of the science in new drug development.

32.11 AYURVEDA – THE SCOPE IN RESEARCH

Ayurveda medical science is based on a raw material base that includes diverse plants and non-plant sources, and this raw material base holds immense promise for exploration and scientific investigations. Diverse diseases and disease conditions both acute and sub-acute find clear mention in the Ayurvedic texts. The Ayurveda knowledge base mentions diverse formulations for various health states and conditions. The Ayurvedic texts also clearly define each herb, herbal part and even purification methodology quite clearly, which can be correlated to modern sciences for definition. The basic principles of *Tridosha* can be easily defined in modern scientific terminology and correlation is already in progress.

32.12 CHALLENGES

There is a lack of knowledge of Ayurveda databases among the modern scientific research fraternity. There is a wealth of elaborate information arranged in a generalised manner with specific references to certain acute conditions, which would be understood with expertise/knowledge of Ayurveda, but the knowledge base may appear to be codified, unorganised and encrypted (Sanskrit or local language), so the definition may require external support. There are significant comprehensive data, but the disease conditions are often mentioned in Sanskrit or a local language and not in modern scientific terminology, which makes it difficult to analyse and decipher. There is also a lack of clinical protocols and scientific methodology, which means that internal research was often not at a par with modern scientific studies.

32.13 METHODOLOGY FOR RESEARCH IN AYURVEDA

Extensive scope exists in leveraging Ayurvedic knowledge with the scientific protocols and tools available today in modern science. Scientific methodology and profiling has become very advanced for analysing, understanding and deciphering the fundamental philosophy and principles of Ayurveda.

32.14 INTEGRATED APPROACH – DIAGNOSIS AND MANAGEMENT

An integrated multi-disciplinary patient-centric approach is required in the diagnosis and management of health conditions. This approach could help create a standardised protocol for the management of various conditions.

32.15 CONCLUSION

Nature is the biggest treasure trove of medicines and can offer solutions for the effective management of preventive and lifestyle disease management, which imposes a big challenge in public healthcare. An integrated approach in healthcare management that blends modern medicine, science and natural medicinal solutions can be a good approach in public healthcare delivery at a lower cost with better effectiveness. Nature already offers that majority of the leads in new drug development, but better understanding and validation utilising modern scientific protocols and methods can help establish the safety and efficacy of the individual drugs and combinations. In conclusion, a new approach in healthcare management and research that synchronises herbal knowledge, research and an integrated approach towards public healthcare could provide significant outcomes in healthcare management at a lower cost.

REFERENCES

Deloitte. (2018). *2018 Global health care outlook: The evolution of smart health care* [white paper]. London, UK: Deloitte. Available from: https://www2.deloitte.com/global/en/pages/about-deloitte/articles/global-health-care-sector-outlook-working-towards-smart-health-care.html.

India. Ministry of AYUSH. (2019). *Ministry of AYUSH*. Available from: http://www.ayush.gov.in.

Kerala. Directorate of Health Services. (2019). *Kerala Directorate of Health Services*. Available from: http://dhs.kerala.gov.in.

Thomas, M. B. and James, K. S. (2014). Changes in mortality and human longevity in Kerala: Are they leading to the advanced stage. *Global Health Action*, **7**(1), 22938. doi:10.3402/gha.v7.22938.

World Health Organization. (2019). *World Health Organization*. Available from: http://www.who.int.

Index

Note: Page numbers in italic and bold refer to figures and tables, respectively.